2016

The Year Book of HAND AND UPPER LIMB SURGERY®

Editors-in-Chief

Jeffrey Yao, MD
Associate Professor, Robert A. Chase Hand & Upper Limb Center, Department of Orthopaedic Surgery, Redwood City, California

Julie Adams, MD
Associate Professor of Orthopedic Surgery, Mayo Clinic Health System, Austin, Minnesota

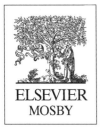

ELSEVIER
MOSBY

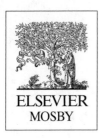

VP Global Medical Reference: Mary E. Gatsch
Senior Clinics Editor: Jennifer Flynn-Briggs
Developmental Editor: Colleen Viola

2016 EDITION

Printed in the United States of America
Composition by TNQ Books and Journals Pvt Ltd, India
Printing/binding by Sheridan Books, Inc.

Editorial Office:
Elsevier
Suite 1800
1600 John F. Kennedy Blvd.
Philadelphia, PA 19103-2899

International Standard Serial Number: 1551-7977
International Standard Book Number: 978-0-323-44684-6

Contributing Editors

Joshua M. Abzug, MD
*Associate Professor, Departments of Orthopedics and Pediatrics, University of
Maryland School of Medicine; Director, University of Maryland Brachial Plexus
Clinic; Director of Pediatric Orthopedics, University of Maryland Medical
Center; Deputy Surgeon-in-Chief, University of Maryland Children's Hospital,
Timonium, Maryland*

Darryl Eugene Barnes, MD
*Consultant; Assistant Professor, Department of Orthopedics and Sports
Medicine, Mayo Clinic Health System, Austin, Minnesota*

Keith A. Bengtson, MD
*Department of Physical Medicine and Rehabilitation, Mayo Clinic, Rochester,
Minnesota*

Philip E. Blazar, MD
*Associate Professor of Orthopaedic Surgery, Harvard Medical School;
Department of Orthopaedic Surgery, Brigham and Women's Hospital,
Boston, Massachusetts*

Deborah C. Bohn, MD
*Orthopaedic Hand & Upper Extremity Surgeon, Tria Orthopaedic Center,
Bloomington, Minnesota*

Jeffrey S. Brault, DO
*Department of Physical Medicine and Rehabilitation, Mayo Clinic, Rochester,
Minnesota*

Brian T. Carlsen, MD
*Consultant, Division of Plastic Surgery and Division of Hand Surgery; Associate
Professor of Orthopedic Surgery and Plastic Surgery, Mayo College of Medicine,
Rochester, Minnesota*

Andre Cheah, MD
*Consultant, Department of Hand & Reconstructive Microsurgery, National
University Hospital, Singapore; Assistant Professor, Department of Orthopaedic
Surgery, National University of Singapore, Singapore*

Neal C. Chen, MD
*Assistant Professor in Orthopaedic Surgery, Massachusetts General Hospital,
Harvard Medical School, Boston, Massachusetts*

Emilie Cheung, MD
*Associate Professor, Department of Orthopedic Surgery, Stanford University,
Redwood City, California*

Matthew Seung Suk Choi, MD
*Associate Professor, Chief, Department of Plastic and Reconstructive Surgery,
Hanyang University Guri Hospital, Guri, Gyunggi-do, Korea*

Alphonsus KS Chong, MD
*Head and Senior Consultant, Department of Hand and Reconstructive
Microsurgery; Assistant Professor, Department of Orthopaedic Surgery, Yong
Loo Lin School of Medicine, National University Hospital, Singapore*

Susan J. Clark, OTR/L, CHT
Certified Hand Therapist, Stanford University Medical Center, Redwood City, California

Catherine Curtin, MD
Associate Professor, Robert A. Chase Hand & Upper Limb Center, Division of Plastic Surgery, Stanford University Medical Center, Stanford, California

Piotr Czarnecki, MD, PhD
Hand Surgery Department, Poznan University of Medical Sciences, Poznan, Poland

John Elfar, MD, FACS
Associate Professor, Department of Orthopaedic Surgery, University of Rochester Medical Center, Rochester, New York

Felicity G. Fishman, MD
Assistant Professor, Department of Orthopaedics and Rehabilitation, Yale University School of Medicine, New Haven, Connecticut

Lori S. Fitton, PhD (c), APN, CNP
Mayo Clinic Orthopedic Surgery, Austin, Minnesota

John M. Froelich, MD
Panorama Orthopedic and Spine Center, Golden, Colorado

R. Glenn Gaston, MD
Hand Fellowship Director, OrthoCarolina; Chief of Hand Surgery, Carolinas Medical Center, Charlotte, North Carolina

Erica Jane Gauger, MD
Department of Orthopaedic Surgery, University of Minnesota, Minneapolis, Minnesota

Erich M. Gauger, MD
Major, USAF; Staff Orthopaedic Surgeon, USAF Academy, 10th MSGS, USAF Academy, Colorado

Ruby Grewal, MD, MSc, FRCS
Associate Professor, Roth\McFarlane Hand and Upper Limb Centre, St Joseph's Health Centre, London, Ontario, Canada

Warren C. Hammert, MD
Professor of Orthopaedic Surgery and Plastic Surgery, Chief, Division of Hand Surgery, Department of Orthopaedics and Rehabilitation, University of Rochester Medical Center, Rochester, New York

Alicia Karin Harrison, MD
Department of Orthopaedic Surgery, University of Minnesota, Minneapolis, Minnesota

Mike Hayton, BSc(Hons) MBChB FRCS(orth) FFSEM(uk)
Consultant Orthopaedic Hand Surgeon, The Wrightington Hospital, Lancashire, United Kingdom

Vincent R. Hentz, MD
Professor of Surgery, Robert A. Chase Hand & Upper Limb Center, Division of Plastic Surgery, Stanford University Medical Center, Stanford, California

Guillaume Herzberg, MD, PhD
Hôpital Édouard Herriot, Orthopaedic Surgery – Shoulder & Elbow, Wrist, Hand, Lyon, France

Pak-Cheong Ho, MD, MBBS, FRCS, FHKCOS, FHKAM (Orthopeadics)
Consultant & Chief, Clinical Professor (Honorary), Division of Hand & Microsurgery, Department of Orthopaedic & Traumatology, Prince of Wales Hospital, Chinese University of Hong Kong, Hong Kong, China

Nathan A. Hoekzema, MD
Assistant Clinical Professor, Department of Orthopaedic Surgery, UCSF – Fresno, Fresno, California

Jerry I. Huang, MD
Associate Professor, Program Director, UW Combined Hand Fellowship, Department of Orthopaedics and Sports Medicine, University of Washington Medical Center, Seattle, Washington

Thomas B. Hughes, MD
Clinical Associate Professor of Orthopaedic Surgery, University of Pittsburgh School of Medicine; Orthopaedic Specialists, UPMC, Pittsburgh, Pennsylvania

Sidney M. Jacoby, MD
Associate Professor in Orthopaedic Surgery, Thomas Jefferson University Hospital, The Philadelphia Hand Center, P.C., Philadelphia, Pennsylvania

Ryosuke Kakinoki, MD, PhD
Professor of Hand Surgery & Microvascular Reconstructive Surgery, Department of Orthopaedic Surgery, Kindai University Hospital, Osaka, Japan

Patrick M. Kane, MD
Assistant Professor of Orthopaedic Surgery, Thomas Jefferson University; The Philadelphia Hand Center, Philadelphia, Pennsylvania

Stephanie Kannas, OTR/L, CHT, CLT-LANA
Mayo Clinic, Rochester, Minnesota

Michael W. Kessler, MD
Chief - Division of Hand & Elbow Surgery, Assistant Professor, Department of Orthopaedic Surgery, MedStar Georgetown University Hospital, Washington, DC

Elspeth Kinnucan, MD
Kaiser Permanente, Roseville, California

Kathleen Kollitz, MD
Department of Orthopaedic Surgery, Mayo Clinic, Rochester, Minnesota

Sonja Kranz, OTR/L, CHT
Department of Physical Medicine and Rehabilitation, Mayo Clinic, Rochester, Minnesota

Amy L. Ladd, MD
Editor-in-Chief, Emeritus, Yearbook of Hand & Upper Limb Surgery; Professor of Orthopaedic Surgery & Plastic Surgery, Robert A. Chase Hand & Upper Limb Center at Stanford University, Palo Alto, California

Ericka Lawler, MD
Clinical Associate Professor of Orthopedic Surgery, University of Iowa, Iowa City, Iowa

Jeffrey Macalena, MD
Assistant Professor, Department of Orthopaedic Surgery, University of Minnesota, Minneapolis, Minnesota

Corey Weston McGee, PhD, MS, OTR/L, CHT
Assistant Professor, Program in Occupational Therapy, University of Minnesota - Rochester, Rochester, Minnesota

Kai Megerle, MD
Assistant Professor, Department of Plastic Surgery and Hand Surgery, Klinikum rechts der Isar, Technische Universitðt Mnchen, Munich, Germany

Amy T. Moeller, MD
Assistant Professor, Department of Orthopaedic Surgery, University of Minnesota, Minneapolis, Minnesota

Peter M. Murray, MD
Professor and Chair, Department of Orthopedic Surgery; Consultant, Orthopedic Surgery and Neurosurgery, Mayo Clinic, Jacksonville, Florida

Virginia H. O'Brien, OTD, OTR/L, CHT
Hand Therapy Residency Coordinator, University Orthopaedics Hand Therapy Center, University of Minnesota Medical Center, Fairview, Minneapolis, Minnesota

Jose A. Ortiz, Jr., MD
Assistant Clinical Professor of Orthopedics, Mayo Clinic College of Medicine, Chief of Medical Staff, Orthopedic Center, Hand and Upper Extremity Service, Eau Claire, Wisconsin

Maureen A. O'Shaughnessy, MD
Mayo Clinic, Rochester, Minnesota

Rick F. Papandrea, MD
Partner, Orthopaedic Associates of WI (OAW), Associate Clinical Professor of Orthopaedic Surgery, Medical College of Wisconsin, Milwaukee, Wisconsin

William T. Payne, MD
Hand and Upper Extremity Surgeon, Northwestern Medicine Regional Medical Group, Warrenville, Illinois

Marc J. Richard, MD
Associate Professor, Hand, Upper Extremity, and Microvascular Surgery, Department of Orthopaedic Surgery, Duke University Medical Center, Durham, North Carolina

Tamara D. Rozental, MD
Chief, Hand and Upper Extremity Surgery; Associate Professor, Harvard Medical School; Beth Israel Deaconess Medical Center, Department of Orthopaedic Surgery, Boston, Massachusetts

Adam Shafritz, MD
Professor of Orthopaedic Surgery, University of Vermont College of Medicine, Burlington, Vermont

Steven Shin, MD
Chief of Hand Surgery, Kerlan-Jobe Orthopaedic Clinic, Los Angeles, California

Juan Pablo Simone, MD
Hospital Alemán, Buenos Aires, Argentina

David J. Slutsky, MD
Department of Orthopedics, Harbor-UCLA Medical Center, Torrance, California

Philipp N. Streubel, MD
Assistant Professor, Shoulder, Elbow and Hand Surgery, Department of Orthopaedic Surgery & Rehabilitation, University of Nebraska Medical Center, Omaha, Nebraska

Jin Bo Tang, MD
Professor and Chair, Department of Hand Surgery, Affiliated Hospital of Nantong University, Chair, Hand Surgery Research Center, Nantong University, Jiangsu, China

Jonathan Tueting, MD
Vice-Chair and Chief, Hand and Upper Extremity Surgery, Department of Orthopedics and Rehabilitation Medicine, University of Wisconsin School of Medicine and Public Health, Madison, Wisconsin

Christina M. Ward, MD
Assistant Professor, Department of Orthopedic Surgery, University of Minnesota, Regions Hospital, Saint Paul, Minnesota

David S. Zelouf, MD
Attending Physician, The Philadelphia Hand Center; Assistant Clinical Professor, Department of Orthopedic Surgery, Thomas Jefferson University Hospital, Philadelphia, Pennsylvania

Table of Contents

JOURNALS REPRESENTED xi

INTRODUCTION xiii

1. Hand and Wrist Arthritis 1
2. Wrist Arthroscopy 33
3. Carpus 35
4. Dupuytren's Contracture 67
5. Compressive Neuropathies 77
6. Nerve 103
7. Brachial Plexus 137
8. Microsurgery 143
9. Tendon 147
10. Trauma 173
11. Distal Radius Fractures 199
12. Diagnostic Imaging 249
13. Elbow: Trauma 259
14. Elbow: Miscellaneous 275
15. Pediatric Trauma 299
16. Congenital 321
17. Shoulder: Rotator Cuff 341
18. Shoulder: Trauma 383
19. Shoulder: Miscellaneous 409
20. Rehabilitation 477
21. Miscellaneous 495

ARTICLE INDEX 521

AUTHOR INDEX 537

Journals Represented

Journals represented in this YEAR BOOK are listed below.

Acta Orthopaedica
American Journal of Sports Medicine
Anesthesiology
Annals of Emergency Medicine
Annals of Plastic Surgery
Archives of Physical Medicine and Rehabilitation
Arthroscopy
Bone and Joint Journal
British Journal of Sports Medicine
Canadian Journal of Surgery
Clinical Biomechanics (BRISTOL, AVON)
Clinical Journal of Pain
Clinical Neurology and Neurosurgery
Clinical Orthopaedics and Related Research
Dermatologic Surgery
Hand
Injury
Journal of Hand Surgery (American Volume)
Journal of Athletic Training
Journal of Applied Physiology
Journal of Bone and Joint Surgery (American)
Journal of Bone Mineral Research
Journal of Hand Surgery
Journal of Hand Therapy
Journal of Manipulative and Physiological Therapeutics
Journal of Orthopaedic and Sports Physical Therapy
Journal of Orthopaedic Research
Journal of Orthopaedic Trauma
Journal of Pediatric Orthopaedics
Journal of plastic, Reconstructive & Aesthetic Surgery
Journal of Reconstructive Microsurgery
Journal of Surgical Research
Journal of Ultrasound in Medicine
Journal of Wrist Surgery
Lancet
Medicine (Baltimore)
Microsurgery
Neurosurgery
Orthopedics
Pediatric Emergency Care
Pediatric Radiology
Plastic and Reconstructive Surgery
Radiology

Regional Anesthesia and Pain Medicine
Skeletal Radiology

STANDARD ABBREVIATIONS

The following terms are abbreviated in this edition: acquired immunodeficiency syndrome (AIDS), cardiopulmonary resuscitation (CPR), central nervous system (CNS), cerebrospinal fluid (CSF), computed tomography (CT), deoxyribonucleic acid (DNA), electrocardiography (ECG), health maintenance organization (HMO), human immunodeficiency virus (HIV), intensive care unit (ICU), intramuscular (IM), intravenous (IV), magnetic resonance (MR) imaging (MRI), ribonucleic acid (RNA), and ultrasound (US).

NOTE

The YEAR BOOK OF HAND AND UPPER LIMB SURGERY® is a literature survey service providing abstracts of articles published in the professional literature. Every effort is made to assure the accuracy of the information presented in these pages. Neither the editors nor the publisher of the YEAR BOOK OF HAND AND UPPER LIMB SURGERY® can be responsible for errors in the original materials. The editors' comments are their own opinions. Mention of specific products within this publication does not constitute endorsement.

To facilitate the use of the YEAR BOOK OF HAND AND UPPER LIMB SURGERY® as a reference tool, all illustrations and tables included in this publication are now identified as they appear in the original article. This change is meant to help the reader recognize that any illustration or table appearing in the YEAR BOOK OF HAND AND UPPER LIMB SURGERY® may be only one of many in the original article. For this reason, figure and table numbers will often appear to be out of sequence within the YEAR BOOK OF HAND AND UPPER LIMB SURGERY®.

Introduction

We are proud to bring you the 32nd edition of the YEAR BOOK OF HAND AND UPPER LIMB SURGERY.

The YEAR BOOK continues to be a comprehensive collection of the most concise, high-yield summaries and commentaries of the previous year's most salient peer-reviewed literature in the field of hand and upper limb surgery. As is the case each year, this YEAR BOOK would not be possible without the invaluable input of our contributing editors. Their critical reviews of the literature are robust and thought-provoking. These contributing editors hail from all over the world, and are all internationally recognized experts in the field of hand and upper extremity surgery. They have generously shared their time and expertise with the readers of the YEAR BOOK and for this we are indebted to them.

We would also like to thank Colleen Viola from Elsevier for her tireless and enthusiastic work to troubleshoot and to bring this edition to fruition.

We hope you continue to learn from and enjoy these cutting edge and thoughtful commentaries as much as we do!

Jeffrey Yao, MD

Julie Adams, MD

1 Hand and Wrist Arthritis

Relationship between Patient Expectations and Clinical Measures in Patients Undergoing Rheumatoid Hand Surgery from the Silicone Arthroplasty in Rheumatoid Arthritis (SARA) Study
Sears ED, Burns PB, Chung KC (Univ of Michigan Health System, Ann Arbor)
Plast Reconstr Surg 136:775e-781e, 2015

Background.—The purpose of this study was to evaluate the relationship between preoperative patient expectations and clinical measures in patients undergoing rheumatoid hand surgery.

Methods.—Patients were recruited as a part of a larger prospective multicenter study to evaluate outcomes of silicone metacarpophalangeal joint arthroplasty (SMPA). Patients in the surgical cohort completed a baseline expectation questionnaire asking about expectations for function, work, pain, and aesthetics after SMPA. Responses were categorized into groups of low, middle, and high expectations for each domain and for cumulative expectations across all domains. Other study measurements were taken at baseline and 1 year, including the Michigan Hand Outcomes Questionnaire (MHQ) and objective clinical measurements (i.e., grip strength, pinch strength, the Jebsen-Taylor Hand Function Test, ulnar drift, and extensor lag).

Results.—Preoperative expectations and clinical measures were complete for 59 patients at baseline and 45 patients at 1-year follow-up. Preoperative expectation level was related to baseline patient-reported domains of activities of daily living and hand satisfaction measured by the MHQ ($p = 0.04$ and $p = 0.07$, respectively). Patients had relatively similar satisfaction with hand function postoperatively regardless of preoperative expectation level. No consistent relationship was seen between preoperative expectations and objective measures at baseline and 1-year follow-up.

Conclusions.—High preoperative expectations were not a risk factor for dissatisfaction postoperatively. Preoperative expectation level may be considered for stratifying baseline patient-reported hand function in patients with similar objective hand function (Table 6).

▶ Although there were significant differences in the activities of daily living (ADL) and satisfaction domains of the Michigan Hand Outcomes

1

TABLE 6.—Clinical Measures across Preoperative Expectations Groups

	Expectations		
	Low	Middle	High
Mean baseline measures ($n = 59$)			
No.	24	28	7
MHQ total	33	38	53
MHQ function	32	39	53
MHQ ADL*	28	35	59
MHQ work	38	42	59
MHQ pain	56	46	32
MHQ aesthetics	34	29	33
MHQ satisfaction[†]	19	29	44
Grip strength, kg	5.4	5.5	5.4
Jebsen-Taylor Hand Function Test, sec	56	53	41
Two-point pinch strength, kg	2.3	2.2	2.7
Mean MCPJ ulnar drift, degrees	36	39	32
Mean MCPJ extensor lag, degrees	60	68	63
Mean 1-yr measures ($n = 45$)			
No.	16	22	7
MHQ total	55	64	71
MHQ function	56	66	76
MHQ ADL	45	59	73
MHQ work	40	54	61
MHQ pain	38	32	28
MHQ aesthetics	68	67	71
MHQ satisfaction	61	67	70
Grip strength, kg	5	6.6	10.1
Jebsen-Taylor Hand Function Test, sec	46	41	45
Two-point pinch strength, kg	1.9	2.7	2.9
Mean MCPJ ulnar drift, degrees	10	14	22
Mean MCPJ extensor lag, degrees	28	24	37

MHQ, Michigan Hand Outcomes Questionnaire; ADL, activities of daily living; MCPJ, metacarpophalangeal joint.
*$p < 0.05$.
[†]$p < 0.10$.
Reprinted from Sears ED, Burns PB, Chung KC. Relationship between patient expectations and clinical measures in patients undergoing rheumatoid hand surgery from the silicone arthroplasty in rheumatoid arthritis (SARA) study. *Plast Reconstr Surg.* 2015;136:775e-781e, with permission from American Society of Plastic Surgeons.

Questionnaire (MHQ), no significant differences were found among the 3 groups at baseline in the objective measures, including 2-point pinch strength, ulnar drift of the wrist, and extensor lag of the fingers. The findings that patients gave good marks in the ADL and satisfaction domains in the MHQ at the baseline and had high expectations were not related to differences in patients' perceptions of disabilities between the expectation groups (Table 6). If people who tend to regard their disabilities as minor have higher expectations for the outcome of the operation, significant differences among the groups would have been found in the 1-year outcomes of the MHQ.

This study indicates that people who have a positive attitude about daily living (considering themselves to be more active and having greater satisfaction against what they could do during daily living) might have had higher expectations for postoperative outcomes. In other words, patients who positively acknowledge their level of disability in daily living may tend to have a positive image of their postoperative daily living. These patients might be able to accept the postoperative outcomes and be satisfied with their postoperative activities. There were fewer patients with high expectations (8 patients) compared with the other groups (28 and 24 patients with middle and low expectations, respectively; Table 6). The results suggest that rheumatoid arthritis, which is often accompanied by depressive mental status, inhibited the patients from forming a positive attitude about daily living.[1]

R. Kakinoki, MD

Reference

1. Lu MC, Guo HR, Lin MC, Livneh H, Lai NS, Tsai TY. Bidirectional associations between rheumatoid arthritis and depression: a nationwide longitudinal study. *Sci Rep.* 2016;6:20647.

Early Osteoarthritis of the Trapeziometacarpal Joint Is Not Associated With Joint Instability During Typical Isometric Loading
Halilaj E, Moore DC, Patel TK, et al (Brown Univ, Providence, RI; The Warren Alpert Med School of Brown Univ, Providence, RI; et al)
J Orthop Res 33:1639-1645, 2015

The saddle-shaped trapeziometacarpal (TMC) joint contributes importantly to the function of the human thumb. A balance between mobility and stability is essential in this joint, which experiences high loads and is prone to osteoarthritis (OA). Since instability is considered a risk factor for TMC OA, we assessed TMC joint instability during the execution of three isometric functional tasks (key pinch, jar grasp, and jar twist) in 76 patients with early TMC OA and 44 asymptomatic controls. Computed tomography images were acquired while subjects held their hands relaxed and while they applied 80% of their maximum effort for each task. Six degree-of-freedom rigid body kinematics of the metacarpal with respect to the trapezium from the unloaded to the loaded task positions were computed in terms of a TMC joint coordinate system. Joint instability was expressed as a function of the metacarpal translation and the applied force. We found that the TMC joint was more unstable during a key pinch task than during a jar grasp or a jar twist task. Sex, age, and early OA did not have an effect on TMC joint instability, suggesting that instability during these three tasks is not a predisposing factor in TMCOA (Figs 4 and 6).

▶ This article provides objective measurements of trapeziometacarpal stability in precision activities of daily living: lateral pinch, grasp, and jar twist. The authors have examined isometric loading, which correlates the effect of a measurable force to a kinematic position. Compared with age-matched controls, the

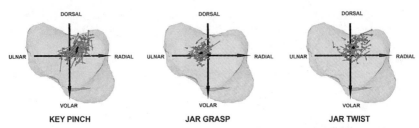

KEY PINCH   JAR GRASP   JAR TWIST

FIGURE 4.—Metacarpal translation. The statistically significant directions of motion in the TMC joint during the execution of the functional tasks were volar translation in key pinch and ulnar and volar translation in jar grasp. Translation of the metacarpal during jar twist did not occur in consistent directions. (Reprinted from Halilaj E, Moore DC, Patel TK, et al. Early osteoarthritis of the trapeziometacarpal joint is not associated with joint instability during typical isometric loading. *J Orthop Res.* 2015;33:1639-1645, with permission from Orthopaedic Research Society.)

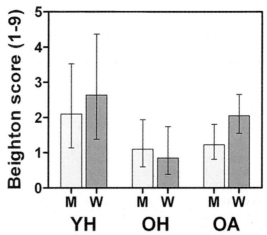

FIGURE 6.—Generalized joint laxity. Mean Beighton scores for generalized joint laxity (with 95% confidence interval bars). Subject groups included young healthy (YH) and older healthy (OH) men (M) and women (W), as well as subject with early stage osteoarthritis (OA). (Reprinted from Halilaj E, Moore DC, Patel TK, et al. Early osteoarthritis of the trapeziometacarpal joint is not associated with joint instability during typical isometric loading. *J Orthop Res.* 2015;33:1639-1645, with permission from Orthopaedic Research Society.)

early arthritis subjects, as determined by symptoms and radiographic changes, did not have significantly different degrees of subluxation in any of the positions. Lateral pinch demonstrated the most "instability," which may reflect a physiologic position of a highly complex joint (Fig 4). Although the trapeziometacarpal joint is, in general, saddle-shaped, its eccentricity precludes identifying 1 axis or center of rotation, which thus changes the definition of "stability" with each position. Note that "laxity" in a traditional sense of ligament looseness and measured by the Beighton and Horan Joint Mobility Index[1,2] did not correlate to the measured findings (Fig 6). This study, along with other biomechanical and kinematic studies of normal and early arthritic states, provides preliminary evidence regarding progression of the common basal joint arthritis. Clues to restoration and prevention based on scientific investigation remain the much larger task for hand surgeons and scientists to tackle.

A. Ladd, MD

References

1. Beighton PH, Horan F. Orthopedic aspects of the Ehlers-Danlos syndrome. *J Bone Joint Surg Br.* 1969;51:444-453.
2. Boyle KL, Witt P, Riegger-Krugh C. Intrarater and interrater reliability of the Beighton and Horan joint mobility index. *J Athl Train.* 2003;38:281-285.

Three-Corner Arthrodesis With Scaphoid and Triquetrum Excision for Wrist Arthritis

Delattre O, Goulon G, Vogels J, et al (Centre Hospitalier Universitaire Pierre Zobda Quitman, Fort-de-France, Martinique; et al)
J Hand Surg Am 40:2176-2182, 2015

Purpose.—To report the clinical and radiographic results of a consecutive series of patients who underwent the 3-corner arthrodesis (3CA) (arthrodesis of capitate, hamate, and lunate with scaphoid and triquetrum excision) procedure for wrist arthritis.

Methods.—This was a retrospective study of 30 consecutive patients who underwent a 3CA between 1994 and 2008. The indications were painful wrist osteoarthritis due to stage 2 or 3 scapholunate advanced collapse, scaphoid nonunion advanced collapse, or scaphoid chondrocalcinosis advanced collapse wrists. The clinical assessment consisted of range of motion, grip strength, and the Disabilities of the Arm, Shoulder, and Hand and Patient-Rated Wrist Evaluation scores. The radiographic assessment parameters consisted of bone fusion, carpal height and translation, lunate tilt, and appearance of the radiolunate joint space.

Results.—The average follow-up was 6 years (± 4 years). The arthrodesis was performed with staples, 2 screws, or a plate and screws. Grip strength was 72% of the contralateral side. The mean range of motion in flexion-extension arc and ulnar-radial deviation arc was 70° and 36°, respectively. The mean Disabilities of the Arm, Shoulder, and Hand and the Patient-Rated Wrist Evaluation scores were 17 (± 11) and 22 (± 24), respectively. The fusion incidence was 90% (27 of 30). The mean difference of radiolunate angle on preoperative and postoperative radiographs was 8° (16°−8° in dorsal direction). The radiolunate joint space had narrowed in 1 patient. Six surgical revisions (20%) were necessary owing to dorsal pain in patients operated using plates, staples, or excessively long screws.

Conclusions.—Three-corner arthrodesis results are comparable with 4-corner arthrodesis and proximal row carpectomy. We feel that it is simpler technically than 4-corner arthrodesis. Although 3CA is more complex than proximal row carpectomy, it preserves the native radiolunate joint. Complications that can be attributed to the dorsal fixation hardware (particularly staples and plates) were noteworthy.

Type of Study/Level of Evidence.—Therapeutic IV.

▶ The optimal management of scapholunate advanced collapse and scaphoid nonunion advanced collapse wrist is a topic of debate with many advocates for proximal row carpectomy and others favoring scaphoid excision with midcarpal fusion. Even among those favoring the latter, there are many technical variations, including 4-corner fusion (4CF), 3-corner fusion (3CF), and isolated capitolunate fusion (CL) with and without triquetral excision. This report is a retrospective review of 30 consecutive patients having undergone 3CF that adds to our body of literature supporting the success of midcarpal fusions, yet highlights that hardware related complications still exist (20% in this series).

The authors have a reasonable sample size with adequate medium-term follow-up for this procedure. They use validated outcome instruments (Disabilities of the Arm, Shoulder, and Hand and Patient-Rated Wrist Evaluation), as well as traditional range of motion (ROM) and grip strength testing. One limiting inclusion by the authors, in my opinion, is patients with scaphoid chondrocalcinosis advanced collapse, which is secondary to gout. These patients differ in many ways to those wrists with changes secondary to trauma. Another limitation is the assessment of fusion with x-rays alone because many studies have recommended CT as the gold standard in determining fusion.

From a surgical technique standpoint, all patients also underwent a posterior interosseous neurectomy neurectomy, which could influence postoperative pain levels (visual analog score). Fixation included staples, screws, and plates, all of which experienced complications. Staples were noted to be placed outside the dorsal cortex without the creation of a trough, likely increasing the rate of hardware impingement they found. The authors had a very aggressive postoperative rehabilitation protocol, immobilizing patients for only 3 weeks before allowing unrestricted ROM, even in the absence of x-ray evidence of fusion.

The authors' results in terms of pain relief, ROM, grip strength, and union rates are similar to other reports of 4CF and CL fusions. Interestingly, no correlation was found between restoration of carpal height and grip strength, which has been assumed by many in the past.

I think the evidence currently supports all methods of midcarpal fusion as relatively equivalent. Certainly isolated CL and 3CF offer technical ease, less bone graft, and equal results to the traditional 4CF and potentially with time savings in the OR. Triquetral excision offers the advantages of eliminated risk of pisotriquetral arthritis late, ease of lunate reduction, and that it serves as a source of bone graft, yet it has been shown to increase the load across the radiolunate joint, potentially leading to future degenerative change.

I personally prefer an isolated capitolunate fusion with memory staples buried in a trough and triquetral retention especially for type 1 lunates. Burying the staples decreases the rate of hardware irritation without affecting fusion in my experience. For type 2 lunates, a 3CF is a nice alternative. Screw back-out has been a problem in my experience.

G. Gaston, MD

Ulnar Head Replacement: 21 Cases; Mean Follow-Up, 7.5 Years
Axelsson P, Sollerman C, Kärrholm J (Univ of Gothenburg, Sweden)
J Hand Surg Am 40:1731-1738, 2015

Purpose.—To report clinical and radiographic outcomes for the Herbert ulnar head prosthesis after a mean of 7.5 years (range, 2.0—12.5 years).

Methods.—We performed 22 Herbert ulnar head prosthesis arthroplasties between 2000 and 2011. Five were primary procedures, and the remaining 17 were done after an average of 2 (range, 1—5) previous operations. The mean age at surgery was 55 years (range, 31—74 years). Follow-up including clinical examination, standardized questionnaires, and radiographic examination was done after mean 7.5 years (range, 2.0—12.5 years) in 21 cases. We used the Disabilities of the Arm, Shoulder, and Hand questionnaire, the Patient-Rated Wrist Evaluation questionnaire, and the Mayo wrist score questionnaire. Pain and satisfaction were evaluated with a 10-cm visual analog scale (VAS). Measurements of range of motion and strength for grip were recorded.

Results.—Wrist range of motion was not affected by the arthroplasty except for supination, which significantly improved from 55° to 70°. At follow-up, grip strength averaged 25 kg (range, 10—48 kg) in the operated wrists and 31 kg (range, 8—74 kg) on the contralateral side. Visual analog scale-pain averaged 2.9 (range, 0—8.7) during activity and 1.7 (range, 0—7) at rest. Satisfaction VAS was 8.9 (range, 4.3—10). Five patients had VAS-pain above 5 during activity, and 1 patient was dissatisfied and regretted having undergone arthroplasty. Mean outcomes were 27 (range, 5—50) for Disabilities of the Arm, Shoulder, and Hand measure, 31 (range, 0—90) for the Patient-Rated Wrist Evaluation score, and 71 (range, 30—90) for the Mayo wrist score. One patient was reoperated with capsuloplasty 9 months after the arthroplasty owing to recurrence of painful instability. Full stability was not achieved but the pain resolved. None of the implants showed any radiographic signs of loosening.

Conclusions.—The Herbert ulnar head prosthesis was a safe method of treatment and provided satisfactory midterm results for selected cases of distal radioulnar joint disorders.

Clinical Relevance.—Increased knowledge of performance for ulnar head implant arthroplasty may aid surgical decision making for distal radioulnar joint disorders.

Type of Study/Level of Evidence.—Therapeutic IV.

▶ Ulnar-sided wrist pain related to disorders of the distal radioulnar joint, specifically instability and arthritis, continues to lead to somewhat unsatisfactory answers. Resection arthroplasties can be successful in low-demand patients, but concerns arise in more active individuals. The Suave-Kapandji procedure has been advocated for younger, active patients, but problems with ulnar stump instability and radial impingement persist.

Ulnar implant arthroplasties, such as that presented here, have been used to address some of these deficiencies. As is evident from this series, they are frequently used in revision cases where resection arthroplasty or other previous surgeries have failed. Only 5 of the 21 cases were done as a primary procedure, and the implants were placed to salvage a variety of procedures.

This is typically a problem with studies of ulnar implant arthroplasties. Because most surgeons still have significant questions regarding the indications, they are used as a procedure of last resort. Therefore, when the studies following their outcomes are published, they are low-powered, poor-quality retrospective reviews performed on patients for a hodgepodge of indications. These studies then fail to elucidate the best cases for implant arthroplasties.

This study does have reasonable follow-up (average 7.5 years) and follows 20 of 21 consecutive patients. It shows good midterm results with few failures. It is underpowered to demonstrate many differences, except for the improvement in supination. I think it is safe to say that it supports the use of this implant in salvage situations but still fails to demonstrate the best indications for its use in either the primary or revision situation.

T. Hughes, MD

First dorsal interosseous muscle contraction results in radiographic reduction of healthy thumb carpometacarpal joint
McGee C, O'Brien V, Van Nortwick S, et al (Univ of Minnesota, Rochester; Univ Orthopaedics Therapy Ctr, Minneapolis, MN; Univ of Minnesota, Minneapolis; et al)
J Hand Ther 28:375-381, 2015

Introduction.—Hand therapists selectively strengthen the first dorsal interosseus (FDI) to stabilize arthritic joints yet the role of the FDI has not yet been radiographically validated.

Purpose.—To determine if FDI contraction reduces radial subluxation (RS) of the thumb metacarpal (MC).

Methods.—Fluoroscopy was used to obtain true anterior-posterior radiographs of non-arthritic CMC joints: 1) at rest, 2) while stressed and 3) while stressed with maximal FDI contraction. Maximal FDI strength during CMC stress and thumb MC RS and trapezial articular width were measured. The ratio of RS to the articular width was calculated.

Results.—Seventeen participants (5 male, 12 female) participated. Subluxation of a stressed CMC significantly reduced and the subluxation to articular width ratio significantly improved after FDI activation.

Conclusions.—Contraction of the FDI appears to radiographically reduce subluxation of the healthy thumb CMC joint. Further exploration on the FDI's reducibility and its carry-over effects in arthritic thumbs is needed.

Level of Evidence.—4.

▶ For many years, our hand therapy clinic has stressed the importance of first dorsal interosseous (FDI) strengthening for stabilization as well as symptom relief for those with thumb CMC osteoarthritis. This study gives us additional clinical evidence for our best practice concerning the FDI strengthening exercises used in treating thumb carpometacarpal (CMC) arthritis. Although this study was done on healthy subjects, the preliminary results of this research suggest that our focus on the FDI has relevance. The authors were able to determine radiographically that subluxation of the thumb was reduced with FDI contraction. Their study also indicated that a stronger FDI may be a factor in preventing the onset of subluxation with improved maintenance of joint congruence. Because FDI strengthening exercises are easy to teach with minimal cost involved, continued use seems to be indicated by this study.

There are limitations of this study, which are well expressed by the authors. They are upfront about the use of a healthy homogeneous population, the lack of a reproducible measure of manual force used, and the fact that they did not attempt to isolate the FDI and may have included co-contraction of other thumb stabilizers in their research. Now that this team of researchers has established a foundation for the study of FDI contraction and its effect on thumb position and stability, they can further their research using a sampling of those in various stages of thumb CMC osteoarthritis. More evidence concerning the role of the FDI both in the healthy and diseased thumb is welcome.

S. J. Clark, OTR/L, CHT

Joint Arthroplasty With Osteochondral Grafting From the Knee for Posttraumatic or Degenerative Hand Joint Disorders
Kodama N, Ueba H, Takemura Y, et al (Shiga Univ of Med Science, Otsu, Japan)
J Hand Surg Am 40:1638-1645, 2015

Purpose.—To describe the operative procedure and report the clinical outcomes of articular surface reconstruction for various hand joint disorders using autologous osteochondral grafts from the knee.

Methods.—Ten patients underwent articular surface reconstruction for hand joint disorders with autologous osteochondral grafts from the patellofemoral joint. Mean patient age was 35 years (range, 15–52 y). The patients were followed for an average of 48 months (range, 16–89 mo).

Arthroplasty was performed on the metacarpophalangeal joint in 4 cases, and on the proximal interphalangeal joint in 6 cases. The patients' clinical outcomes were evaluated with joint range of motion, visual analog scale (0–10 points), and Disabilities of the Arm, Shoulder, and Hand (DASH) score. Histological examination was performed in 3 cases after surgery.

Results.—Graft union was confirmed in all cases without radiographic evidence of resorption or necrosis. Follow-up radiographic examinations showed good graft incorporation without signs of osteoarthritis such as joint space narrowing. The finger flexion-extension arc improved significantly from an average of 21° to 61°. The mean visual analog scale also improved significantly from 7.0 to 1.5. The mean total active motion showed a significant improvement from 151° before surgery to 201° after surgery, and the mean DASH score improved significantly from 33 to 12. There were no significant differences for the arc of finger motion and DASH score between metacarpophalangeal and proximal interphalangeal joint disorders or between hemiarthroplasty and total joint arthroplasty. Histological examination revealed viable chondrocytes in the implanted cartilage.

Conclusions.—Autologous osteochondral grafting from the patellofemoral joint provided satisfactory outcomes and may be a useful option for joint surface reconstruction of traumatic or degenerative hand joint disorders.

Type of Study/Level of Evidence.—Therapeutic IV.

▶ The authors' results in their small (n = 10) series of metacarpophalangeal (MP) and proximal interphalangeal (PIP) joint arthroplasties are encouraging over the intermediate time period. Their patients were relatively young, and an alternative technique, such as silastic implant arthroplasty, would likely need revision over time. The same may be true of these cases because the duration of follow-up averaged 48 months. The use of grafts from non-weight-bearing areas of the knee joint for such problems as scaphoid nonunions is increasing and more hand surgeons are becoming familiar with the anatomy of the area. A major limitation of the report is lack of information regarding which finger was involved. Were any of the MP or PIP joint reconstructions performed for the index finger where lateral stability is a major concern for all other arthroplasty procedures. We are not told the results in terms of lateral stability. The authors state that 4 of the 10 patients required secondary procedures; however, they did not count removal of the external fixator in 3 additional patients as a secondary procedure. Although a much more complicated procedure, this seems to have a role in the management of arthritic joints in younger patients.

V. R. Hentz, MD

Evaluation of Radiographic Instability of the Trapeziometacarpal Joint in Women With Carpal Tunnel Syndrome

Kim JH, Gong HS, Kim YH, et al (Seoul Med Ctr, Korea; Seoul Natl Univ College of Medicine, Korea)
J Hand Surg Am 40:1298-1302, 2015

Purpose.—To determine whether median nerve dysfunction measured by electrophysiologic studies in carpal tunnel syndrome (CTS) is associated with thumb trapeziometacarpal (TMC) joint instability.

Methods.—We evaluated 71 women with CTS and 31 asymptomatic control women. Patients with generalized laxity or TMC joint osteoarthritis were excluded. We classified the electrophysiologic severity of CTS based on nerve conduction time and amplitude and assessed radiographic instability of the TMC joint based on TMC joint stress radiographs. We compared subluxation ratio between patients with CTS and controls and performed correlation analysis of the relationship between the electrophysiologic grade and subluxation ratio.

Results.—Thirty-one patients were categorized into the mild CTS subgroup and 41 into the severe CTS subgroup. There was no significant difference in subluxation ratio between the control group and CTS patients or between the control group and CTS subgroup patients. Furthermore, there was no significant correlation between electrophysiologic grade and subluxation ratio.

Conclusions.—This study demonstrated that patients with CTS did not have greater radiographic TMC joint instability compared with controls, and suggests that TMC joint stability is not affected by impaired median nerve function. Further studies could investigate how to better evaluate proprioceptive function of TMC joint and whether other nerves have effects on TMC joint motor/proprioceptive function, to elucidate the relationship between neuromuscular control of the TMC joint, its stability, and its progression to osteoarthritis.

Type of Study/Level of Evidence.—Diagnostic II.

▶ This study corroborates recent findings that trapeziometacarpal (TMC) arthritis does not require subluxation, nor can subluxation predict arthritis. Furthermore, it supports that subluxation (Fig 1) is a normal occurrence in the population, also reported elsewhere recently.[1-3] The authors conclude that median nerve function does not contribute to TMC stability. I would disagree with that conclusion because each of the peripheral nerves—median, radial, ulnar, and musculocutaneous—contributes capsular innervation in the normal state.[4] We do not specifically know whether additional innervation or denervation exists in the arthritic state. Furthermore, muscle integration from all of the thenar muscles and the first dorsal interosseous (FDI; ulnar innervated) support the TMC joint, with potentially the FDI and the opponens pollicis having the most synergistic support of stabilizing the thumb.[5] Thus, the definition of

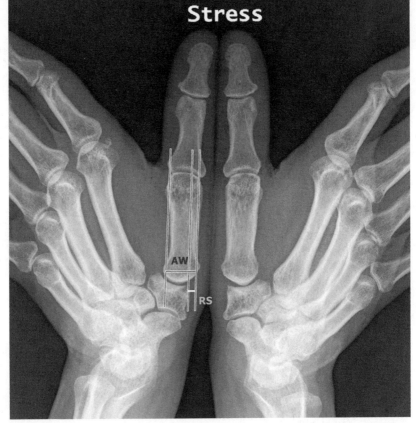

FIGURE 1.—Trapeziometacarpal joint stress view radiograph. Measurement of AW and RS. (Reprinted from Kim JH, Gong HS, Kim YH, et al. Evaluation of radiographic instability of the trapeziometacarpal joint in women with carpal tunnel syndrome. *J Hand Surg Am.* 2015;40:1298-1302, with permission from American Society for Surgery of the Hand.)

thumb stability from a proprioceptive and anatomic standpoint, as well as its role in contributing to arthritis, requires closer scrutiny.

A. Ladd, MD

References

1. Wolf JM, Schreier S, Tomsick S, Williams A, Petersen B. Radiographic laxity of the trapeziometacarpal joint is correlated with generalized joint hypermobility. *J Hand Surg Am.* 2011;36:1165-1169.
2. Ladd AL, Crisco JJ, Hagert E, Rose J, Weiss AP. The 2014 ABJS Nicolas Andry Award: the puzzle of the thumb: mobility, stability, and demands in opposition. *Clin Orthop Relat Res.* 2014;472:3605-3622.
3. Halilaj E, Moore DC, Patel TK, Ladd AL, Weiss AP, Crisco JJ. Early osteoarthritis of the trapeziometacarpal joint is not associated with joint instability during typical isometric loading. *J Orthop Res.* 2015;33:1639-1645.

4. Lorea DP, Berthe JV, De Mey A, Coessens BC, Rooze M, Foucher G. The nerve supply of the trapeziometacarpal joint. *J Hand Surg Br.* 2002;27:232-237.
5. Mobargha N, Esplugas M, Garcia-Elias M, Lluch A, Megerle K, Hagert E. The effect of individual isometric muscle loading on the alignment of the base of the thumb metacarpal: a cadaveric study. *J Hand Surg Eur Vol.* 2016;41:374-379.

Early Osteoarthritis of the Trapeziometacarpal Joint Is Not Associated With Joint Instability During Typical Isometric Loading
Halilaj E, Moore DC, Patel TK, et al (Brown Univ, Providence, RI; et al)
J Orthop Res 33:1639-1645, 2015

The saddle-shaped trapeziometacarpal (TMC) joint contributes importantly to the function of the human thumb. A balance between mobility and stability is essential in this joint, which experiences high loads and is prone to osteoarthritis (OA). Since instability is considered a risk factor for TMC OA, we assessed TMC joint instability during the execution of three isometric functional tasks (key pinch, jar grasp, and jar twist) in 76 patients with early TMC OA and 44 asymptomatic controls. Computed tomography images were acquired while subjects held their hands relaxed and while they applied 80% of their maximum effort for each task. Six degree-of-freedom rigid body kinematics of the metacarpal with respect to the trapezium from the unloaded to the loaded task positions were computed in terms of a TMC joint coordinate system. Joint instability was expressed as a function of the metacarpal translation and the applied force. We found that the TMC joint was more unstable during a key pinch task than during a jar grasp or a jar twist task. Sex, age, and early OA did not have an effect on TMC joint instability, suggesting that instability during these three tasks is not a predisposing factor in TMC OA (Figs 2 and 5).

▶ This excellent study challenges prior understanding of trapeziometacarpal (TMC) osteoarthritis through sound research methodology. The authors assessed joint instability during isometric loading of the TMC joint (Fig 2) with the specific goal of determining whether female sex, older age, and the onset of TMC osteoarthritis were associated with TMC joint instability. High-demand functional tasks that are known to load the TMC joint were examined: key pinch, jar grasp, and jar twist. Significantly, the authors found no differences among the tested groups (young healthy, old healthy, and early-stage osteoarthritis) in trapeziometacarpal instability during these functional tasks (Fig 5). These findings contradict our previous understanding of the disease pathogenesis.

This article advances our understanding of TMC pathology. As the authors acknowledge, further study is warranted to fully understand the relationship between increased mobility and TMC osteoarthritis. I think the inclusion of an older patient cohort and patients with various stages of osteoarthritis at the TMC joint would be beneficial. Additionally, as the authors state, further

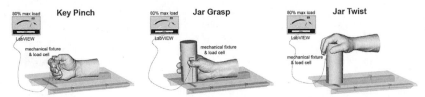

FIGURE 2.—Functional tasks. 3D renderings of the hand of one subject during the functional task positions of key pinch, jar grasp, and jar twist, with the Labview interface that visually assisted the subjects in maintaining 80% of the maximum load for each task during imaging. (Reprinted from Halilaj E, Moore DC, Patel TK, et al. Early osteoarthritis of the trapeziometacarpal joint is not associated with joint instability during typical isometric loading. *J Orthop Res.* 2015;33:1639-1645, with permission from Orthopaedic Research Society.)

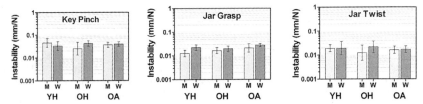

FIGURE 5.—Joint instability. Mean TMC joint instability (with 95% confidence interval bars) during key pinch, jar grasp, and jar twist tasks. Subject groups included young healthy (YH) and older healthy (OH) men (M) and women (W), as well as subjects with early stage osteoarthritis (OA). (Reprinted from Halilaj E, Moore DC, Patel TK, et al. Early osteoarthritis of the trapeziometacarpal joint is not associated with joint instability during typical isometric loading. *J Orthop Res.* 2015;33:1639-1645, with permission from Orthopaedic Research Society.)

understanding of cartilage biology is necessary to better understand this multifactorial disease.

P. Kane, MD

Trapeziometacarpal Arthritis: A Prospective Clinical Evaluation of the Thumb Adduction and Extension Provocative Tests

Gelberman RH, Boone S, Osei DA, et al (Washington Univ School of Medicine, St. Louis, MO)

J Hand Surg Am 40:1285-1291, 2015

Purpose.—To determine the diagnostic performance (ie, sensitivity, specificity, interrater reliability) of the thumb metacarpal adduction and extension tests against traditional examination maneuvers for trapeziometacarpal (TMC) arthritis.

Methods.—This cross-sectional study recruited 129 patients from 2 outpatient offices at a tertiary institution. All patients had radiographic wrist examinations and completed a standardized physical examination consisting of the thumb adduction and extension tests as well as standard examination maneuvers for radial wrist and thumb pain. The physical

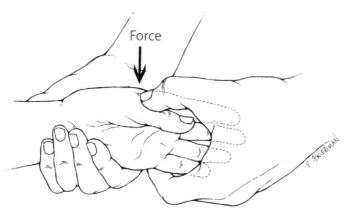

FIGURE 1.—The adduction stress test brings the thumb parallel to the index metacarpal with the arrow indicating the direction of force application. (Reprinted from Gelberman RH, Boone S, Osei DA, et al. Trapeziometacarpal arthritis: a prospective clinical evaluation of the thumb adduction and extension provocative tests. *J Hand Surg Am.* 2015;40:1285-1291, with permission from American Society for Surgery of the Hand.)

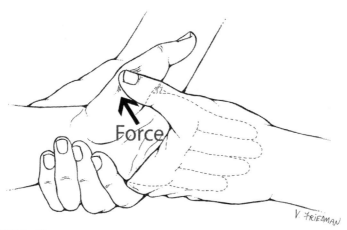

FIGURE 2.—The extension stress test with the arrow indicating the direction of force application that brings the thumb into the plane of the palm. (Reprinted from Gelberman RH, Boone S, Osei DA, et al. Trapeziometacarpal arthritis: a prospective clinical evaluation of the thumb adduction and extension provocative tests. *J Hand Surg Am.* 2015;40:1285-1291, with permission from American Society for Surgery of the Hand.)

examinations were performed by 1 of 2 attending physicians and an independent examiner. Patients were recruited for 3 diagnostic groups: TMC arthritis, radial wrist or hand pain, and nonradial wrist pain controls. Statistical analysis calculated the sensitivity, specificity, and interrater reliability of each physical examination maneuver for detecting TMC arthritis.

Results.—The thumb adduction maneuver was found to have a sensitivity of 0.94 (confidence interval [CI], 0.82—0.98) and a specificity of 0.93

(CI, 0.86–0.97). The thumb extension maneuver had a sensitivity of 0.94 (CI, 0.82–0.98) and a specificity of 0.95 (CI, 0.87–0.98). The interrater reliability was excellent for both the adduction (κ = 0.79) and the extension tests (κ = 0.84). The grind test had a sensitivity of 0.44 (CI, 0.30–0.59), a specificity of 0.92 (CI, 0.84–0.97), and poor interrater reliability (0.31). Point tenderness at the TMC joint had a sensitivity of 0.94 (CI, 0.82–0.98), a specificity of 0.81 (CI, 0.71–0.88) and fair interrater reliability (κ = 0.63).

Conclusions.—The adduction and extension tests each proved to be more sensitive than the grind test for the detection of TMC arthritis. Further, these provocative tests were more specific for basal joint arthrosis than was the elicitation of point tenderness at the joint. The metacarpal adduction and extension maneuvers demonstrated excellent utility as screening tests for the identification of TMC arthritis.

Type of Study/Level of Evidence.—Diagnostic II.

▶ The authors present 2 examination maneuvers which, in their hands, is more sensitive to identifying symptomatic advanced trapeziometacarpal (TMC) arthritis than the commonly cited and used grind test. Similar to the Eaton classification, robust inter- and intraobserver reliability is lacking for the grind test. The maneuvers of adduction and extension are demonstrated here (Figs 1 and 2). The authors investigate the test on subjects with symptomatic advanced Eaton stage II arthritis (referencing Eaton's 1984 classification,[1] not the original 1973 classification, which includes subluxation[2]). The subtleties of the tests suggest that a master class or training video might be helpful in learning how to perform them accurately, as I have not been able to grasp their utility over the grind test in my current efforts to use them. Two recent articles[3,4] have similarly reported sensitive tests for assessing TMC in their respective practices, differing slightly from the adduction and extension tests reported here. Video instruction of all of these might be helpful in discerning their differences and utility to the remote learner. Thereafter, I propose that the next step would be to investigate these sensitive tests on symptomatic subjects with no to minimal radiographic changes because ultimately we would like guidance and better detection/prevention in how to treat this common but enigmatic disease.

A. Ladd, MD

References

1. Eaton RG, Lane LB, Littler JW, Keyser JJ. Ligament reconstruction for the painful thumb carpometacarpal joint: a long-term assessment. *J Hand Surg Am.* 1984;9: 692-699.
2. Eaton RG, Littler JW. Ligament reconstruction for the painful thumb carpometacarpal joint. *J Bone Joint Surg Am.* 1973;55:1655-1666.
3. Choa RM, Parvizi N, Giele HP. A prospective case-control study to compare the sensitivity and specificity of the grind and traction-shift (subluxation-relocation) clinical tests in osteoarthritis of the thumb carpometacarpal joint. *J Hand Surg Eur Vol.* 2014;39:282-285.
4. Model Z, Liu AY, Kang L, Wolfe SW, Burket JC, Lee SK. Evaluation of physical examination tests for thumb basal joint osteoarthritis. *Hand (N Y).* 2016;11: 108-112.

Four-Corner Arthrodesis Versus Proximal Row Carpectomy: A Retrospective Study With a Mean Follow-Up of 17 Years
Berkhout MJL, Bachour Y, Zheng KH, et al (VU Univ Med Ctr, Amsterdam, The Netherlands; et al)
J Hand Surg Am 40:1349-1354, 2015

Purpose.—To compare the long-term outcomes of proximal row carpectomy (PRC) and 4-corner arthrodesis (FCA) in a consecutive series of patients surgically treated between 1989 and 1998 in a single teaching hospital.

Methods.—We included 12 patients (14 wrists) in the PRC group and 8 patients (8 wrists) in the FCA group. Mean follow-up time was 17 years. We compared functional outcome measures (range of motion and grip strength) and patient-reported outcome measures (visual analog score for pain, Mayo Wrist Score, and Michigan Hand Questionnaire). Radiographic evaluation of joint degeneration using the Culp and Jebson scoring system and postoperative complications were assessed for both groups.

Results.—Active range of motion was slightly better after PRC. There were no differences in grip strength and patient-reported outcomes between groups. Severity of degenerative changes did not differ between groups and was not correlated with pain scores. The FCA group showed more postoperative complications.

Conclusions.—Considering the objective and patient-reported outcomes of this study, both types of surgery perform well in the long run. Proximal row carpectomy seems to result in slightly better movement of the wrist with fewer surgical complications and no need for hardware removal. Moreover, postoperative immobilization time was much shorter.

Type of Study/Level of Evidence.—Therapeutic III.

▶ This long-term retrospective study compares the results of 4-corner arthrodesis (FCA) using K-wires with proximal row carpectomy (PRC). They showed statistically better motion in the PRC group with few complications. Other measurements such as radiographic parameters and patient reported outcomes were not significantly different. With an average follow-up of 17 years, this article significantly contributes to the literature regarding these 2 procedures.

The authors correctly mention that previous studies have suggested better grip strength with FCA, although this study did not detect this benefit. Additionally, there is a tendency to favor this operation in younger patients and in laborers. We believe this "makes sense" because the lunate matched the lunate-facet of the distal radius and should hold up better over the longterm. This study contradicts that conventional wisdom. They showed no difference in the radiographic arthritis between groups. This may be because while the lunate does match the radius perfectly, the wrist joint is dramatically changed by the FCA, and this may not be the perfect articulation that we expect.

Although I agree that these data would push me to consider PRCs more often than FCA when the midcarpal joint is preserved, the authors do point out the limitations of the study. These include its retrospective nature, the large number of patients lost to follow-up, and the lack of clear criteria for one procedure over another. Also, it is important with all studies to remember that the lack of a significant difference means just that: there is no significant difference. Therefore, one has to be careful about recommending PRC over FCA because the patient-reported scores were identical. PRC has not been proven worse than FCA, just the same.

T. Hughes, MD

Relationship between Patient Expectations and Clinical Measures in Patients Undergoing Rheumatoid Hand Surgery from the Silicone Arthroplasty in Rheumatoid Arthritis (SARA) Study

Sears ED, Burns PB, Chung KC (Univ of Michigan Health System, Ann Arbor)
Plast Reconstr Surg 136:775e-781e, 2015

Background.—The purpose of this study was to evaluate the relationship between preoperative patient expectations and clinical measures in patients undergoing rheumatoid hand surgery.

Methods.—Patients were recruited as a part of a larger prospective multicenter study to evaluate outcomes of silicone metacarpophalangeal joint arthroplasty (SMPA). Patients in the surgical cohort completed a baseline expectation questionnaire asking about expectations for function, work, pain, and aesthetics after SMPA. Responses were categorized into groups of low, middle, and high expectations for each domain and for cumulative expectations across all domains. Other study measurements were taken at baseline and 1 year, including the Michigan Hand Outcomes Questionnaire (MHQ) and objective clinical measurements (i.e., grip strength, pinch strength, the Jebsen-Taylor Hand Function Test, ulnar drift, and extensor lag).

Results.—Preoperative expectations and clinical measures were complete for 59 patients at baseline and 45 patients at 1-year follow-up.

TABLE 1.—Inclusion and Exclusion Criteria for SARA Study Enrollment

Inclusion criteria
  Diagnosis of rheumatoid arthritis by a rheumatologist
  Age 18–80 yr
  Severe deformity at the metacarpophalangeal joints determined by combined ulnar deviation and extensor lag ≥50 degrees on average for each finger
Exclusion criteria
  Severe medical conditions preventing safe elective surgery
  Existing tendon rupture or swan-neck or boutonnière deformities requiring surgical correction
  Prior metacarpophalangeal joint arthroplasty on the study hand
  Addition of disease-modifying antirheumatic drugs within 3 mo of enrollment

Reprinted from Sears ED, Burns PB, Chung KC. Relationship between patient expectations and clinical measures in patients undergoing rheumatoid hand surgery from the silicone arthroplasty in rheumatoid arthritis (SARA) study. *Plast Reconstr Surg.* 2015;136:775e-781e, with permission from American Society of Plastic Surgeons.

TABLE 2.—Categorization of Preoperative Expectations into High, Middle, and Low Expectations across Function, Work, Pain, and Appearance Domains

Domain	Question	High Expectations	Middle Expectations	Low Expectations
Function	What do you expect to be able to do with your hands 1 yr from now (after surgery)?	"Anything I want."	"More activities than I do now."	"The same kinds of activities I do now." "A little less than I can do now." "A lot less than I can do now."
Work	What do you expect to be able to do in terms of work (including job, housework, and schoolwork) 1 yr from now (after surgery)?	"Everything I need to do."	"More than I can do now."	"The same amount of work I do now." "A little less than I can do now." "A lot less than I can do now."
Pain	How much pain related to your knuckles do you expect to have 1 yr from now (after surgery)?	"No pain."	"Much less pain than I have now."	"A little less pain than I have now." "The same amount of pain I have now." "A little more pain than I have now." "A lot more pain than I have now."
Appearance	What do you expect your hands to look like 1 yr from now (after surgery)?	"Almost perfect."	"Much better than they do now."	"The same as they do now." "A little worse than they do now." "A lot worse than they do now."

Reprinted from Sears ED, Burns PB, Chung KC. Relationship between patient expectations and clinical measures in patients undergoing rheumatoid hand surgery from the silicone arthroplasty in rheumatoid arthritis (SARA) study. *Plast Reconstr Surg.* 2015;136:775e–781e, with permission from American Society of Plastic Surgeons.

Preoperative expectation level was related to baseline patient-reported domains of activities of daily living and hand satisfaction measured by the MHQ ($p = 0.04$ and $p = 0.07$, respectively). Patients had relatively similar satisfaction with hand function postoperatively regardless of preoperative expectation level. No consistent relationship was seen between preoperative expectations and objective measures at baseline and 1-year follow-up.

Conclusions.—High preoperative expectations were not a risk factor for dissatisfaction postoperatively. Preoperative expectation level may be considered for stratifying baseline patient-reported hand function in patients with similar objective hand function (Tables 1 and 2).

▶ The authors in this study are participants in a large National Institutes of Health—funded prospective multicenter study comparing the outcomes of patients treated with silicone metacarpophalangeal joint arthroplasty to patients treated with medical management alone silicone arthroplasty in rheumatoid arthritis (SARA). This operative group was analyzed with respect to pre- and postoperative expectations with the hypothesis that patients with higher preoperative expectations will have better postoperative patient-reported measures including satisfaction. The Michigan Hand Questionnaire (MHQ) was used.

The study did not reach clinical significance in demonstrating better patient-reported outcomes in patients with higher expectations; however, trends were noted with increasing MHQ scores for each domain except aesthetics (this includes function, activities of daily living [ADLs], work, pain, and satisfaction). This large multicenter study, of which the primary author is a participant, is attempting to answer questions about the surgical treatment of rheumatoid arthritis and whether this is actually beneficial to the patient. This particular study provides some insight into treating patients.

What the study does tell us is that patients' preoperative abilities to perform ADLs and preoperative satisfaction with hand function significantly correlated to preoperative expectations. From a practical standpoint, patients who had high preoperative function expected high postoperative function. The study also contradicts the idea that high preoperative expectations may be a risk factor for dissatisfaction after surgery (Tables 1 and 2).

Overall patient satisfaction was not affected by preoperative expectations; however, patient expectations and satisfaction are receiving increasing emphasis as an indicator of quality of care. As practitioners, we need to have open conversations with our patients regarding their expectations, and the development of a validated basic screening tool may be a natural extension of this work.

E. Lawler, MD

First dorsal interosseous muscle contraction results in radiographic reduction of healthy thumb carpometacarpal joint
McGee C, O'Brien V, Van Nortwick S, et al (Univ of Minnesota, Rochester; Univ Orthopaedics Therapy Ctr, Minneapolis, MN; et al)
J Hand Ther 28:375-381, 2015

Introduction.—Hand therapists selectively strengthen the first dorsal interosseus (FDI) to stabilize arthritic joints yet the role of the FDI has not yet been radiographically validated.

Purpose.—To determine if FDI contraction reduces radial subluxation (RS) of the thumb metacarpal (MC).

Methods.—Fluoroscopy was used to obtain true anterior-posterior radiographs of non-arthritic CMC joints: 1) at rest, 2) while stressed and 3) while stressed with maximal FDI contraction. Maximal FDI strength during CMC stress and thumb MC RS and trapezial articular width were measured. The ratio of RS to the articular width was calculated.

Results.—Seventeen participants (5 male, 12 female) participated. Subluxation of a stressed CMC significantly reduced and the subluxation to articular width ratio significantly improved after FDI activation.

Conclusions.—Contraction of the FDI appears to radiographically reduce subluxation of the healthy thumb CMC joint. Further exploration on the FDI's reducibility and its carry-over effects in arthritic thumbs is needed.

Level of Evidence.—4.

▶ This article is an important foundational piece that illustrates the importance of the role of the first dorsal interosseous muscle (FDI) in reducing radial subluxation of the first metacarpal on the trapezium. The sample population was predominantly white, which potentially limits extrapolation to other patient populations.

The authors performed the procedures under fluoroscopy. The results indicated that contraction of the FDI results in statistically significant reduction in radial subluxation of the metacarpal on the trapezium in healthy subjects. A level 5 cadaveric study found that the FDI was the most important stabilizer of the CMC.[1] The results in McGee et al of reducing radial subluxation were large, which may lead to clinical significance, and future studies are needed to determine effects in subjects with osteoarthritis. It remains unknown, however, how much the opponens pollicis (OP) contributed to the reduction of the first metacarpal on the trapezium. Another level 5 cadaveric study found that co-activation of the OP and FDI did the best in reducing radial subluxation and articular width versus contraction of just the OP or the FDI.[2] These authors described the limitations of the study well. Further investigation is needed to understand the influences of ethnicity, age, the dosage of FDI contraction, and possible cocontraction of other dynamic stabilizers including the OP. Because this study only looked at healthy subjects, the reader cannot conclude that the same results will be apparent in people with CMC osteoarthritis. Further research is required to comprehend the benefits of FDI contraction for people with osteoarthritis of the CMC. Further clinical trials are needed to determine the efficacy of dynamic stabilization of the thumb intrinsics on osteoarthritis of the CMC. I am hopeful the authors will continue with this research by studying individuals with carpometacarpal osteoarthritis.

S. Kannas, CHT

References

1. Esplugus M, Morbargha N, Lluch A, Garcias-Elias M, Hagert E. Muscle control of the first carpometacarpal joint. American Association for Hand Surgery 2015 Annual Meeting. Nassau, Bahamas. 2015.
2. Adams JE, O'Brien VH, Magusson E, Rosenstein B. Radiographic analysis of simulated first dorsal interosseous and opponens pollicis activation upon thumb CMC joint subluxation: a cadaver study. American Association for Hand Surgery 2015 Annual Meeting. Nassau, Bahamas. 2015.

Treatment of Digital Mucous Cysts With Intralesional Sodium Tetradecyl Sulfate Injection

Park SE, Park EJ, Kim SS, et al (Hallym Univ College of Medicine, Seoul, Korea)
Dermatol Surg 40:1249-1254, 2014

Background.—Digital mucous cysts (DMCs) are benign myxoid cysts typically involving the distal interphalangeal joint or over the proximal nail fold. There are various treatment modalities for DMCs, and intralesional sodium tetradecyl sulfate injection has been reported as an alternative treatment.

Objective.—To assess the efficacy and safety of intralesional sodium tetradecyl sulfate injection in treating DMCs.

Materials and Methods.—We performed intralesional injection of sodium tetradecyl sulfate in 17 patients (6 men and 11 women) with 20 DMCs. At each session, 1% to 3% sodium tetradecyl sulfate of 0.2 to 0.5 mL was injected into a lesion and repeated every 4 weeks if the cyst persisted. Changes in lesions and adverse reactions were recorded, and therapeutic efficacy was evaluated.

Results.—Of the 20 lesions treated with intralesional sodium tetradecyl sulfate injection, 80% responded. Recurrences were observed in 2 patients, and 2 patients did not respond well to the treatment. No patient reported any major adverse effects.

Conclusion.—Intralesional sodium tetradecyl sulfate injection is a simple, safe, and effective modality for distal mucous cyst. Treatment was well tolerated with few side effects and favorable cure rate. Therefore, we believe that intralesional sodium tetradecyl sulfate injection should be considered an alternative treatment of DMCs.

▶ Nonsurgical alternatives for mucous cysts such as intralesional sodium tetra-decyl sulfate injection could be appealing for those patients who have recurrent cysts after excision or those looking to avoid surgical excision all together. Unfortunately, superficial necrosis, nail deformity, and recurrence are also seen with sodium tetradecyl sulfate (Thromboject). When evaluating the data presented, 9 of the 16 cured lesions have follow-up of less than 12 months and some as few as 2 months. Furthermore, only 3 (50%) of the 6 lesions followed up for more than 24 months were ultimately cured thereby making this adjusted recurrence rate higher than the cited 35% for surgery as well as other modalities like cryosurgery and even drainage. Need for repeated injections, ranging from 1 to 7 sessions, also makes this option seemingly less attractive for most patients. Intralesional injection of sclerosing agents is another modality in our toolbox of treatment options for digital mucoid cysts fraught with similar potential complications.

A. Strohl, MD

Evaluation of Radiographic Instability of the Trapeziometacarpal Joint in Women With Carpal Tunnel Syndrome

Kim JH, Gong HS, Kim YH, et al (Seoul Med Ctr, Korea; Seoul Natl Univ College of Medicine, Korea)
J Hand Surg Am 40:1298-1302, 2015

Purpose.—To determine whether median nerve dysfunction measured by electrophysiologic studies in carpal tunnel syndrome (CTS) is associated with thumb trapeziometacarpal (TMC) joint instability.

Methods.—We evaluated 71 women with CTS and 31 asymptomatic control women. Patients with generalized laxity or TMC joint osteoarthritis were excluded. We classified the electrophysiologic severity of CTS based on nerve conduction time and amplitude and assessed radiographic instability of the TMC joint based on TMC joint stress radiographs. We compared subluxation ratio between patients with CTS and controls and performed correlation analysis of the relationship between the electrophysiologic grade and subluxation ratio.

Results.—Thirty-one patients were categorized into the mild CTS subgroup and 41 into the severe CTS subgroup. There was no significant difference in subluxation ratio between the control group and CTS patients or between the control group and CTS subgroup patients. Furthermore, there was no significant correlation between electrophysiologic grade and subluxation ratio.

Conclusions.—This study demonstrated that patients with CTS did not have greater radiographic TMC joint instability compared with controls, and suggests that TMC joint stability is not affected by impaired median nerve function. Further studies could investigate how to better evaluate proprioceptive function of TMC joint and whether other nerves have effects on TMC joint motor/proprioceptive function, to elucidate the relationship between neuromuscular control of the TMC joint, its stability, and its progression to osteoarthritis.

Type of Study/Level of Evidence.—Diagnostic II.

▶ This article provides evidence that median nerve dysfunction does not directly contribute to trapeziometacarpal (TMC) joint instability. It has been suggested that the muscles around the TMC joint provide dynamic stability, which may be protective against the development of arthritis; however, the association of increased mobility at the TMC joint contributing to the development of arthritis is debatable.

In this article, the authors examine the association of carpal tunnel syndrome with TMC arthritis. Significantly, the authors showed no correlation between electrophysiologic grade and joint instability. Specifically, 102 patients were evaluated: 71 women with carpal tunnel syndrome and 31 asymptomatic controls. Of the 71 patients with carpal tunnel syndrome 31 patients were categorized as having mild and 41 as having severe carpal tunnel syndrome. There was no significant difference in subluxation ratio between the control group and the carpal tunnel patients as a whole and as subgroups. The authors conclude that TMC joint instability is not affected by impaired median nerve function.

The authors acknowledge that limiting the study to the findings from electrophysiologic studies provides an incomplete picture. Further studies are needed to fully appreciate and further examine the contribution of other nerves and muscles effecting TMC joint stability. However, the significance of these findings will still be debatable as the relationship between TMC joint stability and the development of arthritis remains unclear.

P. Kane, MD

What Middle Phalanx Base Fracture Characteristics are Most Reliable and Useful for Surgical Decision-making?
Janssen SJ, on behalf of the Science of Variation Group (Massachusetts General Hosp, Boston; et al)
Clin Orthop Relat Res 473:3943-3950, 2015

Background.—Fracture-dislocations of the proximal interphalangeal joint are vexing because subluxation and articular damage can lead to arthrosis and the treatments are imperfect. Ideally, a surgeon could advise a patient, based on radiographs, when the risk of problems merits operative intervention, but it is unclear if middle phalanx base fracture characteristics are sufficiently reliable to be useful for surgical decision making.

Questions/Purposes.—We evaluated (1) the degree of interobserver agreement as a function of fracture characteristics, (2) the differences in interobserver agreement between experienced and less-experienced hand surgeons, and (3) what fracture characteristics and surgeon characteristics were associated with the decision for operative treatment.

Methods.—Ninety-nine (33%) of 296 hand surgeons evaluated 21 intraarticular middle phalanx base fractures on lateral radiographs. Eighty-one surgeons (82%) were in academic practice and 57 (58%) had less than 10 years experience. Participants assessed six fracture characteristics and recommended treatment (nonoperative or operative: extension block pinning, external fixation, open reduction and internal fixation, volar plate arthroplasty, or hemihamate autograft arthroplasty) for all cases.

Results.—With all surgeons pooled together, the interobserver agreement for fracture characteristics was substantial for assessment of a 2-mm articular step or gap (kappa, 0.73; 95% CI, 0.60−0.86; $p < 0.001$), subluxation or dislocation (kappa, 0.72; 95% CI, 0.58−0.86; $p < 0.001$), and percentage of articular surface involved (intraclass correlation coefficient [ICC], 0.67; 95% CI, 0.54−0.81; $p < 0.001$); moderate for comminution (kappa, 0.55; 95% CI, 0.39−0.70; $p < 0.001$) and stability (kappa, 0.54; 95% CI, 0.39−0.69; $p < 0.001$); and fair for the number of fracture fragments (ICC, 0.39; 95% CI, 0.27−0.57; $p < 0.001$). When recommending treatment, interobserver agreement was substantial (kappa, 0.69; 95% CI, 0.50−0.88; $p < 0.001$) for the recommendation to operate or not to operate, but only fair (kappa, 0.34; 95% CI, 0.21−0.47; $p < 0.001$) for the specific type of treatment, indicating variation in operative techniques. There were no differences in agreement for any of the fracture characteristics or treatment preference between less-experienced and more-experienced surgeons, although statistical power on this comparison was low. None of the surgeon characteristics was associated with the decision for operative treatment, whereas all fracture characteristics were, except for stable and uncertain joint stability. Articular step or gap (β, 0.90; R-squared, 0.89; 95% CI, 0.75−1.05; $p < 0.001$), likelihood of subluxation or dislocation (β, 0.80; R-squared, 0.76; 95% CI, 0.59−1.02; $p < 0.001$), and unstable fractures (β, 0.88; R-squared, 0.81; 95% CI, 0.67−1.1; $p < 0.001$), are most strongly associated with the decision for operative treatment.

Conclusions.—We found that assessment of a step or gap and likelihood of subluxation were most reliable and are strongly associated with the decision for operative treatment. Surgeons largely agree on which fractures might benefit from surgery, and the variation seems to be with the operative technique. Efforts at improving the care of these fractures should focus on the comparative effectiveness of the various operative treatment options.

Level of Evidence.—Level III, diagnostic study.

▶ The authors set out to potentially simplify a set of complicated and vexing questions regarding which middle phalanx base fractures need surgical intervention and what technique should be used to fix them. Unfortunately, there remains variability of optimal repair technique selection (extensive block pinning, external fixation, open reduction and internal fixation, volar plate arthroplasty, or hemi-hamate arthroplasty) among both experienced (> 10 years of practice) and less-experienced (< 10 years of practice) surgeons. We do learn that surgeons mostly agree on characteristics that lead to recommending operative intervention and the radiographic criteria that formulate that basis. Because surgeons cannot agree on how to fix these fracture dislocations, it may be more important to establish guidelines, recommendations, and outcomes measures based on the factors that are in agreement. By focusing on shared decision-making criteria, the outcomes of function, stiffness, and post-traumatic osteoarthritis may be more applicable and useful despite variable treatment specifics.

A. Strohl, MD

The Effect of a Bone Tunnel During Ligament Reconstruction for Trapeziometacarpal Osteoarthritis: A 5-Year Follow-up

Spekreijse KR, Vermeulen GM, Kedilioglu MA, et al (Erasmus Med Ctr, Rotterdam, The Netherlands; Xpert Clinic, Hilversum, The Netherlands)
J Hand Surg Am 40:2214-2222, 2015

Purpose.—To compare in trapeziometacarpal (TMC) osteoarthritis the effects of trapeziectomy with tendon interposition and ligament reconstruction (LRTI) with or without a bone tunnel after a mean follow-up of 5 years.

Methods.—We randomized 79 women (aged 40 years or older) with stage IV TMC osteoarthritis to either trapeziectomy with LRTI using a bone tunnel (Burton-Pellegrini) or a tendon sling arthroplasty (Weilby). Before surgery and at 3 months and 1 year after surgery, patients were evaluated for pain, function, strength, satisfaction, and complications. Of these patients, 72% were evaluated after a mean follow-up of 5 years (range, 3.8–6.4 years).

Results.—There were no significant differences in function and pain (Patient-Rated Wrist and Hand Evaluation) between treatment groups after a mean follow-up of 5 years. In addition, grip and pinch strength, satisfaction, and persisting complications did not differ between groups. Three patients in the Weilby group had repeat surgery (2 for symptomatic scaphotrapezoidal osteoarthritis and 1 elsewhere) and one in the Burton-Pellegrini group operated on again elsewhere. Furthermore, 3 patients who were first conservatively treated for a trigger finger or neuroma were operated on again because conservative therapy failed. Two more patients were operated on again because of de Quervain tendinitis and carpal tunnel syndrome. The overall treatment effect of both groups together showed no significant differences between results at 1 and 5 years after surgery, except for grip strength, which improved for both groups.

Conclusions.—This study showed that improved function, strength, and satisfaction obtained at 1 year after trapeziectomy with LRTI with or without the use of a bone tunnel for stage IV TMC thumb osteoarthritis was maintained after 5 years.

Type of Study/Level of Evidence.—Therapeutic I.

▶ The authors performed a randomized prospective trial comparing standard tendon interposition and ligament reconstruction (LRTI) using a bone tunnel with a tendon sling arthroplasty (Weilby) in 79 women with stage IV trapeziometacarpal arthritis. The patients were evaluated for pain, function, strength, satisfaction, and complications. At a mean follow-up of 5 years, there was no difference between the 2 groups in any of the clinical outcome parameters. This is in contrast to the previous report by the authors on their short-term results at 3 months and 1 year, which found better outcome at 3 months with the bone tunnel patients, suggesting faster recovery. The primary outcome measure was the Patient-Rated Wrist and Hand Evaluation questionnaire for both pain and functionality. The findings in this study are consistent with other studies comparing various procedures for treatment of advanced thumb carpometacarpal (CMC) arthritis, which demonstrate no differences in outcome in those performed with and without ligament reconstruction, and with and without tendon interposition. The Weilby procedure is simpler to perform and avoids the potential complications associated with bone tunnels, including fracture of the tunnel.

Interestingly, despite the published literature demonstrating no difference in outcomes, other than higher complication rates when comparing LRTI with trapeziectomy alone, many hand surgeons still prefer the LRTI for patients with advanced thumb CMC arthritis. In a survey sent to 2536 ASSH members, the treatment of choice was LRTI in 68% of surgeons, regardless of their training and years of experience.[1] Less than 3% of respondents perform a trapeziectomy alone. The majority of hand surgeons (more than 70%) performing surgery for thumb CMC arthritis favored the treatment they have always performed and have not changed their practices.

J. I. Huang, MD

Reference

1. Brunton LM, Wilgis EF. A survey to determine current practice patterns in the surgical treatment of advanced thumb carpometacarpal osteoarthrosis. *Hand.* 2010; 5:415-422.

Revision Proximal Interphalangeal Arthroplasty: An Outcome Analysis of 75 Consecutive Cases
Wagner ER, Luo TD, Houdek MT, et al (Mayo Clinic, Rochester, MN)
J Hand Surg Am 40:1949-1955, 2015

Purpose.—To examine the outcomes and complications associated with revision proximal interphalangeal (PIP) joint arthroplasty.

Methods.—An analysis of 75 consecutive revision PIP joint arthroplasties in 49 patients, performed between 1998 to 2012, was performed. The mean age at the time of surgery was 58 years. Thirty-two patients had a history of prior PIP joint trauma, and 18 patients had rheumatoid arthritis. There were 12 constrained (silicone) implants and 63 nonconstrained implants (34 pyrocarbon and 29 metal-plastic).

Results.—Over the 14-year period, 19 (25%) fingers underwent a second revision surgery. Second revision surgeries were performed for infection, instability, flexion contracture, and heterotopic ossification. The 2-, 5-, and 10-year survival rates were 80%, 70%, and 70%, respectively, for patients requiring a second revision for PIP joint arthroplasty. Worse outcomes were seen with postoperative dislocations, pyrocarbon implants, and when bone grafting was required. Two operations were complicated by intraoperative fractures, but neither required stabilization. Sixteen patients undergoing revision surgery experienced a postoperative complication, including 2 infections, 1 postoperative fracture, 3 cases of heterotopic ossification, and 10 PIP joint dislocations. The volar approach and the use of a pyrocarbon implant were associated with increased rates of heterotopic ossification, whereas preoperative instability increased the rates of PIP joint dislocation following revision. At a mean of 5.3 years (range, 2–10 years) follow-up, 98% of patients had good pain relief but decreased PIP joint total arc of motion.

Conclusions.—Proximal interphalangeal joint arthroplasty in the revision setting represents a challenge for surgeons. Revision arthroplasty was associated with a 70% 5-year survival but with a high incidence of complications. Instability was associated with worse outcomes. In this series, silicone and metal-polyethylene implants had lower rates of implant failure and postoperative complications than ones made from pyrocarbon.

Type of Study/Level of Evidence.—Prognostic III.

▶ This article traces the clinical course of a fairly large cohort of proximal interphalangeal joint (PIPJ) arthroplasty revisions. The authors have had extensive experience with this surgery over a 14-year period and have shown results from the short (1 year) to long (10 years) term. This is an extremely informative article for those of us who have less experience in this challenging procedure.

In their results (Table 2), it is interesting to see that postoperative dislocation, use of pyrocarbon implants, and use of bone graft were all significant risk factors for implant failure after revision surgery. The authors cited poor soft tissue support, implant design limitations, and poor bone stock, respectively, as possible explanations for these observations. It is also noteworthy that the hazard ratios for use of cement or the other implants were below 1, although none of them had a P value $< .05$. These latter results may suggest that cement better compensates for poor bone stock and that the other implants are better suited for use in revisions, although further study would be necessary for a more definitive answer.

Most hand surgeons are aware that reported results of PIPJ arthroplasty are not as predictable as most of us would like. In the setting of revision arthroplasty, these results may become even less favorable, especially when range motion of the PIPJ was shown in this article to decrease, whereas preoperative range of motion is typically maintained after primary PIPJ arthroplasty.

This excellent article would be even better if the authors had analyzed other aspects of this cohort. First, it would be very informative if the risk factors for primary PIPJ arthroplasties to require revision arthroplasty were delineated. This would be especially relevant when it comes to the use of pyrocarbon implants in the primary arthroplasty. Second, it would be educational for our readers to understand the clinical outcomes of the patients who required a second revision. All this information would go a long way in informing both the decision-making process for PIPJ arthroplasty and our counseling of the patients on the risks and benefits of this procedure.

Overall, this article confirms the idea that revision PIPJ arthroplasty should be attempted only by the most experienced of surgeons, because even in their hands, outcomes are variable at best.

A. Cheah, MD

Trapeziectomy With a Tendon Tie-in Implant for Osteoarthritis of the Trapeziometacarpal Joint
Avisar E, Elvey M, Tzang C, et al (Assaf Harofeh Med Ctr, Zerifin, Israel; Univ College London Hosp, United Kingdom)
J Hand Surg Am 40:1292-1297, 2015

Purpose.—To evaluate the early to mid-term clinical and radiological outcomes of trapeziectomy with a tendon tie-in trapezium implant arthroplasty for moderate to severe trapeziometacarpal (TMC) joint osteoarthritis (Eaton stages III to IV).

Methods.—We assessed all patients who underwent trapeziectomy and tendon tie-in trapezium implant arthroplasty stabilized with a Weilby flexor carpi radialis tendon sling for osteoarthritis of the TMC joint between 2008 and 2010 at our institution. Twenty-two patients (28 thumbs) who had had an operation at least 12 months earlier were clinically evaluated at an average follow-up of 18 months. Subjective clinical outcomes evaluation included visual analog scale scores and Disabilities of the Arm, Shoulder, and Hand score questionnaires. Objective clinical evaluation included lateral pinch and grip tests and active thumb range of motion. All patients underwent a radiological assessment by 2 independent musculoskeletal radiologists. In cases of unilateral treatment, we compared clinical results obtained from the operated hands with the contralateral hand.

Results.—The mean preoperative visual analog scale score of the cohort was 7.4. We documented a statistically significant improvement to 1.2 at a mean of 18 months after the operation (range, 12—26 mo). The mean postoperative Disabilities of the Arm, Shoulder, and Hand score was 21. Thumb palmar abduction was 85°; thumb metacarpophalangeal joint flexion and TMC joint extension were 30° and 10°, respectively. There were 2

TABLE 2.—Hazard Ratios for Implant Failure in Revision PIP Arthroplasty

Risk Factor	Hazard Ratio	95% Confidence Interval	P Value
Postoperative dislocation	5.15	1.89–12.97	.002*
Pyrocarbon implant	3.09	1.22–8.81	.02*
Bone graft	2.94	1.03–7.49	.045*
Preoperative instability	1.78	0.69–4.42	.22
Intraoperative fracture	1.66	0.09–8.06	.65
Prednisone use	1.42	0.40–3.96	.55
Diabetes mellitus	1.18	0.18–4.14	.83
Methotrexate use	1.12	0.18–3.92	.88
Posttraumatic arthritis	1.10	0.45–2.72	.83
Osteoarthritis	1.06	0.40–2.65	.90
Female	1.02	0.34–4.41	.97
Body mass index	1.00	0.90–1.07	.94
Age at surgery	1.00	0.97–1.04	.82
Inflammatory arthritis	0.81	0.23–2.22	.69
Surface replacement arthroplasty implant	0.42	0.14–1.11	.08
Silicone implant	0.37	0.02–1.78	.25
Cemented implant	0.41	0.12–1.14	.09

*Statistically significant (P < .05).
Reprinted from Wagner ER, Luo TD, Houdek MT, et al. Revision proximal interphalangeal arthroplasty: an outcome analysis of 75 consecutive cases. *J Hand Surg Am.* 2015;40:1949-1955, with permission from American Society for Surgery of the Hand.

cases of prosthesis removal owing to implant dislocation. No late complications were recorded.

Conclusions.—Good short-term to mid-term results and stability of TMC arthroplasty implant can be achieved with tie-in trapezium implant stabilized with a Weilby flexor carpi radialis tendon sling.

Type of Study/Level of Evidence.—Therapeutic IV.

▶ In this retrospective review, the authors evaluated the early to midterm results of 28 thumbs in 22 patients who were treated with the Weilby FCR tendon silicon implant tie-in technique for treatment of Eaton stage III or IV carpometacarpal arthritis. The authors used lateral pinch and grip strength, clinical evaluation, DASH, and radiographic assessments to evaluate their results of this procedure at a minimum follow-up of 12 months and mean follow-up of 18 months. They suggest that the advantages of this procedure over joint replacement arthroplasty and traditional LRTI are improved thumb biomechanics and less axial displacement after trapeziectomy with less potential fro MCP joint hyperextension.

Although the authors report excellent short-term results, their sample size was small, the review was retrospective and potentially open to bias, and thus it will most likely not significantly change my current practice. The long-term results of traditional LRTI are overwhelmingly favorable and continue to influence my decision to perform this procedure in carefully selected patients. A longer term, prospective, and controlled study evaluating this interesting technique would hopefully address concerns for implant instability, prosthesis-related synovitis, and durability.

J. L. Tueting, MD

Distal Radioulnar Joint Reaction Force Following Ulnar Shortening: Diaphyseal Osteotomy Versus Wafer Resection
Canham CD, Schreck MJ, Maqsoodi N, et al (Univ of Rochester, NY; et al)
J Hand Surg Am 40:2206-2212, 2015

Purpose.—To compare how ulnar diaphyseal shortening and wafer resection affect distal radioulnar joint (DRUJ) joint reaction force (JRF) using a nondestructive method of measurement. Our hypothesis was that ulnar shortening osteotomy would increase DRUJ JRF more than wafer resection.

Methods.—Eight fresh-frozen human cadaveric upper limbs were obtained. Under fluoroscopic guidance, a threaded pin was inserted into the lateral radius orthogonal to the DRUJ and a second pin was placed in the medial ulna coaxial to the radial pin. Each limb was mounted onto a mechanical tensile testing machine and a distracting force was applied across the DRUJ while force and displacement were simultaneously measured. Data sets were entered into a computer and a polynomial was generated and solved to determine the JRF. This process was repeated after ulnar diaphyseal osteotomy, ulnar re-lengthening, and ulnar wafer resection. The JRF was compared among the 4 conditions.

Results.—Average baseline DRUJ JRF for the 8 arms increased significantly after diaphyseal ulnar shortening osteotomy (7.2 vs 10.3 N). Average JRF after re-lengthening the ulna and wafer resection was 6.9 and 6.7 N, respectively. There were no differences in JRF among baseline, relengthened, and wafer resection conditions.

Conclusions.—Distal radioulnar joint JRF increased significantly after ulnar diaphyseal shortening osteotomy and did not increase after ulnar wafer resection.

Clinical Relevance.—Diaphyseal ulnar shortening osteotomy increases DRUJ JRF, which may lead to DRUJ arthrosis.

▶ The purpose of this biomechanical cadaveric study was to compare the effect of diaphyseal ulnar shortening osteotomy and distal ulnar wafer resection on distal radioulnar joint (DRUJ) joint reaction force (JRF). The authors tested 8 fresh frozen cadaveric specimens without preexisting DRUJ pathology. Specimens with Tolat type 3 DRUJ or greater than 1 mm ulnar positive or negative variance were excluded. Each specimen was mounted to a tensile testing apparatus that applied a uniaxial distracting force across the DRUJ while force and displacement were measured. The authors were then able to calculate the JRF across the DRUJ (specific methods previously described in referenced article).[1] Each specimen underwent baseline testing followed by testing after a 3-mm diaphyseal ulnar shortening osteotomy was made and fixed with a 3.5-mm dynamic compression plate. The third test was performed after each specimen underwent relengthening of the previously made osteotomy to confirm return to baseline. The 4th test was performed after a 3-mm distal ulnar wafer resection. There was a statistically significant increase in DRUJ JRF after diaphyseal ulnar shortening osteotomy that returned to baseline after relengthening. Distal ulnar wafer resection did not increase the JRF. Previous reports have shown a 16% to 50% rate of radiographic changes at the DRUJ 2 to 5 years after diaphyseal ulnar shortening osteotomy; however, the rate of symptomatic DRUJ arthrosis is uncertain. This is likely because of increased JRF across the DRUJ and also joint surface incongruity after ulnar osteotomy. The major limitation of this study is that specimens with greater than 1-mm ulnar positive or negative variation were excluded. Clinically, ulnar shortening osteotomies are performed on patients with ulnar positive variance, and therefore the changes seen across the DRUJ may differ after shortening osteotomy in those patients. Additionally, having separate specimens for the distal wafer resection and diaphyseal osteotomies could have further validated the results. This article provides valuable insight into the development of DRUJ arthrosis after ulnar shortening osteotomy and leads the reader to critically evaluate which osteotomy may be better suited to each individual patient. However, further clinical studies would be needed to help determine the rates of symptomatic arthrosis after each procedure before instituting large practice changes. Additionally, it would be interesting to see changes in DRUJ JRF after osteotomy in an ulnar positive specimen.

E. J. Gauger, MD

Reference

1. Canham CD, Schreck MJ, Maqsoodi N, Doolittle M, Olles M, Elfar JC. A nondestructive, reproducible method of measuring joint reaction force at the distal radioulnar joint. *J Hand Surg Am.* 2015;40:1138-1144.

2 Wrist Arthroscopy

Arthroscopic Skills Acquisition Tools: An Online Simulator for Arthroscopy Training
Gandhi MJ, Anderton MJ, Funk L (Orthopaedic Inst, Oswestry, England; Royal Blackburn Hosp, England; Wrightington Hosp, Wigan, England)
Arthroscopy 31:1671-1679, 2015

Purpose.—To evaluate correlations between objective performances measured by a new online arthroscopic skills acquisition tool (ASAT, in which "shape match" with inverted controls requires lifting shapes and releasing them into their corresponding silhouettes) and a validated virtual reality (VR) shoulder arthroscopy simulator (Insight Arthro VR; GMV, Madrid, Spain).

Methods.—Forty-nine medical students familiarized themselves with 5 ASATs. They were then assessed using a sixth ASAT (shape match with inverted controls) and 4 VR tasks (operating room, visualize, locate and palpate, and pendulum) on the VR simulator. Correlations were assessed between 11 ASAT measures and 15 VR measures using Pearson correlation coefficients.

Results.—Time taken and delta distance (actual distance minus minimum distance traveled) were the most frequent and correlated ASAT measures. Time taken correlated with the VR locate-and-palpate time ($r = 0.596$, $P < .001$), visualize time ($r = 0.381$, $P = .007$), and pendulum time ($r = 0.646$, $P < .001$), whereas delta distance correlated with the locate-and-palpate camera distance ($r = 0.667$, $P < .001$), instrument distance ($r = 0.664$, $P < .001$), visualize distance ($r = 0.4$, $P = .004$), pendulum camera distance ($r = 0.538$, $P < .001$), and instrument distance ($r = 0.539$, $P < .001$).

Conclusions.—There were significant correlations between performance measures on the ASAT and a validated arthroscopic VR simulator.

Clinical Relevance.—Arthroscopic simulators are available but are limited by their high cost and availability. ASATs may overcome these limitations by using widely available Internet-based software and basic input devices.

▶ The acquisition of arthroscopic skills poses a special challenge in orthopedic surgery training. The learning curve for even basic skills can be time consuming and costly when only performed in the clinical setting, apart from posing a potential safety risk for patients. Cadaver-based simulation most closely reproduces the anatomic complexity found in the living patient. However, cadaver laboratories are expensive and require an extended infrastructure. Several simulators have been developed for teaching basic arthroscopic skills, including knot-tying boards and anatomy models. More recently, virtual reality—based simulators are increasingly popular for the transition in training from basic models to advanced cadaver-based sessions. However, virtual reality—based simulation requires the acquisition of expensive equipment.

The study by Gandhi et al presents the validation of an arthroscopic skills assessment tool developed by the authors. The tool provides an attractive alternative to more expensive virtual reality—based simulators, as it is based on widely available hardware with comparatively low costs of purchase and maintenance. As the authors point out, their tool will be most effective in the familiarization and core skill acquisition phases of arthroscopic training.

P. Streubel, MD

3   Carpus

Force in the Scapholunate Interosseous Ligament During Active Wrist Motion

Dimitris C, Werner FW, Joyce DA, et al (SUNY Upstate Med Univ, Syracuse, NY)
J Hand Surg Am 40:1525-1533, 2015

Purpose.—To examine the force experienced by the scapholunate interosseous ligament (SLIL) during movements of the wrist.

Methods.—Six fresh-frozen cadaveric wrists were freed of soft tissue and tested in a computer controlled, servohydraulic simulator. Each wrist was tested cyclically through simulated active arcs of flexion-extension and dart throw motion. Tensile forces were recorded across the scapholunate joint with the SLIL cut through a cable placed through the scaphoid to the lunate and fixed to a force transducer external to the wrist.

Results.—The average recorded maximal tensile force across the scapholunate joint during all tested motions was 20 N. During wrist flexion-extension and the dart throw motion, SLIL force was greater at maximum extension than at maximum flexion. No significant differences among the different motions at maximum flexion or extension or for maximal force during motion were found.

Conclusions.—Forces during the flexion-extension and dart throw motions were significantly higher in extension than in flexion. However, during simple unresisted wrist motions, the force did not exceed 20 N.

Clinical Relevance.—This information can be used to evaluate surgical methods used for SLIL repairs and thus provide better outcomes for patients.

▶ This biomechanical study examined the force through a cable approximating the scapholunate ligament during simulated wrist motion. The bulk of this article describes the biomechanical setup. In brief, the authors placed a cable between the scaphoid and lunate of a cadaver wrist, stripped most of the soft tissues except the wrist flexors and extensors, sectioned the scapholunate ligament, and then used the intact tendons to move the wrist through flexion and extension and dart-throwing motion. Using this arrangement, the authors found relatively low forces through the cable (average maximal tensile force of 20 N) and that the force was slightly higher in wrist extension than in other motions.

In this model, the cable was passed approximately along the center axis of sca-pholunate interval (much like a screw would be placed for an RASL), and that single cable is used to approximate the forces of the proximal, dorsal, and volar components of the scapholunate ligament. One might guess that forces would be lower in this central position than ligaments placed more peripherally. The authors suggest that one clinical application would be to avoid wrist extension during rehabilitation of the scapholunate ligament, but clear evidence support-ing that recommendation is lacking.

C. M. Ward, MD

Accuracy of enhanced and unenhanced MRI in diagnosing scaphoid proximal pole avascular necrosis and predicting surgical outcome
Fox MG, Wang DT, Chhabra AB (Univ of Virginia, Charlottesville; Univ of Virginia Health System, Charlottesville; et al)
Skeletal Radiol 44:1671-1678, 2015

Purpose.—Determine the sensitivity, specificity and accuracy of unen-hanced and enhanced MRI in diagnosing scaphoid proximal pole (PP) avascular necrosis (AVN) and correlate whether MRI can help guide the selection of a vascularized or nonvascularized bone graft.

Methods.—The study was approved by the IRB. Two MSK radiologists independently performed a retrospective review of unenhanced and enhanced MRIs from 18 patients (16 males, 2 females; median age, 17.5 years) with scaphoid nonunions and surgery performed within 65 days of the MRI. AVN was diagnosed on the unenhanced MRI when a diffusely decreased T1-W signal was present in the PP and on the enhanced MRI when PP enhancement was less than distal pole enhancement. Surgical absence of PP bleeding was diagnostic of PP AVN. Postoperative osseous union (OU) was assessed with computed tomography and/or radiographs.

Results.—Sensitivity, specificity and accuracy for PP AVN were 71, 82 and 78% for unenhanced and 43, 82 and 67% for enhanced MRI. Patients with PP AVN on unenhanced MRI had 86% (6/7) OU; 100% (5/5) OU with vascularized bone grafts and 50% (1/2) OU with nonvascularized grafts. Patients with PP AVN on enhanced MRI had 80% (4/5) OU; 100% (3/3) OU with vascularized bone grafts and 50% (1/2) OU with nonvascularized grafts. Patients with viable PP on unenhanced and enhanced MRI had 91% (10/11) and 92% (12/13) OU, respectively, all but one with nonvascularized graft.

Conclusions.—When PP AVN is evident on MRI, OU is best achieved with vascularized grafts. If PPAVN is absent, OU is successful with nonvas-cularized grafts.

▶ This study investigates the predictive value of enhanced and unenhanced MRI scans to assess viability of the proximal pole of the scaphoid and, ultimately, clinical outcome. The authors conclude that MRI scans can accurately predict intraoperative perfusion and that osseous union is achieved most reliably by using vascularized bone grafts in patients with avascular necrosis of the proximal pole. Although, apart from the small number of patients, this study is generally well designed, there are some other weaknesses: surgeons were not blinded to the radiologists' assessments, it remains unclear how the grafts were chosen, and quite a few patients were not assessed by CT scans postoperatively. Its first aim is not quite new, but this study adds some evidence that preoperative MRI scans are a valuable predictive tool in determining the vascularity of the scaphoid. However, considering the small patient population and arbitrary allocation to treatment options, the conclusion concerning the choice of grafts does not seem justified. It also seems bold to suggest that preoperative MRI predicts clinical outcome better than the intraoperative assessment of vascularity. Our group has found the opposite result in a prospective study of 60 patients,[1] and unfortunately our study is not discussed in this article. Vascularity of the proximal pole is an important, but certainly not the only critical determinant in scaphoid reconstruction. In my opinion, MRI scans may help in discussing possible options with the patient, but, as a surgeon, I think that the ultimate decision of whether to use a vascularized bone graft should be made intraoperatively.

K. Megerle, MD

Reference

1. Megerle K, Worg H, Christopoulos G, Schmitt R, Krimmer H. Gadolinium-enhanced preoperative MRI scans as a prognostic parameter in scaphoid nonunion. *J Hand Surg Eur Vol.* 2011;36:23-28.

Surgical Treatments for Scapholunate Advanced Collapse Wrist: Kinematics and Functional Performance
Wolff AL, Garg R, Kraszewski AP, et al (Hosp for Special Surgery, New York)
J Hand Surg Am 40:1547-1553, 2015

Purpose.—The purpose of this investigation was to compare kinematic motion and functional performance during 2 tasks in patients following 4-corner fusion (4CF) or proximal row carpectomy (PRC) and to compare these data with those from healthy asymptomatic individuals.

Methods.—Twenty men (10 4CFs and 10 PRCs, ages, 43–82 y) were recruited for 3-dimensional wrist motion analysis testing. Kinematic coupling (the ratio of wrist flexion/extension to radialulnar deviation), kinematic path length (a measure of total angle distance), clinical measures, and performance measures were collected during 2 tasks: dart throwing and hammering. For each outcome, between-group comparisons employed a 1-way analysis of variance with post hoc analysis using the Fisher least significant difference test.

Results.—All clinical measures (flexion-extension, radial-ulnar deviation, and grip strength) were decreased for 4CF and PRC patients compared with healthy subjects. Coupling, kinematic path length, and performance were all significantly reduced in 4CF and PRC patients compared with healthy subjects during both tasks. Reduced coupling and a shorter kinematic path length are indicative of less global and combined wrist motion. There were no differences identified in coupling patterns or performance between the surgical groups for the dart-throwing task. However, in hammering, the kinematic path length and performance (time and total strikes) were worse in 4CF than in PRC.

Conclusions.—Differences in wrist kinematics and performance were identified between the groups. PRC subjects performed better on kinematic and performance variables. As expected, both groups demonstrated decreased wrist kinematic motion and functional performance compared with individuals with normal wrists. These results require confirmation and while they cannot be used to determine the benefits of one procedure over the other, they are an important step in quantifying differences in motion and function between procedures.

Type of Study/Level of Evidence.—Therapeutic II.

▶ This article summarizes results for the use of a motion analysis system that captures motion in 3 dimensions using skin-based markers in an important group of patients. The authors examine 20 patients who have undergone salvage wrist procedures for scapholunate advanced collapse. Ten of the patients underwent a 4-corner fusion, and the other 10 underwent a proximal row carpectomy. They compared the motion in these patients, all of whom underwent salvage procedure in the dominant hand, to control patients.

They examined motion during 2 interesting tasks. The first task is a dart-throwing motion task that invokes a discussion of coupling. Coupling is the linked relationship between flexion-extension and radioulnar deviation in the wrist. By way of review, radial deviation of the wrist flexes the proximal carpal row and ulnar deviation does the opposite. This coupling of motion allows for the definition of a somewhat idealized, albeit probably not terribly important, kind of motion that is embodied in the dart thrower's task. When this task is undertaken, the wrist essentially flexes and ulnarly deviates, and this could theoretically occur in just the right amounts so that the flexion of the wrist and, therefore, the proximal row is counteracted perfectly by the ulnar deviation of the wrist and its concurrent extension of the same proximal row. Coupling is therefore ideally studied in the dart-throwers motion where flexion is counteracted by ulnar deviation and a single dart thrower on a single trial might theoretically be able to hold his or her proximal row relatively still while launching the dart. In these patients, the dart-throwing motion is done several times, and an actual target is used. All of this is done while motion in the wrist is measured with great precision. The second task used in this study is hammering, where subjects were instructed to strike a nail repeatedly until the head was flush with a wood surface or until the nail was irreparably bent.

Motion analysis during normal tasks is novel in and of itself, and yet the authors are able to add this to the study of patients who have undergone salvage procedures that are motion sparing in nature. They compare the results in 4-corner fusion patients to proximal row carpectomy patients, and in so doing, they enter the fray of discussion among hand surgeons as to the relative merits of one of these procedures over the other. Classical studies have shown that both of these procedures lead to roughly the same amount of wrist motion and some have suggested that 4-corner fusion patients fare better when it comes to strength in the hand. Others have noted that proximal row carpectomy patients fare better in the postoperative period and have a lower complication rate. Still others have noted that proximal row carpectomy may have a shorter longevity than 4-corner fusion because of the inevitable onset of arthritis. The debate is ongoing as to which patients are best suited for which procedure. What is notable is that no single study has addressed wrist kinematics using these types of sensors in these patients. All patients included in the study had undergone wrist salvage-type procedures more than 6 months earlier, and all 4-corner fusion patients had gone on to complete union.

The results of the study are very interesting. As is perhaps expected, all clinical measurements, including the flexion extension and radial ulnar deviation arcs, were smaller for 4-corner fusion and proximal row carpectomy patients as compared with healthy patients, as was grip strength compared with healthy subjects. The kinematic path length, which is an aggregate measure of flexion-extension and radial and ulnar deviation, as well as coupling and all other parameters of motion measured were smaller for 4-corner fusion and proximal row carpectomy patients. Most notably, there were no differences identified in coupling patterns or performance between surgical groups for the dart-throwing task; however, in hammering, the kinematic path length and performance were worse for 4-corner fusion patients than for proximal row carpectomy patients.

This result is enlightening. Those who favor 4-corner fusion in patients requiring salvage procedures have often believed that the 4-corner fusion results in a more natural wrist with the lunate resting in its own fossa and range of motion, therefore, theoretically being greater. The idea of having a capitate bone sitting in the lunate fossa with 2 corresponding surfaces that have different radii of curvature has been unattractive to some surgeons. And yet in this study, it appears as if proximal row carpectomy fared at least as well as 4-corner fusion in all testing and may have fared better in the hammering task.

Although conclusions drawn from a study like this are difficult to apply in the simple, day-to-day assessment and decision-making process for patients, the study has merit on multiple levels. First, it allows a new and relatively noninvasive way to analyze postoperative motion in patients for whom functional outcome has always been statically assessed. The role of dynamic assessment is only now emerging in its importance and relevance in hand surgery. If dynamic assessment can reproducibly reveal differences between proximal row carpectomy and 4-corner fusion patients, then it may be applied elsewhere in hand surgery, and this may have clear implications for the assessment of function even outside the realm of surgery. Additionally, the importance of the result and the seemingly never-ending debate between practitioners who favor one or another salvage procedure cannot be overlooked. Perhaps those who favor the simpler proximal row carpectomy, with its more reliable healing time, may derive some satisfaction from this study, which shows that characteristics of motion in proximal row carpectomy patients are equally impaired compared with those who have undergone 4-corner fusion. The authors are to be congratulated in all cases for a novel approach to noninvasive assessment and its creative application to address what is becoming an age-old question in hand surgery.

J. Elfar, MD

Wafer Resection of the Distal Ulna

Griska A, Feldon P (Orthopedic Associates of Lancaster, PA; New England Baptist Hosp, Boston, MA)
J Hand Surg Am 40:2283-2288, 2015

The wafer procedure is an effective treatment for ulnar impaction syndrome, which decompresses the ulnocarpal junction through a limited open or arthroscopic approach. In comparison with other common decompressive procedures, the wafer procedure does not require bone healing or internal fixation and also provides excellent exposure of the proximal surface of the triangular fibrocartilage complex. Results of the wafer procedure have been good and few complications have been reported.

▶ This article essentially describes a surgical technique used to resect the distal pole of the ulna. The authors describe the use of this technique to treat ulna impaction syndrome as well as symptomatic tears of the triangular fibro cartilage complex (TFCC). Both open and arthroscopic approaches are described. The outcomes compare favorably with open ulnar shortening osteotomies. The technique allows for direct inspection of the TFCC with possible debridement and repair as indicated. The advantages and disadvantages are well delineated, as are the indications and contraindications. The surgical approach is also well described.

I have been quite satisfied with the results of this procedure in my own patients. I favor only 2-week postoperative immobilization with early range of motion unless triangular fibro cartilage repair is performed.

All and all, this is a well-done review of distal ulna resection. It is complete with thorough delineation of pearls and pitfalls.

J. A. Ortiz, Jr, MD

Multiplanar wrist joint proprioception: The effect of anesthetic blockade of the posterior interosseous nerve or skin envelope surrounding the joint
Taylor KF, Meyer VM, Smith LB, et al (Penn State Milton S. Hershey Med Ctr, PA; Brooke Army Med Ctr, Fort Sam Houston, TX; US Army Res Inst of Environmental Medicine, Natick, MA; et al)
J Hand Ther 28:369-374, 2015

Study Design.—Randomized clinical trial.

Purpose.—Contribution of the posterior interosseous nerve (PIN) and surrounding skin envelope to wrist proprioception is a topic of debate and the primary focus of this research.

Methods.—We performed a double-blinded, placebo control study in which subjects underwent baseline multiplanar testing of wrist proprioception. They were randomized to receive either anesthetic blockade of the PIN within the fourth dorsal compartment, or circumferential topical anesthetic blockade of skin surrounding the wrist. Corresponding opposite wrists underwent placebo intervention with saline injection or inert ultrasound gel. Subjects repeated proprioceptive testing.

Results.—Eighty subjects, 45 male and 35 female, mean age 33 years (range, 19—64 years), completed testing. The percentage of measurements falling outside a $\pm 18°$ range did not differ between pre-treatment and post-treatment PIN blockade or for circumferential skin anesthesia.

Conclusions.—Wrist proprioception appears to be a multifactorial phenomenon. Surgeons may sacrifice the PIN without concern for effect on joint proprioception.

Level of Evidence.—Level I.

▶ This article provides a good exploration of wrist joint proprioception effect by the terminal capsular branch of the posterior interosseous nerve (PIN). The PIN is the most common nerve innervating the wrist capsule. The aim of this study was to develop an objective standardized tool that could be used in the clinical setting to assess if the terminal capsular branch of the PIN does have cause and effect on wrist proprioception. Often the PIN is excised to decrease postoperative dorsal wrist pain, improve measured grip strength, and return clients back to employment. Studies have been performed on proprioception feedback effects in the shoulder, knee, and ankle, which do impact joint stability. For the wrist, therapeutic exercise includes stabilizing effect of wrist using proprioception by using, as the article described, dynamic reactive muscle activation and voluntary type movements used in mirror box therapy. The authors were forthcoming in stating the study limitations but did come to the conclusion that the capsular branch of the PIN, if resected in surgery, has no bearing on wrist proprioception. It is my opinion that studies like this can be beneficial in hand rehabilitation, to reassure therapist and the client that procedures like PIN resections will not affect proprioception or return to function of the wrist.

S. Kranz, OTR/L, CHT

Cost-Effectiveness of Diagnostic Strategies for Suspected Scaphoid Fractures

Yin Z-G, Zhang J-B, Gong K-T (Tianjin Hosp, China)
J Orthop Trauma 29:e245-e252, 2015

Objectives.—The aim of this study was to assess the cost effectiveness of multiple competing diagnostic strategies for suspected scaphoid fractures.

Methods.—With published data, the authors created a decision-tree model simulating the diagnosis of suspected scaphoid fractures. Clinical outcomes, costs, and cost effectiveness of immediate computed tomography (CT), day 3 magnetic resonance imaging (MRI), day 3 bone scan, week 2 radiographs alone, week 2 radiographs—CT, week 2 radiographs—MRI, week 2 radiographs—bone scan, and immediate MRI were evaluated. The primary clinical outcome was the detection of scaphoid fractures. The authors adopted societal perspective, including both the costs of healthcare and the cost of lost productivity. The incremental cost-effectiveness ratio (ICER), which expresses the incremental cost per incremental scaphoid fracture detected using a strategy, was calculated to compare these diagnostic strategies. Base case analysis, 1-way sensitivity analyses, and "worst case scenario" and "best case scenario" sensitivity analyses were performed.

Results.—In the base case, the average cost per scaphoid fracture detected with immediate CT was $2553. The ICER of immediate MRI and day 3 MRI compared with immediate CT was $7483 and $32,000 per scaphoid fracture detected, respectively. The ICER of week 2 radiographs—MRI was around $170,000. Day 3 bone scan, week 2 radiographs alone, week 2 radiographs—CT, and week 2 radiographs—bone scan strategy were dominated or extendedly dominated by MRI strategies. The results were generally robust in multiple sensitivity analyses.

Conclusions.—Immediate CT and MRI were the most cost-effective strategies for diagnosing suspected scaphoid fractures.

Level of Evidence.—Economic and Decision Analyses Level II. See Instructions for Authors for a complete description of levels of evidence.

▶ The purpose of this study by Yin et al was to assess the cost-effectiveness of various diagnostic strategies for suspected scaphoid fractures. This study, published in the *Journal of Orthopedic Trauma*, was a statistical analysis using 2013 Medicare data and evaluated multiple diagnostic strategies in the setting of various clinical scenarios regarding "lost productivity per week immobilized," which would clearly vary based on the patient's occupation. The bottom line was that immediate CT and MRI were the most "cost-effective" strategies for diagnosing suspected scaphoid fractures, except in cases where wrist immobilization only "slightly" influenced the patient's productivity.

In this age of rising medical costs, we must constantly evaluate our diagnostic and treatment strategies for the common scenario of a patient with negative plain x-rays and radial-sided wrist tenderness after a fall on the outstretched hand. It should be remembered that it is crucial to avoid "missing" a scaphoid fracture in such a patient, who may go on to nonunion despite negative plain x-rays initially. On the basis of prior studies, as well as this study and my own clinical experience, I do favor early MRIs in those patients with negative x-rays and significant radial-sided wrist tenderness, particularly if the patient would otherwise be out of work if casted or splinted. Most important, a patient should not be discharged with ongoing snuff box tenderness and negative plain films until either a CT or MRI is obtained.

D. Zelouf, MD

Midterm Outcome of Bone-Ligament-Bone Graft and Dorsal Capsulodesis for Chronic Scapholunate Instability

Gray A, Cuénod P, Papaloïzos MY (Centre Hospitalier du Valais Romand (CHVR), Sierre, Switzerland; Ctr for Hand Surgery and Therapy, Geneva, Switzerland)
J Hand Surg Am 40:1540-1546, 2015

Purpose.—To assess midterm outcomes of our bone-ligament-bone (BLB) grafts for chronic scapholunate (SL) instability and better define criteria for their use.

Methods.—We conducted a retrospective review of 26 patients treated with BLB grafts and dorsal capsulodesis between 1997 and 2009. Twenty-four patients were reviewed. Mean follow-up was 8.2 years. Two patients had dynamic lesions, 7 had SL dissociation, 14 had a dorsal intercalated segment instability lesion, and 1 had SL advanced collapse stage 1. Mean age at surgery was 46 years. All patients presented with pain and 14 had lack of strength. Results were reviewed clinically and radiologically. Images were assessed by 4 surgeons and 1 radiologist for radial styloid, radioscaphoid, radiolunate, midcarpal, and scaphotrapezio-trapezoid degenerative changes.

Results.—Five patients needed subsequent 4-corner arthrodesis. Of the remaining 19 patients at follow-up, both extension and flexion decreased to 73% of the contralateral side. Postoperative grip strength improved from 78% to 90% of the nonsurgical wrist. Quick Disabilities of the Arm, Shoulder, and Hand score was 10 of 100 and the Patient-Rated Wrist Evaluation score was 10 of 100. Radiologically, the SL gap was improved and maintained at follow-up. The SL angle (mean before surgery, 79°) was initially corrected to 69° but returned to preoperative values at follow-up. Eleven of the 19 cases had signs of midcarpal arthritis.

Conclusions.—Bone-ligament-bone grafts with SL dorsal capsulodesis were able to restore and maintain an improved SL interval in all patients. The technique achieved good clinical results and high patient satisfaction, but it did not stop the progression of arthritis, particularly at the midcarpal level. This technique is an option for isolated unrepairable lesion of the dorsal SL ligament with an easily correctable lunate and especially when restoration of grip strength is important.

Type of Study/Level of Evidence.—Therapeutic IV.

▶ The Study. The bone ligament bone reconstruction of the scapholunate interosseous ligament (SLIL) was initially met with great hope and enthusiasm and was proposed as an alternative to tenodesis procedures. This was modeled after the successful bone ligament bone reconstruction described for anterior cruciate ligament reconstruction in the knee. A number of donor sites have been described, but they all share in common the harvesting of 2 bone plugs, which are united by a soft tissue bridge. Weiss et al[1] described a bone retinaculum bone autograft that was harvested from Lister's tubercle, and the midportion of the bone plug was resected to provide 2 bone plugs bridged by extensor retinaculum. Others have used a capitohamate bone-ligament-bone (BLB) substitute.[2,3] The authors of the present study used a BLB graft from the trapezoid-to-second metacarpal (23 cases) and the capitate-to-trapezoid ligaments (2 cases) based on their previous biomechanical study, which showed that these 2 intracarpal bone-ligament-bone grafts shared similar mechanical properties with the dorsal component of the scapholunate ligament.[4] The reconstruction was supplemented with a dorsal intercarpal ligament capsulodesis as described by Szabo et al.[5] Scapholunate and scaphocapitate pins were left in place for 8 to 10 weeks followed by wrist motion.

Twenty-four patients with a mean age of 46 years (range 22-69 years) were reviewed at a mean follow-up of 8.2 years (range 3-13 years). Two patients had dynamic lesions, 7 had scapholunate (SL) dissociation, 14 had a dorsal intercalated segment instability (DISI) deformity, and 1 had radial styloid osteoarthritis. The average QuickDASH score was 10 of 100, and the Patient-Rated Wrist Evaluation score was 10 of 100 for patients who underwent BLB grafting. Five patients required a 4-corner fusion (4 CF) because of persistent pain. A visual analog pain scale was not used, but 12/19 patients reported pain with weather change and 12 reported pain after heavy activity. Wrist extension and flexion were both 73% of the uninjured side. Grip strength improved from 78% before surgery to 90% at follow-up. Radiographically, the SL angle was corrected from 79 to 69 degrees ($P < .001$) after surgery, but at follow-up, the average angle returned to 78 degrees. A clenched-fist SL gap was reduced from 5.2 to 3.5 mm in the postoperative period and was 3.1 mm at follow-up. The mean SL gap on plain radiographs measured 3 mm (SD 1.41) before surgery and 2.1 mm (SD 1.34) at follow-up ($P = .0174$). Eleven of the 19 cases had some signs of midcarpal arthritis, which was not clinically symptomatic.

Study Limitations. The study was retrospective and the BLB graft was combined with a dorsal capsulodesis, which made it difficult to separate out the respective contribution of each component. Detailed patient data are not included; therefore, the poor results tend to be smoothed out by the better outcomes. The authors defined failure as a need for a 4 CF, but pain was still present in 12 of 19 patients. The results were not tabulated separately for each cohort, and hence it is not possible to determine who is the best candidate for this BLB graft and whether a preexisting DISI deformity is a contraindication to this type of procedure. The authors stated, however, that the 2 dynamic lesions had excellent outcomes, but that the results were comparable between the groups with SL dissociations compared with those with a DISI deformity.

Study Benefits. SL instability remains an unsolved problem. There is no 1 procedure that provides complete long-term relief from a chronic scapholunate ligament injury. Similar rates of failure have been demonstrated with midterm and long-term follow-up for treatment of complete SLIL tears following an isolated capsulodesis,[6] SLIL repair and capsulodesis,[7] or tenodesis procedures.[8] The BLB procedure described in this report does provide pain relief in the midterm follow-up of 8.2 years in roughly 50% of patients despite the radiographic abnormalities and does not preclude the conversion to a salvage procedure for progressive pain.

Author's experience. No one procedure can be used for every case of SL instability. The degree of SL joint instability, rather than the size of the ligament tear, should determine the type of reconstructive procedure. The type of repair or reconstruction should be tailored to the individual patient, based on his or her specific pathology. Wrist arthroscopy is an ideal method to assess the degree of SL instability, but only milder degrees of SLIL instability can be treated with arthroscopic methods. Lesser degrees of SL instability typically do well with any type of repair. Complete SLIL tears require open treatment. Those with intact secondary joint stabilizers will present without a DISI deformity and should be treated differently from those patients with a DISI. In these patients, there is attenuation of the secondary SL joint stabilizers, so that both the sagittal and coronal plane stability must be addressed by also stabilizing the scaphotrapezial ligaments. Most of the popular SLIL reconstructions only stabilize the dorsal SLIL, including the BLB graft. Newer procedures that reconstruct both the volar and dorsal components of the SL ligament separately may show better long-term outcomes. Ligament healing may require protection for 6 months or more[9]; therefore, the use of a temporary scapholunate screw should be considered.[10]

D. Slutsky, MD

References

1. Weiss AP. Scapholunate ligament reconstruction using a bone-retinaculum-bone autograft. *J Hand Surg Am.* 1998;23:205-215.
2. Nakamura T, Abe K, Iwamoto T, Ochi K, Sato K. Reconstruction of the scapholunate ligament using capitohamate bone-ligament-bone. *J Wrist Surg Am.* 2015; 4:264-268.
3. van Kampen RJ, Bayne CO, Moran SL, Berger RA. Outcomes of capitohamate bone-ligament-bone grafts for scapholunate injury. *J Wrist Surg Am.* 2015;4: 230-238.
4. Cuenod P, Charriere E, Papaloizos MY. A mechanical comparison of bone-ligament-bone autografts from the wrist for replacement of the scapholunate ligament. *J Hand Surg Am.* 2002;27:985-990.
5. Szabo RM, Slater RR Jr, Palumbo CF, Gerlach T. Dorsal intercarpal ligament capsulodesis for chronic, static scapholunate dissociation: clinical results. *J Hand Surg Am.* 2002;27:978-984.
6. Gajendran VK, Peterson B, Slater RR Jr, Szabo RM. Long-term outcomes of dorsal intercarpal ligament capsulodesis for chronic scapholunate dissociation. *J Hand Surg Am.* 2007;32:1323-1333.

7. Pomerance J. Outcome after repair of the scapholunate interosseous ligament and dorsal capsulodesis for dynamic scapholunate instability due to trauma. *J Hand Surg.* 2006;31:1380-1386.
8. Moran SL, Ford KS, Wulf CA, Cooney WP. Outcomes of dorsal capsulodesis and tenodesis for treatment of scapholunate instability. *J Hand Surg.* 2006;31: 1438-1446.
9. Short WH, Werner FW, Green JK, Sutton LG, Brutus JP. Biomechanical evaluation of the ligamentous stabilizers of the scaphoid and lunate: part III. *J Hand Surg.* 2007;32:297-309.
10. Fok MW, Fernandez DL. Chronic scapholunate instability treated with temporary screw fixation. *J Hand Surg.* 2015;40:752-758.

Dart-Splint: An innovative orthosis that can be integrated into a scapholunate and palmar midcarpal instability re-education protocol
Braidotti F, Atzei A, Fairplay T (Fenice Hand Surgery and Rehabilitation Team, Treviso, Italy; Studio Fairplay — Private Professional Functional Rehabilitation of the Upper Extremity Clinic, Bologna, Italy; et al)
J Hand Ther 28:329-335, 2015

The Authors describe a novel hinged orthosis that permits selective midcarpal mobilization along the plane of the dart throwing motion. This orthotic device can be used to assist rehabilitation protocols aimed to limit radiocarpal joint mobility and scapho-lunate ligament overload and to accelerate wrist functional recovery after ligamentous injuries around the proximal carpal row. — VICTORIA W. PRIGANC, PhD, OTR, CHT, CLT, Practice Forum Editor.

▶ This article describes a cutting-edge orthosis designed by a team comprising therapists and a physician from Italy. The authors begin this article with a valuable review of carpal kinematics to establish the need for an orthosis that promotes the dart thrower's motion (DTM). Once established that midcarpal motion may protect healing tissue in the proximal carpal row while allowing early wrist motion, the authors then describe in detail the orthosis they developed. Their step-by-step guide to the fabrication of the Dart-Splint is comprehensive and clear. However, the fabrication of the hinge component is a somewhat complicated procedure and calls for the use of a product (Plast-O-Fit) that is no longer manufactured.

The authors suggest use of flouroscan to confirm the correct placement of the rivets on the hinges. This may be a limiting factor because many hand therapists do not have access to a flouroscan. They also suggest that this orthosis can be used early in the rehab process, eliminating up to 2 weeks of full immobilization postsurgery. However, the time to fabricate this orthosis followed by the need to determine correct motion and hinge placement with fluoroscopy may incur a large additional expense to the patient to gain a few weeks of partial wrist mobility.

Because this is an early prototype of a DTM orthosis, it is necessary now to follow up with some actual studies to determine the efficacy of this splint design. If the results of early protected mobility are promising, then the expense of using a DTM orthosis may well be offset by improved outcomes and potentially fewer therapy sessions. Future DTM orthotic designs that reduce the complexity of fabrication and use readily available products may enhance use of this innovative orthosis.

S. J. Clark, OTR/L, CHT

The Missed Scaphoid Fracture—Outcomes of Delayed Cast Treatment
Grewal R, Suh N, MacDermid JC (Univ of Western Ontario, London, Canada)
J Wrist Surg 4:278-283, 2015

Background.—The purpose of this study is to evaluate outcomes (report union rates and times based on CT) for subacute scaphoid fractures, defined as those presenting between 6 weeks and 6 months from injury.

Questions.—1) What are the expected union rates for subacute scaphoid fractures? 2) What are the expected union times for subacute scaphoid fractures? 3) Is it worth trialing a period of cast immobilization for these patients?

Methods.—All isolated sub-acute scaphoid fractures that presented at our institution between 2006 and 2010 were identified. Each subject's health record, CT scans and X-rays were retrospectively reviewed.

Results.—There were 20 males and 8 females, with a mean age of 30, treated with casting alone. There were 20 waist, 7 proximal and 1 distal pole fracture. The mean casting time was 11 (waist) and 14 (proximal pole) weeks with a union rate of 82% (23/28). Diabetes, comminution and a humpback deformity increased the non-union risk in this cohort. Exclusion of these cases resulted in a 96% union rate (23/24).

Conclusion.—Subacute scaphoid fractures (presenting within 6 months from injury) can be expected to successfully heal with casting alone, even if the initial diagnosis is delayed. The expected time frame for union with cast treatment is shorter than previously reported.

Level of Evidence.—IV.

▶ Grewal and colleagues report on an interesting cohort of patients: those with a previously neglected scaphoid fracture diagnosed in the subacute setting (6 weeks to 6 months). Traditionally these patients are thought to be at a higher risk of nonunion, and therefore typically operative treatment is chosen. In this series, patients with a scaphoid fracture not previously treated and diagnosed between 6 weeks and 6 months from injury were chosen. A CT scan was performed at initial presentation, and those patients with sclerotic borders or humpback deformity per surgeon preference were given operative treatment. Of the 28 patients in the study, there were 7 proximal pole fractures, 20 waist, and 1 distal pole fracture (Fig 1, Tables 1 and 2). An impressive 82% union rate at average of 11 and 14 weeks (waist and proximal pole, respectively) was noted. Most important, early CT scan at 7 weeks after initiation of immobilization was predictive of those who would go on to union. Those

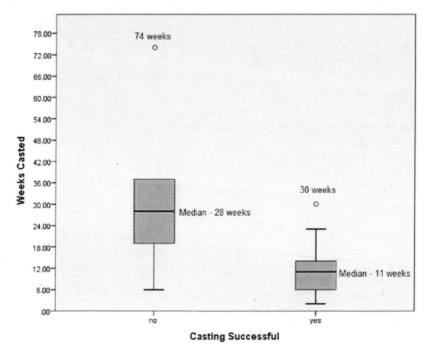

FIGURE 1.—Comparison of casting times for patients who did and did not heal with casting. (Reprinted from Grewal R, Suh N, MacDermid JC. The missed scaphoid fracture—outcomes of delayed cast treatment. *J Wrist Surg.* 2015;4:278-283, with permission from Thieme Medical Publishers, Inc.)

TABLE 1.—Potential Risk Factors Associated With Failure of Casting

	Casting Failed	Casting Successful	P-Value
Diabetics	2	0	0.03
Non-Diabetics	3	23	
Humpback	4	4	0.02
No Humpback	1	19	
Comminution	3	3	0.05
No Comminution	2	20	
Cysts	1	15	0.09
No Cysts	4	8	

Reprinted from Grewal R, Suh N, MacDermid JC. The missed scaphoid fracture—outcomes of delayed cast treatment. *J Wrist Surg.* 2015;4:278-283, with permission from Thieme Medical Publishers, Inc.

ultimately achieving union had 38% increase in union at 7 weeks, whereas those who did not had only an 11% increase at 7 weeks. Thus, if only 10% of the fracture unites as determined by CT by 6 to 7 weeks of immobilization, complete union is unlikely. Risk factors for nonunion included humpback deformity, comminution, and presence of diabetes. If patients with these risk factors were excluded, the union rate rose to 96%. This study is helpful for practice because it

TABLE 2.—Patient and Scaphoid Fracture Characteristics and Outcome

		Patient Factors			Fracture Characteristics					Outcome	
	Age/Sex	Smoker	DM	Displaced	Cysts	Comminution	Sclerosis	Union (%) After 1st Cast	Total Weeks Casted	Final Union
Proximal Pole	42f	Y	N	N	Y	N	N	88% (6w)	No cast	70%
	17m	?	N	Y (2 mm)	N	Y	N	40% (6w)	6	88%
	26f	N	N	N	Y	N	N	75% (8w)	8	80%
	24m	N	N	N	Y	N	N	15% (6w)	8	90%
	16m	?	N	Y (3 mm)	Y	Y	N	40% (10w)	15*	60%
	21m	?	N	N	Y	Y	N	10% (7w)	26	50%
	29m	N	N	Y (2 mm, H)	N	N	N	50% (4w)	ORIF + bone graft	50%
Waist	18m	?	N	Y (2 mm)	N	N	N	100% (4w)	4	50%
	12m	N	N	N	Y	N	N	50% (4w)	4	100%
	55m	?	N	N	N	Y	N	30% (4w)	6	50%
	65f	N	N	H	N	N	N	35% (6w)	6	50%
	53f	Y	N	Y (1 mm)	Y	N	N	30% (6w)	9	55%
	28f	N	N	N	Y	N	N	30% (6w)	9	100%
	16m	N	N	N	Y	N	N	65% (7w)	9	50%
	23m	?	N	Y (1 mm)	N	N	N	No interim CT	9	65%
	52m	?	N	Y (4 mm, H)	Y	Y	N	50% (4w)	11	100%
	22m	N	N	H	N	N	N	0% (5w)	11	65%
	15m	N	N	Y (1 mm, H)	N	N	N	40% (7.5w)	12	75%
	55m	N	N	N	Y	N	N	15% (4w)	14	80%
	17m	N	N	N	Y	N	N	40% (6w)	14	77%
	26m	Y	N	N	Y	N	N	40% (6w)	14	65%
	19m	?	N	N	N	N	N	60% (20w)	20	90%
	46m	N	N	N	Y	Y	N	30% (6w)	24+	85%
	49f	N	Y	Y (2 mm, H)	N	Y	N	20% (9w)	Never casted, Asymptomatic nonunion accepted	
	19m	N	N	N	N	N	N	20% (8w)	ORIF, no bone graft	
	17m	?	N	H	Y	N	N	0% (11w)	ORIF + bone graft	
Distal	54f	Y	Y	Y (2 mm, H)	N	Y	N	15% (8w)	Failed ORIF + bone graft, required fusion	
	13f	N	N	N	Y	N	N	80% (2.5w)	2.5	80%

Abbreviations: ?, unknown; DM, diabetes; f, female; H, humpback; m, male; mm, millimeters; n, no; w, weeks; y, yes.

*patient had multiple lower extremity injuries and was casted for a lengthy time as it helped with weightbearing.
+patient wanted to avoid surgery.

Reprinted from Grewal R, Suh N, MacDermid JC. The missed scaphoid fracture–outcomes of delayed cast treatment. *J Wrist Surg*. 2015;4:278-283, with permission from Thieme Medical Publishers, Inc.

demonstrates that even in the setting of delayed diagnosis of up to 6 months, a trial of immobilization in a short arm thumb spica cast for 6 to 7 weeks is reasonable. Getting a CT at that time to evaluate for interval healing can help the surgeon determine whether a continued course of immobilization is likely to be successful.

J. E. Adams, MD

Results of Perilunate Dislocations and Perilunate Fracture Dislocations With a Minimum 15-Year Follow-Up
Krief E, Appy-Fedida B, Rotari V, et al (CHU Amiens-Picardie, Site Sud, France)
J Hand Surg Am 40:2191-2197, 2015

Purpose.—To evaluate the long-term clinical, functional, and radiological outcomes in 30 patients with at least 15 years of follow-up.

Methods.—We performed a retrospective study that identified 73 patients. Thirty patients agreed to participate and were included. The mean follow-up was 18 years (range, 15—24 years). There were 14 cases of perilunate dislocation and 16 cases of perilunate fracture-dislocation (including 13 transscaphoid perilunate fracture-dislocations). At the last follow-up, the clinical and functional evaluation was based on the range of motion, grip strength, the Mayo wrist score, the Quick Disabilities of the Arm Shoulder and Hand score, and the Patient-Rated Wrist Evaluation score. Radiological abnormalities, according to the Herzberg classification, were 5 type A1 cases, 7 type B, 16 type B1, and 2 type C.

Results.—The mean flexion—extension arc, radial—ulnar abduction arc, and pronation—supination arc were, respectively, 68%, 67%, and 80%, relative to the contralateral side. The mean grip strength was 70%, relative to the contralateral side. The mean Mayo wrist score was 70, and the mean Quick Disabilities of the Arm Shoulder and Hand and Patient-Rated Wrist Evaluation scores were, respectively, 20 and 21. Five patients had secondary procedure. Six patients had a complex regional pain syndrome type 1.

Conclusions.—Although arthritis occurred in 70% of cases, its clinical and functional impact appeared to be low. However, the 2 lowest Mayo wrist scores corresponded to the patients with the most advanced arthritis. Complex regional pain syndrome appeared to have an impact on long-term outcomes.

Type of Study/Level of Evidence.—Therapeutic IV.

▶ This article provides long-term (minimum, 15 years) follow-up of 30 patients with perilunate dislocations (PLD) and perilunate fracture dislocations (PLFD). At final follow-up, 80% of patients reported some pain, but for most (16 of 30), the pain was occasional with everyday activities. Half of patients had a good or excellent result based on the Mayo wrist score. Two patients underwent proximal row carpectomy for lunate necrosis, and 3 patients underwent bone grafting for scaphoid nonunion. Not surprisingly, 21 of 30 patients (70%) had radiographic evidence of arthritis.

Interestingly, 12 of 30 patients were treated with either closed reduction and casting or closed reduction and pinning. Although the authors note that current standard of care treatment would involve open reduction and ligament repair, they did not correlate outcome with the treatment approach. The authors reported a rather low incidence of carpal tunnel syndrome (2 of 30), compared with other reports of median nerve dysfunction in up to 47% of patients.[1] Complex regional pain syndrome (CRPS) occurred in 20% of patients in this study, leading to the question of whether failure to recognize and treat median nerve compression may have contributed to the high incidence of CRPS. Alternatively, CRPS may have been underreported in prior series.

This article provides further long-term results of PLD and PLFD and finds similar functional results as previous shorter-term follow-up studies with progression of radiographic arthritis.

C. M. Ward, MD

Reference

1. Wickramasinghe NR, Duckworth AD, Clement ND, Hageman MG, McQueen MM, Ring D. Acute median neuropathy and carpal tunnel release in perilunate injuries. *J Hand Microsurg.* 2015;7:237-240.

Delayed Avascular Necrosis and Fragmentation of the Lunate Following Perilunate Dislocation
Wilke B, Kakar S (Mayo Clinic, Rochester, MN)
Orthopedics 38:e539-e542, 2015

Perilunate and perilunate fracture dislocations are high-energy injuries with the wrist loaded in extension, ulnar deviation, and intercarpal supination. The force vector travels from a radial to a ulnar direction and can result in complex carpal instability. The diagnosis is often delayed, which can result in suboptimal outcomes. Nonoperative management can produce inferior results, with patients experiencing pain and weakness. Therefore, early treatment with open reduction and internal fixation is recommended to assess the osteochondral and ligamentous disruption and to achieve anatomic reduction of the carpus. Despite this, these patients can develop radiographic degenerative joint disease, which can be seen in up to 90% of cases. This can be due to difficulty in holding and maintaining carpal reduction. Increased radiodensity of the lunate following these injuries has been observed but is believed to be a transient phenomenon without risk of progression to avascular necrosis. This may be due to the blood supply of the lunate, which has varied patterns of intraosseous and extraosseous vascularity. The authors report a patient who developed avascular necrosis and delayed lunate fragmentation following a Mayfield Type IV perilunate dislocation. This finding highlights the importance of long-term follow-up with these patients.

▶ The authors report the first case of delayed avascular necrosis (AVN) of the lunate following a Mayfield IV perilunate dislocation.

Perilunate dislocations are high-energy injuries that are a result of complex carpal instability. The diagnosis is often delayed, and nonoperative management can lead to inferior outcomes, which makes early recognition and treatment important. Standard treatment is open reduction and internal fixation to hold the carpus reduced anatomically. Complications following perilunate dislocation include posttraumatic arthritis, which is seen in up to 90% of cases.

Postinjury, a transient radiodensity can be seen within the lunate and has been reported to be present in 12.5% of perilunate dislocations.[1] This finding is thought to be a benign, self-limited process related to a temporary ischemia in the traumatic period and is not thought to be a risk factor for AVN.

The authors present a case of a 30-year-old mechanic who sustained a closed Mayfield IV dislocation in a motorcycle accident. He underwent successful closed reduction and subsequent open reduction with internal fixation using temporary k-wires using a combined dorsal/volar approach. He did well and returned to labor 2 months after wire removal. At 14 months postoperatively he returned to the clinic for routine follow-up. Radiographs showed AVN with coronal fragmentation of the lunate and preserved carpal height. He was completely asymptomatic and elected no intervention. At most recent follow-up 23 months after injury, radiographs show lunocapitate arthritis, yet the patient remains asymptomatic and elected conservative management.

The importance of this case report is that it is believed to be the first episode of AVN following a perilunate dislocation. Subsequently, patients and providers should be advised to continue long-term follow-up to monitor for this potential complication.

M. O'Shaughnessy, MD

Reference

1. White RE Jr, Omer GE Jr. Transient vascular compromise of the lunate after fracture-dislocation or dislocation of the carpus. *J Hand Surg Am.* 1984;9:181-184.

The Effect of Midcarpal Versus Total Wrist Fusion on the Hand's Load Distribution During Gripping
Mühldorfer-Fodor M, Reger A, Schoonhoven Jv, et al (Rhön Klinikum AG, Bad Neustadt/Saale, Germany; Univ of Rostock, Germany)
J Hand Surg Am 40:2183-2190, 2015

Purpose.—To analyze the total grip force and load distribution of the hand with midcarpal fusion (MCF) and total wrist fusion (TWF).

Methods.—Twelve patients with unilateral TWF and 12 patients with unilateral MCF were assessed at an average 64 months (range, 19-100 months) postoperatively. The total grip force and load distribution of both hands were measured by the Manugraphy system using 3 cylinder sizes. The load applied to 7 anatomical areas of the hand during cylinder grip was analyzed, comparing the operated and the nonsurgical hands.

Results.—For the 100 mm and 150 mm cylinders, a significantly lower total grip force was found in hands operated with either TWF or MCF. For the 200 mm cylinder, there was a significant difference between nonsurgical hands and those with MCF but not between nonsurgical hands and those with TWF. For the 100 mm cylinder, the difference between nonsurgical and operated hands was greater in hands with TWF than those with MCF. For the load distribution of the hand, no differences between the operated and the nonsurgical hand were found for either MCF or TWF.

Conclusions.—MFC and TWF resulted in a reduced cylinder grip force. With respect to the load distribution, neither procedure influenced the relative contribution that each area of the hand produced during cylinder grip.

Type of Study/Level of Evidence.—Therapeutic III.

▶ The Study: The purpose of this study was to analyze the total grip force and load distribution of the hand after either a scaphoidectomy and midcarpal fusion (MCF) or a total wrist fusion (TWF), using 3 cylinders of 100-, 150-, and 200-mm circumferences wrapped with electronic pressure sensor matrices. They also examined the site-specific loads for the thumb and each finger as well as the thenar and hypothenar areas.

The average age of the patients at the time of surgery was 41 years (range 25-56 years) in the TWF group and 38 years (range 24-51 years) in the MCF group. In both groups, 11 of 12 patients were men with the dominant hand involved in 10 of 12 patients. The average follow-up was 57 months (range 19-100 months) after TWF and 71 months (range 20-98 months) after scaphoid excision and MCF. Radiographs revealed an average wrist position of 14 degrees extension (range 0-18 degree) and 7-degree ulnar deviation (range 0-10) for patients with a TWF. The residual wrist motion after MCF averaged 30 degrees of wrist extension (range 15-50), 27 degrees of flexion (range 5-50), 9 degrees of ulnar deviation (range 0-20), and 14 degrees of radial deviation (range 5-20). The average patient-rated pain scale, was 3.4 of 10 (range 0-8) after a TWF and 4.3 (range 0-8) following an MCF. In general, both groups had smaller grip strength compared with the normal hand. The grip also progressively diminished with increasing cylinder size for both groups. For the 100-mm cylinder, the average grip force loss of the operated hand was 35% with TWF compared with that of the nonsurgical hand and 25% with MCF, statistically significant differences. For the 150-mm cylinder, the grip force loss was 24% with TWF and 25% with MCF, statistically significant differences. For the 200-mm cylinder, the grip force loss averaged 21% compared with the nonsurgical hand for both kinds of fusions.

According to the authors, as the object to grip becomes smaller, the wrist extends further to allow an optimal power grip, whereas ulnar deviation is not affected by the size of the object. Unfortunately, because of the heterogenous range of wrist extension in each group, it is not possible to determine whether the degree of wrist extension influenced the grip strength. Comparing the operated hand with TWF or MCF and the nonsurgical opposite hand, the contribution of each of the 7 sections differed by 3% or less in each case.

Study Limitations: The authors do not provide the preoperative diagnosis and reason for choosing a TWF over a MCF. This introduces possible surgeon bias in patient selection, in that more severe deformities may have been treated with a TWF and may be a factor in the overall lower grip strengths versus an MCF. TWF patients also had a higher VAS than the MCF patients, which could account for the diminished grip strengths. Grip strength was not analyzed with respect to residual pain.

The size of the patient's hand might affect the grip strength, but this information is not included. Grip strengths were not age adjusted because younger patients would typically have higher grip strengths. Previous studies have shown a wide range of wrist positions for maximum grip from 0 to 45 degrees extension and 0 to 15 degrees ulnar deviation.[1-4] The position of the wrist fusion, however, was not specifically studied as to whether it influenced the grip strength. The authors did not measure the wrist position during grip force testing with MCF and could not measure to what extent the reduced wrist motion contributed to the grip force loss.

It makes sense that the grip strength is less than the opposite side with both TWF and MCF regardless of the cylinder size. Although the authors claimed statistical significance in the differences, this is intuitive and not new information. The authors' data did not prove their hypothesis that TWF reduces grip strength more than MCF. The small number of patients enrolled in this study also limited a direct comparison of the TWF and MCF groups.

Authors' Experience: Although the authors could not demonstrate a statistical difference, there was a universal trend that the patients with a TWA had more residual pain and a weaker grip than an MCF. This information is potentially useful in counseling patients who might then choose an MCF over a TWA to retain some wrist motion. In my practice, I prefer to proceed with a motion-sparing procedure first because a TWF can always then be done for persistent or recurrent wrist pain as a salvage procedure, whereas the reverse cannot be done.

D. J. Slutsky, MD

References

1. Ambike SS, Paclet F, Latash ML, Zatsiorsky VM. Grip-force modulation in multi-finger prehension during wrist flexion and extension. *Exp Brain Res.* 2013;227: 509-522.
2. Bhardwaj P, Nayak SS, Kiswar AM, Sabapathy SR. Effect of static wrist position on grip strength. *Indian J Plast Surg.* 2011;44:55-58.
3. Haque S, Khan AA. Effects of ulnar deviation of the wrist combined with flexion/extension on the maximum voluntary contraction of grip. *J Hum Ergol.* 2009;38:1-9.

4. Pryce JC. The wrist position between neutral and ulnar deviation that facilitates the maximum power grip strength. *J Biomech.* 1980;13:505-511.

Hybrid Russe Procedure for Scaphoid Waist Fracture Nonunion With Deformity
Lee SK, Byun DJ, Roman-Deynes JL, et al (Weill Med College of Cornell Univ, New York; New York Univ Hosp for Joint Diseases)
J Hand Surg Am 40:2198-2205, 2015

Purpose.—To assess the results of a hybrid Russe procedure using a corticocancellous strut, cancellous autologous nonvascularized bone graft, and cannulated headless compression screw to reduce the deformity reliably from a collapsed scaphoid nonunion, provide osteoinductive stimulus, and stabilize the fracture for predictable union.

Methods.—A hybrid Russe procedure was performed for scaphoid waist fracture nonunions with humpback deformity and no evidence of avascular necrosis. A volar distal radius autologous bone graft was harvested and a strut of cortical bone was fashioned and placed into the nonunion site to restore length and alignment. We packed cancellous bone graft in the remainder of the nonunion site and fixed the scaphoid was with a headless compression screw. Union was determined by radiographs or computed tomography, and intrascaphoid, scapholunate, and radiolunate angles were calculated on final radiographs. We recorded wrist range of motion, grip strength, pinch strength, pain, and complications.

Results.—Fourteen male and 3 female patients (average age, 32 years; range, 16—78 years), with a mean follow-up of 32 months, were examined clinically and radiographically. All 17 scaphoids united with a mean time for union of 3.6 months. The mean postoperative intrascaphoid angle was significantly reduced from 65° preoperatively to 35° postoperatively. The mean radiolunate angle was significantly improved from 20° from neutral (lunate tilted dorsally) preoperatively to 0° postoperatively. The scapholunate angle also demonstrated significant improvement from 70° preoperatively to 56° postoperatively. Grip strength improved from 70% of the contralateral hand to 89% after the procedure. All patients were satisfied with the functional outcome and no donor site morbidity or hardware issues were identified.

Conclusions.—This straightforward hybrid Russe technique predictably restored radiolunate, scapholunate, and intrascaphoid angles with a 100% union incidence. The technique provides excellent functional results in patients with a challenging clinical problem, and we recommend it for scaphoid fracture waist nonunions with dorsal intercalated segment instability deformity.

Type of Study/Level of Evidence.—Therapeutic IV.

▶ Scaphoid nonunions remain a vexing problem in hand surgery. The treatment evolution continues, and the authors report their experience with a hybrid technique including both old and new concepts. This technique is conceptually appealing in its simplistic nature and the outstanding results reported by the authors. The small number of patients and narrow scope to only include waist nonunions without any evidence of dysvascularity leave some future questions as to its true efficacy to be answered.

The strengths of the manuscript include the use of multiple validated outcome instruments, the majority of patients having CT confirmation of fusion, the impressive restoration of radiographic parameters in all patients and reasonable midterm follow-up. A subtle technical point mentioned in the body of the article but not highlighted in the abstract is that in addition to the inlay Russe bone graft, autograft cancellous bone graft, and compression screw, patients with significant preoperative dorsal intercalated segmental instability also had a radiolunate pin kept in place initially to maintain the radiolunate reduction.

Weaknesses of the study include primarily the small number of patients (any study with a 100% union rate is likely underpowered) but also the confounding use of so many techniques must be remembered when interpreting the results (inlay graft, autograft cancellous graft, compression screw, and temporary pinning). Also its use in proximal pole nonunions or any signs of dysvascularity cannot be assessed. The authors have selected those malunions most amenable to surgical correction and not reported any cases of the more challenging proximal pole fractures or early AVN.

All factors considered, I will likely consider adding the Russe inlay graft into the nonunion site in the future. It conceptually would be a simple addition to my current technique, which otherwise is almost identical to that reported by the authors.

G. Gaston, MD

Results of Perilunate Dislocations and Perilunate Fracture Dislocations With a Minimum 15-Year Follow-Up
Krief E, Appy-Fedida B, Rotari V, et al (CHU Amiens-Picardie, Amiens, France)
J Hand Surg Am 40:2191-2197, 2015

Purpose.—To evaluate the long-term clinical, functional, and radiological outcomes in 30 patients with at least 15 years of follow-up.

Methods.—We performed a retrospective study that identified 73 patients. Thirty patients agreed to participate and were included. The mean follow-up was 18 years (range, 15–24 years). There were 14 cases of perilunate dislocation and 16 cases of perilunate fracture-dislocation (including 13 transscaphoid perilunate fracture-dislocations). At the last follow-up, the clinical and functional evaluation was based on the range of motion, grip strength, the Mayo wrist score, the Quick Disabilities of the Arm Shoulder and Hand score, and the Patient-Rated Wrist Evaluation score. Radiological abnormalities, according to the Herzberg classification, were 5 type A1 cases, 7 type B, 16 type B1, and 2 type C.

Results.—The mean flexion–extension arc, radial–ulnar abduction arc, and pronation–supination arc were, respectively, 68%, 67%, and 80%, relative to the contralateral side. The mean grip strength was 70%, relative to the contralateral side. The mean Mayo wrist score was 70, and the mean Quick Disabilities of the Arm Shoulder and Hand and Patient-Rated Wrist Evaluation scores were, respectively, 20 and 21. Five patients had secondary procedure. Six patients had a complex regional pain syndrome type 1.

Conclusions.—Although arthritis occurred in 70% of cases, its clinical and functional impact appeared to be low. However, the 2 lowest Mayo wrist scores corresponded to the patients with the most advanced arthritis. Complex regional pain syndrome appeared to have an impact on long-term outcomes.

Type of Study/Level of Evidence.—Therapeutic IV.

▶ The study describes the long-term results of perilunate fracture dislocations with mean follow-up of 18 years. The authors mainly focused on range of motion, grip strength, the Mayo wrist score, the Quick Disabilities of the Arm

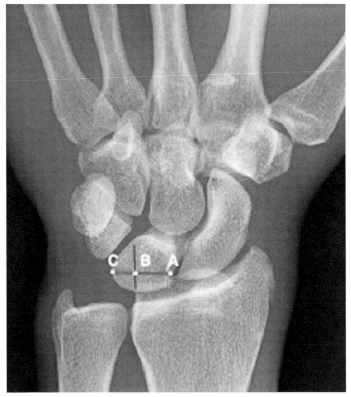

FIGURE 1.—Schuind et al[13] method of measuring the ulnar translocation ratio. The distance B–C (uncovered lunate) is divided by the distance A–C (length of the lunate). *Editor's Note*: Please refer to original journal article for full references. (Reprinted from Krief E, Appy-Fedida B, Rotari V, et al. Results of perilunate dislocations and perilunate fracture dislocations with a minimum 15-year follow-up. *J Hand Surg Am.* 2015;40:2191-2197, with permission from American Society for Surgery of the Hand.)

Shoulder and Hand score, and the Patient-Rated Wrist Evaluation score assessment. These long-term studies are important for giving us information about "real" results and the impact of these injuries on patients' lives. The observed mean motion arc was 89%, and grip strength was approximately 70% of the contralateral side. More important was the evaluation of arthritic changes, which occurred in 70% cases, and their correlation to the patient-rated evaluation scores.

What I really miss is the influence of these injuries and treatment on the patients' lives. When long-term follow-up is analyzed, I am especially curious about a patient's abilities related to work, sports, and hobbies, not just the biomechanical parameters that we know will be altered after such an injury.

In my practice, I treat these kinds of injuries with open reduction and stabilization, mostly from the dorsal approach. I use K-wires for reduction and fixation and compression screws for scaphoid fractures (Fig 1). Unfortunately, we still have some late presentations of nondiagnosed dislocations, which are difficult to reduce and sometimes need proximal row carpectomy. Interestingly, we have seen situations of volar lunate subluxation that can produce carpal tunnel symptoms and in later cases need lunate excision, which surprisingly result in functional ranges of motion. Despite many problems and different patterns of these injuries, most of the patients can still return to manual work with a functional range of motion and acceptable pain level, which is mostly confirmed by this study.

P. Czarnecki, MD

The Palpable Scaphoid Surface Area in Various Wrist Positions

Giugale JM, Leigey D, Berkow K, et al (Univ of Pittsburgh Med Ctr, PA; et al)
J Hand Surg Am 40:2039-2044, 2015

Purpose.—To determine the theoretical amount of surface area available for palpation of the scaphoid in various wrist positions and to provide a guide depicting which wrist position will expose proximal pole, waist, and distal pole fractures.

Methods.—Using 3 fresh-frozen male cadaver wrists, we digitized palpable surface areas (dorsal, volar, and snuffbox) of the scaphoid in several wrist positions. The entire scaphoid was then excised and a digitized 3-dimensional reconstruction of the entire scaphoid was obtained. The 2 images were superimposed and the surface area was calculated.

Results.—The maximum palpable area of the scaphoid was achieved with the wrist in neutral extension and maximum ulnar deviation and the wrist in maximum flexion and neutral deviation. Neutral wrist extension and ulnar deviation exposed all but the most proximal portion of the proximal pole and the distal pole, which made this the ideal position to detect tenderness from a scaphoid waist fracture and larger proximal pole fractures. Maximum wrist flexion with neutral wrist deviation exposed the entire proximal pole, which made this the ideal position to detect tenderness from a proximal pole scaphoid fracture.

Conclusions.—Wrist position influences the amount of scaphoid surface area available for palpation and should be considered when examining a patient with a suspected scaphoid fracture.

Clinical Relevance.—The scaphoid should be palpated in 3 anatomic regions with the wrist placed in different positions to maximally expose the anatomical region being palpated.

▶ The authors performed a study on 3 cadaveric wrists to determine the maximum palpable area of the scaphoid with the wrist in various positions. Classically, physical examination for suspected scaphoid fracture includes assessment of tenderness over the anatomic snuffbox and over the scaphoid tubercle. The authors performed measurements to determine the amount of exposed surface area of the scaphoid dorsally, over the anatomic snuffbox, and volarly with the wrist in different positions. At the anatomic snuffbox, positioning of the wrist in ulnar deviation significantly increased the amount of the scaphoid available for direct palpation. For the scaphoid tubercle, wrist extension increased the available area for direct palpation by 168%.

The authors are to be commended for designing this simple but very clinically relevant study. Current descriptions for physical examination of the wrist do not include wrist positioning. Based on the authors' findings, standard palpation for suspected scaphoid fractures should include (1) anatomic snuffbox tenderness with wrist in ulnar deviation, (2) scaphoid tubercle tenderness with wrist extension, and (3) dorsoradial wrist tenderness with wrist flexion. It would be interesting to follow-up this cadaveric study with a clinical study to determine sensitivity and specificity of each of these examination maneuvers.

J. I. Huang, MD

Treatment of Scaphoid Nonunion: A Systematic Review of the Existing Evidence

Pinder RM, Brkljac M, Rix L, et al (Castle Hill Hosp, Cottingham, United Kingdom; Univ of Manchester Med School, Greater Manchester, United Kingdom; et al)

J Hand Surg Am 40:1797-1805, 2015

Purpose.—To determine by systematic review the optimal treatment of scaphoid nonunion.

Methods.—We conducted a systematic review of the literature with a meta-analysis of proportions to investigate the comparative effectiveness of different surgical techniques.

Results.—A total of 48 publications (1,602 patients) met the eligibility criteria. Vascularized and nonvascularized bone grafts had an estimated union incidence of 92% and 88%, respectively. Distal radius and iliac crest bone grafts had similar union rates (89% and 87%, respectively) but harvesting of iliac crest bone grafts had more complications. Both screw and K-wire fixation had a higher incidence of union (88% and

91%, respectively) than no fixation (79%). No approach was statistically different. Patients fixed with screws were mobilized earlier than those with K-wire fixation.

Conclusions.—Current evidence does not demonstrate a significantly superior method for the treatment of scaphoid nonunion. A multicenter randomized trial would be ideal but the large numbers that would be required may make this unrealistic. We recommend the continued reporting of series with specific assessments and outcome measures to optimize future comparisons in an attempt to determine the best management of scaphoid nonunion.

Clinical Relevance.—The use of bone grafts and the methods of their fixation for scaphoid nonunion are debated issues in hand and wrist surgery, with multiple methods employed. There is no current consensus on optimal treatment. A meta-analysis of proportions of available data from recent studies was deemed the most appropriate way to assimilate the available evidence with the view to inform surgeons of the optimal treatment according to the evidence base.

▶ The study presents results from a meta-analysis of 48 studies determining optimal treatment rates for scaphoid nonunions with a primary outcome of radiographic bony union. The authors report similar union rates and time to union for vascularized and nonvascularized grafts and for different methods of fixation (screws vs K-wires). The analysis of complications was limited but suggested an increased risk for vascularized grafts.

The analysis is helpful in that it pools data for 1602 patients treated for scaphoid nonunions and thus presents a large patient population to study. Like many meta-analyses, however, conclusions are limited given the heterogeneity of the data presented. Furthermore, the study group is not well defined in terms of the types of nonunions, prior treatment methods, and other factors. With so many kinds of fixation and bone grafts, it is a challenging and daunting task to draw meaningful conclusions in terms of the optimal treatment method. Lastly, the authors state that in most studies, plan radiographs were used to determine union, but many investigators would consider CT to be a superior modality for this purpose.

The authors conclude with an invaluable list of key outcome reporting criteria for scaphoid nonunions. If future investigators make efforts to include all of these reporting criteria in their studies, additional meta-analyses on this topic are likely to be more fruitful.

As noted by this study, treatment algorithms for scaphoid nonunions are varied, and my practice is no exception. I assess the anatomy of the nonunion with a CT scan and determine the optimal bone graft based on the presence or absence of a humpback deformity as well as the likely vascularity of the proximal fragment. For nonunions at the waist, I prefer nonvascularized bone grafts from the radius or iliac crest, whereas I am more likely to treat proximal nonunions with vascularized options. Lastly, I always assess healing with a CT because plain radiographs can be unpredictable.

T. D. Rozental

Fixation and Grafting After Limited Debridement of Scaphoid Nonunions
McInnes CW, Giuffre JL (Univ of Manitoba, Winnipeg, Canada)
J Hand Surg Am 40:1791-1796, 2015

Purpose.—To evaluate a surgical technique of treating nondisplaced waist and proximal pole scaphoid nonunions without avascular necrosis (AVN).

Methods.—We performed a retrospective review of all patients with nondisplaced, scaphoid waist or proximal pole nonunions without AVN treated with the following technique. Two K-wires are positioned along the scaphoid axis to stabilize the proximal and distal poles. Debridement with a curette or burr is performed parallel to the nonunion site until the K-wires are visualized and punctate bleeding of the proximal and distal fragments is encountered. The volar, radial fibrous union is left intact. Distal radius cancellous bone graft is packed into the nonunion site. A headless screw is placed perpendicular to the fracture and the K-wires are removed.

Results.—Between 2012 and 2014, 12 patients (ages 13—29 y) with clinical and radiographic evidence (10 had computed tomography or magnetic resonance imaging; 2 had radiographs only) of scaphoid nonunion were identified (10 transverse waist and 2 proximal pole fractures). Median interval from injury to surgery was 38 weeks (range, 3 mo to 9 y). Four patients were active smokers and 2 had failed previous iliac crest bone grafting. All patients healed as confirmed by computed tomography. Average time to union was 14 weeks (range, 6—31 wk). Four patients had delayed union requiring a bone stimulator. All patients had resolution of pain and there were no complications.

Conclusions.—The technique described is an effective and efficient method of treating nondisplaced scaphoid nonunions without AVN. We suggest that complete debridement of the nonunion is not essential to achieve union. In addition, pinning the proximal and distal scaphoid poles initially and maintaining the volar fibrous union of the scaphoid nonunion stabilizes the fracture fragments, increasing the technical ease of grafting and fixation.

Type of Study/Level of Evidence.—Therapeutic IV.

▶ This study evaluates the outcomes for scaphoid reconstruction with limited debridement. The authors demonstrate osseous healing in all 12 patients treated with their technique.

Scaphoid reconstruction remains a challenging operation with many important technical details, and there are numerous battles going on regarding the best treatment strategy: radical open debridement versus minimally invasive reconstruction; vascularity versus stability (arguing that the use of vascularized bone grafts often compromises fixation); etc. We will probably not know most of the answers any time soon. However, it is safe to say that not all scaphoid nonunions should be treated the same. I therefore think that this study is especially valuable by demonstrating that not all patients require vascularized bone grafts, even after failed primary reconstruction. Simple, less invasive techniques should be preferred under favorable circumstances. From a technical point of view, a second K-wire may not even be necessary in cases such as the ones discussed in this article because rotational stability may be maintained by preserving parts of the fibrous union.

K. Megerle, MD

Force in the Scapholunate Interosseous Ligament During Active Wrist Motion
Dimitris C, Werner FW, Joyce DA, et al (SUNY Upstate Med Univ, Syracuse, NY)
J Hand Surg Am 40:1525-1533, 2015

Purpose.—To examine the force experienced by the scapholunate interosseous ligament (SLIL) during movements of the wrist.

Methods.—Six fresh-frozen cadaveric wrists were freed of soft tissue and tested in a computer controlled, servohydraulic simulator. Each wrist was tested cyclically through simulated active arcs of flexion-extension and dart throw motion. Tensile forces were recorded across the scapholunate joint with the SLIL cut through a cable placed through the scaphoid to the lunate and fixed to a force transducer external to the wrist.

Results.—The average recorded maximal tensile force across the scapholunate joint during all tested motions was 20 N. During wrist flexion-extension and the dart throw motion, SLIL force was greater at maximum extension than at maximum flexion. No significant differences among the different motions at maximum flexion or extension or for maximal force during motion were found.

Conclusions.—Forces during the flexion-extension and dart throw motions were significantly higher in extension than in flexion. However, during simple unresisted wrist motions, the force did not exceed 20 N.

Clinical Relevance.—This information can be used to evaluate surgical methods used for SLIL repairs and thus provide better outcomes for patients.

▶ The Study. The authors' purpose was to examine the force experienced by the scapholunate interosseous ligament (SLIL) during wrist motion, which would then have implications with regards to the strength needed for an SLIL repair or reconstruction. They tested 6 cadaver arms with an average age of 70 years, with minimal SLIL instability (2 Geissler grade I wrists and 4 Geissler grade II wrists). Their experimental model included potting the forearm and then inserting a wire between drill holes in the scaphoid and lunate and attached to a bolt in the lunate on one end and an external force transducer assembly on the other. Tensile forces between the scaphoid and the lunate were thus measured as a compressive force in the load washer while the wrist was moved using sequential force applied to the wrist flexors and extensor tendons with a computer driven algorithm.

The average force for all 6 specimens in a small arc with a maximum flexion/ extension range of 30 and 30 degrees averaged 4.1 N (SD 0.6) in flexion and 17.6 N (SD 5.7) in extension. With a large arc of motion with a maximum flexion of 30 degrees and maximum extension of 50 degrees, this average pressure increased by only 2 N to 4.3 N (SD 0.6) in flexion and dropped slightly to 17.5 N (SD 5.8) in extension. Dart-throwing motion in a small arc and large motion arc were essentially the same with 4.3 N (SD 1.6) and 4.1 N (SD 1.7) in flexion and 17.1 N (SD 5.1) and 17.0 N (SD 5.2) in extension, respectively. There was no statistical difference between these forces, however.

Study Limitations. Berger et al[1] reported the failure force for the dorsal, palmar, and proximal aspects of the SLIL to be 260 N (± 118), 118 N (± 21), and 63 N (± 32), respectively, which suggests that the SLIL ligament experiences much more force than observed in this study. This may be because this study used a single interosseous cable to represent the dorsal, proximal, and palmar components of the SLIL, and assumed that the measured force reflected the force in the 3 components of the SLIL. This model does not take into account the increased forces needed during grip and high-speed loading. Muscle forces contribute significantly to the SL joint stability, which explains how a 150-lb gymnast can perform a handspring without immediately tearing the SLIL, which can only seemingly tolerate 20 N, which is roughly 4.5 lbs of force.

Implications for Treatment. There are some useful observations from this study. There was much less force across the SL joint with the wrist in flexion. This perhaps explains why the dorsal SLIL is thicker and stronger than the volar SLIL because axial load is rarely applied to the flexed wrist so the ligament does not need to be as strong. The SL joint forces are greater in extension, which is the usual position of the wrist with an axial load such as a pushup or falling onto the outstretched hand. The implications are that any dorsal SLIL repair or reconstruction must be at least 4 times as strong as any volar reconstruction such as the long radiolunate capsulodesis described by van Kampen et al,[2] in which the ligament-suture for the capsulodesis interface had an average strength of 43.5 N. This volar reconstruction could therefore still be effective even though it was less than the strength of the native SLIL.

Surprisingly, the SL joint forces during dart-throwing motion were similar to other motions, even though dart throwing motion is a mostly pure midcarpal motion without and significant proximal row motion.[3] If this were the case, patients who underwent a SLIL repair or reconstruction could start early dart-throwing exercises without the risk of pulling the sutures apart. The present study refutes this notion, however. This has also been demonstrated by Garcia-Elias et al.[4] They analyzed the carpal behavior of 6 normal wrists and 6 wrists with scapholunate instability during dart-throwing motion. In the normal wrists, the scaphoid and lunate did not flex or extend but translated along the frontal plane an average 5.9 and 5.6 mm, respectively. When the scapholunate ligaments were torn, the scaphoid shifted toward the radial styloid considerably more than the lunate (12.8 mm vs 4.8 mm; $P = 0.005$), inducing a scapholunate gap. Based on these findings, they could not recommend dart-throwing exercises after scapholunate ligament repair, unless the joint is stabilized with wires or screws.

D. J. Slutsky, MD

References

1. Berger RA, Imeada T, Berglund L, An KN. Constraint and material properties of the subregions of the scapholunate interosseous ligament. *J Hand Surg Am.* 1999; 24:953-962.
2. van Kampen RJ, Bayne CO, Moran SL. A new technique for volar capsulodesis for isolated palmar scapholunate interosseous ligament injuries: a cadaveric study and case report. *J Wrist Surg.* 2015;4:239-245.
3. Moritomo H, Apergis EP, Herzberg G, Werner FW, Wolfe SW, Garcia-Elias M. 2007 IFSSH committee report of wrist biomechanics committee: biomechanics of the so-called dart-throwing motion of the wrist. *J Hand Surg Am.* 2007;32: 1447-1453.
4. Garcia-Elias M, Alomar Serrallach X, Monill Serra J. Dart-throwing motion in patients with scapholunate instability: a dynamic four-dimensional computed tomography study. *J Hand Surg Eur Vol.* 2014;39:346-352.

A comparative study on autologous bone grafting combined with or without posterior interosseous nerve neurectomy for scaphoid nonunion treatment
Xiong L, Harhaus L, Heffinger C, et al (Univ of Heidelberg, Ludwigshafen, Germany)
J Plast Reconstr Aesthet Surg 68:1138-1144, 2015

Background and Aim.—Scaphoid nonunion (SN) is a challenging state after scaphoid fracture. The posterior interosseous nerve neurectomy (PINN) is often performed adjunctively with scaphoid reconstruction using autologous bone grafts. However, it remains unclear whether PINN has a prophylactic or therapeutic value, and thus it results superior to patients with SN without PINN.

Methods.—A retrospective study was performed to evaluate patients with SN who were treated with autologous bone grafts with (cohort 1) or without PINN (cohort 2) between 1996 and 2010. Clinical outcomes, Mayo-wrist score, quality of life by Short Form (SF)-36 questionnaire, and analysis of risk factors were included.

Results.—A total of 151 patients with SN met the inclusion criteria, and 48 were lost in follow-up. The mean follow-up was 71.3 ± 39.0 months. Out of the remaining 103 patients, the union rate was without a statistical difference ($P = 0.847$) between cohorts 1 and 2. Functional results and the Mayo score were comparable in patients with bone union between both cohorts ($P > 0.05$). The results of wrist-pain measurements, including visual pain scales and wrist tenderness, were found to be similar ($P > 0.05$). Additionally, there was no significant difference in the quality of life.

Conclusion.—The comparative study on autologous bone grafts for scaphoid reconstruction revealed comparable results for both patients with and without PINN independent from the choice of bone graft. We anticipate a prophylactic value of PINN due to a potential injury or an irritation during dissection of the wrist capsule. Further research on PIN, its sensory characteristics, and its impact on wrist function is required.

Levels of Evidence.—III.

▶ Painful scaphoid nonunion is an important clinical problem. The most widely used method of treatment is bone grafting and fixation of the scaphoid to achieve union and concomitant symptom relief. Wrist neurectomy is a surgical procedure usually performed as a salvage procedure for the complications of scaphoid nonunion. In limited wrist neurectomy, the anterior and posterior interosseous nerves are resected. Other nerves supplying the wrist capsule are also excised or transected for more extensive neurectomies.

This article reports the study of the role of posterior interosseous nerve (PIN) neurectomy for pain relief in scaphoid nonunion. This procedure was done in addition to and at the same time as bone grafting and fixation. The authors found no differences in union or patient-reported outcomes between the 2 groups.

The difficulty in extrapolating these data to other clinical populations is a result of limitations in the study methodology. This is a retrospective study, and it is unclear from the article as to how patients were allocated between the 2 groups.

From a surgical perspective, a variety of surgical approaches, fixation techniques (including wires and screws), as well as different bone-grafting choices (site as well as type), makes each group heterogeneous. In addition, only the PIN was excised. This is very limited compared to the usual wrist neurectomies done for the salvage of such conditions.

The findings are consistent with what we know about the pathoanatomy and natural course of the condition.

A. Chong, MD

The Missed Scaphoid Fracture—Outcomes of Delayed Cast Treatment
Grewal R, Suh N, MacDermid JC (Univ of Western Ontario, London, Canada)
J Wrist Surg 4:278-283, 2015

Background.—The purpose of this study is to evaluate outcomes (report union rates and times based on CT) for subacute scaphoid fractures, defined as those presenting between 6 weeks and 6 months from injury.

Questions.—1) What are the expected union rates for subacute scaphoid fractures? 2) What are the expected union times for subacute scaphoid fractures? 3) Is it worth trialing a period of cast immobilization for these patients?

Methods.—All isolated sub-acute scaphoid fractures that presented at our institution between 2006 and 2010 were identified. Each subject's health record, CT scans and X-rays were retrospectively reviewed.

Results.—There were 20 males and 8 females, with a mean age of 30, treated with casting alone. There were 20 waist, 7 proximal and 1 distal pole fracture. The mean casting time was 11 (waist) and 14 (proximal pole) weeks with a union rate of 82% (23/28). Diabetes, comminution and a humpback deformity increased the non-union risk in this cohort. Exclusion of these cases resulted in a 96% union rate (23/24).

Conclusion.—Subacute scaphoid fractures (presenting within 6 months from injury) can be expected to successfully heal with casting alone, even if the initial diagnosis is delayed. The expected time frame for union with cast treatment is shorter than previously reported.

Level of Evidence.—IV.

▶ Delayed presentation of scaphoid fractures is a frequent occurrence and often poses a challenge to the managing clinicians in the assessment and decision making. Often symptoms vary and do not necessarily correlate with the radiologic findings. A relative lack of pain and tenderness in a patient presenting with a radiologically poor union of the scaphoid may signify an ongoing healing process and can be a good indicator for predicting union. Limited by the retrospective nature of the study design, this important factor was unfortunately not taken into account.

It is interesting to see the large number of patients with a missed diagnosis of scaphoid fracture and delay in treatment of an average 10.5 weeks in one single center, which reflected the service provision of the primary health care in the area. It was equally interesting to see a significant proportion of cases with known humpback deformity, comminution, and cystic formation to be included in the conservative treatment regime. In many centers, including my practice, these sorts of cases are operated on once they present. The risk of conservative treatment, apart from persistent nonunion, is the problem of malunion and functional impairment caused by prolonged immobilization. Although the authors could show that despite the delay in treatment, 82% of the whole group or 96% of the patients without diabetes, humpback, or comminution could achieve a union at the end, they failed to produce data on the radiologic outcome in terms of scaphoid and carpal alignment or as the functional outcome of the patients. The authors could also have underestimated the impact of immobilization for an average of 11 to 14 weeks in this group who had already been bothered by the fracture problem for more than 2 months prior to the treatment. They did not discuss the advantage of operative treatment, which would usually bring forth a more anatomic reduction of the scaphoid and allow earlier mobilization and rehabilitation.

Nevertheless, this report did provide updated information about the chance of union with conservative treatment under such a circumstance for the patients and clinicians to consider. The reference value of this article will be increased if there is more information on the radiologic and functional outcomes.

P. C. Ho, MD

4 Dupuytren's Contracture

Collagenase Clostridium Histolyticum versus Limited Fasciectomy for Dupuytren's Contracture: Outcomes from a Multicenter Propensity Score Matched Study
Zhou C, Hovius SER, Slijper HP, et al (Hand Surgery and Rehabilitation Medicine, Erasmus, MC; Xpert Clinic, Rotterdam, Hilversum, The Netherlands)
Plast Reconstr Surg 136:87-97, 2015

Background.—Controversy exists about the relative effectiveness of injectable collagenase (collagenase clostridium histolyticum) and limited fasciectomy in the treatment of Dupuytren's contracture. The authors compared the effectiveness of both techniques in actual clinical practice.

Methods.—This study evaluated all subjects treated with collagenase clostridium histolyticum or limited fasciectomy for metacarpophalangeal and/or proximal interphalangeal joint contractures between 2011 and 2014 at seven practice sites. The authors compared the degree of residual contracture (active extension deficit), Michigan Hand Outcomes Questionnaire scores, and adverse events at follow-up visits occurring between 6 and 12 weeks after surgery or the last injection with the use of propensity score matching.

Results.—In 132 matched subjects who were treated with collagenase (n = 66) or fasciectomy (n = 66), the degree of residual contracture at follow-up for affected metacarpophalangeal joints was not significantly different (13 degrees versus 6 degrees; $p = 0.095$) and affected proximal interphalangeal joints had significantly worse residual contracture in the collagenase group compared with those in the fasciectomy group (25 degrees versus 15 degrees; $p = 0.010$). Collagenase subjects experienced fewer serious adverse events than did fasciectomy subjects and reported larger improvements in the Michigan Hand Outcomes Questionnaire subscores evaluating satisfaction with hand function, activities of daily living, and work performance.

Conclusions.—This propensity score–matched study showed that collagenase clostridium histolyticum was not significantly different from limited fasciectomy in reducing metacarpophalangeal joint contractures, whereas proximal interphalangeal joint contractures showed slightly better reduction following limited fasciectomy. Collagenase provided a more rapid recovery of hand function than did fasciectomy and was associated with fewer serious adverse events.

Clinical Question/Level of Evidence.—Therapeutic, III.

▶ This Dutch study is a prospective, randomized trial. Partial, open, palmar fasciectomy was compared with collagenase injection for the treatment of single-digit Dupuytren's contracture. The patients were collected between 2011 and 2014 with the goal of evaluating the early clinical results of both treatments.

The primary outcome measurement was residual contracture assessed at clinical follow-up between 6 and 12 weeks. The secondary outcomes included "clinical improvement" (which was defined as > 50% contracture reduction), adverse events, and the Michigan Hand Questionnaire. I was a bit surprised that the authors intentionally left out pain as an outcome measurement. Their stated rationale for this was that restoration of function was the primary treatment objective.

The open group was treated with surgery followed by 2 weeks of splinting and then 3 months of night splinting. The collagenase group was given up to 3 injections offered at 4-week intervals. The digit was manipulated 24 to 72 hours after the injection.

After statistical analysis, the 2 groups had similar results at the metacarpophalangeal joints. The proximal interphalangeal joint correction averaged 10 degrees better in the open treatment, but the open patients had a higher incidence of adverse events. In patients who were being treated for recurrent disease, the results were the same as in primary disease patients.

The conclusion is that a patient may trade a straighter digit for a quicker return to function and less of a chance for adverse event.

I found this article to be well thought out and presented. I would have liked a more standardized postoperative protocol because 1 group was splinted for 3 months while the other group was not. However, I believe this mirrors current practice.

This article shines a spotlight on some of the differences in these 2 treatment options, providing more information to both surgeons and patients.

N. A. Hoekzema, MD

Factors affecting functional recovery after surgery and hand therapy in patients with Dupuytren's disease
Engstrand C, Krevers B, Kvist J (County Council of Östergötland, Linköping, Sweden; Linköping Univ, Sweden)
J Hand Ther 28:255-260, 2015

Study Design.—Prospective cohort study.
Introduction.—The evidence of the relationship between functional recovery and impairment after surgery and hand therapy are inconsistent.

Purpose of the Study.—To explore factors that were most related to functional recovery as measured by DASH in patients with Dupuytren's disease.

Methods.—Eighty-one patients undergoing surgery and hand therapy were consecutively recruited. Functional recovery was measured by the Disability of the Arm, Shoulder and Hand (DASH) questionnaire. Explanatory variables: range of motion of the finger joints, five questions regarding safety and social issues of hand function, and health-related quality of life (Euroqol).

Results.—The three variables "need to take special precautions", "avoid using the hand in social context", and health-related quality of life (EQ-5D index) explained 62.1% of the variance in DASH, where the first variable had the greatest relative effect.

Discussion.—Safety and social issues of hand function and quality of life had an evident association with functional recovery.

Level of Evidence.—IV.

▶ The authors aimed to study the correlation between the Disability of the Arm, Shoulder and Hand (DASH) questionnaire and quality-of-life outcomes for clients after fasciectomy for Dupuytren's disease. The study population was Swedish speaking and 88% men and 12% women. Outcome measures included the DASH score before and after surgery, total active flexion range of motion, total active extension range of motion, 5 questions related to safety and social issues, and the Euroqol (EQ-5D). Measures were done before surgery and 3 months after surgery. The reduction in total active extension showed a small correlation between the DASH scores. As the authors continued to analyze the data, total active extension became less important in understanding functional recovery after fasciectomy. Often in the clinic I become more focused at the impairment level and want to treat the deficits in extension with range of motion and orthosis. However, this study found that there is only a small correlation between total active extension and functional activities. The article reminds me that I must look at patient performance of daily activities and be patient centered in treatment.

The most important statement in this article is:

"Although interventions in hand surgery and therapy often target physical function, the overall goal is to enhance the individual's ability to execute tasks and to participate fully in life situations. From the patients' perspective, performance of daily activities, interaction with others, or quality of life may be more important outcomes than the degree of impairment." (p. 258)

Occupational performance is the ultimate goal of hand therapy. The therapist wants the patient to participate fully in meaningful and purposeful activities. The authors found that total active extension impairment is important to remediate in therapy sessions; however, the therapist must also be mindful of occupational performance barriers to the client. A patient-centered approach will allow the therapist to make the greatest impact on quality of life for each patient.

S. Kannas, CHT

Collagenase Clostridium Histolyticum versus Limited Fasciectomy for Dupuytren's Contracture: Outcomes from a Multicenter Propensity Score Matched Study

Zhou C, Hovius SER, Slijper HP, et al (Erasmus MC, Rotterdam, The Netherlands; Xpert Clinic, Hilversum, The Netherlands)
Plast Reconstr Surg 136:87-97, 2015

Background.—Controversy exists about the relative effectiveness of injectable collagenase (collagenase clostridium histolyticum) and limited fasciectomy in the treatment of Dupuytren's contracture. The authors compared the effectiveness of both techniques in actual clinical practice.

Methods.—This study evaluated all subjects treated with collagenase clostridium histolyticum or limited fasciectomy for metacarpophalangeal and/or proximal interphalangeal joint contractures between 2011 and 2014 at seven practice sites. The authors compared the degree of residual contracture (active extension deficit), Michigan Hand Outcomes Questionnaire scores, and adverse events at follow-up visits occurring between 6 and 12 weeks after surgery or the last injection with the use of propensity score matching.

Results.—In 132 matched subjects who were treated with collagenase ($n = 66$) or fasciectomy ($n = 66$), the degree of residual contracture at follow-up for affected metacarpophalangeal joints was not significantly different (13 degrees versus 6 degrees; $p = 0.095$) and affected proximal interphalangeal joints had significantly worse residual contracture in the collagenase group compared with those in the fasciectomy group (25 degrees versus 15 degrees; $p = 0.010$). Collagenase subjects experienced fewer serious adverse events than did fasciectomy subjects and reported larger improvements in the Michigan Hand Outcomes Questionnaire subscores evaluating satisfaction with hand function, activities of daily living, and work performance.

Conclusions.—This propensity score—matched study showed that collagenase clostridium histolyticum was not significantly different from limited fasciectomy in reducing metacarpophalangeal joint contractures, whereas proximal interphalangeal joint contractures showed slightly better reduction following limited fasciectomy. Collagenase provided a more rapid recovery of hand function than did fasciectomy and was associated with fewer serious adverse events.

Clinical Question/Level of Evidence.—Therapeutic, III.

▶ The authors sought to compare the outcomes of collagenase and limited fasciectomy at 3 months, finding limited fasciectomy had statistically better correction of the proximal interphalangeal (PIP) joint and collagenase had better subjective outcomes and fewer adverse events. The difference in correction of the contracture at the PIP joint (15 degrees vs 25 degrees residual contracture) was statistically significant, but the clinical significance of this difference is unclear. This study was not randomized, which gives the potential for bias based on surgeon preference. The biggest limitation of the study is the short follow-up of 3 months because this is a condition one for which long-term follow-up is essential to determine whether there is a preferred treatment. There are other variables that may affect outcomes in the surgical group, such as anesthetic choice and tourniquet use. The authors did not assess return to work or activities for either group. In addition, the cost of each procedure was not discussed, which may make one treatment preferred over the other.

Given our published literature on this topic, we know both collagenase and limited fasciectomy can produce good results. Recurrence rates are higher after treatment with collagenase, but satisfaction is also higher and complication rates lower. The outcomes for both treatments are more favorable for the metacarpophalangeal joints than the PIP joints. Hopefully, current or future research will lead to finding a cure with gene modulation rather than our current efforts to treat the end result, which is the contracture.

W. C. Hammert, MD

The Efficacy and Safety of Concurrent Collagenase Clostridium Histolyticum Injections for 2 Dupuytren Contractures in the Same Hand: A Prospective, Multicenter Study
Gaston RG, Larsen SE, Pess GM, et al (OrthoCarolina, Inc., Charlotte, NC; Odense Univ Hosp, Denmark; Central Jersey Hand Surgery, Eatontown, NJ; et al)
J Hand Surg Am 40:1963-1971, 2015

Purpose.—To evaluate efficacy and safety of concurrent administration of 2 collagenase clostridium histolyticum (CCH) injections to treat 2 joints in the same hand with Dupuytren fixed flexion contractures (FFCs).

Methods.—Patients with 2 or more contractures in the same hand caused by palpable cords participated in a 60-day, multicenter, open-label, phase 3b study. Two 0.58 mg CCH doses were injected into 1 or 2 cords in the same hand (1 injection per affected joint) during the same visit. Finger extension was performed approximately 24, 48, or 72 or more hours later. Changes in FFC and range of motion, incidence of clinical success (FFC ≤ 5°), and adverse events (AEs) were summarized.

Results.—The study enrolled 715 patients (725 treated joint pairs), and 714 patients (724 joint pairs) were analyzed for efficacy. At day 31, mean total FFC (sum of 2 treated joints) decreased 74%, from 98° to 27°. Mean total range of motion increased from 90° to 156°. The incidence of clinical success was 65% in metacarpophalangeal joints and 29% in proximal interphalangeal joints. Most treatment-related AEs were mild to moderate, resolving without intervention; the most common were swelling of treated extremity, contusion, and pain in extremity. The incidence of skin lacerations was 22% (160 of 715). Efficacy and safety were similar regardless of time to finger extension.

Conclusions.—Collagenase clostridium histolyticum can be used to effectively treat 2 affected joints concurrently without a greater risk of AEs than treatment of a single joint, with the exception of skin laceration.

The incidence of clinical success in this study after 1 injection per joint was comparable to phase 3 study results after 3 or more injections per joint. Two concurrent CCH injections may allow more rapid overall treatment of multiple affected joints, and the ability to vary the time between CCH injection and finger extension may allow physicians and patients greater flexibility with scheduling treatment.

Type of Study/Level of Evidence.—Therapeutic III.

▶ This article answers a key question regarding use of collagenase clostridium histolyticum (CCH) for Dupuytren contractures (DC), and the answer is clearly a positive for hand surgeons using CCH. The question: Is it safe and effective to treat multiple joints and/or fingers simultaneously with CCH? A large percentage of patients with indications for treatment for DC present with 2 or more digits on the same hand with indications for intervention. Early on in the use of CCH, I personally wondered whether this group with multiple affected fingers and joints a good match for CCH treatment. Certainly the authors avoided a moderate to large hand surgery procedure, but under the original treatment protocol that lead to Food and Drug Administration approval, a patient with 5 joints with contractures of > 30 degrees in 3 fingers, for example, might need 6 injections and at least a dozen visits to complete treatment of 1 hand. Having treated patients under this protocol in the past, in real life this takes at least 6 months. This article showed that whether 2 joints were in the same finger, different fingers, 2 metacarpophalangeal, 2 proximal interphalangeal, or a combination, patients averaged correction of at least 55 degrees. There was no increased risk of complication except a higher rate of skin tearing than patients with 1 joint treated, which is an expected phenomenon. The study also confirmed the expected finding that there was no apparent difference in performing the extension procedure at 24, 48, or 72 hours. This study confirms what my clinical experience over time has shown: it is a rare patient with DC who will need more than 1 visit for injection(s) and 1 visit for manipulation.

P. Blazar

Dupuytren Contracture Recurrence Following Treatment With Collagenase Clostridium Histolyticum (CORDLESS [Collagenase Option for Reduction of Dupuytren Long-Term Evaluation of Safety Study]): 5-Year Data
Peimer CA, Blazar P, Coleman S, et al (Michigan State Univ, East Lansing; Brigham and Women's Hosp, Boston, MA; Hand and Upper Limb Clinic, Brisbane, Queensland, Australia; et al)
J Hand Surg Am 40:1597-1605, 2015

Purpose.—Collagenase Option for Reduction of Dupuytren Long-Term Evaluation of Safety Study was a 5-year noninterventional follow-up study to determine long-term efficacy and safety of collagenase clostridium histolyticum (CCH) treatment for Dupuytren contracture.

Methods.—Patients from previous CCH clinical studies were eligible. Enrolled patients were evaluated annually for contracture and safety at 2, 3, 4, and 5 years after their first injection (0.58 mg) of CCH. In successfully treated joints (≤ 5° contracture following CCH treatment), recurrence was defined as 20° or greater worsening (relative to day 30 after the last injection) with a palpable cord or any medical/surgical intervention to correct new/worsening contracture. A post hoc analysis was also conducted using a less stringent threshold (≥ 30° worsening) for comparison with criteria historically used to assess surgical treatment.

Results.—Of 950 eligible patients, 644 enrolled (1,081 treated joints). At year 5, 47% (291 of 623) of successfully treated joints had recurrence (≥ 20° worsening)—39% (178 of 451) of metacarpophalangeal and 66% (113 of 172) of proximal interphalangeal joints. At year 5, 32% (198 of 623) of successfully treated joints had 30° or greater worsening (metacarpophalangeal 26% [119 of 451] and proximal interphalangeal 46% [79 of 172] joints). Of 105 secondary interventions performed in the successfully treated joints, 47% (49 of 105) received fasciectomy, 30% (32 of 105) received additional CCH, and 23% (24 of 105) received other interventions. One mild adverse event was attributed to CCH treatment (skin atrophy [decreased ring finger circumference from thinning of Dupuytren tissue]). Antibodies to clostridial type I and/or II collagenase were found in 93% of patients, but over the 5 years of follow-up, this did not correspond to any reported clinical adverse events.

Conclusions.—Five years after successful CCH treatment, the overall recurrence rate of 47% was comparable with published recurrence rates after surgical treatments, with one reported long-term treatment-related adverse event. Collagenase clostridium histolyticum injection proved to be an effective and safe treatment for Dupuytren contracture. For those receiving treatment during follow-up, both CCH and fasciectomy were elected options.

Type of Study/Level of evidence.—Therapeutic II.

▶ These 950 eligible subjects have to be the best studied Dupuytren patients ever. (Full disclosure: I was a participant in this study.) The 5-year data are quite compelling in supporting the contention of many collagenase users that the rate of recurrence after successful contracture correction would correspond more closely to "average" (if there indeed is such a thing) reported postsurgical rates rather than reported rates of recurrence after needle aponeurectomy. These findings should be interpreted in the context of the study's chosen definition of recurrence. A palpable new cord leading to 20 degrees or greater of contracture in a previously successfully treated joint is a more strict definition than that used in most published studies, at least those that actually defined recurrence. Importantly, only a third of patients with recurrence, as defined, chose to undergo any treatment. The subjects in this study had every joint of both hands examined yearly for 5 years. This has resulted in a wealth of data to be mined for information beyond the specific goal of the study. Wouldn't it be great if the industry sponsor willingly made the raw data available to qualified investigators who could use their time and energy to see what else could be learned from such a well-controlled study?

V. R. Hentz, MD

Factors affecting functional recovery after surgery and hand therapy in patients with Dupuytren's disease
Engstrand C, Krevers B, Kvist J (County Council of Östergötland, Linköping, Sweden; Linköping Univ, Sweden)
J Hand Ther 28:255-260, 2015

Study Design.—Prospective cohort study.

Introduction.—The evidence of the relationship between functional recovery and impairment after surgery and hand therapy are inconsistent.

Purpose of the Study.—To explore factors that were most related to functional recovery as measured by DASH in patients with Dupuytren's disease.

Methods.—Eighty-one patients undergoing surgery and hand therapy were consecutively recruited. Functional recovery was measured by the Disability of the Arm, Shoulder and Hand (DASH) questionnaire. Explanatory variables: range of motion of the finger joints, five questions regarding safety and social issues of hand function, and health-related quality of life (Euroqol).

Results.—The three variables "need to take special precautions", "avoid using the hand in social context", and health-related quality of life (EQ-5D index) explained 62.1% of the variance in DASH, where the first variable had the greatest relative effect.

Discussion.—Safety and social issues of hand function and quality of life had an evident association with functional recovery.

Level of Evidence.—IV.

▶ Factors affecting functional recovery after any type of surgery are of much interest to those providing the postoperative care. We can certainly learn from our patients what they feel is most important in their recovery and daily function. The authors of this article put together a fairly comprehensive cohort study of 81 participants who underwent surgical intervention for Dupuytren contractures to determine the patient's perspective on functional recovery. The study focused on outcome measures, which included the Swedish version of the DASH, range of motion (ROM) measurements, and the Swedish version of the Euroqol (EQ-5D). In addition, the authors wrote 5 questions that they used to investigate safety and social issues of hand function. Although all patients had clinically objective improvements with ROM, it was noted that they had variations in their final DASH scores (Table 2). The authors were able to determine that emotional functions as reported on their outcome measures explained the variation in the DASH scores. It is not surprising to find that patients are quite concerned with social and safety issues concerning use of their hands. As treating therapists and physicians, we know that

TABLE 2.—Physical Measurement and Self-reported Outcomes Before Surgery and at Three Months Follow Up, Presented as Mean (*m*), Standard Deviation (SD) or Median (md), and Interquartile Range (Iqr)

Variables	n	Before Surgery $m \pm$ SD	n	3 months $m \pm$ SD
Functional recovery				
DASH score[a]	81	21 ± 14	81	12 ± 13
Range of motion				
Total active extension deficit in degrees[b]	81	109 ± 32	81	33 ± 19
Total active finger flexion in degrees[c]	81	239 ± 16	81	222 ± 26
Quality of life				
EQ-VAS[d]	79	80 ± 15	76	79 ± 17
EQ-5D index[e]	79	0.82 ± 0.13	79	0.86 ± 0.17

Variables	n	md (Iqr)	n	md (Iqr)
Safety & social issues of hand function[f]				
1. Worry about not trusting in hand function	79	5 (3−7)	79	8 (6−10)
2. Need to take special precautions due to hand function	78	6 (4−8)	79	8 (6−10)
3. Fear of hurting the hand	80	5 (4−8)	78	9 (7−10)
4. Concerned about appearance of the hand	80	8 (5−10)	79	10 (10−10)
5. Avoid using the hand in social context	80	9 (5−10)	79	10 (10−10)

[a]DASH score: 0 = no disability, 100 = severest disability.
[b]Total active extension deficit: Calculated as the sum of the extension deficit of the MCP, PIP and DIP joint in the affected finger. Higher scores indicate worse extension deficit.
[c]Total active finger flexion: Calculated as the sum of the active flexion of the MCP, PIP and DIP joint in the affected finger. Higher scores indicate better finger flexion.
[d]EQ VAS: 100 = best imaginable health state, 0 = worst imaginable health state.
[e]EQ-5D index: 1 = full health, −0.594 = worst imaginable health state.
[f]Safety and social issues: 1 = to a large degree, 10 = not at all.
Reprinted from Engstrand C, Krevers B, Kvist J. Factors affecting functional recovery after surgery and hand therapy in patients with Dupuytren's disease. *J Hand Ther.* 2015;28:255-260, with permission from Hanley & Belfus, an imprint of Elsevier.

regaining mobility is an important aspect of hand therapy. However, this study reminds us that quality of life for our patients includes much more than improved ROM.

S. J. Clark, OTR/L, CHT

5 Compressive Neuropathies

Biomechanical Role of the Transverse Carpal Ligament in Carpal Tunnel Compliance
Li Z-M, Marquardt TL, Evans PJ, et al (Cleveland Clinic, OH)
J Wrist Surg 3:227-232, 2014

The transverse carpal ligament (TCL) is a significant constituent of the wrist structure and forms the volar boundary of the carpal tunnel. It serves biomechanical and physiological functions, acting as a pulley for the flexor tendons, anchoring the thenar and hypothenar muscles, stabilizing the bony structure, and providing wrist proprioception. This article mainly describes and reviews our recent studies regarding the biomechanical role of the TCL in the compliant characteristics of the carpal tunnel. First, force applied to the TCL from within the carpal tunnel increased arch height and area due to arch width narrowing from the migration of the bony insertion sites of the TCL. The experimental findings were accounted for by a geometric model that elucidated the relationships among arch width, height, and area. Second, carpal arch deformation showed that the carpal tunnel was more flexible at the proximal level than at the distal level and was more compliant in the inward direction than in the outward direction. The hamate-capitate joint had larger angular rotations than the capitate-trapezoid and trapezoid-trapezium joints for their contributions to changes of the carpal arch width. Lastly, pressure application inside the intact and released carpal tunnels led to increased carpal tunnel cross-sectional areas, which were mainly attributable to the expansion of the carpal arch formed by the TCL. Transection of the TCL led to an increase of carpal arch compliance that was nine times greater than that of the intact carpal tunnel. The carpal tunnel, while regarded as a stabile structure, demonstrates compliant properties that help to accommodate biomechanical and physiological variants such as changes in carpal tunnel pressure.

▶ Carpal tunnel syndrome is associated with elevated carpal tunnel pressure and with bowing of the transverse carpal ligament (TCL) and narrowing of the carpal arch. The authors review several of their own recent investigations that describe the mechanics of the carpal tunnel and TCL to better understand the mechanics of the wrist in carpal tunnel syndrome and after surgical release.

The carpal tunnel is formed by a bony arch composed of the proximal and distal carpal rows that form the medial, lateral, and dorsal borders and the TCL, which forms the volar boundary. The TCL inserts on the proximal and distal carpal rows at the scaphoid tuberosity and trapezial ridge radially and the pisiform and hook of the hamate ulnarly. Its contents include 9 tendons of the finger and thumb flexors, the median nerve, and other connective tissues. It also serves as an attachment site for the thenar and hypothenar muscles.

The first set of experiments focused on the response of the carpal tunnel when force is applied to the TCL. The authors found that the force-deformation relationship was direction and location dependent. A palmarly directed force applied to the TCL from within the tunnel increased the volume of the carpal tunnel by pulling the TCL insertion sites together, thereby producing a narrower and higher arch. The TCL itself was found to bow, but its length remained constant. The carpal tunnel narrowed when a compressive force was applied in a radial-ulnar direction to the TCL insertion sites but did not widen when a distracting force was applied to the same locations. The proximal portion of the tunnel was more compliant than the distal portion.

The authors next describe an investigation into the relationship between pressure and morphologic changes to the carpal arch using a custom balloon device in a cadaveric wrist to produce increasing pressure from 0 to 200 mm Hg (Fig 2). Cross-sectional MRI was used to examine carpal tunnel morphology. They demonstrated considerable compliance, with increase in distal cross-sectional area of 9% and 15% at 100 and 200 mm Hg, respectively, with most of the increase in

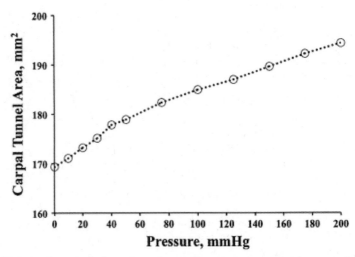

FIGURE 2.—Change in total carpal tunnel area with respect to carpal tunnel pressure. (Reprinted from Li Z-M, Marquardt TL, Evans PJ, et al. Biomechanical role of the transverse carpal ligament in carpal tunnel compliance. *J Wrist Surg*. 2014;3:227-232, with permission Thieme Medical Publishers, Inc.)

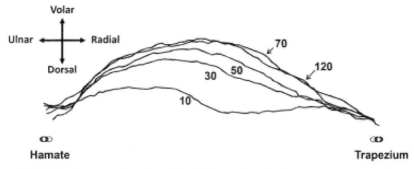

FIGURE 5.—Representative outlines of the TCL volar boundary in response to pressure changes. (Reprinted from Li Z-M, Marquardt TL, Evans PJ, et al. Biomechanical role of the transverse carpal ligament in carpal tunnel compliance. *J Wrist Surg.* 2014;3:227-232, with permission Thieme Medical Publishers, Inc.)

tunnel area attributable to bowing of the TCL. The tunnel itself took on a rounder morphology, although the perimeter distance remained unchanged.

To understand the mechanics after surgical release of the TCL, Kim et al used ultrasound scan to evaluate morphology as water infusion was used to increase pressure in the carpal tunnel to 120 mm Hg. They found that the released carpal arch area increased linearly at lower pressures and plateaued at 70 mm Hg, showing that the released carpal tunnel is relatively compliant at low pressures and then becomes more rigid at higher pressures (Fig 5). The released carpal tunnel had 9 times greater compliance than the intact carpal tunnel because of the cut edges of the TCL separating further with increased pressure.

Based on their experimental results, the authors created a high-fidelity computation model of the wrist that can be used to simulate pathology, the effect of surgical procedures, and patient-specific simulations. Further studies should explore wrist function in vivo.

K. Kollitz, MD

Longitudinal Gliding of the Median Nerve in the Carpal Tunnel: Ultrasound Cadaveric Evaluation of Conventional and Novel Concepts of Nerve Mobilization

Meng S, Reissig LF, Beikircher R, et al (Kaiser-Franz-Josef Hosp, Vienna; Med Univ of Vienna; Univ of Applied Sciences, Krems)
Arch Phys Med Rehabil 96:2207-2213, 2015

Objective.—To evaluate median nerve excursion during conventional nerve gliding exercises and newly developed exercises, primarily comprising abduction and adduction of the fingers.

Design.—Descriptive study.

Setting.—Anatomical dissection facility.

Cadavers.—Random sample of upper extremities of fresh whole-body human cadavers (N = 18). Cadavers with neuromuscular diseases in the medical record or anatomic variations were excluded.

Intervention.—Conventional and new nerve gliding exercises.

Main Outcome Measures.—Distances between markers applied into the nerve and markers in the periosteum were visualized with ultrasound and measured. Comparisons of nerve excursions between different exercises were performed.

Results.—Conventional exercises led to substantial nerve gliding proximal to the carpal tunnel and between the head of the pronator teres (12 and 13.8 mm, respectively), but it led to far less in the carpal tunnel (6.6 mm). With our novel exercises, we achieved nerve gliding in the carpal tunnel of 13.8 mm. No substantial marker movement could be detected during lateral flexion of the cervical spine.

Conclusions.—Although conventional nerve gliding exercises only lead to minimal nerve excursions in the carpal tunnel, our novel exercises with the abduction and adduction of the fingers result in substantial longitudinal gliding throughout the arm. Clinical trials will have to deliver the clinical evidence.

▶ The authors of this study went to enormous lengths to study nerve gliding at the carpal tunnel. They designed a beautiful study to measure the movement of the median nerve at the carpal tunnel. Unfortunately, they completely miss the point of the technique of nerve gliding.

Nerve gliding exercises are meant to move the median nerve (or other affected nerves) proximally and distally at the sight of irritation or compression (in this case, the carpal tunnel). In order to move the median nerve proximally, one would put as much slack as possible on the median nerve distally by flexing the wrist (and according to these authors adducting the fingers). At the same time, one would put as much tension or pull on the nerve proximal to the carpal tunnel by extending the elbow, retracting and adducting the shoulder to 90 degrees, and laterally flexing the neck to the contralateral side. To move the nerve distally, one would do the opposite at each joint. In this study, the authors performed each of these maneuvers at each joint in isolation and measured the movement of the nerve at the carpal tunnel. As such, very little movement was seen.

K. Bengston, MD

Carpal Tunnel Syndrome Pathophysiology: Role of Subsynovial Connective Tissue
Werthel J-DR, Zhao C, An K-N, et al (Mayo Clinic, Rochester, MN)
J Wrist Surg 3:220-226, 2013

Carpal tunnel syndrome (CTS) is a very common pathology. Its most common diagnosis is idiopathic. Although it is accepted that chronic increase in pressure within the carpal tunnel is responsible for median nerve neuropathy, the exact pathophysiology leading to this pressure increase remains unknown. All the histological studies of the carpal tunnel in the CTS find a noninflammatory thickening of the subsynovial connective tissue (SSCT), which seems to be a characteristic of this pathology. Numerous animal models have been developed to recreate CTS in vivo to develop and improve preventive strategies and effective conservative treatments by a better understanding of its pathophysiology. The creation of a shear injury of the SSCT in a rabbit model induced similar modifications to what is observed in CTS, suggesting that this could be a pathway leading to idiopathic CTS.

▶ The authors present a Special Focus article highlighting the most current research regarding the basic science and pathophysiology of carpal tunnel syndrome (CTS), with a special emphasis on the development of a shear injury rabbit model.

CTS is most commonly attributed to idiopathic causes, and the commonly accepted theory is that a chronic increase in pressure in the carpal tunnel leads to median nerve ischemia with resultant demyelination. The exact pathophysiology that leads to increased pressure in the canal is not yet proven. The authors underscore that the creation of accurate animal models to recreate CTS could lead to the development of new therapeutic or preventative modalities.

Subsynovial connective tissue (SSCT) seems to play a pivotal role. The SSCT within the tunnel is called the *microvacuolar collagenous dynamic absorbing system* (MVCAS) and envelops the flexor tendons. The MVCAS has a unique dual purpose within the carpal canal, facilitating tendon excursion by assisting with gliding function by contributing both a viscoelastic and synovial fluid lubrication component. Fig 3 shows electromicroscopy of the SSCT in the flexed and resting positions.

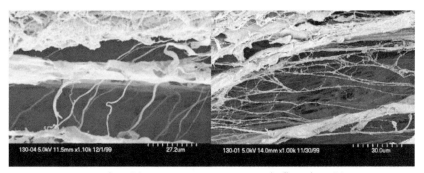

a. neutral position   b. flexed position

FIGURE 3.—Vertical fibers between different layers in the SSCT are loose (a) in neutral position and (b) become stretched as the tendon slides. (SEM original magnification, a: ×1.10k b: ×1.00k.) (Reprinted from Werthel J-DR, Zhao C, An K-N, et al. Carpal tunnel syndrome pathophysiology: role of subsynovial connective tissue. *J Wrist Surg.* 2013;3:220-226, with permission from Thieme Medical Publishers, Inc.)

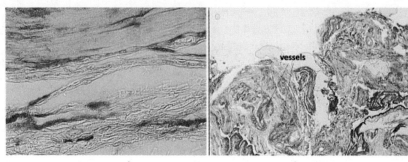

a. normal   **b. CTS**

FIGURE 4.—Collagen type VI staining (a) in normal and (b) CTS SSCT. Fibrosis and increased vascularization are observed in CTS. (Reprinted from Werthel J-DR, Zhao C, An K-N, et al. Carpal tunnel syndrome pathophysiology: role of subsynovial connective tissue. *J Wrist Surg.* 2013;3:220-226, with permission from Thieme Medical Publishers, Inc.)

The authors report that all histologic studies of the SSCT in CTS find a consistent noninflammatory thickening. It is thought that the noninflammatory thickening leads to the characteristic increase in volume and pressure within the tunnel. The thickening also decreases the SSCT permeability, which results in tenosynovial ischemia. Collagen IV is the predominant fiber in normal SSCT, yet recent studies by Ettema et al[1] found a predominance of type III collagen in the SSCT of pathologic samples and increased diameter of the subsynovial fibers. Fig 4 shows the pathologic change of the SSCT between normal and pathologic tissue with increased fibrosis and increased blood vessels with thickened, obstructed lumen. The pathologic changes of SSCT are likely the primary pathophysiologic change leading to CTS.

The next question to answer is what exactly triggers the SSCT changes? Rabbit models have been used to attempt to answer this question and show promise, as the SSCT changes are similar between humans and rabbits. The current hypothesis is that of microtears, or shear injury, leading to SSCT alteration. This finding is in keeping with the commonly accepted observation that repetitive use can result in CTS. Studies find in cadaver studies and animal models that repetitive use leads to increased friction on the SSCT. This friction could trigger the wound healing response, which is supported by the high levels of tumor necrosis factor beta noted in CTS SSCT.

This hypothesis was successfully shown in a rabbit model in which an in vivo rabbit had the flexor digitorum superficialis tendon fixed in a stretched position resulting in SSCT changes consistent with CTS (Fig 3). The authors conclude that this model strengthens the hypothesis that SSCT shear injury is the first event ultimately leading to CTS.

M. O'Shaughnessy, MD

Reference

1. Ettema AM, Amadio PC, Zhao C, et al. Changes in the functional structure of the tenosynovium in idiopathic carpal tunnel syndrome: a scanning electron microscope study. *Plast Reconstr Surg.* 2006;118:1413-1422.

Carpal Tunnel Release: Do We Understand the Biomechanical Consequences?

Morrell NT, Harris A, Skjong C, et al (The Warren Alpert Med School of Brown Univ, Providence, RI)
J Wrist Surg 3:235-238, 2013

Carpal tunnel release is a very common procedure performed in the United States. While the procedure is often curative, some patients experience postoperative scar sensitivity, pillar pain, grip weakness, or recurrent median nerve symptoms. Release of the carpal tunnel has an effect on carpal anatomy and biomechanics, including increases in carpal arch width and carpal tunnel volume and changes in muscle and tendon mechanics. Our understanding of how these biomechanical changes contribute to postoperative symptoms is still evolving. We review the relevant morphometric and biomechanical changes that occur following release of the transverse carpal ligament.

▶ Carpal tunnel release (CTR) may lead to biomechanical changes in the hand and wrist that we do not fully understand. The authors present a Special Focus article highlighting the most current research regarding the biomechanical alterations that follow release of the transverse carpal ligament (TCL).

Anatomically, the TCL is 10 times thicker than the antebrachial fascia and has broader insertions distally than proximally. It serves at least 3 primary functions: to provide transverse stability to the carpus, to anchor the thenar and hypothenar muscles, and to serve as a pulley for the extrinsic flexor tendons.

Cadaveric studies found that sectioning of the TCL alone leads to diastasis of the carpal arch of 1.3 mm but when combined with sectioning of the distal aponeurosis diastasis measured 6.6 mm.[1] A radiographic analysis found that post-CTR patients had an average 14% (2.9 mm) increase in carpal arch widening on carpal tunnel radiographs 20 months postoperatively and found a statistically significant decrease in grip strength of 26% when arch was increased more than 20%.[2] No significant effect was noted with change of less than 10%, and there was no correlation with postoperative wrist pain and arch width.[2]

Advanced imaging studies (CT, MRI) have evaluated the volume of the carpal tunnel before and after CTR. Several studies verify that the volume of the tunnel increases postoperatively, but the increase is transient and generally returns to the preoperative state, suggesting a certain amount of recoil inherent to the carpus. The greatest increase is noted in the volar-dorsal plane rather than the radioulnar plane, suggesting that increase in carpal arch width may not play a major role.[3] There is consensus in the literature that not only does the carpal volume increase but, importantly, the geometry of the tunnel changes after CTR.

A cadaveric study evaluating stiffness of the carpal arch showed decreased stiffness of only 7.5% with TCL sectioning, concluding that intercarpal ligaments provide the critical support of the arch.[4] This finding suggests that there may be a subset of patients undergoing CTR who have underlying injury or weakness of the intercarpal ligaments, putting them at increased risk of arch diastasis and, therefore, greater risk for symptomatic biomechanical changes.

The authors remark that although the implications of these changes are not well understood, it is reasonable to conclude that the changes are not inconsequential and may explain the pillar pain and decreased grip strength seen after CTR.

Considering the TCL serves as the origin for thenar and hypothenar musculature, sectioning of the ligament may lead to altered mechanics of opposition and pinch. A cadaveric study found significant muscle shortening and loss of pull after TCL sectioning; the authors suggested that this would significantly alter hand biomechanics leading to decreased strength.[5]

Injury to superficial nerves with the "critical pillar rectangle" described by Wilson may be a culprit of scar sensitivity and pillar pain. Additionally, postoperative edema may play a critical role in pain. The slight relaxation of the carpal arch may place increased tension on the surgical scar and lead to sensitivity and pain. No studies are cited to confirm these conjectures.

Some argue that the TCL is an important pulley in the flexor tendon system, and TCL sectioning may result in increased flexor tendon excursion and bowstringing, which may lead to postoperative grip strength weakness in flexion.

The morphologic changes that occur after sectioning of the TCL—increased width of the carpal arch, increased tunnel volume and altered geometry, effect on thenar and hypothenar muscles, and the flexor pulley system—all appear to have biomechanical consequences and may help explain the etiologies of postoperative pain and decreased grip strength.

M. O'Shaughnessy, MD

References

1. Tanabe T, Okutsu I. An anatomical study of the palmar ligamentous structures of the carpal canal. *J Hand Surg Br.* 1997;22:754-757.
2. Gartsman GM, Kovach JC, Crouch CC, Noble PC, Bennett JB. Carpal arch alteration after carpal tunnel release. *J Hand Surg Am.* 1986;11:372-374.
3. Kato T, Kuroshima N, Okutsu I, Ninomiya S, et al. Effects of endoscopic release of the transverse carpal ligament on carpal canal volume. *J Hand Surg Am.* 1994;19:416-419.
4. Garcia-Elias M, An KN, Cooney WP 3rd, Linscheid RL, Chao EY. Stability of the transverse carpal arch: an experimental study. *J Hand Surg Am.* 1989;14:277-282.
5. Fuss FK, Wagner TF. Biomechanical alterations in the carpal arch and hand muscles after carpal tunnel release: a further approach toward understanding the function of the flexor retinaculum and the cause of postoperative grip weakness. *Clin Anat.* 1996;9:100-108.

Carpal tunnel syndrome and prediabetes: Is there a true association?
Sousa Vasconcelos JT, Freitas Paiva ÂM, Cavalcanti MF, et al (Piauí State Univ, Brazil; Getulio Vargas Hosp, Teresina, Piauí, Brazil; et al)
Clin Neurol Neurosurg 137:57-61, 2015

Background.—Carpal tunnel syndrome (CTS) is probably associated with diabetes mellitus, but its link to prediabetes (PD) is unknown.

Objective.—To determine prevalence of PD and others risk factors in CTS.

Methods.—A cross-sectional study including 115 idiopathic CTS patients and 115 age-, gender-and body mass index (BMI)-matched controls was performed. Clinical, laboratory and neurophysiological evaluations were conducted in all subjects to confirm CTS diagnosis. CTS severity was graded on a standardized neurophysiological scale. PD was defined using strict criteria.

Results.—The prevalence of PD was similar in CTS and control groups (27% vs. 21.7%, respectively $P = 0.44$). Nocturnal symptoms (91.3%) and moderate CTS (58.3%) were most frequently observed in CTS patients. In logistic regression analysis, PD was significantly correlated with age (odds ratio [OR] 1.05, 95% confidence interval [CI] 1.01−1.09; $P = 0.006$) and BMI (OR 1.08. 95% CI 1.01−1.16; $P = 0.026$), but not with CTS (OR 0.82, 95% CI 0.43−1.53; $P = 0.537$). CTS patients with PD had a significantly higher mean age compared to those without PD (53.8 ± 10.2 vs. 49.5 ± 8.6 years, respectively $P = 0.027$). The frequency of age >60 years was significantly higher in CTS with PD than in CTS without PD (29.0% vs. 8.3%, respectively $P = 0.04$) as was BMI >30 kg/m^2 (64.5% vs. 33.3%, respectively $P = 0.03$). No significant differences were observed between the two CTS groups with respect to gender, BMI, symptoms, and neurophysiological severity of CTS.

Conclusions.—Our findings indicated that CTS is not associated with PD, but that PD is closely linked to age and overweight.

▶ This is a cross-sectional study of 115 patients, ages 25 to 74 years, with a diagnosis of idiopathic carpal tunnel syndrome (CTS) based on clinical examination and nerve conduction studies. The study patients were then compared with 115 age, sex, and body mass index (BMI)—matched controls without CTS with the purpose of comparing the prevalence of prediabetes (PD) and its risk factors among the groups. All patients underwent blinded clinical examination and nerve conduction studies (NCS) to confirm the presence or absence of CTS. All subsequently underwent a 12-hour fasting oral glucose tolerance test to evaluate for the presence of either impaired fasting glucose (IFG) or impaired glucose tolerance (IGT). Prediabetes was defined as the presence of either IFG or IGT or both. Results showed no statistically significant differences among groups save for a lower proportion of nonwhites in CTS groups compared with controls, which is of uncertain significance. There was no difference in the frequency of PD among groups; however, PD was correlated with increased age and BMI. There was also no difference in symptoms or severity of CTS on NCS when comparing subjects with and without PD. These results were different than those of previous studies, suggesting a higher rate of CTS in patients with PD; however, the testing for PD was more specific and standardized in the current study. Strengths of the study include the large sample of patients, matching for age, sex, and BMI as well as the simultaneous clinical and neurophysiologic evaluation to diagnose CTS. I believe this study convincingly shows that PD is associated with advancing age and increasing BMI, however, does not show a clear link between PD and CTS as there is between diabetes mellitus and carpal tunnel syndrome. Nonetheless, it remains a wise idea to evaluate patients for comorbid conditions when evaluating and treating CTS.

E. J. Gauger, MD

Multidimensional Ultrasound Imaging of the Wrist: Changes of Shape and Displacement of the Median Nerve and Tendons in Carpal Tunnel Syndrome
Filius A, Scheltens M, Bosch HG, et al (Erasmus MC Univ Med Ctr, Rotterdam, Netherlands; Erasmus MC, Rotterdam, The Netherlands; et al)
J Orthop Res 33:1332-1340, 2015

Dynamics of structures within the carpal tunnel may alter in carpal tunnel syndrome (CTS) due to fibrotic changes and increased carpal tunnel pressure. Ultrasound can visualize these potential changes, making ultrasound potentially an accurate diagnostic tool. To study this, we imaged the carpal tunnel of 113 patients and 42 controls. CTS severity was classified according to validated clinical and nerve conduction study (NCS) classifications. Transversal and longitudinal displacement and shape (changes) were calculated for the median nerve, tendons and surrounding tissue. To predict diagnostic value binary logistic regression modeling was applied. Reduced longitudinal nerve displacement ($p \leq 0.019$), increased nerve cross-sectional area ($p \leq 0.006$) and perimeter ($p \leq 0.007$), and a trend of relatively changed tendon displacements were seen in patients. Changes were more convincing when CTS was classified as more severe. Binary logistic modeling to diagnose CTS using ultrasound showed a sensitivity of 70—71% and specificity of 80—84%. In conclusion, CTS patients have altered dynamics of structures within the carpal tunnel.

▶ This prospective study by Filius et al addresses the issue of complementary and potentially disruptive diagnostic methods of diagnosing carpal tunnel syndrome (CTS) by using musculoskeletal ultrasound techniques to statically and dynamically measure anatomic structures within the carpal tunnel. Their findings support those of previous studies showing that the static cross-sectional area of the median nerve directly correlates with the severity of CTS determined clinically or by nerve conduction study. In addition, this group observed the differences in longitudinal plane displacement median nerve, flexor digitorum superficialis of the middle finger, and flexor digitorum profundus of the middle finger with surrounding tissue but no significant difference in transversal displacement of these structures. Some association of shape was also noted. I am a major proponent of the clinical use of musculoskeletal ultrasound scan and especially of disruptive diagnostic methods that decrease the invasiveness and cost while increasing its accuracy. After reading this article, I wonder if in the case of carpal tunnel syndrome, we could accept the accuracy of clinical judgment and increased cross-sectional areas of the median nerve measure by ultrasound scan to make the diagnosis[1,2] and create better methods of treating CTS based on biomechanical insights provided by this and other similar studies.

D. Barnes, MD

References

1. Fowler JR, Cipolli W, Hanson T. A comparison of three diagnostic tests for carpal tunnel syndrome using latent class analysis. *J Bone Joint Surg Am.* 2015;97: 1958-1961.
2. Fowler JR, Maltenfort MG, Ilyas AM. Ultrasound as a first-line test in the diagnosis of carpal tunnel syndrome: a cost-effectiveness analysis. *Clin Orthop Relat Res.* 2013;471:932-937.

Enhanced Expression of Wnt9a in the Flexor Tenosynovium in Idiopathic Carpal Tunnel Syndrome
Yamanaka Y, Menuki K, Zenke Y, et al (Univ of Occupational and Environmental Health, Kitakyushu Fukuoka, Japan)
J Orthop Res 33:1531-1536, 2015

This study aimed to clarify the association between abnormal Wnt signaling and the cause of idiopathic carpal tunnel syndrome (ICTS) and whether an association exists between Wnt signaling and cell proliferation in the flexor tenosynovium. The subjects included nine patients with ICTS; the controls were nine patients with distal radius fractures without any symptoms of carpal tunnel syndrome. We extracted mRNA from the flexor tenosynovium and compared the expression levels of genes encoding 17 types of Wnt in both subjects and controls via quantitative real-time polymerase chain reaction (PCR). Expression levels of factors involved in cell proliferation, such as estrogen-responsive finger protein, epidermal growth factor receptor, heparin binding-epidermal growth factor-like growth factor, insulin-like growth factor-1, and vascular endothelial growth factor (VEGF) were also measured using quantitative real-time PCR. In addition, we compared the Wnt and MIB-1 protein expression levels to clarify the effect of Wnt on cell proliferation. Quantitative real-time PCR revealed significantly greater expression of the gene encoding Wnt9a in subjects with ICTS than in controls and also revealed a positive correlation between the expression of genes encoding Wnt9a and VEGF in subjects with ICTS. Quantitative evaluation using immunohistochemical staining also indicated more marked Wnt9a expression in subjects than in controls. However, there was no relationship between the expression of Wnt9a and the cell proliferation index MIB-1. These results indicate that Wnt9a expression is enhanced in ICTS and that Wnt9a may be involved in VEGF expression in ICTS.

▶ Idiopathic carpal tunnel syndrome (ICTS) is a familiar yet mysterious condition. ICTS is common in the clinics, with an effective surgical treatment; yet the underlying etiology and pathophysiology that initiates and controls its progression is still relatively unclear.

We understand that the interactions among genetics, anatomy, dynamic wrist and hand motion, and other factors result in intermittent or continuous compression of the median nerve within the carpal tunnel. This leads to ischemia, nerve scarring, demyelination, and ultimately axonal loss. The differences in each of these end-point components for a particular patient are thought to account for the variation in clinical and neurophysiological findings in patients with this diagnosis.

Previous work has shown that changes related to neuronal vasculature and perfusion are involved in the development of ICTS. This article provides a further glimpse into the mechanisms behind this. It suggests that Wnt signaling, and in particular Wnt9a, may be involved in the causation of ICTS via vascular endothelial growth factor signaling. The findings are congruent with current knowledge of the condition.

There are limitations in the study, such as the choice of distal radius fracture patients as a control group. This group of patients has a higher rate of carpal tunnel syndrome, and this may affect the findings. It is also unclear whether there was blinding in the assessments, so some bias may remain. Finally, it remains to be determined whether this association at the molecular biological level is of any clinical importance.

Our understanding of this condition from cellular and biochemical perspectives is still patchy and incomplete. It will take much more work before we can hope to manipulate these processes nonsurgically to treat this condition.

A. Chong, MD

Carpal Tunnel Release: Do We Understand the Biomechanical Consequences?

Morrell NT, Harris A, Skjong C, et al (Brown Univ, Providence, RI)
J Wrist Surg 3:235-238, 2013

Carpal tunnel release is a very common procedure performed in the United States. While the procedure is often curative, some patients experience postoperative scar sensitivity, pillar pain, grip weakness, or recurrent median nerve symptoms. Release of the carpal tunnel has an effect on carpal anatomy and biomechanics, including increases in carpal arch width and carpal tunnel volume and changes in muscle and tendon mechanics. Our understanding of how these biomechanical changes contribute to postoperative symptoms is still evolving. We review the relevant morphometric and biomechanical changes that occur following release of the transverse carpal ligament.

▶ Although carpal tunnel release (CTR) is a commonly performed procedure with a relatively low risk of associated complications, a subset of patients experiences postoperative problems. This study reviews the existing evidence, and the authors explore possible etiologies for these symptoms. The authors describe the ligamentous, muscular, neurogenic, and edematous changes that occur after CTR and their biomechanical consequences. They conclude that any insufficiency of intercarpal ligaments during the release of the transverse carpal ligament could contribute to pillar pain and decreased grip strength. Other biomechanical changes proposed to produce such symptoms include shortening of the thenar and hypothenar muscles, and volar displacement of the flexor tendons traversing the carpal tunnel. However, these studies used simulated grasp models and cadaveric wrists, and it is difficult to interpret the clinical significance of these results. Unfortunately, with limited high-quality evidence to support these theories, a more rigorous systematic review or meta-analysis is not possible. However, any further knowledge allowing surgeons to predict who is at risk of developing complications after this procedure is a step in the right direction.

Paul Kooner, BSc contributed to the writing of this review under the direction of Ruby Grewal, MD, MSc, FRCSCP.

R. Grewal, MD, MSc, FRCSC

The Effect of Moving Carpal Tunnel Releases Out of Hospitals on Reducing United States Health Care Charges
Nguyen C, Milstein A, Hernandez-Boussard T, et al (Stanford Univ School of Medicine, CA; et al)
J Hand Surg Am 40:1657-1662, 2015

Purpose.—To better understand how perioperative care affects charges for carpal tunnel release (CTR).

Methods.—We developed a cohort using ICD9-CM procedure code 04.43 for CTR in the National Survey of Ambulatory Surgery 2006 to test perioperative factors potentially associated with CTR costs. We examined factors that might affect costs, including patient characteristics, payer, surgical time, setting (hospital outpatient department vs. freestanding ambulatory surgery center), anesthesia type, anesthesia provider, discharge status, and adverse events. Records were grouped by facility to reduce the impact of surgeon and patient heterogeneity. Facilities were divided into quintiles based on average total facility charges per CTR. This division allowed comparison of factors associated with the lowest and highest quintile of facilities based on average charge per CTR.

Results.—A total of 160,000 CTRs were performed in 2006. Nearly all patients were discharged home without adverse events. Mean charge across facilities was $2,572 (SD, $2,331–$2,813). Patient complexity and intraoperative duration of surgery was similar across quintiles (approximately 13 min). Anesthesia techniques were not significantly associated with patient complexity, charges, and total perioperative time. Hospital outpatient department setting was strongly associated with total charges, with $500 higher charge per CTR. Half of all CTRs were performed in hospital outpatient departments. Facilities in the lowest quintile charge group were freestanding ambulatory surgery centers.

Conclusions.—Examination of charges for CTR suggests that surgical setting is a large cost driver with the potential opportunity to lower charges for CTRs by approximately 30% if performed in ASCs.

Type of Study/Level of Evidence.—Economic/decision analysis II.

▶ This article is significant in that the authors investigate which perioperative factors might be most correlated with increased charges in carpal tunnel release (CTR) surgery, including where the surgery was performed: hospital outpatient department (HOPD) versus ambulatory surgery center (ASC). The authors note that spending on CTR exceeds $2 billion in the United States alone; therefore, finding areas to cut costs in this common procedure could help decrease the overall costs of health care in this country.

The authors used a database called the National Survey of Ambulatory Surgeries from 2006 to evaluate the perioperative factors in 160 000 CTRs. The study was well constructed: the authors used 1 clear *International Classification of Diseases* (9th Revision, clinical modification) procedure code, 04.43 (for CTR), and studied several variables, such as patient characteristics, payer, surgical time, surgical setting, anesthesia type, and adverse events. They found that the surgical setting was a major factor in the charges associated with CTR surgery, with ASCs outperforming HOPDs by about 30%.

Although the 04.43 code may capture all of the CTRs reported in the survey, it may not be representative of all of the CTRs performed in the United States. Rather than coding the surgery as a CTR, some surgeons code it as a "flexor tenosynovectomy" or "neuroplasty of a major peripheral nerve." This study was also unable to evaluate CTRs performed in the office-based procedure room, because these data are not captured in the NSAS data set. As the authors stated, in 1 study at a single US institution, there was "a large cost difference in the cost of care between CTRS performed in a procedure room and those done in an operating room." The term "charges" also does not equate exactly to "costs," and this distinction may be especially apparent in the out-of-network facility where charges are often a high multiple of the costs actually paid for by the payer.

I perform almost 100% of my surgeries in the ASC setting, and this includes my CTRs, which I perform both open and endoscopic. I am not surprised at all that this study found the surgical setting to be the major factor in costs related to CTR surgery. In fact, studies looking at other common outpatient procedures would likely come to the same conclusion. One significant factor that would affect costs in the ASC is surgeon ownership in the center. The surgeon who owns shares in an ASC may have more of a stake in making sure costs are minimized, versus the HOPD, where he or she may have no ownership and no control over costs.

S. S. Shin, MD, MMSc

Pathophysiology and Etiology of Nerve Injury Following Peripheral Nerve Blockade

Brull R, Hadzic A, Reina MA, et al (Univ of Toronto, Ontario, Canada; Columbia Univ, New York; Monteprincipe Univ Hosp, Madrid, Spain; et al)
Reg Anesth Pain Med 40:479-490, 2015

This review synthesizes anatomical, anesthetic, surgical, and patient factors that may contribute to neurologic complications associated with peripheral nerve blockade. Peripheral nerves have anatomical features unique to a given location that may influence risk of injury. Peripheral nerve blockade-related peripheral nerve injury (PNI) is most severe with intrafascicular injection. Surgery and its associated requirements such as positioning and tourniquet have specific risks. Patients with preexisting neuropathy may be at an increased risk of postoperative neurologic dysfunction. Distinguishing potential causes of PNI require clinical assessment and investigation; a definitive diagnosis, however, is not always possible. Fortunately, most postoperative neurologic dysfunction appears to resolve with time, and the incidence of serious long-term nerve injury directly attributable to peripheral nerve blockade is relatively uncommon. Nonetheless, despite the use of ultrasound guidance, the risk of block-related PNI remains unchanged.

What's New.—Since the 2008 Practice Advisory, new information has been published, furthering our understanding of the microanatomy of peripheral nerves, mechanisms of peripheral nerve injection injury, toxicity of local anesthetics, the etiology of and monitoring methods, and technologies that may decrease the risk of nerve block-related peripheral nerve injury.

▶ This is a narrative review in which the MEDLINE search database was used to identify articles in which the complications associated with peripheral nerve block were assessed. All of the articles were reviewed by the authors individually, and an emphasis was placed on those published since 2008 when a practice advisory based on the same kinds of search criteria was published in the Regional Anesthesia and Pain Medicine journal.

The story is complex. This review underlines the point that nerve complications associated with peripheral nerve block are caused by may factors, including issues with the patient, anesthetic chosen, surgery planned, and perioperative processes. The authors cite the variability of location of peripheral nerves as a key factor in making them prone to injury during peripheral nerve block placement, and they also note that the main source of peripheral nerve block-mediated neurologic complications is likely mechanical fascicular injury or injection of local anesthetic into an actual fascicle in the nerve. Intrafascicular injections cause myelin injury and axonal degeneration the avoidance of intraneural injection is a key safety principle for regional anesthesia. The authors find no evidence that ultrasound guidance or any other form of localization method reduces the actual risk of peripheral nerve injury in the setting of peripheral nerve blockade, and they also note that peripheral nerve block does not increase the risk of peripheral nerve injury following major surgery. They further note that the primary determinant of prognosis after these injuries is likely the integrity of axons, a fact that is hard to confirm using modern imaging or diagnostic techniques. Complications are also probably underreported in the literature.

The authors summarize many possible mechanisms of injury to nerves even in the absence of regional anesthesia, including chemical injury and inflammatory injury as well as injury mechanisms that are specifically related to peripheral nerve block including anesthetic factors, intraneural injection factors, and factors associated with needle type and nerve structure. The authors also reviewed the effect of surgical factors, such as positioning and the effects of the pneumatic tourniquet. They note with regard to tourniquet effects in particular that wider tourniquets and the use of lower cuff pressures as well as limiting the duration of inflation seem to reduce the risk of permanent damage, and they also cite a study that shows that tourniquet compression results in increased vascular permeability and intraneural edema in 1 nonhuman model of tourniquet-mediated injury. The authors also include a clear discussion of injection pressure monitoring and peripheral nerve stimulation as methods to possibly alter the course of peripheral nerve injury after peripheral nerve blockade.

Finally, the authors spend part of their work focusing on patient factors, including preoperative neural compromise in the evolution of peripheral nerve injury and lumbar spinal canal stenosis. Notable results on this important matter include the fact that lumbar spinal canal stenosis is an independent risk factor for common peroneal palsy after total hip arthroplasty. This lends credence to the somewhat antiquated notion of double-crush syndrome as a mechanism for injury. They do not, in their work, cite any information specifically related to cervical canal stenosis as it relates to predisposing patients to upper extremity nerve injury in the setting of peripheral nerve blockade; but it is also quite clear that the same mechanism may apply in the upper extremity as in the lower extremity. Spinal issues likely predispose patients to nerve complications in limb surgery.

Taken together, this special article in *Regional Anesthesia and Pain Medicine* may provide some insights for the review of the risks of peripheral nerve blockade for patients undergoing upper extremity procedures.

J. Elfar, MD

Effects of Metabolic Syndrome on the Outcome of Carpal Tunnel Release: A Matched Case-Control Study
Roh YH, Lee BK, Noh JH, et al (Gachon Univ School of Medicine, Incheon, Korea; Kangwon Natl Univ Hosp, Gangwon-do, Korea; et al)
J Hand Surg Am 40:1303-1309, 2015

Purpose.—To compare outcomes of carpal tunnel release in patients with or without metabolic syndrome.

Methods.—In a prospective consecutive series, 35 patients with metabolic syndrome and surgically treated carpal tunnel syndrome (CTS) were age- and sex- matched with 37 control patients without metabolic syndrome. Grip, pinch strength, perception of touch with Semmes-Weinstein monofilament, and Boston Carpal Tunnel Questionnaires (BCTQ) were assessed preoperatively and at 3, 6, and 12 months postoperatively.

Results.—Patients with metabolic syndrome had more severe electrophysiologic grade of CTS than those without metabolic syndrome, but the 2 groups had similar preoperative grip/pinch strength and BCTQ scores. The BCTQ symptom score for the metabolic syndrome group was significantly greater than that of the control group at 3 months, and the BCTQ function score of the metabolic syndrome group was significantly greater than that of the control group at 3 and 6 months' follow-up. However, there was no significant difference in BCTQ symptom or functional scores between groups at 12 months' follow-up. There was no significant difference in grip strength between groups through 12 months' follow-up whereas the pinch strength of the control group was significantly greater than that of the metabolic syndrome group at 12 months' follow-up. Semmes-Weinstein monofilament test results were significantly greater in the control group than in the metabolic syndrome group at 3 and 6 months' follow-up but were similar at 12 months.

Conclusions.—Patients with CTS and metabolic syndrome have delayed functional recovery after carpal tunnel release, but noteworthy improvements in symptom severity and hand function are similar to those in patients without metabolic syndrome 1 year after surgery.

Type of Study/Level of Evidence.—Prognostic II.

▶ In this study, patients with metabolic syndrome were compared with control cohorts without metabolic syndrome. Metabolic syndrome, for the purposes of this study and this commentary, is the presence of 3 of 5 criteria including the following: (1) a clinical diagnosis of diabetes with dietary, oral, or insulation treatment; (2) an arterial blood pressure of greater than 130/85 or the current use of antihypertensive medication; (3) a plasma triglyceride level of greater than 150 mg/dL; (4) a high-density lipoprotein cholesterol level of less than 50 mg/dL for females or less than 40 mg/dL for males; and (5) a waist size higher than 80 cm for females or higher than 90 cm for males in the Asian population or a body mass index of greater than 30. In essence, by this definition, metabolic syndrome represents a growing segment of the American population, and the prevalence is increasing dramatically all over the world. The metabolic syndrome is a correlate of obesity, and its presence has multiple implications for the general health of patients. This syndrome increases the rate of peripheral nerve impairment, and this has direct bearing on the results of this study.

In this well-performed examination, 2 groups of about 35 patients, 1 with and 1 without metabolic syndrome, were treated for surgically correctable carpal tunnel syndrome. Parameters of hand surgery outcome including grip and pinch strengths and sensibility of Semmes-Weinstein monofilament testing were used and Boston Carpal Tunnel Questionnaire outcomes were obtained at 3, 6, and 12 months postoperatively.

The results were interesting. Although patients with metabolic syndrome had more severe carpal tunnel syndrome by electrodiagnostic criteria, both groups had similar preoperative pinch and grip strengths and questionnaire scores. At 3 months, the metabolic syndrome patients fared more poorly on the symptom portion of the questionnaire; however, there was no significant difference in the questionnaire results on symptom or functional domains between the 2 groups at 1-year follow-up. Grip strengths were not different between the 2 groups at 12 months; however, the pinch strength was greater in the unaffected group at the 12-month time point. Sensibility testing was better in the control group but only at early times points.

The conclusion of the study was that patients with carpal tunnel syndrome and metabolic syndrome have some delay in functional recovery, but it is notable that at 1 year, most results are similar. This study is informative with regard to patient expectations. Can patients with metabolic syndrome, obesity, diabetes, or other such related conditions expect the same recovery after surgery for carpal tunnel release as other patients who are unaffected? The answer is yes from this study's results. This is useful in the normal clinical practice of hand surgery. It is clear that the importance of being able to predict outcome in these patients is increasing along with the size of this subpopulation, and it is helpful to have every indication that we can about their future outcomes.

J. Elfar, MD

Endoscopic vs Open Decompression of the Ulnar Nerve in Cubital Tunnel Syndrome: A Prospective Randomized Double-Blind Study
Schmidt S, Kleist Welch-Guerra W, Matthes M, et al (Ernst Moritz Arndt Univ, Greifswald, Germany; et al)
Neurosurgery 77:960-970, 2015

Background.—Prospective randomized data for comparison of endoscopic and open decompression methods are lacking.

Objective.—To compare the long- and short-term results of endoscopic and open decompression in cubital tunnel syndrome.

Methods.—In a prospective randomized double-blind study, 54 patients underwent ulnar nerve decompression for 56 cubital tunnel syndromes from October 2008 to April 2011. All patients presented with typical clinical and neurophysiological findings and underwent preoperative nerve ultrasonography. They were randomized for either endoscopic (n = 29) or open (n = 27) surgery. Both patients and the physician performing the follow-up examinations were blinded. The follow-up took place 3, 6, 12, and 24 months postoperatively. The severity of symptoms was measured by McGowan and Dellon Score, and the clinical outcome by modified Bishop Score. Additionally, the neurophysiological data were evaluated.

Results.—No differences were found regarding clinical or neurophysiological outcome in both early and late follow-up between both groups. Hematomas were more frequent after endoscopic decompression ($P = .05$). The most frequent constrictions were found at the flexor carpi ulnaris (FCU) arch and the retrocondylar retinaculum. We found no compressing structures more than 4 cm distal from the sulcus in the endoscopic group. The outcome was classified as "good" or "excellent" in 46 out of 56 patients (82.1%). Eight patients did not improve sufficiently or had a relapse and underwent a second surgery.

Conclusion.—The endoscopic technique showed no additional benefits to open surgery. We could not detect relevant compressions distal to the FCU arch. Therefore, an extensive far distal endoscopic decompression is not routinely required. The open decompression remains the procedure of choice at our institution.

▶ This prospective, randomized study from Greifswald, Germany, was published in the journal *Neurosurgery*. The authors designed an elegant trial to compare mini open in situ cubital tunnel release with endoscopic release.

Fifty-four patients were randomized to have either a 3-cm open procedure or an endoscopic procedure that was also performed through a 3-cm skin incision. The patients were evaluated preoperatively with electromyography/nerve conduction study and nerve ultrasound to assess for compression location. The patients were followed for 2 years including clinical examination and nerve conduction velocity.

On statistical analysis of the results, there was no difference in patient outcomes with regard to short- or long-term recovery. Both groups looked similar at follow-up with the exception of the endoscopic group having more wound hematomas.

The authors also paid close attention to see if there were any constrictive structures greater than 4 cm distal or proximal to the cubital tunnel. One of the proposed benefits of the endoscopic technique is the ability to achieve a release farther away from the small incision. These investigators found no significant compression greater than 4 cm from the cubital tunnel.

The final conclusion was that mini-open cubital tunnel release was as efficacious as endoscopic release. The endoscopic surgery took longer to perform and had a higher rate of surgical site hematoma.

This study mirrors my personal experience with endoscopic cubital tunnel release. I no longer perform endoscopic releases at the elbow. I feel there is actually greater visibility with a well-placed 3-cm open incision, an Army-Navy retractor, and a headlight than with an endoscope. I have felt that the clinical results are identical at both short- and long-term follow-up, and this paper is further proof.

N. A. Hoekzema, MD

The Management of Cubital Tunnel Syndrome
Boone S, Gelberman RH, Calfee RP (Washington Univ in St. Louis School of Medicine, MO)
J Hand Surg Am 40:1897-1904, 2015

Symptomatic cubital tunnel syndrome is a condition that frequently prompts patients to seek hand surgical care. Although cubital tunnel syndrome is readily diagnosed, achieving complete symptom resolution remains challenging. This article reviews related anatomy, clinical presentation, and current management options for cubital tunnel syndrome with an emphasis on contemporary outcomes research.

▶ This article presents a nice summary of the challenges and the shifts in the management of cubital tunnel syndrome. The article specifically discusses the pros and cons of the major treatment methodologies for cubital tunnel syndrome and adds value to the literature in that it attempts to address 2 areas often neglected: posttraumatic and pediatric ulnar nerve abnormalities. This is a great review for anyone who treats this condition intermittently or daily, as the data presented are timely and well organized to help elevate the level of care provided for these patients.

J. M. Froelich, MD

Surgical Treatment of Cubital Tunnel Syndrome: Trends and the Influence of Patient and Surgeon Characteristics
Adkinson JM, Zhong L, Aliu O, et al (Ann and Robert H. Lurie Children's Hosp of Chicago, IL; Univ of Michigan Health System, Ann Arbor)
J Hand Surg Am 40:1824-1831, 2015

Purpose.—To examine trends in and determinants of the use of different procedures for treatment of cubital tunnel syndrome.

Methods.—We performed a retrospective cross-sectional analysis of the Healthcare Cost and Utilization Project Florida State Ambulatory Surgery Database for 2005 to 2012. We selected all patients who underwent *in situ* decompression, transposition, or other surgical treatments for cubital tunnel syndrome. We tested trends in the use of these techniques and performed a multivariable analysis to examine associations among patient characteristics, surgeon case volume, and the use of different techniques.

Results.—Of the 26,164 patients who underwent surgery for cubital tunnel syndrome, 80% underwent *in situ* decompression, 16% underwent transposition, and 4% underwent other surgical treatment. Over the study period, there was a statistically significant increase in the use of *in situ* release and a decrease in the use of transposition. Women and patients treated by surgeons with a higher cubital tunnel surgery case volume underwent *in situ* release with a statistically higher incidence than other techniques.

Conclusions.—In Florida, surgeon practice reflected the widespread adoption of *in situ* release as the primary treatment for cubital tunnel syndrome, and its relative incidence increased during the study period. Patient demographics and surgeon-level factors influenced procedure selection.
Type of Study/Level of Evidence.—Therapeutic III.

▶ This retrospective cross-sectional analysis reviewed the Florida State Ambulatory Surgery Database looking for trends in the surgical treatment of cubital tunnel syndrome. Evidence shows no significant difference in the clinical outcomes when comparing in situ decompression and anterior transposition of the ulnar nerve. However, surgical trends continue to change. Similar to the study by Soltani et al,[1] the incidence of cubital tunnel surgery and, specifically, the rate of in situ decompression is increasing. Recent studies show a lower incidence of complications with in situ decompression,[2] and the vascular insult to the ulnar nerve is also lessened. The highest-volume surgeons in this study were more likely to perform in situ decompression, which the authors believe is secondary to those surgeons' awareness of the expanding role and known effectiveness of in situ decompression. One may also surmise that in situ decompression is more amenable to a high-volume surgical practice because of decreased operating time.

In my practice, an in situ decompression is the procedure of choice for primary ulnar nerve decompression. For revision surgery, ulnar nerve subluxation, and in the setting of osseous deformities at the elbow, a transposition is performed.

A. T. Moeller, MD

References

1. Soltani AM, Best MJ, Francis CS, et al. Trends in the surgical treatment of cubital tunnel syndrome: an analysis of the national survey of ambulatory surgery database. *J Hand Surg Am.* 2013;38:1551-1556.
2. Chen H-W, Ou S, Liu G-D, et al. Clinical efficacy of simple decompression versus anterior transposition of the ulnar nerve for treatment of cubital tunnel syndrome: a meta-analysis. *Clin Neurol Neurosurg.* 2014;126:150-155.

Ulnar Nerve Transposition at the Elbow under Local Anesthesia: A Patient Satisfaction Study
Roberti del Vecchio PM, Christen T, Raffoul W, et al (Univ Hosp of Lausanne (CHUV), Switzerland)
J Reconstr Microsurg 31:187-190, 2015

Background.—Ulnar nerve decompression at the elbow traditionally requires regional or general anesthesia. We wished to assess the feasibility of performing ulnar nerve decompression and transposition at the elbow under local anesthesia.
Methods.—We examined retrospectively the charts of 50 consecutive patients having undergone ulnar nerve entrapment surgery either under

general or local anesthesia. Patients were asked to estimate pain on post-operative days 1 and 7 and satisfaction was assessed at 1 year.

Results.—On day 1, pain was comparable among all groups. On day 7, pain scores were twice as high when transposition was performed under general anesthesia when compared with local anesthesia. Patient satisfaction was slightly increased in the local anesthesia group. These patients were significantly more willing to repeat the surgery.

Conclusion.—Ulnar nerve decompression and transposition at the elbow can be performed under local anesthesia without added morbidity when compared with general anesthesia.

▶ Increasingly, hand and upper extremity surgeons are performing surgical procedures under local anesthesia. The reasons for this are multifactorial, including reduced cost to the patient and the medical system, increased safety, and higher satisfaction for the patient and physician. The authors of this study are commended for investigating their outcomes of release of the ulnar nerve elbow under local anesthesia. This is a common upper extremity procedure, and the results of this study will be of interest to many hand and upper extremity surgeons.

This study is a retrospective review of 50 consecutive patients who had ulnar nerve decompression or transposition surgery by a single surgeon. Over a 2-year period, the surgeon transitioned from using general anesthesia to using local anesthesia for release of the ulnar nerve. The general and local anesthesia

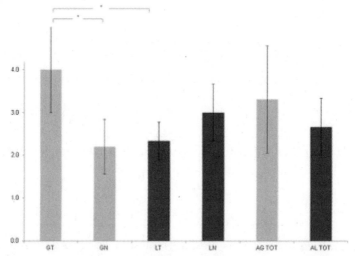

FIGURE 1.—Postoperative pain at day 7. Patients undergoing ulnar nerve decompression with transposition under general anesthesia showed the highest pain scores. $*p < 0.05$; GT, general anesthesia and ulnar nerve transposition; GN, general anesthesia without ulnar nerve transposition; LT, local anesthesia and ulnar nerve transposition; LN, local anesthesia without ulnar nerve transposition, AG TOT = GT + GN, AL TOT = LT + LN. (Reprinted from Roberti del Vecchio PM, Christen T, Raffoul W, et al. Ulnar nerve transposition at the elbow under local anesthesia: a patient satisfaction study. *J Reconstr Microsurg.* 2015;31:187-190, with permission from Thieme Medical Publishers, Inc.)

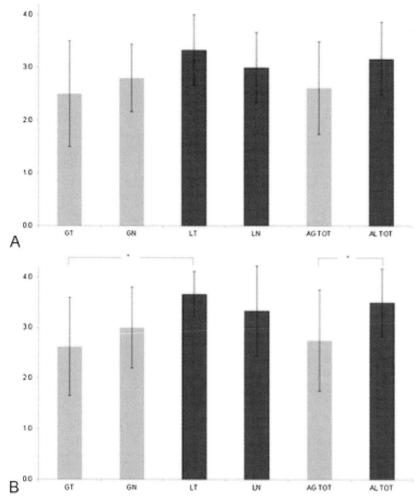

FIGURE 2.—Patient satisfaction. (A) Patient satisfaction with surgery was comparable among groups. When asked if they were willing to repeat surgery, significantly higher scores were found in patients who had nerve decompression under local anesthesia. (B) Nerve decompression with transposition under general anesthesia was associated with the lowest satisfaction. $*p < 0.05$; GT, general anesthesia and ulnar nerve transposition; GN, general anesthesia without ulnar nerve transposition; LT, local anesthesia and ulnar nerve transposition; LN, local anesthesia without ulnar nerve transposition; AG TOT = GT + GN; AL TOT = LT + LN. (Reprinted from Roberti del Vecchio PM, Christen T, Raffoul W, et al. Ulnar nerve transposition at the elbow under local anesthesia: a patient satisfaction study. *J Reconstr Microsurg.* 2015;31:187-190, with permission from Thieme Medical Publishers, Inc.)

groups were similar in size, and both decompression and transposition procedures were performed in each group. The primary outcomes were pain and patient satisfaction, which are relevant when choosing a mode of anesthesia.

The study reports superior pain control in the first week after surgery in the local anesthesia group undergoing ulnar nerve transposition. Unfortunately,

TABLE 1.—Patient Demographics

	GT Group	GN Group	LT Group	LN Group
Number of patients	17	10	12	11
Mean age (y)	49	46	49	44
Female-to-male ratio	7:10	3:7	7:5	9:2
Dominant hand	14	5	7	7
Posttraumatic	7	3	2	3
Number of consultations first 6 mo	3.6	3.5	2.2	3

Abbreviations: GN = general anesthesia without ulnar nerve transposition; GT, general anesthesia and ulnar nerve transposition; LN = local anesthesia without ulnar nerve transposition; LT = local anesthesia and ulnar nerve transposition.
Reprinted from Roberti del Vecchio PM, Christen T, Raffoul W, et al. Ulnar nerve transposition at the elbow under local anesthesia: a patient satisfaction study. *J Reconstr Microsurg.* 2015;31:187-190, with permission from Thieme Medical Publishers, Inc.

several possible confounding variables were not addressed. Did the choice to perform the surgery under local anesthesia influence the size of the incision and amount of dissection performed? Was a tourniquet used in the general anesthesia group? Was local anesthetic infiltrated about the incision in the general anesthesia group? Did postoperative pain management differ between the 2 groups?

There was also more willingness to repeat the surgery in the local anesthesia group. The authors attributed increased satisfaction in this group to better early pain control. It would be interesting to know if there were other factors that may have influenced patient satisfaction, such as perceived risk of the procedure, operating time, postoperative recovery time, and postoperative nausea and vomiting. The authors note that the study lacks power, and it many have been difficult to detect differences in these factors.

It is helpful to learn that the patients in this study had a good experience with ulnar nerve decompression and transposition under local anesthesia (Figs 1 and 2, Table 1). Furthermore, local anesthesia appears to be a safe option for this surgery; no increase in complications was reported. As more studies look at this technique, there is a real potential that the practice patterns of many surgeons may shift toward the use of local anesthesia for these procedures.

E. Kinnucan, MD

Patient education for carpal tunnel syndrome: analysis of readability
Eberlin KR, Vargas CR, Chuang DJ, et al (Harvard Med School, Boston, MA)
Hand (N Y) 10:374-380, 2015

Background.—The National Institutes of Health and American Medical Association recommend a sixth grade reading level for patient-directed content. This study aims to quantitatively evaluate the readability of the most commonly used resources for surgical treatment of carpal tunnel syndrome.

Methods.—A web search for "carpal tunnel surgery" was performed using an Internet search engine, and the 13 most popular sites were identified. Relevant, patient-directed articles immediately accessible from the main site were downloaded and formatted into plain text. A total of 102 articles were assessed for readability using ten established analyses: first overall, then by website for comparison.

Results.—Patient information about carpal tunnel surgery had an overall average reading level of 13.1. Secondary analysis by website revealed a range of mean readability from 10.8 (high school sophomore level) to 15.3 (university junior level). All sites exceeded the recommended sixth grade reading level.

Conclusions.—Online patient resources for carpal tunnel surgery uniformly exceed the recommended reading level. These are too difficult to be understood by a large portion of American adults. A better understanding of readability may be useful in tailoring more appropriate resources for average patient literacy.

▶ This quantitative study aims to determine the readability level of common online resource sites for surgical consideration of carpal tunnel syndrome. In the article, it was suggested that with the increased availability of the Internet, patients are turning to online resources to help decide on possible methods of treatment for carpal tunnel syndrome. According to the National Institutes of Health and American Medical Association, a sixth grade reading level for patient-directed content material is recommended. However, online patient resources overall did exceed this recommended reading grade level. Identification of popular online resources was also the aim, and searches were performed by a single investigator to rule out search bias. A total of 102 articles were collected from 13 sites and were determined to have a mean reading level of 13.1 grade level, using Readability Studio Professional Edition software (Oleander Software, Ltd, Vandalia, OH). Authors recognized that carpal tunnel syndrome or Web site searches for "carpal tunnel surgery" may be more common to the general population than other hand surgery conditions, thus affecting the web sites used for analysis. The reader should examine his or her current patient education practice and consider offering sixth-grade reading level material on Internet/computer-based learning methods.

S. Kranz, OTR/L, CHT

6 Nerve

Intraneural Ganglion in Superficial Radial Nerve Mimics de Quervain Tenosynovitis

Haller JM, Potter MQ, Sinclair M, et al (Univ of Utah, Salt Lake City)
J Wrist Surg 3:262-264, 2013

Background.—Intraneural ganglions in peripheral nerves of the upper extremity are extremely rare and poorly understood.

> *Case Description.*—We report a patient with symptoms consistent with de Quervain tenosynovitis who was found to have an intraneural ganglion in the superficial radial nerve. The ganglion did not communicate with the wrist joint. We removed the intraneural ganglion, and the patient's symptoms resolved. At her 6-month postoperative follow-up, she remained asymptomatic.

Literature Review.—There is only one case report of intraneural ganglion in the superficial radial nerve. In that case, the patient had symptoms consistent with nerve irritation, including radiating pain and paresthesias. In contrast to that previous report, the patient in the current case had only localized pain, no paresthesias, and a physical exam consistent with de Quervain tenosynovitis.

Clinical Relevance.—This case demonstrates that an intraneural ganglion cyst can mimic the symptoms of de Quervain tenosynovitis without the more usual presentation of painful paresthesias.

▶ The authors in this article present a case that reminds us to be vigilant in evaluating our patients, even when the diagnosis seems to be straightforward.

We often say "common things are common because they're common." Thus, we tend to look for the obvious when we evaluate our patients. This case report reminds us to look beyond the common. As physicians we need to maintain a high index of suspicion and be prepared to recognize that conditions may not always be what they seem to be. I had the experience of treating a patient sent to me with a diagnosis of carpal tunnel syndrome. Although she did have some of the symptoms, it turns out that her real diagnosis was a schwannoma of the median nerve approximately 5 cm proximal to the carpal tunnel. Treatment was excision of the lesion; no carpal tunnel release was necessary.

We need to look at the whole patient and not have tunnel vision. Often, we evaluate the patient simply from the standpoint of what we think they have instead of taking the physical examination at full value and identifying the true cause of their condition. As one of my early mentors was fond of saying, "listen to the patient ... they'll tell you what's wrong."

J. A. Ortiz, Jr, MD

Low profile radial nerve palsy orthosis with radial and ulnar deviation
Peck J, Ollason J (Creighton Univ Med Ctr, Omaha, NE)
J Hand Ther 28:421-424, 2015

Individuals who sustain damage to the radial nerve experience a significant loss in functional use of the hand. Traditional orthoses have been effective in providing assistance with wrist stabilization and finger/thumb MP extension. These authors adapted a low profile orthosis to provide the necessary support while allowing radial and ulnar deviation of the wrist, thus increasing functional use of the hand. —VICTORIA PRIGANC, PhD, OTR, CHT, CLT, Practice Forum Editor.

▶ This article outlines a unique and more simplified approach to the fabrication of a dynamic radial nerve palsy orthosis. An orthosis for radial nerve palsy (RNP) is essential to support the healing radial nerve, to prevent overstretching of the dorsal wrist ligaments, contracturing of the wrist and finger flexors, and to allow the person to maintain the functional sensorimotor input to the injured extremity.

Traditional approaches to the fabrication of RNP orthoses span a wide gamut: from the static wrist orthosis, custom or over the counter, to the complex dynamic orthosis. The simple wrist orthosis does not supply finger extension support. More complex orthoses, which have been described in several publications, support the wrist and fingers and can include high profile outriggers with the necessary delicate balance of finger extension slings to provide the lost function and which may draw even more attention to the injured arm. This orthosis seeks to solve the difficult problem of RNP without extensive time to fabricate it yet seems to provide functional use without the unsightly outriggers. The design described in this article not only provides for stable wrist extension and elastic extension support of the fingers, it adds the necessary ulnar and radial deviation for even greater functional hand use.

Although this remains a complex diagnosis for which to fabricate an orthosis, this design is well described such that the attentive hand therapist should have no difficulty in fabricating it.

V. H. O'Brien, OTD, OTR/L, CHT

Targeted Muscle Reinnervation of the Brachium: An Anatomic Study of Musculocutaneous and Radial Nerve Motor Points Relative to Proximal Landmarks

Renninger CH, Rocchi VJ, Kroonen LT (Naval Med Ctr San Diego, CA; Southern California Permanente Med Group, San Diego)
J Hand Surg Am 40:2223-2228, 2015

Purpose.—Targeted muscle reinnervation (TMR) offers enhanced prosthetic use by harnessing additional neural control from unused nerves in the amputated limb. The purpose of this study was to document the location and number of motor end plates to each muscle commonly used in TMR in the brachium relative to proximally based bony landmarks.

Methods.—We dissected 18 matched upper limbs (9 fresh-frozen cadavers). The locations of each of the nerves' muscular insertions into the medial biceps and brachialis were measured relative to the anterolateral tip of the acromion. The terminal branches to the lateral triceps were measured relative to the posterolateral tip of the acromion. Both the number of branches and the location of the muscular insertions were documented. Common descriptive statistics were used to describe the data.

Results.—There was a median of 2 branches to the medial biceps located 19.6 cm from the anterolateral tip of the acromion (range, 15−25 cm). There was a median of 3.5 branches to the brachialis located 24.2 cm from the anterolateral tip of the acromion (range, 19−27.5 cm). There was a median of 2.5 branches to the lateral triceps located 21.6 cm from the posterolateral tip of the acromion (range, 11−29 cm). The mean distances to the primary branch muscle and the number of smaller branches were not significantly different when compared by sex or side.

Conclusions.—Motor points for the medial biceps, brachialis, and lateral triceps can be identified reliably using proximal landmarks in targeted muscle reinnervation.

Clinical Relevance.—The data obtained from this study may assist the surgeon in localizing the nerve branches and muscular insertions for the commonly used muscles for TMR of the brachium.

▶ This is a cadaver study aimed at clarifying the branch points of the musculocutaneous nerve to the medial biceps and the radial nerve branch to the lateral head of the triceps. The goal is to assist surgical planning for targeted muscle reinnervation (TMR). The study used 18 limbs and skin markings from the acromion to identify the branch points with the goal of decreasing the extent of surgical dissection for these procedures. Figs 1 and 2 demonstrate the findings.

TMR is an exciting new area for hand and nerve surgeons and can potentially address the major problem with current prosthetics: low rates of user acceptance.[1] Many amputees discard their prostheses when they return to everyday life, and a primary reason such patients cite is lack of functionality. The myoelectric prosthetics are also limited by a slight delay in responsiveness because of the computer processing and increased weight. TMR addresses the lack of

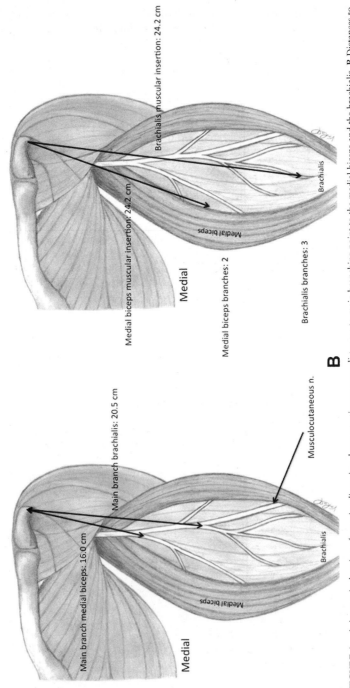

FIGURE 1.—A Anatomic drawing of anterior dissection demonstrating average distances to main branching point to the medial biceps and the brachialis. B Distances to the muscular insertions and median number of branches for both the medial biceps and brachialis. (Reprinted from Renninger CH, Rocchi VJ, Kroonen LT. Targeted muscle reinnervation of the brachium: an anatomic study of musculocutaneous and radial nerve motor points relative to proximal landmarks. *J Hand Surg Am.* 2015;40:2223-2228, with permission from the American Society for Surgery of the Hand.)

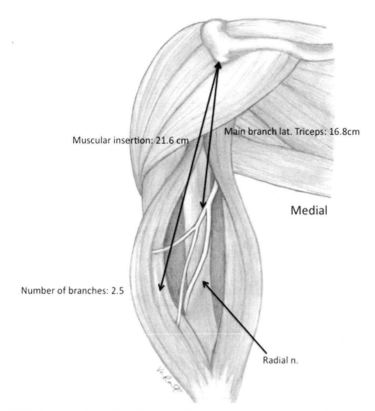

Muscular insertion: 21.6 cm

Main branch lat. Triceps: 16.8cm

Medial

Number of branches: 2.5

Radial n.

FIGURE 2.—Anatomic drawing of posterior dissection demonstrating average distances to main branches and muscular insertions and median number of branches for the lateral triceps branch. (Reprinted from Renninger CH, Rocchi VJ, Kroonen LT. Targeted muscle reinnervation of the brachium: an anatomic study of musculocutaneous and radial nerve motor points relative to proximal landmarks. *J Hand Surg Am.* 2015;40:2223-2228, with permission from the American Society for Surgery of the Hand.)

functionality because this technique provides more functional options and thus allows more complex movements. Thus, as materials improve (making the prosthetics lighter) and computing becomes more powerful (increased responsiveness), barriers to acceptance will recede. Surgeons need to be prepared to provide the foundation for these prosthetics.

C. Curtin, MD

Reference

1. Biddiss E, Chau T. Upper-limb prosthetics: critical factors in device abandonment. *Am J Phys Med Rehabil.* 2007;86:977-987.

Comparative Study of Nerve Grafting versus Distal Nerve Transfer for Treatment of Proximal Injuries of the Ulnar Nerve

Flores LP (Hosp das Forças Armadas, Brasília, Distrito Federal, Brazil)
J Reconstr Microsurg 31:647-653, 2015

Background.—The prognosis for motor recovery associated with ulnar nerve injuries at a level proximal to the elbow is usually considered poor. Nerve transfers techniques were introduced as an alternative for the management of nerve lesions of the upper limb, aiming to improve the surgical results of those nerves for which direct reconstruction has not historically yielded good outcomes.

Methods.—A retrospective chart review was conducted to compare the outcomes obtained using nerve grafting (20 cases) with those of distal nerve transfer (15 patients) for the treatment of proximal injuries of the ulnar nerve. Nerve transfer combined the suture of the anterior interosseous nerve to the motor branch of the ulnar nerve and the cooptation of its sensory branch to the third common digital nerve via an end-to-side suture.

Results.—The Medical Research Council M3/M4 outcomes were observed significantly more often in the nerve transfer group (80 vs. 22%), and the mean values for handgrip strength were higher (31.3 ± 5.8 vs. 14.5 ± 7.2 kg). The groups were similar in attaining good sensory recovery (40 vs. 30%) and mean two-point-discrimination (grafting: 11 ± 2 mm; nerve transfer: 9 ± 1 mm). The mean value of the disabilities of arm, shoulder, and hand for the nerve transfer group (23.6 ± 6.7) was significantly lower than for grafting (34.2 ± 8.3).

Conclusions.—Distal nerve transfer resulted in better motor and functional outcomes than nerve grafting. Both techniques resulted in similar sensory outcomes, and nerve grafting was demonstrated to be a better technique for managing the painful symptoms associated with the nerve injury.

▶ High ulnar nerve injuries too often result in poor function. Distal nerve transfers offer the possibility of improved outcomes through shorter regenerative distances for the nerve to its end organs. This retrospective chart review assessed functional outcomes of 35 high ulnar nerve injuries some treated with primary nerve graft (20). The other group was treated with anterior interosseous nerve to ulnar motor and third common digital to the ulnar sensory branch (15).

The authors found that the motor recovery was superior in the nerve transfer group, and sensory outcomes were comparable.

The primary weakness of this study is the retrospective nature and the significant selection bias. The author reports that clean acute injuries were treated with grafting, whereas delayed presentation (greater than 8 months) or mangled nerve inures were treated with distal sensory and motor transfers. Indeed the mean time to surgery was significantly longer in the nerve transfer group. This increased delay to care would result in worse outcomes for the transfer group (delay to surgery has consistently been linked to poorer outcomes in other nerve repair studies). Thus, the better functional outcomes seen in the nerve transfer group could be even more robust than found in this study if earlier intervention was included.

Another interesting finding in this article was the increased pain found in the transfer-only group. This finding that leaving the ulnar nerve unreconstructed increases the risk of painful neuroma formation makes sense. There have been multiple studies suggesting that repairing a damaged nerve gives the axons a path to their end organs reducing the risk of painful neuroma.

This article provides convincing data that for high ulnar nerve injuries, distal motor transfers should be considered. In addition, the surgeon may consider a mixed approach: reconstructing the nerve with graft to minimize painful neuroma as well as distal nerve transfer(s) to improve function.

C. Curtin, MD

Ulnar Nerve Repair With Simultaneous Metacarpophalangeal Joint Capsulorrhaphy and Pulley Advancement

Atiyya AN, Nassar WAM (Ain Shams Univ, Cairo, Egypt)
J Hand Surg Am 40:1818-1823, 2015

Purpose.—To evaluate the validity of performing a static anti-claw procedure (metacarpophalangeal joint volar capsulorrhaphy and A1 and A2 pulley release) at the time of ulnar nerve repair for acute or chronic lacerations to prevent development of claw hand deformity and disability or to correct them.

Methods.—We present a case series of 14 patients for whom metacarpophalangeal joint capsulorrhaphy and pulley advancement were done at the time of ulnar nerve management. Direct nerve repair was performed in 10 patients, nerve grafting in 2, neurolysis in 1, and combined direct repair and anterior interosseous nerve transfer in 1. Outcome measurements included assessment of claw hand correction and sequence of phalangeal flexion according to modified evaluation criteria of Brand and motor recovery of ulnar nerve function using the British Medical Research Council (MRC) scale.

Results.—Average follow-up was 39 months. At 3 months, 12 patients had good and 2 had fair claw hand correction. At 6 months, 2 patients had excellent, 10 patients had good, and 2 patients had fair correction. At final follow-up, 13 patients had good to excellent correction and 1 had fair correction. Motor recovery of the intrinsic muscles was rated from 2 to 5 according to the MRC scale.

Conclusions.—This technique is simple and effective. It acts as an internal orthosis during recovery of sufficient strength of the intrinsic muscles. In cases of incomplete recovery of the intrinsic muscles (up to MRC grade 2), it may eliminate the need for secondary surgery to correct a claw hand deformity.

Type of Study/Level of Evidence.—Therapeutic IV.

▶ Because the patients in this study had an ulnar nerve lesion in the forearm, the flexor digitorum profundus (FDP) branches of the ulnar nerve were intact or were expected to be innervated immediately after the neurorrhaphy. Ulnar nerve lesions with a functioning FDP cause a more severe claw finger deformity than do those with ineffective FDP branches. From the perspective of FDP function, correction of the claw finger deformity might have been essential in this study.

The authors performed the metacarpophalangeal (MP) joint capsulorrhaphy combined with removal of the A1 and A2 pulleys. Removal of the pulleys strengthened the MP joint flexion strength, and it may have helped keep the MP joint flexed, which would help prevent recurrence of the claw finger deformity, even though plication was performed using polypropylene sutures only on the volar capsule of the MP joint.

The authors mentioned that they removed the entire A1 pulley and proximal A2 pulley just distal to the proximal finger flexion crease. According to Gordon et al, who studied the relationship between the anatomic location of the finger flexor pulleys and the skin surface landmarks of the hand,[1] the proximal finger flexion crease corresponds to just over the midpoint of the A2 pulley. This indicates that the entire A1 pulley and at least the proximal 50% of the A2 pulley were excised. Previous authors have reported that as much as 50% excision of the A2 pulley may be feasible because the resultant decrease in the range of motion is small and within the range required for normal function activity.[2,3] They also reported that the bony attachment strength of the distal 25% of the A2 pulley is stronger than the proximal 25% A2 pulley, which indicates that leaving the distal half of the A2 pulley is also advantageous from the perspective of the pulley failure.[2]

The patients' ages in this study varied from 4 to 53 years. Only neurorrhaphy should have been performed on the 4-year-old patient because good nerve regeneration would have been expected with this procedure alone. There would be an option to perform pulley advancement and MP joint capsulorrhaphy as an additional operation after the neurorrhaphy, if it were to fail, in patients for whom good nerve regeneration can be expected after neurorrhaphy.

R. Kakinoki, MD

References

1. Gordon JA, Stone L, Gordon L. Surface markers for locating the pulleys and flexor tendon anatomy in the palm and fingers with reference to minimally invasive incisions. *J Hand Surg Am.* 2012;37:913-918.
2. Tanaka T, Amadio PC, Zhao C, Zobit ME, An KN. The effect of partial A2 pulley excision on gliding resistance and pulley strength in vitro. *J Hand Surg Am.* 2004; 29:877-883.
3. Hume MC, Gellman H, McKellop H, Brumfield RH Jr. Functional range of motion of the joints of the hand. *J Hand Surg Am.* 1990;15:240-243.

Targeted Muscle Reinnervation of the Brachium: An Anatomic Study of Musculocutaneous and Radial Nerve Motor Points Relative to Proximal Landmarks

Renninger CH, Rocchi VJ, Kroonen LT (Naval Med Ctr San Diego, CA; Southern California Permanente Med Group, San Diego)
J Hand Surg Am 40:2223-2228, 2015

Purpose.—Targeted muscle reinnervation (TMR) offers enhanced prosthetic use by harnessing additional neural control from unused nerves in the amputated limb. The purpose of this study was to document the location and number of motor end plates to each muscle commonly used in TMR in the brachium relative to proximally based bony landmarks.

Methods.—We dissected 18 matched upper limbs (9 fresh-frozen cadavers). The locations of each of the nerves' muscular insertions into the medial biceps and brachialis were measured relative to the anterolateral tip of the acromion. The terminal branches to the lateral triceps were measured relative to the posterolateral tip of the acromion. Both the number of branches and the location of the muscular insertions were documented. Common descriptive statistics were used to describe the data.

Results.—There was a median of 2 branches to the medial biceps located 19.6 cm from the anterolateral tip of the acromion (range, 15–25 cm). There was a median of 3.5 branches to the brachialis located 24.2 cm from the anterolateral tip of the acromion (range, 19–27.5 cm). There was a median of 2.5 branches to the lateral triceps located 21.6 cm from the posterolateral tip of the acromion (range, 11–29 cm). The mean distances to the primary branch muscle and the number of smaller branches were not significantly different when compared by sex or side.

Conclusions.—Motor points for the medial biceps, brachialis, and lateral triceps can be identified reliably using proximal landmarks in targeted muscle reinnervation.

Clinical Relevance.—The data obtained from this study may assist the surgeon in localizing the nerve branches and muscular insertions for the commonly used muscles for TMR of the brachium.

▶ As targeted muscle reinnervation (TMR) gains popularity, more surgeons are performing this operation to improve myoelectric prosthetic control. As surgeons gain experience, technical obstacles are encountered. Historically, surgeons cared little about what happened to any particular motor nerve between its branching from the main nerve until it reached the muscle. However, with the advent of TMR, this anatomy has become critically important. It not only is helpful with regard to finding the nerves for transfer, but if these nerves are not attended to (either by denervation/transection alone or by transfer), and the native innervation is left intact, then the transferred nerve signal will be lost in the stronger and more powerful native innervation. This study documents well the complexity of the motor nerve anatomy after it has branched from the main nerve. The appreciation of the complexity alone makes this study valuable. Adding some data with regard to the median number of motor nerves and locations make it a valuable resource and must-read for the surgeon preparing to do a TMR procedure for the transhumeral amputee.

B. T. Carlsen, MD

Targeted Muscle Reinnervation in the Upper Extremity Amputee: A Technical Roadmap
Gart MS, Souza JM, Dumanian GA (Northwestern Memorial Hosp, Chicago, IL)
J Hand Surg Am 40:1877-1888, 2015

Targeted muscle reinnervation (TMR) offers the potential for improved prosthetic function by reclaiming the neural control information that is lost as a result of upper extremity amputation. In addition to the prosthetic control benefits, TMR is a potential treatment for postamputation neuroma pain. Here, we present our surgical technique for TMR nerve transfers in transhumeral and shoulder disarticulation patients.

▶ Targeted muscle reinnervation is increasing in popularity with surgeons around the country performing this operation for both improved prosthetic control and as a treatment for (or prophylaxis against) neuroma-related pain. The lead author, Dr Dumanian, previously published the techniques for both transhumeral and shoulder disarticulation amputation with the goal of improved prosthetic control. Although very helpful, these previous publications lacked some important details regarding the technical execution of the procedures. This report in the *Journal of Hand Surgery* is afforded more space and detail that make this article the main reference for those looking to perform this operation. For those individuals, this article should be read repeatedly to gather a deep appreciation for the technique. However, I must iterate that reading the article alone is insufficient preparation for performing the operation.

I must disagree with the authors on one point, and that is that these operations are technically easy. Some important points deserve special attention. First, an understanding of brachial plexus anatomy is very important. With an amputation, the targets of these nerves are lost or only partially present; therefore, one must determine which nerve is which without the benefit of a distal target or a nerve stimulator to see what moves with stimulation as a guide. Add to that the distorted anatomy that resulted from the (usually traumatic) amputation, and this can be a tedious operation. Second, the dissection of the targeted motor nerves is critically important and can also be tedious. Any native innervation must not be left intact and should be used as a common target with the transferred nerve to that portion of the muscle, as the native innervation will surely be more powerful than the transferred innervation.

B. T. Carlsen, MD

Management of Acute Postoperative Pain in Hand Surgery: A Systematic Review
Kelley BP, Shauver MJ, Chung KC (Univ of Michigan Med School, Ann Arbor)
J Hand Surg Am 40:1610-1619, 2015

Purpose.—To conduct a systematic review to guide hand surgeons in an evidenced-based approach in managing postoperative pain.

Methods.—We performed a literature review for primary research articles on management of postoperative pain in hand surgery patients using Medical Literature Analysis and Retrieval System Online (MEDLINE; PubMed), Excerpta Medica database (EMBASE), and the Cochrane Collaboration Library. Inclusion criteria were primary journal articles examining treatment of acute postoperative pain based on any modality. Data related to pain assessment, postoperative recovery, and total postoperative analgesic consumption were extracted.

Results.—A total of 903 publications were reviewed; 184 publications underwent abstract review. After applying inclusion and exclusion criteria, 10 primary articles were selected for inclusion in this review. Data were noted to be heterogeneous and findings were compiled. Results were divided into groups evaluating postoperative pain medications or pain infusion catheters.

Conclusions.—Although this review did not demonstrate a best practices model for postoperative pain management, it provides evidence for alternative medications and treatment strategies. The evidence available suggests that postoperative pain control should begin before surgery and that combining multiple strategies for pain treatment is beneficial. Given the increasing attention paid to narcotic prescriptions and the potential for abuse, surgeons should adopt evidence-based pain management practices. We provide an example algorithm for pain treatment in hand surgery based on available data and the authors' experience.

Type of Study/Level of Evidence.—Therapeutic III.

▶ This systematic review of research on postoperative analgesia after hand surgery only includes a few studies that are heterogeneous. Although we can not draw any conclusions about the best treatment, the authors provide a nice summary of the available data in Table 3.

C. M. Ward, MD

TABLE 3.—Oral Medications in Hand Surgery

	Study	Comparison	Rescue	Significant Findings
Acetaminophen	Rawal et al[18]	Tramadol or metamizole	DXP	Fewer acetaminophen tablets consumed vs tramadol or metamizole ($P < .001$). Significantly lower nausea up to 24 h ($P < .050$) and 48 h ($P < .001$) postoperatively vs tramadol.
	Spagnoli et al[19]	Acetaminophen	NR	Acetaminophen alone showed higher mean VAS scores vs combined with tramadol up to 24 h postoperatively ($P < .005$); however, no difference up to POD 7. Significantly more rescue drug consumption vs combined with tramadol ($P < .005$). No difference in adverse events.
Arnica	Stevinson et al[25]	NR	Acetaminophen/diclofenac	No significant difference in pain scores ($P = .790$) up to POD 4.
Ampiroxicam	Sai et al[27]	Placebo	Diclofenac PR	Preoperatively administered ampiroxicam. Significantly less rescue medication ($P < .0001$), lower median VAS pain scores ($P < .001$) vs placebo given preoperatively.
Gabapentin	Turan et al[22]	Placebo	Diclofenac	Prolonged time to first rescue drug request ($P < .050$) and lower total rescue drug usage ($P < .050$) with preoperative gabapentin vs placebo.
Melatonin	Mowafi and Ismail[31]	Placebo	Acetaminophen/diclofenac	Decreased postoperative anxiety for melatonin vs placebo ($P = .023$). Prolonged time to first postoperative rescue drug for melatonin vs placebo ($P < .001$). Decreased total diclofenac use postoperatively in melatonin group vs placebo ($P = .007$).
Metamizole	Rawal et al[18]	Acetaminophen or tramadol	DXP	Significantly higher percentage of patient satisfaction vs tramadol ($P < .050$). No difference vs acetaminophen. Significantly lower nausea up to 24 h ($P < .05$) and 48 h ($P < .001$) postoperatively vs tramadol.
Opiate*	Rawal et al[18]	Acetaminophen or metamizole	DXP	Tramadol: Significantly higher consumption of rescue medication vs metamizole ($P < .050$) or acetaminophen ($P < .001$) up to 24 h postoperatively. Higher incidence of nausea in first 48 h ($P < .05$). Lower patient satisfaction vs metamizole ($P < .05$).
	Spagnoli et al[19]	Acetaminophen	NR	Tramadol: Significantly improved VAS pain scores up to 24 h ($P < .005$) and lower consumption of rescue medication ($P < .005$) with acetaminophen vs acetaminophen alone. No difference in adverse events. Supports multimodal medication regimen.
	Rodgers et al[11]	NR	NR	Variable opiate*: More tablets consumed if undergoing bone-related vs soft tissue procedure ($P = .010$). Tablets prescribed significantly differed based on payer status (private insurance, Medicare, or Medicaid), but only 2% used Medicaid. Five of 150 patients were not prescribed a narcotic, and all reported getting these from alternative sources (spouse leftover medications).

Editor's Note: Please refer to original journal article for full references.

DXP, dextropropoxyphene; NR, none recorded; PR, per rectum; VAS, visual analog scale (pain); POD, postoperative day.

*Opiates included tramadol, hydrocodone, oxycodone, propoxyphene, and codeine.

Reprinted from Kelley BP, Shauver MJ, Chung KC. Management of acute postoperative pain in hand surgery: a systematic review. *J Hand Surg Am.* 2015;40:1610-1619, with permission from American Society for Surgery of the Hand.

Comparative Study of Nerve Grafting versus Distal Nerve Transfer for Treatment of Proximal Injuries of the Ulnar Nerve

Flores LP (Hosp das Forças Armadas, Brasília, Distrito Federal)
J Reconstr Microsurg 31:647-653, 2015

Background.—The prognosis for motor recovery associated with ulnar nerve injuries at a level proximal to the elbow is usually considered poor. Nerve transfers techniques were introduced as an alternative for the management of nerve lesions of the upper limb, aiming to improve the surgical results of those nerves for which direct reconstruction has not historically yielded good outcomes.

Methods.—A retrospective chart review was conducted to compare the outcomes obtained using nerve grafting (20 cases) with those of distal nerve transfer (15 patients) for the treatment of proximal injuries of the ulnar nerve. Nerve transfer combined the suture of the anterior interosseous nerve to the motor branch of the ulnar nerve and the cooptation of its sensory branch to the third common digital nerve via an end-to-side suture.

Results.—The Medical Research Council M3/M4 outcomes were observed significantly more often in the nerve transfer group (80 vs. 22%), and the mean values for handgrip strength were higher (31.3 ± 5.8 vs. 14.5 ± 7.2 kg). The groups were similar in attaining good sensory recovery (40 vs. 30%) and mean two-point-discrimination (grafting: 11 ± 2 mm; nerve transfer: 9 ± 1 mm). The mean value of the disabilities of arm, shoulder, and hand for the nerve transfer group (23.6 ± 6.7) was significantly lower than for grafting (34.2 ± 8.3).

Conclusions.—Distal nerve transfer resulted in better motor and functional outcomes than nerve grafting. Both techniques resulted in similar sensory outcomes, and nerve grafting was demonstrated to be a better technique for managing the painful symptoms associated with the nerve injury.

▶ Although single surgeon reviews can be criticized, they should have an inherent control of a very important variable (surgical technique). This is a single surgeon, retrospective review of high ulnar nerve injuries comparing nerve transfer (anterior interosseous nerve [AIN], third web space common digital nerve) and nerve grafting. Nerve grafting for these lesions has notoriously bad motor outcomes, and this study again demonstrates this. There is little comparative work done in these types of nerve injury cases; therefore, this study has value. The important finding of improved motor function with nerve transfer suggests this may be the preferred treatment for these high injuries. However, based on the findings, it seems that nerve reconstruction is still indicated to treat the pain-related symptoms and really makes sense to avoid neuroma pain at the site of injury. Given the equivalent sensory outcomes, sensory nerve transfer may not be indicated, as it requires sacrifice of sensation the noncritical nature of which is debatable.

B. T. Carlsen, MD

End-to-side neurorrhaphy for nerve repair and function rehabilitation
Gao W, Liu Q, Li S, et al (The First Affiliated Hosp of Zhengzhou Univ, China; Zhengzhou Central Hosp Affiliated to Zhengzhou Univ, China)
J Surg Res 197:427-435, 2015

Background.—End-to-side neurorrhaphy is a promising procedure for nerve repair in peripheral nerve injury. However, in previous studies, this technique was limited to somatic nerves. The present study was designed to investigate the feasibility of nerve regeneration after end-to-side neurorrhaphy between autonomic nerve and somatic nerve.
Materials and Methods.—Thirty adult male Sprague—Dawley rats were randomly divided into the following three groups ($n = 10$ per group) for different treatments: (1) end-to-side neurorrhaphy group, the left L6 and S1 spinal nerves were transected in the dura, and the distal stump of L6 ventral root (L6VR) was sutured to the lateral face of L4 ventral root (L4VR) through end-to-side coaptation; (2) no repair group, the rats received the same operation as the end-to-side neurorrhaphy group but without coaptation; (3) control group, the rats received the same operation as the end-to-side neurorrhaphy group but the L6VR was preserved. After 4 month, the origin and mechanism of nerve regeneration were evaluated by retrograde nerve tracing. Morphologic and functional properties of the regenerated nerve were investigated by morphologic examination and intravesical pressure measurement.
Results.—Retrograde nerve tracing indicated that the new neural reflex pathway was successfully established, and the main regeneration mechanism was axon collateral sprouting. Morphologic examination and intravesical pressure measurement indicated prominent axonal regeneration and good bladder functional rehabilitation in the neurorrhaphy group. Wet weight and morphology of left extensor digitorum longus muscles appeared no detrimental effect on the donor nerve.
Conclusions.—These results indicated that the somatic motor axons growth into autonomic nerve may be achieved through axon collateral sprouting for nerve repair and function rehabilitation after end-to-side neurorrhaphy of autonomic nerve and somatic nerve without apparent impairment of the donor somatic nerve.

▶ This study comes from the urology literature where they are most interested in restoring bladder function. Because there are limited donor nerves available, the authors explored the use of somatic nerve to restore autonomic nerve deficit. The authors were successful in achieving outsprouting of donor nerves via end-to-side neurorrhaphy with restoration of bladder function after 4 months. Of course, as hand surgeons we are interested in restoration of the somatic nervous system with less concern regarding the autonomic nervous system. The study, therefore, is likely of limited applicability for those of us interested in restoring hand function. Certainly, the reverse nerve transfer would not be successful given the need for cerebral (not autonomic) control of our motor nerves for hand and upper extremity function.

B. T. Carlsen, MD

Bionic reconstruction to restore hand function after brachial plexus injury: a case series of three patients

Aszmann OC, Roche AD, Salminger S, et al (Med Univ of Vienna, Austria; et al)
Lancet 385:2183-2189, 2015

Background.—Brachial plexus injuries can permanently impair hand function, yet present surgical reconstruction provides only poor results. Here, we present for the first time bionic reconstruction; a combined technique of selective nerve and muscle transfers, elective amputation, and prosthetic rehabilitation to regain hand function.

Methods.—Between April 2011, and May 2014, three patients with global brachial plexus injury including lower root avulsions underwent bionic reconstruction. Treatment occurred in two stages; first, to identify and create useful electromyographic signals for prosthetic control, and second, to amputate the hand and replace it with a mechatronic prosthesis. Before amputation, the patients had a specifically tailored rehabilitation programme to enhance electromyographic signals and cognitive control of the prosthesis. Final prosthetic fitting was applied as early as 6 weeks after amputation.

Findings.—Bionic reconstruction successfully enabled prosthetic hand use in all three patients. After 3 months, mean Action Research Arm Test score increased from $5 \cdot 3$ (SD $4 \cdot 73$) to $30 \cdot 7$ ($14 \cdot 0$). Mean Southampton Hand Assessment Procedure score improved from $9 \cdot 3$ (SD $1 \cdot 5$) to $65 \cdot 3$ ($19 \cdot 4$). Mean Disabilities of Arm, Shoulder and Hand score improved from $46 \cdot 5$ (SD $18 \cdot 7$) to $11 \cdot 7$ (SD $8 \cdot 42$).

Interpretation.—For patients with global brachial plexus injury with lower root avulsions, who have no alternative treatment, bionic reconstruction offers a means to restore hand function.

▶ This article represents a unique and creative approach to restoring function to patients with one of the most devastating injuries, brachial plexus avulsion injuries. Despite advances in nerve transfer reconstruction, tendon transfers, and functional muscle transfers, restoring hand function in this population is the exception rather than the rule. The authors present an "out-of-the-box" approach to restoring some degree of hand function in the form of grasp using a prosthetic. The foundation of this work comes from targeted muscle reinnervation in which nerves are transferred to muscles for the sole purpose of improving prosthetic control. This same principle, in these cases, is used to provide independent control of the prosthetic hand (presumably open and close functions) while maintaining intact elbow control. Only slight muscle activity is required to generate a signal that can be captured by the myoelectric prosthesis. Therefore, a muscle that may not be strong enough to move the biological hand may work just fine to control the prosthesis. This was the case in one of the three patients reported on here. The other two patients required free functioning muscle transfer for the sole purpose of providing a myoelectric signal for prosthetic control.

This bionic approach requires the full spectrum of upper extremity knowledge, surgical skill, and technologic prowess. It is a salvage approach and should not be the first option that comes to mind when faced with a patient with a severe brachial plexus injury. Success in these complicated scenarios requires more than surgical expertise. One must work closely with a prosthetist to optimize muscle position, innervation, and cognitive control. The patient must have access to a highly functional prosthetic (Michelangelo prosthetic hand by Ottobock in these cases), the cost of which is no small consideration. However, if these stars align, this approach can, as documented here, lead to improvement in patient function and independence.

B. T. Carlsen, MD

Intra-articular and portal infiltration *versus* wrist block for analgesia after arthroscopy of the wrist: A prospective RCT
Agrawal Y, Russon K, Chakrabarti I, et al (Rotherham NHS Foundation Trust, United Kingdom)
Bone Joint J 97-B:1250-1256, 2015

Wrist block has been used to provide pain relief for many procedures on the hand and wrist but its role in arthroscopy of the wrist remains unexplored. Chondrotoxicity has been a concern with the intra-articular infiltration of local anaesthetic. We aimed to evaluate and compare the analgesic effect of portal and wrist joint infiltration with a wrist block on the pain experienced by patients after arthroscopy of the wrist.

A prospective, randomised, double-blind trial was designed and patients undergoing arthroscopy of the wrist under general anaesthesia as a day case were recruited for the study. Levo-bupivacaine was used for both techniques. The effects were evaluated using a ten-point visual analogue scale, and the use of analgesic agents was also compared. The primary outcomes for statistical analyses were the mean pain scores and the use of analgesia post-operatively.

A total of 34 patients (63% females) were recruited to the portal and joint infiltration group and 32 patients (59% males) to the wrist block group. Mean age was 40.8 years in the first group and 39.7 years in the second group ($p > 0.05$). Both techniques provided effective pain relief in the first hour and 24 hours post-operatively but wrist block gave better pain scores at bedtime on the day of surgery ($p = 0.007$) and at 24 hours post-operatively ($p = 0.006$).

Wrist block provides better and more reliable analgesia in patients undergoing arthroscopy of the wrist without exposing patients to the risk of chondrotoxicity.

▶ Wrist arthroscopy is a common procedure and allows surgeons to treat a variety of wrist pathology. It can be used for diagnostic and therapeutic purposes and is a relatively low-risk procedure. The authors have evaluated two adjunctive anesthetic techniques with regard to postoperative pain and analgesic requirements. In an appropriately powered study, the patients were prospectively randomized to receive either local anesthesia with intraarticular and portal site infiltration or a wrist block. All patients also received general anesthesia. The patients with supplemental anesthesia in the form of a wrist block reported less pain and lower analgesia requirements. Furthermore, the concern for chondrotoxicity associated with intraarticular injection of some local anesthetics is obviated with this method.

The one potential variable that is not addressed in the study design is the type of procedure being performed. The duration of the procedure was evaluated, and there was no difference in mean tourniquet times between the two groups. Furthermore, the wrist block group received 50% more lidocaine by volume compared with the infiltration and intra-articular group. Although the study was well done and answers a clinical question that improves patient care, it is not generally relevant to my practice. The overwhelming majority of patients that I treat with wrist arthroscopy undergo a regional brachial plexus block. These patients avoid general anesthesia and do not require any supplemental anesthetic techniques. In my practice, this has proven to be a successful mode of anesthetic care for patients undergoing wrist arthroscopy. Occasionally, patients will not choose or be candidates for regional anesthesia techniques. In these patients, I would choose a supplemental wrist block to augment the general anesthesia based on the results of this study.

M. J. Richard

Vitamin C to Prevent Complex Regional Pain Syndrome in Patients With Distal Radius Fractures: A Meta-Analysis of Randomized Controlled Trials

Evaniew N, McCarthy C, Kleinlugtenbelt YV, et al (McMaster Univ, Hamilton, Ontario, Canada)
J Orthop Trauma 29:e235-e241, 2015

Objective.—To determine whether vitamin C is effective in preventing complex regional pain syndrome (CRPS) in patients with distal radius fractures.

Data Sources.—MEDLINE (1946 to present), EMBASE (1974 to present), and The Cochrane Library (no date limit) were systematically searched up to September 6, 2014, using MeSH and EMTREE headings with free text combinations.

Study Selection.—Randomized trials comparing vitamin C against placebo were included. No exclusions were made during the selection of eligible trials on the basis of patient age, sex, fracture severity, or fracture treatment.

Data Extraction.—Two reviewers independently screened articles, extracted data, and applied the Cochrane Risk of Bias tool. Evidence was graded using the Grading of Recommendations Assessment, Development, and Evaluation approach.

Data Synthesis.—Heterogeneity was quantified using the χ^2 test and the I^2 statistic. Outcome data were combined with a random effects model.

Results.—Across 3 trials (n = 890) of patients with distal radius fractures, vitamin C did not reduce the risk for CRPS (risk ratio = 0.45; 95% confidence interval, 0.18–1.13; $I^2 = 70\%$). This result was confirmed in sensitivity analyses to test the importance of missing data because of losses to follow-up under varying assumptions. Heterogeneity was explained by diagnostic criteria, but not regimen of vitamin C or fracture treatment.

Conclusions.—The evidence for vitamin C to prevent CRPS in patients with distal radius fractures fails to demonstrate a significant benefit. The overall quality of the evidence is low, and these results should be interpreted in the context of clinical expertise and patient preferences.

▶ The authors have performed a meta-analysis of the three randomized controlled trials (RCTs) looking at the efficacy of vitamin C in the prevention of complex regional pain syndrome (CRPS) after distal radius fractures. The two initial trials indicated a benefit with statistically significant decrease in the incidence of CRPS after treatment of distal radius fractures and subsequent clinical practice guidelines produced by the American Academy of Orthopaedic Surgeons recommended the use of vitamin C after distal radius fractures based on the published evidence. A subsequent randomized trial did not find a benefit, so the current study pooled the data in effort to determine whether there is a benefit to using vitamin C in prevention of CRPS.

This article is important because it helps us understand the limitations of conflicting evidence after RCTs. Even Level I studies can have flaws because no study is perfect. The meta-analysis is only as good as the literature being reviewed, and even well designed studies are imperfect. Although this article suggests that there is not a benefit from vitamin C after distal radius fractures, there does not appear to be any harm either, and the cost is low.

W. C. Hammert, MD

Management of Acute Postoperative Pain in Hand Surgery: A Systematic Review

Kelley BP, Shauver MJ, Chung KC (Univ of Michigan Med School, Ann Arbor)
J Hand Surg Am 40:1610-1619, 2015

Purpose.—To conduct a systematic review to guide hand surgeons in an evidenced-based approach in managing postoperative pain.

Methods.—We performed a literature review for primary research articles on management of postoperative pain in hand surgery patients using Medical Literature Analysis and Retrieval System Online (MEDLINE; PubMed), Excerpta Medica database (EMBASE), and the Cochrane Collaboration Library. Inclusion criteria were primary journal articles examining treatment of acute postoperative pain based on any modality. Data related to pain assessment, postoperative recovery, and total postoperative analgesic consumption were extracted.

Results.—A total of 903 publications were reviewed; 184 publications underwent abstract review. After applying inclusion and exclusion criteria, 10 primary articles were selected for inclusion in this review. Data were noted to be heterogeneous and findings were compiled. Results were divided into groups evaluating postoperative pain medications or pain infusion catheters.

Conclusions.—Although this review did not demonstrate a best practices model for postoperative pain management, it provides evidence for alternative medications and treatment strategies. The evidence available suggests that postoperative pain control should begin before surgery and that combining multiple strategies for pain treatment is beneficial. Given the increasing attention paid to narcotic prescriptions and the potential for abuse, surgeons should adopt evidence-based pain management practices. We provide an example algorithm for pain treatment in hand surgery based on available data and the authors' experience.

Type of Study/Level of Evidence.—Therapeutic III.

▶ This is a systematic review of clinical studies of trials that tested various acute pain management interventions after hand surgery. The authors provide a nice discussion highlighting the tension surgeons face when treating pain: the humanistic goal of pain control versus not contributing to the epidemic of prescription drug abuse.

This article's most striking finding is the lack of studies assessing efficacy of pain interventions after hand surgery. After a thorough search, the authors found only a handful of studies; despite postoperative pain being an enormous issue for surgeons and patients. The limited data availability prevented this study from performing any statistical analysis or generating any evidence-based recommendations. The authors did provide their pain treatment algorithm based on their experience and examples in the literature (Fig 2).

Although studies within hand surgery are limited, many more general studies on surgical pain exist, often in the anesthesia literature. For example, a recent meta-analysis of preoperative gabapentin administration showed benefit on

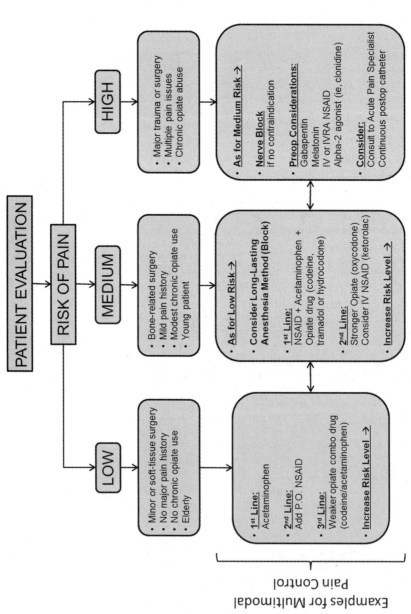

FIGURE 2.—Example algorithm for hand surgery patient with acute postoperative pain. This suggested algorithm reflects current knowledge and is an evidence-based approach to postoperative pain treatment. P.O., orally; IV, intravenously; combo, combination; preop, preoperative; postop, postoperative. (Reprinted from Kelley BP, Shauver MJ, Chung KC. Management of acute postoperative pain in hand surgery: a systematic review. *J Hand Surg Am.* 2015;40:1610-1619, with permission from American Society for Surgery of the Hand.)

postsurgical pain.[1] To improve our treatment of pain, future studies on pain interventions in hand surgery are needed. In addition, there need to be more studies such as this pooling all of the available literature on treatment of pain and presenting it to the hand surgery audience.

C. Curtin, MD

Reference

1. Doleman B, Heinink TP, Read DJ, Faleiro RJ, Lund JN, Williams JP. A systematic review and meta-regression analysis of prophylactic gabapentin for postoperative pain. *Anaesthesia*. 2015;70:1186-1204.

Effect of Time Interval Between Tumescent Local Anesthesia Infiltration and Start of Surgery on Operative Field Visibility in Hand Surgery Without Tourniquet

Bashir MM, Qayyum R, Saleem MH, et al (King Edward Med Univ, Lahore, Punjab, Pakistan; Univ of Tennessee College of Medicine at Chattanooga)
J Hand Surg Am 40:1606-1609, 2015

Purpose.—To determine the optimal time interval between tumescent local anesthesia infiltration and the start of hand surgery without a tourniquet for improved operative field visibility.

Methods.—Patients aged 16 to 60 years who needed contracture release and tendon repair in the hand were enrolled from the outpatient clinic. Patients were randomized to 10-, 15-, or 25-minute intervals between tumescent anesthetic solution infiltration (0.18% lidocaine and 1:221,000 epinephrine) and the start of surgery. The end point of tumescence anesthetic infiltration was pale and firm skin. The surgical team was blinded to the time of anesthetic infiltration. At the completion of the procedure, the surgeon and the first assistant rated the operative field visibility as excellent, fair, or poor. We used logistic regression models without and with adjustment for confounding variables.

Results.—Of the 75 patients enrolled in the study, 59 (79%) were males, 7 were randomized to 10-minute time intervals (further randomization was stopped after interim analysis found consistently poor operative field visibility), and 34 were randomized to the each of the 15- and 25-minute groups. Patients who were randomized to the 25-minute delay group had 29 times higher odds of having an excellent operative visual field than those randomized to the 15-minute delay group. After adjusting for age, sex, amount of tumescent solution infiltration, and duration of operation, the odds ratio remained highly significant.

Conclusions.—We found that an interval of 25 minutes provides vastly superior operative field visibility; 10-minute delay had the poorest results.

Type of Study/Level of Evidence.—Therapeutic I.

▶ WALANT hand surgery has changed how many of us do a variety of operations, but like many changes in practice, maximizing its utility requires further study and experience. This study investigates a key surgical question: How long after injection of tumescent local anesthesia must one wait to have a clear, bloodless field? Using an average of 50 cc of tumescent solution, procedures lasting almost two hours were performed with a subjectively graded excellent field in 91% of patients. The answer to the question of the time interval after injection is longer than 15 minutes. The study group at 25 minutes after injection had a significantly clearer field than at 15 minutes. Twenty minutes, as proposed by others, was not studied.

For a surgeon and a patient waiting 20 or 25 minutes after injection requires changing some of the mechanics of how these procedures are done. In the past, hand surgery done under local anesthesia with a tourniquet, with or without sedation, the incision has begun almost instantaneously after injection. To ensure a bloodless field with this investigated technique, it almost requires that the surgeon, if he or she is doing the injection, inject before positioning, prepping, and draping because waiting 25 minutes after injection is a long time before incision. It should be noted that this group studied 75 patients with tendon or burn contracture release surgery, so it is fair to assume there is a significant amount of experience with this technique; novice WALANT practitioners may want to begin with less complex surgeries to gain experience.

P. Blazar, MD

Light-Activated Sealing of Nerve Graft Coaptation Sites Improves Outcome Following Large Gap Peripheral Nerve Injury
Fairbairn NG, Ng-Glazier J, Meppelink AM, et al (Massachusetts General Hosp, Boston; Walter Reed Natl Military Med Ctr, Bethesda, MD)
Plast Reconstr Surg 136:739-750, 2015

Background.—Nerve repair using photochemically bonded human amnion nerve wraps can result in superior outcomes in comparison with standard suture. When applied to nerve grafts, efficacy has been limited by proteolytic degradation of bonded amnion during extended periods of recovery. Chemical crosslinking of amnion before bonding may improve wrap durability and efficacy.

Methods.—Three nerve wraps (amnion, cross-linked amnion, and cross-linked swine intestinal submucosa) and three fixation methods (suture, fibrin glue, and photochemical bonding) were investigated. One hundred ten Lewis rats had 15-mm left sciatic nerve gaps repaired with isografts. Nine groups (n = 10) had isografts secured by one of the aforementioned wrap/fixation combinations. Positive and negative control groups (n = 10) were repaired with graft and suture and no repair, respectively. Outcomes

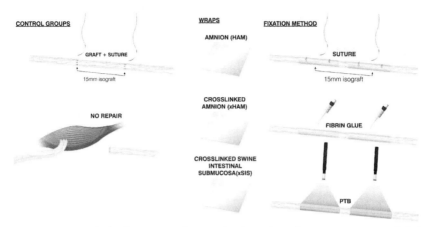

FIGURE 2.—Methods of nerve repair for control and experimental groups. Positive controls had nerves repaired using isografts secured with standard epineurial suture. Negative controls had 15-mm sections of nerve excised and no repair. Proximal nerve ends were buried into adjacent muscle and secured with two 10-0 nylon sutures. Nine experimental groups were composed of different combinations of the three different nerve wraps and three different fixation methods illustrated. (Reprinted from Fairbairn NG, Ng-Glazier J, Meppelink AM, et al. Light-activated sealing of nerve graft coaptation sites improves outcome following large gap peripheral nerve injury. *Plast Reconstr Surg.* 2015;136:739-750, with permission from the American Society of Plastic Surgeons.)

were assessed using sciatic function index, muscle mass retention, and histomorphometry. Statistical analysis was performed using analysis of variance and the post hoc Bonferroni test ($p < 0.05$).

Results.—Cross-linking improved amnion durability. Photochemically bonded crosslinked amnion recovered the greatest sciatic function index, although this was not significant in comparison with graft and suture. Photochemically bonded crosslinked amnion recovered significantly greater muscle mass (67.3 ± 4.4 percent versus 60.0 ± 5.2 percent; p = 0.02), fiber diameter, axon diameter, and myelin thickness (6.87 ± 2.23 μm versus 5.47 ± 1.70 μm; 4.51 ± 1.83 μm versus 3.50 ± 1.44 μm; and 2.35 ± 0.64 μm versus 1.96 ± 0.47 μm, respectively) in comparison with graft and suture.

Conclusion.—Light-activated sealing of cross-linked human amnion results in superior outcomes when compared with conventional suture (Fig 2).

▶ In this study, Fairbairn et al have provided compelling evidence for the potential clinical utility of photochemical bonding of human cross-linked amnion nerve wraps to facilitate nerve repair in a rat model. In his study comparing this technique to conventional suture coaptation of nerve grafting technique, superior muscle mass was observed in the experimental group (Fig 2).

The conventional means of nerve graft reconstruction using suture requires repeated handling of the nerve, which can lead to scarring and neuroma formation. Photochemical bonding of the nerve using human nerve wrap material theoretically limits the amount of handling of the nerve and provides an attractive alternative to nerve reconstruction.

Additional studies would further enhance our understanding of the clinical potential of this technique. For example, a study of repair strength of the photochemical bonding technique would be of interest, as would a study looking only at primary nerve repair (without interposed grafting), comparing photochemical bonding of nerve wraps and simple suture techniques.

P. Murray, MD

Effects of a dynamic orthosis in an individual with claw deformity
Sousa GGQ, de Macêdo MP (4 Hands Rehabilitation Ctr, Maceió, AL, Brazil)
J Hand Ther 28:425-428, 2015

These authors describe their utilization of a dynamic orthosis to correct a strong claw deformity in a patient with a median and ulnar laceration. After 4 weeks of wearing the dynamic orthosis, these authors noted that the patient was able to actively extend all his fingers orthosis-free, with no evidence of claw. —VICTORIA PRIGANC, PhD, OTR, CHT, CLT, Practice Forum Editor.

▶ I applaud the authors for being creative in a treatment to allow for patient-centered care. The traditional lumbrical bar orthosis did not enable the patient to have enough hand function. Instead, the authors fabricated an orthosis with the dynamic pull from the volar wrist region to the proximal phalanx using rubber bands. This limits metacarpal joint (MCP) extension and increases hand function in daily activities. I find that the rubber band pull in the palm of the hand may limit functional use of the hand. Based on the article, it appears close supervision is required by a hand therapist to assess the pull of the rubber bands and make modifications to limit MCP extension on a consistent basis. With health care reform, close supervision by a therapist is not always possible. Distance of the patient from a knowledgeable hand therapist may be a barrier in close supervision. A patient needs to have explicit instructions to make any modifications at home with the tension of the rubber band pull on the MCP.

The other concern with this orthosis is the timing of possible reinnervation of the ulnar nerve. There is a possibility that the patient had reinnervation of the ulnar nerve and by 20 weeks would not have needed any orthosis. I would like to see future studies use electromyography to examine if this type of orthosis is beneficial for neuromuscular re-education after reinnervation, a biomechanical balance of de-innervated intrinsics, or both.

S. Kannas, CHT

The optimization of peripheral nerve recovery using cortical reorganization techniques: A retrospective study of wrist level nerve repairs
Walbruch B, Kalliainen L (Regions Hosp, St. Paul, MN)
J Hand Ther 28:341-346, 2015

Study Design.—Retrospective case series.
Introduction.—Outcomes following peripheral nerve repairs have not significantly improved over the past few decades. A new protocol using cortical reorganization techniques was developed with the goal of improving nerve recovery in the hand.
Purpose of the Study.—To determine if early sensory re-education using cortical reorganization techniques improved sensory outcomes in the hand after repair of wrist-level nerve injuries.
Methods.—A retrospective study was completed of wrist-level peripheral nerve repairs in patients who underwent a sensory re-education protocol which included cutaneous anesthesia, tactile stimulation, and sensory and motor imagery. Data for static 2-point discrimination, Semmes Weinstein monofilament assessments and the shortened version of the Disabilities of the Arm, Shoulder and Hand (QuickDASH) scores were collected.
Results.—At four months post-repair, three of seven of the median nerve lacerations had static 2-point discrimination of 7 mm or less in at least one digit. Using the Semmes Weinstein monofilaments, 9 of 11 nerve repairs felt the 4.31 filament (protective) or better by eleven months with five able to perceive the 2.83 filament (normal) in that time frame.
Conclusions.—This limited retrospective study suggests that early sensory re-education using cortical reorganization techniques may improve sensory outcomes. A larger scale study is indicated to confirm our findings.
Level of Evidence.—IV.

▶ The traditional sensory re-education approaches described by Dellon and Wynn-Parry, now more commonly referred to as *phase two*, have remained a mainstay in rehabilitation after wrist-level nerve lacerations since the 1970s. In this approach, sensory re-education is not initiated until vibration sense has returned. More recently, there is neuroscientific evidence to support that changes in the brain's sensorimotor strip occur within minutes of being deprived of sensorimotor stimuli in that those sensorimotor intact regions in the affected limb assume the affected region's homunculus representation.[1] This evidence has altered the manner in which rehabilitation therapists conduct sensory re-education after nerve laceration in that they are now intervening to, in theory, preserve cortical representation of the affected region of the limb during a period of absent sensorimotor input from the periphery. This is now commonly referred to as *phase 1* sensory re-education, and the interventions used during this phase are referred to as *cortical reorganization techniques*. These techniques include, but are not limited to, imagining the experience of touch/movement of the insensate hand, observing touch and movement of a mirror reflection of the contralateral uninvolved limb, and use of a local anesthetic to the region proximal to the nerve laceration.

The authors of this small retrospective study (n = 10) sought to investigate if, among persons with median, radial, or ulnar nerve repairs, early introduction of cortical reorganization techniques (ie, anesthetizing the region proximal to the injury combined with tactile input to insensate area,[2] motor/sensory imagery and mirror therapy), resulted in improved touch perception and discrimination outcomes relative to previously published research on traditional Dellon and Wynn-Parry[3] approaches to re-education. The authors built upon the work of Rosen et al[2] who, through use of a placebo-controlled prospective trial, studied the effectiveness of using local anesthesia to the region proximal to the nerve repair and traditional phase 2 sensory re-education at an average of 22 months postrepair. Beyond this, the authors sought to investigate if patients perceive clinically meaningful improvements in upper limb function after participating in this early-intervention approach.

The authors reported their sensory outcomes to be descriptively better than the outcomes of traditional sensory re-education programs. Touch threshold was restored to normal (as per Semmes Weinstein Monofilaments) in 3 participants (2 median, 1 radial), whereas no previous studies had reported returns to normal following sensory re-education.[4] Likewise, 2-point discrimination improved to 7 mm or less in 42% of the subjects at 4 months, whereas previous studies had reported discrimination to return to values no greater than 7 mm at 18+ months after repairs.[5,6] These findings, however, could not be compared to those of Rosen et al[2] who implemented delayed (ie, approximately 22 months) cortical reorganization strategies given that these authors only reported change scores in 2-point discrimination and touch perception scores.

Lastly, 9 of 10 participants experienced clinically meaningful improvements (>18)[7] in upper limb function as per the shortened version of the Disabilities of the Arm, Shoulder and Hand Questionnaire at the conclusion of therapy. However, this finding, in addition to the improvements in sensation would carry additional validity if they were attained via use of prospective controlled trials.

Other limitations to external and internal validity include variance in approaches to surgical repairs, no controls for the effects of comorbidities and age, variable data collection time points, small sample size, undocumented therapy adherence, and the use of multiple reorganizing interventions.

Nonetheless, although of a lower level of evidence, these findings illustrate improvements not previously documented in the literature after nerve repair, and sensory re-education and should be the impetus for further study. Additional research should include feasibility and larger scale prospective controlled deigns in which there are controls for age, surgical approach, comorbidities, and concomitant injuries. Follow-ups to this might include comparative effectiveness trials to tease out which components and intensities of the program are most effective.

C. McGee, PhD, OTR/L, CHT

References

1. Stavrinou ML, Penna SD, Pizzella V, et al. Temporal dynamics of plastic changes in human primary somatosensory cortex after finger webbing. *Cerebral Cortex.* 2007;17:2134-2142.
2. Rosen B, Bjorkman A, Lundborg G. Improved sensory relearning after nerve repair induced by selective temporary anaesthesia e a new concept in hand rehabilitation. *J Hand Surg Br.* 2006;31:126-132.
3. Dellon AL. *Evaluation of Sensibility and Re-education of Sensation in the Hand.* Baltimore, MD: Williams and Wilkins; 1981.
4. Imai H, Tajima T, Natsuma Y. Interpretation of cutaneous pressure threshold (Semmes Weinstein Monofilament Measurement) following median nerve repair and sensory reeducation in the adult. *Microsurgery.* 1989;10:142-144.
5. Bjorkman A, Rosen B, van Westen D, Larsson EM, Lundborg G. Acute improvement of contralateral hand function after deafferentation. *Eur J Neurosci.* 2004; 15:1861-1865.
6. Bjorkman A, Rosen B, Lundborg G. Enhanced function in nerve-injured hands after contralateral deafferentation. *Eur J Neurosci.* 2005;16:517-519.
7. Mintken P, Glynn P, Cleland J. Psychometric properties of the shortened disabilities of the Arm, Shoulder, and Hand Questionnaire (QuickDASH) and Numeric Pain Rating Scale in patients with shoulder pain. *J Shoulder Elbow Surg.* 2009; 18:920-926.

Nerve Regeneration: Is There an Alternative to Nervous Graft?

Sabongi RG, De Rizzo LALM, Fernandes M, et al (Universidade Federal de São Paulo, Brazil)

J Reconstr Microsurg 30:607-616, 2014

Background.—In nerve injury with nervous gap, no restitution method was found better than the autograft, however, it has the disadvantage of damaging a normal nerve to be used as a graft. Platelet-rich plasma (PRP) is a possible filler material for vein grafts used as conduits for nerve regeneration, preventing its collapse, and providing growth factors and osteoconductive proteins.

Methods.—Isogenic rats were randomly divided into three groups. They received nerve autografts (GRF), PRP-containing vein grafts or a sham operation. Outcomes were evaluated by the sciatic functional index (SFI), morphometric, and morphologic analyses of the nerve distal to the lesion, and the number of spinal cord motoneurons positive for retrograde Fluoro-Gold (Santa Cruz Biotechnology, Inc., Dallas, TX) tracer.

Results.—The PRP and GRF groups had lower SFI values than the control animals throughout the postoperative period. The SFI was significantly higher in the PRP group than the GRF group at 90 days postoperatively ($p = 0.011$). Fiber diameter and number of motoneurons were significantly decreased in both the PRP and GRF groups, as compared with the control.

Conclusion.—PRP within a vein conduit may be an effective alternative or adjuvant to GRF, the current preferred treatment for nerve injury with a nerve gap, and further investigations are required to fully define the role of PRP in nerve regeneration.

▶ In this well-controlled and well-analyzed study, Sabongi et al expand on the concept of nerve regeneration by offering another method of nerve reconstruction. Although the concept of vein wrapping of nerve defects has met with mixed results, particularly for long gaps, the authors propose that the issue of vein collapse can be prevented with the use of platelet-rich plasma (PRP) placed in the vein tube. The authors also theorize that PRP placed in the vein wrap could also potentially augment nerve regeneration through the release of diverse growth factors, which enhance collagen synthesis, stimulate angiogenesis, and promote vascular ingrowth. Two experimental groups and one control group were carefully analyzed postprocedure using rat sciatic nerve index and morphometric and fluorogold tracer analysis. The authors conclude that the use of PRP within a vein wrap has possible clinical merit. Such a substrate would be of clinical interest given the elimination of nerve autograft donor site morbidity and time for autograft harvest. Overall, cost of this technique and the ultimate functional outcome from this alternative to nerve graft reconstruction are questions that would need further scrutiny prior to translation into the clinical setting.

P. Murray, MD

Light-Activated Sealing of Nerve Graft Coaptation Sites Improves Outcome Following Large Gap Peripheral Nerve Injury

Fairbairn NG, Ng-Glazier J, Meppelink AM, et al (Massachusetts General Hosp, Boston; Walter Reed Natl Military Medical Ctr, Bethesda, MD)
Plast Reconstr Surg 136:739-750, 2015

Background.—Nerve repair using photochemically bonded human amnion nerve wraps can result in superior outcomes in comparison with standard suture. When applied to nerve grafts, efficacy has been limited by proteolytic degradation of bonded amnion during extended periods of recovery. Chemical cross-linking of amnion before bonding may improve wrap durability and efficacy.

Methods.—Three nerve wraps (amnion, cross-linked amnion, and cross-linked swine intestinal submucosa) and three fixation methods (suture, fibrin glue, and photochemical bonding) were investigated. One hundred ten Lewis rats had 15-mm left sciatic nerve gaps repaired with isografts. Nine groups ($n = 10$) had isografts secured by one of the aforementioned wrap/fixation combinations. Positive and negative control groups ($n = 10$) were repaired with graft and suture and no repair, respectively. Outcomes were assessed using sciatic function index, muscle mass retention, and histomorphometry. Statistical analysis was performed using analysis of variance and the post hoc Bonferroni test ($p < 0.05$).

Results.—Cross-linking improved amnion durability. Photochemically bonded crosslinked amnion recovered the greatest sciatic function index, although this was not significant in comparison with graft and suture.

Photochemically bonded crosslinked amnion recovered significantly greater muscle mass (67.3 ± 4.4 percent versus 60.0 ± 5.2 percent; $p = 0.02$), fiber diameter, axon diameter, and myelin thickness (6.87 ± 2.23 μm versus 5.47 ± 1.70 μm; 4.51 ± 1.83 μm versus 3.50 ± 1.44 μm; and 2.35 ± 0.64 μm versus 1.96 ± 0.47 μm, respectively) in comparison with graft and suture.

Conclusion.—Light-activated sealing of cross-linked human amnion results in superior outcomes when compared with conventional suture.

▶ This is an elegant and well-designed experimental study on a new method of nerve coaptation. Light-activated sealing is described as novel form of nerve coaptation that can eliminate weaknesses of fibrin glue and foreign body influence that is present in the standard suture technique. In light of these innovations, the process of harvesting and preparing human amnion and swine submucosa is described. The methods of evaluation are standards and well described.

The authors conclude that nerves repaired with cross-linked human amnion and photochemical tissue bonding showed the greatest functional recovery after 5 months, as well as significantly greater muscle mass retention and significantly increased nerve fiber diameter, axon diameter, and myelin thickness. Therefore, all 3 evaluated parameters were better in cross-linked human amnion and photochemical tissue bonding. The control groups showed inferior results, which make the study more reliable. The authors are also aware of the high capability of rodent recovery and use nerve graft from another animal, which is less common but better for the scientific purposes.

At this time, practical issues of this technique remain in question. It requires 2 elements: specifically prepared tissue and equipment, which are apparently expensive. Second, the authors suggest that it can be used by less skilled surgeons; it avoids microsurgical methods and thus is more easy to apply. From my perspective, this may be true in bigger nerves, but its special skills are still required.

Generally, when looking at new surgical techniques, I try to find the points that will convince me the option is better for my patients. In this case, I cannot say it is faster or cheaper, or that there is less morbidity (we still use nerve graft for the gap), but there may be superior regeneration, which remains to be proven in humans, which perhaps we will see in the follow-up of this elegant study.

P. Czarnecki, MD

Decellularized Nerves for Upper Limb Nerve Reconstruction: A Systematic Review of Functional Outcomes
Deslivia MF, Lee H-J, Adikrishna A, et al (Korea Inst of Science and Technology, Seoul; Kyungpook Natl Univ Hosp, Daegu, Korea; Univ of Ulsan, Seoul, Korea; et al)
J Reconstr Microsurg 31:660-667, 2015

Background.—This is a systematic review for evaluating the evidence for functional outcomes after decellularized nerve use in clinical setting.

Decellularized nerves are allografts whose antigenic components have been removed, leaving only a scaffold that promotes the full regeneration of axons.

Methods.—Literature research was performed using the PubMed/MEDLINE database for English language studies with the keywords "decellularized nerve" and "processed nerve allograft." Inclusion criteria were prospective and retrospective case reviews in clinical settings. Exclusion criteria were case reports and case series.

Results.—We retrieved six level VIII studies and one level VI study (classified according to the Jovell and Navarro—Rubio scale) with a total of 131 reconstructions. The basic data ranges of the studies were as follows: patient age, 18 to 86 years; duration between initial injury and nerve reconstruction procedure, 8 hours to 4 years; and follow-up period, 40 days to 2 years. The maximum lengths of the nerve gap for chemically washed decellularized nerves and cryopreserved decellularized nerves were 50 and 100 mm, respectively. Quantitatively, the functional outcome ranges were as follows: static two-point discrimination, 3 to 5 mm; and moving two-point discrimination, 2 to 15 mm. For motor assessment, all patients had a > M3 Medical Research Council score. It is also important to notice that a large variability occurs in almost every factor in the reviewed studies.

Conclusion.—Our study is the first to summarize the clinical results of decellularized nerves. Decellularized nerves have been used to bridge nerve gaps ranging from 5 to 100 mm with associated satisfactory outcomes in static and moving two-point discriminations.

▶ The authors performed a systematic review of the available literature to determine the effectiveness of acellular nerve allografts for reconstruction of nerve defects. The published evidence is primarily retrospective reviews and case series, which limits the usefulness of this information because the quality of the review is based on the quality of existing evidence. In addition, the heterogeneity of the group, with nerve gaps from 5 to 100 mm and the inclusion of sensory, mixed, and motor nerves makes it difficult to understand the true outcomes for a given scenario. Finally, 2 of the 7 articles included are from a registry hosted by the manufacturer of the allograft nerve, and although there is no reason to believe these data are not accurate, it is a potential source of bias.

Given the total body of literature evaluating outcomes of autograft, allograft, and nerve conduits, I think allograft nerves are a reasonable treatment for some nerve injuries. There is basic science literature to indicate autograft is better than allograft for motor nerve injuries,[1] but also clinical reports of good outcome for use on motor nerve reconstruction, so again, the literature is unclear.

My personal opinion is allograft nerve is a reasonable option for sensory nerves with defects less than 50 mm and probably equivalent to conduits for defects less than 15 mm, but again, this is opinion and not evidence.

W. C. Hammert, MD

Reference

1. Giusti G, Willems WF, Kremer T, Friedrich PF, Bishop AT, Shin AY. Return of motor function after segmental nerve loss in a rat model: comparison of autogenous nerve graft, collagen conduit, and processed allograft (AxoGen). *J Bone Joint Surg Am.* 2012;94:410-417.

Comparison of Nerve, Vessel, and Cartilage Grafts in Promoting Peripheral Nerve Regeneration

Firat C, Geyik Y, Aytekin AH, et al (Inonu Univ School of Medicine, Malatya, Turkey)

Ann Plast Surg 73:54-61, 2014

Peripheral nerve injury primarily occurs due to trauma as well as factors such as tumors, inflammatory diseases, congenital deformities, infections, and surgical interventions. The surgical procedure to be performed as treatment depends on the etiology, type of injury, and the anatomic region. The goal of treatment is to minimize loss of function due to motor and sensory nerve loss at the distal part of the injury. Regardless of the cause of the injury, the abnormal nerve regeneration due to incomplete nerve regeneration, optimal treatment of peripheral nerve injuries should provide adequate coaptation of proximal and distal sides without tension, preserving the neurotrophic factors within the repair line. The gold standard for the treatment of nerve defects is the autograft; however, due to denervation of the donor site, scarring, and neuroma formation, many studies have aimed to develop simpler methods, better functional results, and less morbidity. In this study, a defect 1 cm in length was created on the sciatic nerve of rats. The rats were treated with the following procedures: group 1, autograft; group 2, allogeneic aorta graft; group 3, diced cartilage graft in allogeneic aorta graft; and group 4, tubularized cartilage graft in allogeneic aorta graft. Group 5 was the control group. The effects of cartilage tissue in nerve regeneration were evaluated by functional and histomorphological methods.

Group 1, for which the repair was performed with an autograft, was evaluated to be the most similar to the control group. There was not a statistically significant difference in myelination and Schwann cell rates between group 2, in which an allogeneic aorta graft was used, and group 3, in which diced cartilage in an allogeneic aorta graft was used. In group 4, myelination and Schwann cell formation were observed; however, they were scattered and irregular, likely due to increased fibrosis.

In all of the groups, nerve regeneration at various rates was observed both functionally and histomorphologically. This study demonstrates that cartilage tissue has promoting effects in nerve regeneration.

▶ The authors have reported on a laboratory study comparing nerve regeneration with autograft, allograft aorta as a conduit and with autograft cartilage,

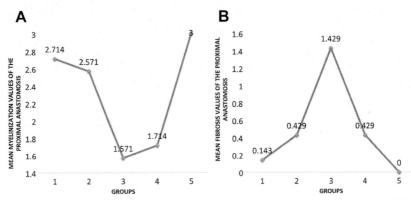

FIGURE 2.—A, B, Mean myelination and fibrosis values of proximal anastomoses. (Reprinted from Firat C, Geyik Y, Aytekin AH, et al. Comparison of nerve, vessel, and cartilage grafts in promoting peripheral nerve regeneration. *Ann Plast Surg.* 2014;73:54-61, with permission from Lippincott Williams & Wilkins.)

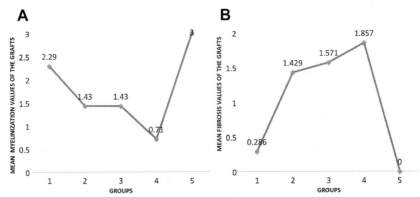

FIGURE 4.—A, B: Mean myelination and fibrosis values of grafts. (Reprinted from Firat C, Geyik Y, Aytekin AH, et al. Comparison of nerve, vessel, and cartilage grafts in promoting peripheral nerve regeneration. *Ann Plast Surg.* 2014;73:54-61, with permission from Lippincott Williams & Wilkins.)

and a tubularized cartilage graft. They used a standard rat model, and their results were best in the autograft group. Other groups have demonstrated mylenization across the proximal neuropathy site as well as the entire graft, but also increased fibrosis (Figs 2A, B and 4A, B). The search for an alternative to autograft for nerve reconstruction remains elusive. Allograft nerve is promising but still does not appear to be equivalent to autograft, at least in motor recovery.[1] The lack of donor site morbidity is appealing, but for critical nerves, the compromise of recovery may be too great for many situations. Continued search for other materials is important to advance the science of nerve regeneration. Although cartilage autografts demonstrate some myelin across the graft site, there is also increased fibrosis. Further research is necessary to determine whether this is a potential clinical alternative.

W. Hammert, MD

Reference

1. Giusti G, Willems WF, Kremer T, Friedrich PF, Bishop AT, Shin AY. Return of motor function after segmental nerve loss in a rat model: comparison of autogenous nerve graft, collagen conduit, and processed allograft (AxoGen). *J Bone Joint Surg Am.* 2012;94:410-417.

7   Brachial Plexus

Spinal Accessory Nerve Transfer Outperforms Cervical Root Grafting for
Suprascapular Nerve Reconstruction in Neonatal Brachial Plexus Palsy
Seruya M, Shen SH, Fuzzard S, et al (Royal Children's Hosp Melbourne,
Victoria, Australia)
Plast Reconstr Surg 135:1431-1438, 2015

Background.—The authors evaluated long-term shoulder function in patients with neonatal brachial plexus palsy undergoing suprascapular nerve reconstruction with cervical root grafting or spinal accessory nerve transfer.

Methods.—A retrospective review was performed on all infants presenting with neonatal brachial plexus palsy between 1994 and 2010. Functional outcomes were compared by type of suprascapular nerve reconstruction.

Results.—Seventy-four patients met the inclusion criteria (46 transfers, 28 grafts). Both groups presented with an active movement scale score of 2.0 for shoulder abduction and 0.0 for external rotation. Postoperative follow-up was 9.0 years for the graft group and 6.7 years for the transfer group. Both groups achieved an active movement scale score of 5.0 for shoulder abduction at 12, 24, and 36 months postoperatively. Active movement scale scores for shoulder external rotation were 1.0, 2.0, and 2.5 for the graft group versus 2.0, 2.0, and 3.0 for the transfer group at 12, 24, and 36 months postoperatively. None of these differences reached statistical significance. Composite Mallet scores were 13.0 for the graft group versus 15.0 for the transfer group at 3 years ($p = 0.06$) and 13.0 for the graft group versus 16.0 for the transfer group at 5 years postoperatively ($p = 0.07$). Secondary shoulder surgery was performed on 57.1 percent (16 of 28) of patients with grafts compared with 26.1 percent (12 of 46) of patients with transfers (OR, 3.17; $p = 0.02$).

Conclusion.—Suprascapular nerve reconstruction by cervical root grafting results in poorer shoulder function and a two-fold increase in secondary shoulder surgery compared with spinal accessory nerve transfer.

Clinical Question/Level of Evidence.—Therapeutic, III.

▶ Seruya et al reviewed, in a level 4 retrospective study, the comparative results of suprascapular nerve root reconstruction via C5 nerve root grafting verses spinal accessory to suprascapular nerve transfer in infant brachial plexus palsy patients. The authors found that patients with suprascapular nerve root reconstruction by C5 nerve root nerve grafting had poorer shoulder function and required more secondary shoulder surgeries than those patients receiving the nerve transfer procedure. Although these results are intriguing, particularly given the more straightforward nature of nerve transfer surgery, what is unclear from the study is the average length of the grafts used in the C5 reconstruction cases. Also of note is that the average age of the C5 nerve root reconstruction patients was almost 10 months at time of surgery, whereas the age of the nerve transfer patients was 8 months. The reader is left to wonder whether the results would have been more similar if the C5 nerve root reconstruction cases would have been closer to 6 months. Nevertheless, this study highlights the growing enthusiasm for nerve transfer surgery as a first-line treatment option for infants with brachial plexus palsy.

P. Murray, MD

Free functioning gracilis transplantation for reconstruction of elbow and hand functions in late obstetric brachial plexus palsy
El-Gammal TA, El-Sayed A, Kotb MM, et al (Assiut Univ School of Medicine, Egypt)
Microsurgery 35:350-355, 2015

Background.—In late obstetric brachial plexus palsy (OBPP), restoration of elbow and hand functions is a difficult challenge. The use of free functioning muscle transplantation in late OBPP was very scarcely reported. In this study, we present our experience on the use of free functioning gracilis transfer for restoration of elbow and hand functions in late cases of OBPP.

Patients and Methods.—Eighteen patients with late OBPP underwent free gracilis transfer for reconstruction of elbow and/or hand functions. The procedure was indicated when there was no evidence of reinnervation on EMG and in the absence of local donors. Average age at surgery was 102.5 months. Patients were evaluated using the British Medical Research Council (MRC) grading system and the Toronto Active Movement Scale. Hand function was evaluated by the Raimondi scoring system.

Results.—The average follow-up was 65.8 ± 41.7 months. Contraction of the transferred gracilis started at an average of 4.5 ± 1.03 months. Average range of elbow flexion significantly improved from 30 ± 55.7 to 104 ± 31.6 degrees $(P < 0.001)$. Elbow flexion power significantly increased with an average of 3.8 grades $(P = 0.000147)$. Passive elbow range of motion significantly decreased from an average of 147 to 117 degrees $(P = 0.003)$. Active finger flexion significantly improved from 5 ± 8.3 to 63 ± 39.9 degrees $(P < 0.001)$. Finger flexion power significantly increased with an average 2.7 grades $(P < 0.001)$. Only 17% achieved useful hand (grade 3) on Raimondi hand score. Triceps reconstruction resulted in an average of M4 power and 45 degrees elbow extension.

Conclusion.—Free gracilis transfer may be a useful option for reconstruction of elbow and/or hand functions in late OBPP.

▶ The use of free functioning muscle transfer for infantile brachial plexus palsy was reviewed in study of 18 patients by El-Gammal et al and represents the largest cohort of patients with this condition. At an average follow-up of almost 66 months in a patient population with an average age of more than 8 years, the authors determine that free functioning muscle transfer for elbow animation is a reliable procedure in late-presenting infantile brachial plexus palsy. Although this finding has been established by other authors, this study represents the largest published series to date on the subject. A study comparing the results of latissimus or flexor-pronator flexorplasty with free functioning muscle transfer would be of interest.

P. Murray, MD

Short-term and Long-term Clinical Results of the Surgical Correction of Thumb-in-Palm Deformity in Patients With Cerebral Palsy
Alewijnse JV, Smeulders MJC, Kreulen M (Academic Med Ctr, Amsterdam, The Netherlands; Red Cross Hosp, Beverwijk, The Netherlands)
J Pediatr Orthop 35:825-830, 2015

Background.—Thumb-in-palm deformity disturbs a functional grip of the hand in patients with cerebral palsy. Reported recurrence rates after surgical correction are contradicting and earlier studies are limited to short-term follow-up. Therefore, the aim of this retrospective clinical outcome study is to evaluate the success rate of surgical correction of thumb-in-palm deformity around 1 year and at a minimum of 5 years follow-up. In addition, long-term patient satisfaction of the treatment is evaluated.

Methods.—Patients with cerebral palsy who underwent a surgical correction for their thumb-in-palm deformity between April 2003 and April 2008 at the Academic Medical Center in Amsterdam were included. All patients were classified into 4 categories according to the assessment system of the Committee on Spastic Hand Evaluation. The result of surgery was considered "short-term successful" and "long-term successful" when, respectively, short-term and long-term classification was better compared with preoperative. The association between the patient satisfaction outcomes and the long-term clinical outcomes were statistically analyzed.

Results.—Data were collected from 39 patients and their charts. The success rate was 87% at short-term follow-up, which in the long term decreased to 80%. Interestingly, thumb position deteriorated in 29% of the patients between short-term and long-term follow-up. In the long term, 74% of the patients were satisfied with the position of their thumb and 87% would undergo the surgery again. Both these outcomes were statistically significant associated with the long-term success rate (*P* < 0.05).

Conclusions.—The surgical correction of thumb-in-palm deformity has a high clinical success rate and patient satisfaction in the long term. However, it should be taken into account that the clinical result around 1 year postoperative cannot be considered final.

Level of Evidence.—Level IV.

▶ This is a retrospective review of 39 patients who underwent surgical release of thumb-in-palm deformity as a result of cerebral palsy. The surgical procedures were performed by the same surgeon. Assessments preoperatively and at 1 year postoperatively were performed by an independent physiatrist; however, the long-term follow-up was performed using photographs assessed by 2 trainees. This method would make accurate assessment of the long-term outcomes difficult, especially because one could not assess for overcorrection. The authors did note that the results deteriorate over time. However, most patients did appear to improve from baseline. Patient satisfaction assessment has substantial recall bias and, therefore, this information should be used cautiously. My preference is to treat these patients to aid them in grip but also to permit acquisition of larger objects. Often a first webspace deepening is added to my procedures to allow for acquisition of large objects.

J. M. Abzug, MD

Spinal Accessory Nerve Transfer Outperforms Cervical Root Grafting for Suprascapular Nerve Reconstruction in Neonatal Brachial Plexus Palsy
Seruya M, Shen SH, Fuzzard S, et al (Royal Children's Hosp Melbourne, Australia)
Plast Reconstr Surg 135:1431-1438, 2015

Background.—The authors evaluated long-term shoulder function in patients with neonatal brachial plexus palsy undergoing suprascapular nerve reconstruction with cervical root grafting or spinal accessory nerve transfer.

Methods.—A retrospective review was performed on all infants presenting with neonatal brachial plexus palsy between 1994 and 2010. Functional outcomes were compared by type of suprascapular nerve reconstruction.

Results.—Seventy-four patients met the inclusion criteria (46 transfers, 28 grafts). Both groups presented with an active movement scale score of 2.0 for shoulder abduction and 0.0 for external rotation. Postoperative follow-up was 9.0 years for the graft group and 6.7 years for the transfer group. Both groups achieved an active movement scale score of 5.0 for shoulder abduction at 12, 24, and 36 months postoperatively. Active movement scale scores for shoulder external rotation were 1.0, 2.0, and 2.5 for the graft group versus 2.0, 2.0, and 3.0 for the transfer group at 12, 24, and 36 months postoperatively. None of these differences reached statistical significance. Composite Mallet scores were 13.0 for the graft group versus 15.0 for the transfer group at 3 years ($p = 0.06$) and 13.0 for the graft group versus 16.0 for the transfer group at 5 years postoperatively ($p = 0.07$). Secondary shoulder surgery was performed on 57.1 percent (16 of 28) of patients with grafts compared with 26.1 percent (12 of 46) of patients with transfers (OR, 3.17; $p = 0.02$).

Conclusion.—Suprascapular nerve reconstruction by cervical root grafting results in poorer shoulder function and a two-fold increase in secondary shoulder surgery compared with spinal accessory nerve transfer.

Clinical Question/Level of Evidence.—Therapeutic, III.

▶ This article is a retrospective review assessing shoulder function after either nerve grafting or nerve transfer to the suprascapular nerve in infants with brachial plexus birth palsy (BPBP). The authors noted no difference in shoulder abduction or external rotation between the two groups. They did note an improvement in composite Mallet scores when performing the nerve transfer; however, this was not statistically significant. The one metric that showed a statistically significant difference between the two groups was the need for secondary shoulder procedures. It is important to note that we do not know how patients were chosen to undergo a secondary shoulder procedure. It is plausible that the authors were biased and performed those procedures more commonly in the nerve-grafting group and then reported it. It is also possible that their practice evolved over time, and these differences are a result of that. Despite these limitations, I do agree that nerve transfers are an excellent alternative to nerve grafting. The need for only one coaptation site and ability to be close to the target muscle are obvious advantages. Future studies with larger patient numbers are needed to truly assess whether nerve transfers are superior to nerve grafting of the suprascapular nerve for BPBP patients.

J. M. Abzug, MD

8   Microsurgery

Predictors of Proximal Interphalangeal Joint Flexion Contracture After Homodigital Island Flap
Nakanishi A, Omokawa S, Iida A, et al (Takita Hosp, Nara, Japan; Nara Med Univ, Japan)
J Hand Surg Am 40:2155-2159, 2015

Purpose.—To identify independent predictors of postoperative proximal interphalangeal (PIP) joint contracture after direct-flow homodigital island flap transfer.

Methods.—Forty-four fingertip amputations in 39 patients treated with oblique triangular flaps were evaluated at a minimum of 1 year after surgery. Five variables were examined: patient age, injured finger, mechanism of injury, flap advancement distance, and time required for wound healing. Univariate and multivariate linear regression analyses were performed to identify the extent to which these variables affected the flexion contracture of the PIP joint.

Results.—The average reduction in the passive extension angle of the PIP joint was 16° at final follow-up. Univariate analysis indicated significant correlations of PIP joint flexion contracture with age, injured finger, and time for wound healing, but no significant correlation with the distance the flap was advanced. Multivariate analysis indicated that the age and duration of wound healing were independent predictors of the flexion contracture of the PIP joint.

Conclusions.—Elderly people and cases with delayed wound healing are at risk for postoperative PIP joint contracture after homodigital flap transfer. Intervention with early hand therapy and orthotics may be useful in elderly patients with delayed wound healing.

Type of Study/Level of Evidence.—Prognostic II.

▶ It is interesting that the patients' age and duration of the wound healing were significantly related to flexion contracture of the proximal interphalangeal (PIP) joint after treatment of the fingertip injuries using homodigital triangular island flaps. It is necessary to keep the fingers in a slightly flexed posture postoperatively until the blood circulation of the flaps stabilizes. In elderly people, one can easily imagine that keeping the PIP joint flexed or prohibiting PIP joint motion for several weeks can lead to the flexion contracture.

In my opinion, there may have been several confounding factors affecting wound healing in this study. The neurovascular bundle is elastic and can be stretched. If the neurovascular bundle is stretched over a limited distance, the vascularity of the flap begins to be compromised, and a flap with compromised vascularity would delay wound healing. If the bundle is stretched until it can be stretched no further, the neurovascular bundle would flex the PIP joint. We suspect that there may have been a flap advancement distance at which the stretched neurovascular bundle did not generate flexion of the PIP joint but compromised the vascularity of the flap. The delayed wound healing may have been related to the flap advancement distance.

R. Kakinoki, MD

A Comparative Study of Attitudes Regarding Digit Replantation in the United States and Japan
Nishizuka T, Shauver MJ, Zhong L, et al (Nagoya Univ Graduate School of Medicine, Japan; Univ of Michigan, Ann Arbor)
J Hand Surg Am 40:1646-1656, 2015

Purpose.—To compare the societal preferences for finger replantation between the United States (US) and Japan and to investigate factors influencing the preferences.

Methods.—A sample of the general population without current hand disease or condition was recruited via flyers posted in public areas of 2 major academic centers in the US and Japan. The recruited subjects completed a survey presenting finger amputation scenarios and various factors that may affect treatment decisions. We performed univariate analysis using treatment preference as the outcome and all other factors as possible predictors using the chi-square test.

Results.—Most respondents in both countries preferred replantation and there was no significant difference between the US and Japan. Treatment preference was significantly associated with the importance of appearance, recovery time, and the chance of survival of the replanted digit. There was no association between treatment preference and attitudes regarding body integrity or estimate of stigma toward finger amputees. Japanese participants agreed more with statements of body integrity, and Japanese respondents rated appearance, sensation, and chance of survival of the replant as more important than did American participants.

Conclusions.—Patient preference is not driving the decrease in finger replantations in the US. The general public in both countries prefer replantation over wound closure for digit amputations.

Type of Study/Level of Evidence.—Economic and decision analysis III.

▶ As a Japanese hand surgeon who is familiar with hand surgery in the United States, I believe that Japanese patients tend to place great importance on body integrity, especially the number of fingers. Imagine a person who had a middle finger amputated at the proximal interphalangeal joint level. The middle finger looks abnormal, and the hand function is impaired, which affects the person's daily living (eg, cannot scoop water using both hands to wash). It is usual to transfer the index finger ray to the base of the third metacarpal after removal of the middle finger stump. In our experience, many Japanese patients with this injury often refuse the ray-transfer operation because they do not wish to lose a finger. The same tendency can also be seen in patients with a congenital abnormality. In Japan, many parents of infants who have hypoplastic thumbs, such as type 3b or 4 (modified Blauth classification), often ask the surgeon to preserve the original thumbs, even though we explain repeatedly that the hand function would be improved with pollicization after removal of the hypoplastic thumbs. We may have more opportunities to perform metatarsal or toe transfer to thumb and fingers on these patients than do American hand surgeons.

I am concerned about the ratio of male-to-female participants in this study. There were 2.5 times more females than males in the US sample, but the ratio was equal in the Japanese sample. Males are more likely than females to experience finger amputation injuries. The outcomes might have provided a more accurate reflection of the actual situation if the study had included only manual workers.

R. Kakinoki, MD

Innervated Digital Artery Perforator Propeller Flap for Reconstruction of Lateral Oblique Fingertip Defects

Shen XF, Xue MY, Mi JY, et al (Wuxi Ninth People's Hosp, Jiangsu, China; et al)

J Hand Surg Am 40:1382-1388, 2015

Purpose.—To report our experience with the use of a digital artery perforator propeller flap based on a constant distal perforator in the middle phalanx for resurfacing of lateral oblique fingertip amputations.

Methods.—Twelve fingertips in 10 patients underwent reconstruction, with a mean follow-up of 8 months (range, 8—12 mo). The size of the flaps ranged from 2.5 × 1.5 cm to 3.0 × 2.0 cm.

Results.—All flaps survived entirely and restored a rounded fingertip contour. Mean static 2-point discrimination was 5 mm (range, 4—6 mm). With the exception of 1 patient with an amputation at the distal interphalangeal joint, the distal interphalangeal joint was preserved in all patients and had 30° to 60° of motion at final follow-up. No patients complained of cold intolerance or residual joint contracture. No hooked nail deformity occurred in patients who had remaining nailbed.

Conclusions.—The digital artery perforator propeller flap is particularly suited to coverage of a lateral oblique fingertip defect, because only a 90° rotation is required when inset, and the bulk of the flap serves to restore the rounded contour of the fingertip. The skin over the entire dorsal surface of the middle phalanx can be elevated as a flap, providing adequate tissue to resurface the defect and restore a rounded contour to the fingertip.

Type of Study/Level of Evidence.—Therapeutic IV.

▶ The authors present a new pedicled perforator flap for the coverage for oblique fingertip defects. The perforator, on which the flap is based, is located at the distal part of the middle phalanx. The flap can be reinnervated by including the dorsal digital nerve of the contralateral side and suturing this nerve to the palmar digital nerve stump. Excellent sensory recovery (mean static 2-PD = 5 mm) is reported.

In a series of 12 flaps there was no case of cold intolerance. The authors believe that the flap is superior in this aspect to reverse-flow homodigital island flaps based on a proper digital artery because the latter can lead to cold intolerance due to the sacrifice of a proper digital artery. We should not forget, however, that cold intolerance is not only a consequence of vessel sacrifice during reconstructive surgery, but also of vessel and nerve damage due to the primary trauma.

The rotation of the flap described in this report is 90 degrees. Unlike previously described digital artery perforator flaps that require a rotation of 180 degrees, the smaller degree of rotation produces less torsion on the vulnerable venous system, which may result in less venous congestion.

This flap may enrich our flap armamentarium for the coverage of fingertip defects.

M. Choi, MD

9 Tendon

Effect of wrist and interphalangeal thumb movement on zone T2 flexor pollicis longus tendon tension in a human cadaver model
Rappaport PO, Thoreson AR, Yang T-H, et al (Mayo Clinic, Rochester, MN; et al)
J Hand Ther 28:347-355, 2015

Introduction.—Therapy after flexor pollicis longus (FPL) repair typically mimics finger flexor management, but this ignores anatomic and biomechanical features unique to the FPL.

Purpose of the study.—We measured FPL tendon tension in zone T2 to identify biomechanically appropriate exercises for mobilizing the FPL.

Methods.—Eight human cadaver hands were studied to identify motions that generated enough force to achieve FPL movement without exceeding hypothetical suture strength.

Results.—With the carpometacarpal and metacarpophalangeal joints blocked, appropriate forces were produced for both passive interphalangeal (IP) motion with 30° wrist extension and simulated active IP flexion from 0° to 35° with the wrist in the neutral position.

Discussion.—This work provides a biomechanical basis for safely and effectively mobilizing the zone T2 FPL tendon.

Conclusion.—Our cadaver study suggests that it is safe and effective to perform early passive and active exercise to an isolated IP joint.

Level of Evidence.—NA.

▶ Rappaport et al studied the kinetics of the flexor pollicis longus (FPL) tendon at zone T2 in 8 human cadaveric specimens with the intent of better understanding the wrist and thumb joint positioning and movements, which most optimally promote FPL glide within an effective and safe margin of tension (ie, safe and effective zone)[1,2] following FPL repair at zone T2. The authors expanded on the earlier work of Brown and McGrouther[3] who reported improved FPL glide with isolated IP movement when compared with composite interphalangeal (IP)/metacarpophalangeal (MP) flexion to better understand (1) the amount of tendon tension created at the repair site during passive IP flexion/extension across varying thumb carpometacarpal (CMC) and wrist positions, (2) how varying positions of the thumb CMC and wrist influence zone T2 FPL glide and repair site tension (ie, the effects of tenodesis and

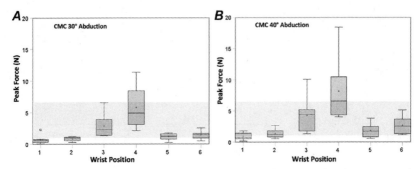

FIGURE 5.—Box-and-whisker plots showing estimated mean (plus sign), median (line), interquartile range (box) and range of peak forces across 8 specimens when performing IP passive motion for all wrist positions (1 = flexion 30°, 2 = neutral, 3 = extension 30°, 4 = extension 60°, 5 = radial deviation 20° and 6 = ulnar deviation 40°). A) CMC at 30° abduction; B) CMC at 40° abduction. The safe and effective zone (SEZ) of forces between 1.3 N and 7 N is highlighted. (Reprinted from Rappaport PO, Thoreson AR, Yang T-H, et al. Effect of wrist and interphalangeal thumb movement on zone T2 flexor pollicis longus tendon tension in a human cadaver model. *J Hand Ther.* 2015;28:347-355, with permission from Hanley & Belfus.)

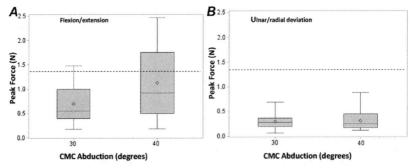

FIGURE 6.—Box-and-whisker plots showing estimated mean (diamond), median (line), interquartile range (box) and range of peak forces (N) for synergistic arc of wrist motion. Dashed line represents the lower threshold of SEZ (1.3 N). A) Flexion/extension arc of motion; B) Ulnar/radial deviation arc of motion. (Reprinted from Rappaport PO, Thoreson AR, Yang T-H, et al. Effect of wrist and interphalangeal thumb movement on zone T2 flexor pollicis longus tendon tension in a human cadaver model. *J Hand Ther.* 2015;28:347-355, with permission from Hanley & Belfus.)

thumb positioning) sans IP motion, and (3) how the repair site tension varied across the arc of IP active motion with the joints proximal to the IP fixated. Exploring these aims will assist in the design of early passive and active mobilization protocols, which are grounded in FPL mechanics and not based on inferences made from biomechanical studies of finger flexor tendon repairs.

The authors' main findings are as follows (Figs 5-9):

1. Passive IP motion with the MP extended, CMC in 30° or 40° of radial abduction, and wrist in 30° of extension will generate sufficient forces to create tendon glide yet not exceed the strength of FPL repairs performed using a modified Kessler suture technique. Positioning of the wrist in

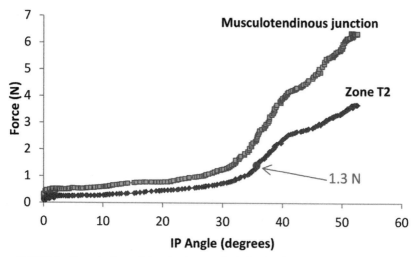

FIGURE 7.—Example of recorded tendon forces as the IP flexed in response to gentle graduated force applied at the musculotendinous junction. For this trial, the 1.3 N threshold in zone T2 was crossed at a measured IP flexion angle of 36° (red dot). (For interpretation of the references to color in this figure legend, the reader is referred to the web version of this article.) (Reprinted from Rappaport PO, Thoreson AR, Yang T-H, et al. Effect of wrist and interphalangeal thumb movement on zone T2 flexor pollicis longus tendon tension in a human cadaver model. *J Hand Ther.* 2015;28:347-355, with permission from Hanley & Belfus.)

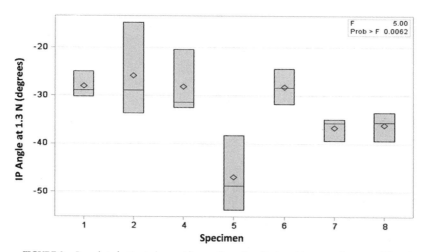

FIGURE 8.—Box plot of estimated mean (diamond), median (line), and interquartile range of IP angles (box) at which each specimen crossed the lower SEZ threshold of 1.3 N during induced active IP motion. (Reprinted from Rappaport PO, Thoreson AR, Yang T-H, et al. Effect of wrist and interphalangeal thumb movement on zone T2 flexor pollicis longus tendon tension in a human cadaver model. *J Hand Ther.* 2015;28:347-355, with permission from Hanley & Belfus.)

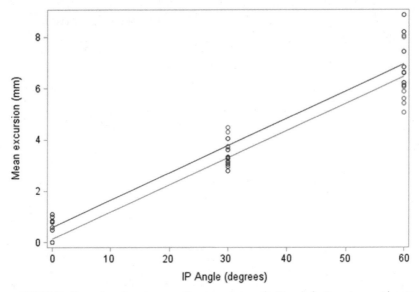

FIGURE 9.—Regression of specimen-specific mean values on the IP angle for 8 specimens with wrist neutral (blue) and wrist 30° extension (red). (For interpretation of the references to color in this figure legend, the reader is referred to the web version of this article.) (Reprinted from Rappaport PO, Thoreson AR, Yang T-H, et al. Effect of wrist and interphalangeal thumb movement on zone T2 flexor pollicis longus tendon tension in a human cadaver model. *J Hand Ther.* 2015;28:347-355, with permission from Hanley & Belfus.)

flexion or deviation did not allow for force generation necessary to overcome passive resistance to glide and 60° of wrist extension resulted in forces that exceed the tensile strength of modified Kessler suturing.

2. In the absence of IP joint motion, the effect of tenodesis (ie, wrist posturing in flexion/extension or ulnar/radial deviation) on FPL tension at T2 did not appear to exceed the forces required to exceed passive resistance to gliding; however, the position of the CMC joint in greater radial abduction (40° vs 30°) did have a significant effect on the forced acting on the FPL with an extension/flexion arc of wrist motion.

3. With the wrist and thumb MP in neutral and thumb CMC in 30° radial abduction, the FPL would, on average, actively generate enough force to exceed passive resistance to gliding on reaching 33° of IP active flexion.

4. With tension within the safe and effective zone, FPL excursion at T2 would exceed the gliding distance believed to sufficiently prevent adhesion development[4,5] (2 mm) when the IP joint passively flexed to 30° in a neutral or slightly extended (30°) wrist. Excursion of the FPL did not appear to be impacted by more or less (40° vs 30°) radial abduction; however, when the wrist was placed in 30° of extension, tendon glide was, on average, 0.5 mm greater than when the wrist was placed in neutral.

Based on the findings the authors recommend the following rehabilitative protocol:

1. Full passive IP range of motion (0° ext → flexion → 0° ext) with the wrist in 30° of extension, the CMC in 30° of radial abduction, and the MP in full extension. This would be accomplished within the confines of a forearm-based dorsal blocking orthosis with a thumb MP blocking component. Care should be taken to avoid IP hyperextension.

2. A tenodesis-style orthosis, like what is used in early active motion protocols[6,7] for finger flexor tendon repairs, in which the wrist is hinged but limited to 60° of extension, and the thumb IP, MP, and CMC joints are placed in a relaxed position will not necessarily result in the tension needed to overcome frictional resistance to gliding.

3. Early active motion of the IP joint should be initiated 3 to 5 days postoperatively up until 4 weeks. With these exercises, the CMC should be placed in 30° of radial abduction and the MP in full extension. Unlike the IP passive motion exercises, the wrist should be placed into a neutral position during active IP flexion, and the arc of movement should be limited from 0° extension to 30° flexion. This might be also be accomplished within the confines of a dorsal blocking orthosis with a hinged wrist to accommodate the variable wrist positions needed to perform passive and active IP exercises.

This cadaveric study proposes new rehabilitation strategies for consideration after zone T2 FPL repairs involving use of a modified Kessler suturing technique. Protocols involving a stronger repair might vary in terms of the permitted arc of IP active motion. Future study in human subjects is justified and might include comparative effectiveness trials in which the novel program is compared with other standard approaches.

C. McGee, PhD, OTR/L, CHT

References

1. Kutsumi K, Amadio PC, Zhao C, Zobitz ME, An KN. Gliding resistance of the flexor pollicis longus tendon after repair: does partial excision of the oblique pulley affect gliding resistance? *Plast Reconstr Surg.* 2006;118:1423-1428 [discussion: 1429-30].
2. Buonocore S, Sawh-Martinez R, Emerson JW, Mohan P, Dymarczyk M, Thomson JG. The effects of edema and self-adherent wrap on the work of flexion in a cadaveric hand. *J Hand Surg Am.* 2012;37:1349-1355.
3. Brown CP, McGrouther DA. The excursion of the tendon of flexor pollicis longus and its relation to dynamic splintage. *J Hand Surg Am.* 1984;9:787-791.
4. Gelberman RH, Boyer MI, Brodt MD, Winters SC, Silva MJ. The effect of gap formation at the repair site on the strength and excursion of intrasynovial flexor tendons. An experimental study on the early stages of tendon-healing in dogs. *J Bone Joint Surg Am.* 1999;81:975-982.
5. Silva MJ, Boyer MI, Gelberman RH. Recent progress in flexor tendon healing. *J Orthop Sci.* 2002;7:508-514.
6. Elliot D, Moiemen NS, Flemming AS, Harris SB, Foster AJ. The rupture rate of acute flexor tendon repairs mobilized by the controlled active motion regimen. *J Hand Surg Am.* 1994;19B:607-612.
7. Silverskiöld K, May E. Flexor tendon repair in zone II a new suture technique and an early mobilization program combining passive and active flexion. *J Hand Surg Am.* 1994;19A:53-60.

Stenosing flexor tenosynovitis: Validity of standard assessment tools of daily functioning and quality of life
Langer D, Luria S, Bar-Haim Erez A, et al (Hadassah and Hebrew Univ, Jerusalem, Israel; Hadassah-Hebrew Univ Med Ctr, Jerusalem, Israel; Ono Academic College, Kiryat-Ono, Israel; et al)
J Hand Ther 28:384-388, 2015

Study Design.—Cross-sectional.
Introduction.—Stenosing flexor tenosynovitis (SFT) is a common hand disease, yet there is a lack of valid standard assessments for this population.
Purpose of the Study.—Validation of assessment for the evaluation of disability and quality of life related to SFT clinical severity.
Methods.—Sixty five participants with SFT were matched to 71 controls. Participant's symptoms were graded using the Quinnell classification. Disability and quality of life were evaluated using the DASH and WHOQOL-BREF questionnaires.
Results.—Small to moderate correlations were found between SFT grade and the DASH and WHOQOL-BREF. Both questionnaires differentiated between the first and third clinical grades and between SFT and healthy groups.
Discussion.—Both questionnaires are useful tools to distinguish between participants with SFT and controls and between mild and severe clinical grades.
Conclusion.—The DASH and WHOQOL-BREF may be implemented in the clinical management and research of SFT.
Level of Evidence.—Diagnostic III.

▶ The authors of this study sought to establish if an upper limb disability index (Disabilities of the Arm, Shoulder, and Hand questionnaire [DASH]) and a quality-of-life (QOL) measure (short version of The World Health Organization Quality of Life questionnaire [WHOQOL-BREF]) can produce composite scores that reflect differences (1) between those with and without stenosing flexor tenosynovitis (SFT) and (2) among those with variable condition severity. The authors do not describe the criteria by which a diagnosis was rendered but used the Quinnell grading system to describe the severity of those with the condition. It is presumed that those with normal movement of all digits, or a Quinnell score of zero for each digit, were those without the condition and all of those who had at least 1 digit with a Quinnell score of 1 or greater carried the diagnosis.

The authors report statistically significant differences in QOL and upper limb disability between persons with SFT and their age- and gender-matched controls. Beyond this, the authors report that the WHOQOL-BREF could distinguish (1) between a person with "uneven movement" (Quinnell grade 1) and one with "passively correctable locking" (Quinnell grade 3) and (2) between those with "actively correctable locking" (Quinnell grade 2) and Quinnell grade 3. Additionally, they report that the DASH can distinguish between those with Quinnell grades 1 and 3. These findings validate that these tools are responsive to change as SFT progresses, most notably as the condition advances from an early to late phase. Of some importance, although of lesser emphasis in the article, is that SFT disease advancement has large effects (2 > 0.138) on QOL and medium (2 > 0.059) effects on upper limb disability as per Cohen.[1] Although omitted in the discussion, it should be noted that the differences in DASH scores between those with grade 1 and 3 Quinnell scores exceed the DASH's average minimal clinically important difference (MCID) of 18 points[2]; this would imply that there are clinically meaningful differences in disability as the condition progresses from early to later stages; however, a cohort study would better substantiate this observation. Currently, the MCID is not known for the WHOQOL-BREF, and thus, the clinically meaningfulness of these QOL differences is unknown.

There is now evidence to support that these tools might be used to measure the intended constructs in persons with SFT. Moreover, it seems that the WHOQOL-BREF survey may be more responsive to differences between intermediate and later stages of the condition than is the DASH. Lastly, there is now descriptive evidence to support that QOL is largely negatively impacted with progression of SFT. Future research should include testing the tool's psychometrics in this population (eg, MCID, and response stability) and cohort studies and intervention trials so as to measure these tools' within-patient responsiveness to change.

In terms of study limitations, it should be acknowledged that the authors use a condition severity scale that is not commonly accepted as being gold standard and do not report on the QOL and upper limb disability of persons with fixed deformities related to SFT (Quinnell grade 4). Additionally, the sample sizes for the Quinnell grades 1 and 3 strata were notably smaller than was the sample size for the grade 2 strata and, thus, the findings should be interpreted with some caution.

C. McGee, PhD, OTR/L, CHT

References

1. Cohen J. *Statistical Power Analysis for the Behavioral Sciences.* 2nd ed. Hillsdale, NJ: Erlbaum Associates; 1988:567.
2. Beaton DE, Katz JN, Fossel AH, Wright JG, Tarasuk V, Bombardier C. Measuring the whole or the parts? Validity, reliability, and responsiveness of the disabilities of the arm, shoulder, and hand outcome measure in different regions of the upper extremity. *J Hand Ther.* 2001;14:128-146.

Single-Stage Flexor Tendon Grafting: Refining the Steps
Fletcher DR, McClinton MA (MedStar Union Memorial Hosp, Baltimore, MD)
J Hand Surg Am 40:1452-1460, 2015

Single-stage tendon grafting for reconstruction of zone I and II flexor tendon injuries is a challenging procedure in hand surgery. Careful patient selection, strict indications, and adherence to sound surgical principles are mandatory for return of digital motion.

▶ Flexor tendon grafting remains a challenging procedure but is a useful technique. The authors offer guidance for appropriate indications, patient selection, and surgical technique to improve outcomes.

Indications for single-stage flexor tendon grafting are narrow. Delayed presentation of either flexor digitorum superficialis (FDS) or flexor digitorum profundus (FDP) laceration beyond 3 weeks, either intentional or unintentional, accompanied by degeneration of the cut tendon ends or myostatic contraction of the muscle belly may be treated with single-stage grafting. The authors also recommend the procedure be considered in patients with isolated FDP injuries who perform complex finger motions (eg, musicians). Finally, segmental tendon loss of the FDP or FDS will require tendon grafting.

Equally important is appropriate patient selection. The authors describe the ideal surgical candidate as possessing the following traits: (1) highly motivated to comply with postoperative rehabilitation, (2) injury severity of Boyes grade 1, (3) supple joints on the injured digit with full passive range of motion, (4) supple and adequate soft tissue coverage of all vital structures of the finger, (5) a well-perfused digit with at least 1 proper digital nerve intact, and (6) an intact flexor tendon sheath with minimal scarring and intact pulleys. If any of these conditions are absent, the authors recommend a 2-stage tendon reconstruction.

The technique is described in detail (p 1453). The authors prefer to secure the tendon graft outside of the tendon sheath on both ends, over the distal

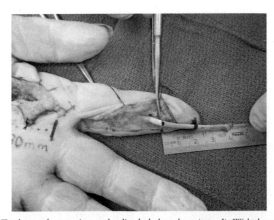

FIGURE 8.—Tendon graft excursion at the distal phalanx base (zone I). With the proximal tenorrhaphy completed, a reference skin mark is made adjacent to the insertion point of the Mini Micro Mitek anchors. Next, with the wrist in neutral position, the finger straight, and the muscle-tendon graft unit in its relaxed position, the tendon graft is marked at the level of the reference skin marking. The muscle-tendon graft unit is then maximally stretched in a distal fashion and a second tendon marking is made at the level of the skin reference point. The interval length between the first (distal) and second (proximal) tendon markings denotes the degree of excursion at the distal juncture. The length of muscle-tendon graft unit excursion at the level of the distal phalanx base is typically 20 mm. (Reprinted from Fletcher DR, McClinton MA. Single-stage flexor tendon grafting: refining the steps. *J Hand Surg Am.* 2015;40:1452-1460, with permission from American Society for Surgery of the Hand.)

phalanx and in the palm or at the wrist, to mitigate the risk of adhesion formation. Midlateral incision is recommended whenever possible. The tendon sheath should be preserved. Undamaged FDS tendons are left alone, and damaged FDS tendons are excised, leaving the distal 1.5 cm as a gliding bed for the tendon graft. The A5 pulley is divided, and a 1-cm stump of FDP is preserved.

The preferred donor tendons and graft harvesting techniques are detailed (p 1454). A chilled pediatric catheter is passed from proximal to distal, and the tendon graft is sutured to the proximal end and drawn distally until the graft is positioned within the flexor sheath. The authors first secure the proximal juncture, preferring the Pulvertaft tendon weave and 5 passes. The tendon excursion is then estimated by marking the tendon at the skin when the muscle is fully relaxed and the wrist is in neutral. The muscle-tendon unit is then maximally stretched, and a second mark is made at the level of the palmar skin. The excursion is approximately half the distance between the 2 marks. Optimal motor function is obtained if the estimated excursion is at least 30 mm (Fig 8).

The distal juncture is then secured using 2 small bone anchors with a modified Bunnell suture technique. The graft is tensioned to maximize functional tendon excursion. A dorsal blocking splint is applied and the postoperative rehab protocol is described (p 1458). Complications and their management are discussed in detail (p 1459).

K. Kollitz, MD

Zone III flexor tendon injuries — A proposed modification to rehabilitation
Chinchalkar SJ, Pipicelli JG, Agur A, et al (St. Joseph's Health Care, London, Ontario, Canada; The Univ of Toronto, Canada; et al)
J Hand Ther 28:319-324, 2015

In this manuscript, these authors have utilized years of clinical experience to suggest rehabilitation modifications for Zone III flexor tendon injuries.

▶ The authors of study sought to reproduce, in cadaveric specimens, the complications experienced by hand therapists and surgeons following zone III flexor tendon repairs. Historically, zone III repairs are treated postsurgically as if they are no different than a zone I or II injury; however, based on the authors' clinical experiences, there seems to be some pathomechanical nuances to consider following a zone III repair. These nuances, specifically limitations in proximal interphalangeal (PIP)/distal interphalangeal (DIP) extension and tethered long and ring finger flexion/extension, are presumed to be related to (1) lumbrical and flexor digitorum superficialis (FDS)/flexor digitorum profundus (FDP) adherence and (2) long and ring finger FDS adherence, respectively; however, these mechanisms had not yet been validated via cadaveric study.

As expected, simulating adhesions resulting from a distal zone III repair through suturing a lumbrical muscle to the FDS and FDP tendons proximal to the A1 pulley resulted in restricted digital PIP and DIP passive extension. Likewise, simulating adhesions resulting from a proximal zone III repair through suturing together long and ring finger FDS tendons resulted in the inability of these 2 digits to independently flex or extend relative to the other. The functional consequences of such are likely (1) limited capacity to grasp large-diameter objects because of limited extension and (2) challenges with motoric separation of the ulnar and radial sides of the hand during prehension and isolating the long finger for a faux pas gesture of hostility!

Based on these validations, for distal zone III repairs, the authors propose gradual adjustments to wrist and metacarpophalangeal positioning within a dorsal blocking orthosis for the first 4 to 6 weeks to gradually promote increased glide of the long finger flexors. In addition, they suggest a tenodesis/place-and-hold program combined with gradually incorporating active and later resisted digital extension exercises within confines of the blocking orthosis to recruit the lumbricals to offer tension to any forming musculotendonous adhesions 4 to 8 weeks post repair.

For proximal zone III repairs, the authors also recommend gradual weekly progression of wrist positioning from 30° of flexion into slight extension through serial modifications to dorsal blocking orthosis. In addition to tenodesis/place-and-hold exercises, the authors recommend use of isolated finger active extension within the confines of orthosis in the first month, progressing into composite wrist and digital active range of motion within orthosis in month number 2, and later progressing into resisted isolated digital extension and flexion exercises.

These protocols differ from others in that there are serial adjustments made to a dorsal blocking orthosis up until orthosis discontinuation to better enhance tendon glide and lumbrical muscle tension to prevent musculo-tendious and intertendinous adhesions. Beyond this, additional focus is placed on facilitating the excursion of the lumbrical muscle and differential tendon glide of the long finger flexors through exercise within the blocking orthosis.

These are novel recommendations and are deserving of additional exploration. Additional study should include comparative effectiveness trials in which more traditional zone I through III protocols are compared with a zone III—specific protocol such as was proposed by the authors.

C. McGee, PhD, OTR/L, CHT

Biomechanical Study of the Digital Flexor Tendon Sliding Lengthening Technique

Hashimoto K, Kuniyoshi K, Suzuki T, et al (Chiba Univ, Japan)
J Hand Surg Am 40:1981-1985, 2015

Purpose.—To compare the mechanical properties of sliding lengthening (SL) and Z-lengthening (ZL) for flexor tendon elongation used for conditions such as Volkmann contracture, cerebral palsy, and poststroke spasticity.

Methods.—We harvested 56 flexor tendons, including flexor pollicis longus tendons, flexor digitorum superficialis tendons (zones II to IV), and flexor digitorum profundus tendons (zones II to V) from 24 upper limbs of 12 fresh cadavers. Each tendon was harvested together with its homonymous tendon from the opposite side of the cadaver and paired. We used 28 pairs of tendons and divided them randomly into 4 groups depending on the lengthening distance (20 or 30 mm) and type of stitching (single or double mattress sutures). Then we divided each pair into either the SL or ZL group. Each group was composed of 7 specimens. The same surgeon lengthened all tendons and stitched them with 2-0 polyester sutures. We tested biomechanical tensile strength immediately after completing lengthening and suturing in each group.

Results.—Ultimate tensile strengths were: 23 N for the SL 20-mm lengthening and single mattress suture and 7 N for the ZL; 25 N for the SL 20-mm lengthening and double mattress suture and 10 N for the ZL; 15 N for the SL 30-mm lengthening and single mattress suture and 8 N for the ZL; and 18 N for the SL 30-mm lengthening and double mattress suture and 10 N for the ZL.

Conclusions.—The SL technique may be a good alternative to the ZL technique because it provides higher ultimate tensile strength.

Clinical Relevance.—Because of its higher ultimate tensile strength, the SL technique may allow for earlier rehabilitation and reduced risk of postoperative complications.

▶ The authors have shown that if some intratendinous connections are left intact, the ultimate tensile strength of what they refer to as a sliding-lengthening technique, reinforced by either 1 or 2 sutures, is increased over a more standard z-lengthening with 1 or 2 sutures. However, the tensile strength of the sliding-lengthening does not give confidence that this procedure will safely tolerate early active movement. The authors refer to articles describing tendon repair techniques that provide, ex vivo, more resistance to rupture, but these techniques are more designed for end-to-end repair of lacerated flexor tendons. They fail to refer to the study of Friden and Lieber,[1] which described a suture technique very appropriate for tendon lengthening and with a much higher rupture resistance.

V. R. Hentz, MD

Reference

1. Brown SH, Hentzen ER, Kwan A, Ward SR, Fridén J, Lieber RL. Mechanical strength of the side-to-side versus Pulvertaft weave tendon repair. *J Hand Surg Am.* 2010;35:540-545.

The Effect of 1-Ethyl-3-(3-Dimethylaminopropyl) Carbodiimide Suture Coating on Tendon Repair Strength and Cell Viability in a Canine Model

Thoreson AR, Hiwatari R, An K-N, et al (Mayo Clinic, Rochester, MN)
J Hand Surg Am 40:1986-1991, 2015

Purpose.—To determine if impregnating a suture with a cross-linking agent, 1-ethyl-3-(3-dimethylaminopropyl) carbodiimide hydrochloride (EDC), improved suture pull-out strength and cell viability.

Methods.—Canine flexor digitorum profundus tendons were cut in canine zone D, and a single suture loop was placed in each end, with sutures soaked in either saline or an EDC solution with a concentration of 1%, 10%, or 50%. Suture pull-out strength, stiffness, and elongation to failure was determined by pulling the loop until failure. Cytotoxicity of the EDC treatment was evaluated by suspending treated sutures over cultured tenocytes.

Results.—Mechanical properties for the EDC-treated side were improved over controls when treated with the 10% and 50% EDC solutions. The ratio of dead to live cells was significantly increased at all distances from the suture for the 50% EDC-treated group.

Conclusions.—Suture treated with a 10% EDC solution provided the best combination of mechanical reinforcement and limited toxicity.

Clinical Relevance.—Sutures so treated may improve the ability of a tendon repair to sustain early mobilization.

▶ Tendon rupture during rehabilitation after repair is still a concern in flexor tendon surgery. Methods to increase the repair strength provide a higher theoretical safety margin for rehabilitation. The usual methods to achieve this are by modifying the repair technique and adding more sutures across the repair site.

This work takes a different tack. It explores a chemical adjunctive method to improve tendon repair, while leaving the option for combination with biological adjuncts such as cell therapy still open. Their findings provide a useful start point for future work. The authors found an improvement in repair strength for both the 10% and 50% 1-ethyl-3-(3-dimethylaminopropyl) carbodiimide hydrochloride (EDC) groups. The 10% EDC group did not appear to have an effect on viability of cells. This suggested that 10% EDC provided the best balance of effects.

Although pull-through strength is increased, this method does not address the issue of suture breakage. It is also not clear how this technique affects other conditions such as the gliding resistance. Because this is an in vitro study, the biological changes that might affect this treatment are also unknown.

A. Chong, MD

Biomechanical Analysis of the Modified Kessler, Lahey, Adelaide, and Becker Sutures for Flexor Tendon Repair

Jordan MC, Schmitt V, Jansen H, et al (Univ Hosp, Wuerzburg, Germany)

J Hand Surg Am 40:1812-1817, 2015

Purpose.—To compare the biomechanical properties of the modified Kessler, Lahey, Adelaide, and Becker repairs, which are marked by either a locking-loop or a cross-lock configuration.

Methods.—Ninety-six lacerated porcine flexor tendons were repaired using the respective core suture and an epitendinous repair. Biomechanical testing was conducted under static and cyclic loads. Parameters of interest were 2-mm gap formation force, displacement during different loads, stiffness, maximum force, and mode of failure.

Results.—The meaningful gap formation occurred in all 4 repairs at similar tension loads without any significant differences. Maximum force was highest in the Becker repair with a considerable difference compared with the modified Kessler and Lahey sutures. The Adelaide repair showed the highest stiffness. Overall, the displacement during cyclic loading demonstrated similar results with an exception between the Lahey and the Adelaide repairs at 10 N load. Failure by suture pull-out occurred in 42% in the modified Kessler, in 38% in the Lahey, and in 4% in the Adelaide repairs. The Becker repair failed only by suture rupture.

Conclusions.—The results of our study suggest that the difference between the 4-strand repairs with a cross-lock or a locking-loop configuration is minor in regard to gap formation. A strong epitendinous suture and the application of core suture pretension might prevent differences in gapping. However, the modified Kessler and Lahey repairs had an inferior maximum tensile strength and were prone to early failure caused by the narrow locking loops with their limited locking power.

Clinical Relevance.—We suggest that surgeons should use pre-tension in repaired tendons to improve gap resistance and should avoid narrow locking loop anchoring to the tendon.

▶ In 2012, my colleague Ya Fang Wu and I published a study showing the role of pretensioning of the tendon repair site in minimizing gapping.[1] This was followed by several studies in which the effect of pretensioning was confirmed and reemphasized. Adding pretension to the repair site has become an important consideration in tendon repair, perhaps as important as placing a peripheral suture. The present study by Jordon et al reconfirmed this important point, and this is the most important message of the article.

I strongly believe that some degree of pretension at the repair site is necessary and even vital to tendon healing. In performing an end-to-end tendon repair, surgeons cannot avoid slight bulkiness at the repair site, which actually does not greatly interfere with tendon gliding. However, tendon twisting and more notable bulkiness at the repair site should be avoided. Clinically, I suggest about 10% shortening of the length of the tendon segment after placement of core suture strands into it. This degree of shortening generates pretension to resist gapping, but it will not cause remarkable bulkiness at the repair site. I perform zone 1 to 3 primary repairs with this degree of pretension. A tension-free approach is harmful because the repair site can gap easily (or be caught on pulley edges) when the tendon is tensioned by muscle contracture and gliding during early active digital motion.

In repairing tendon, it is good repair principles that should matter, not a particular suture configuration. Different surgeons actually use different suture configurations. In other words, many methods can yield a good repair if the design fulfills several essential requirements: (1) sufficient number of core suture across the repair site; (2) sufficient core suture purchase at each site; (3) core suture caliber is either 4-0 or 3-0; (4) pretension added at the repair site; (5) not too bulky; and (6) sufficient size of locked area when a locking suture is used. The findings by Jordon et al show nicely that different suture configurations can all create reliable repairs if the preceding requirements are met.

I should also draw the attention of readers to a finding of this study: a higher rate of suture pullout in repairs with locking tendon-suture anchors with small locks in the tendon, which indicates these locks were actually too small and not secure enough to hold the tendon. This finding highlights the importance of sufficient lock size. In other words, we should not be fooled by using a locking suture if the lock size is too small; it cannot secure the tendon substance! A locking suture can add strength to a repair only when it is large and deep enough. This is a vital technical point in making a secure lock in the tendon.

J. B. Tang, MD, PhD

Reference

1. Wu YF, Tang JB. Effects of tension across the tendon repair site on tendon gap and ultimate strength. *J Hand Surg Am.* 2012;37:906-912.

A Mechanical Evaluation of Zone II Flexor Tendon Repair Using a Knotless Barbed Suture Versus a Traditional Braided Suture

Nayak AN, Nguyen D-V, Brabender RC, et al (Foundation for Orthopaedic Res & Education, Tampa, FL; Florida Orthopaedic Inst, Tampa; et al)
J Hand Surg Am 40:1355-1362, 2015

Purpose.—To determine repair site bulk, gliding resistance, work of flexion, and 1-mm gap formation force in zone II flexor tendon lacerations repaired with knotless barbed or traditional braided suture.

Methods.—Transverse zone II lacerations of the flexor digitorum profundus (FDP) tendon were created in 36 digits from 6 matched human cadaveric pairs. Repair was performed with 2-0 barbed suture ($n = 18$) or 3-0 polyethylene braided suture ($n = 18$). Pre- and postrepair cross-sectional area was measured followed by quantification of gliding resistance and work of flexion during cyclic flexion-extension loading at

10 mm/min. Thereafter, the repaired tendons were loaded to failure. The force at 1 mm of gap formation was recorded.

Results.—Repaired FDP tendon cross-sectional area increased significantly from intact, with no difference noted between suture types. Gliding resistance and work of flexion were significantly higher for both suture repairs; however, we identified no significant differences in either nondestructive biomechanical parameters between repair types. Average 1-mm gap formation force with the knotless barbed suture (52 N) was greater than that of the traditional braided suture (43 N).

Conclusions.—We identified no significant advantage in using knotless barbed suture for zone II FDP repair in our primary, nondestructive mechanical outcomes in this *in vitro* study.

Clinical Relevance.—*In vivo* studies may be warranted to determine if one suture method has an advantage with respect to the parameters tested at 4, 6, and 12 plus weeks postrepair and the degree of adhesion formation. The combined laboratory and clinical data, in additional to cost considerations, may better define the role of barbed knotless suture for zone II flexor tendon repair.

▶ Barbed suture materials were first developed half a century ago, but they have never been popular in tendon repair. This study examined gap resistance and ultimate strength of a tendon repaired with a knotless barbed suture material and compared them with those repaired using a conventional braided suture material. I am not surprised at the results: no significant difference in the bulkiness of the repair site, gliding resistance, or gap resistance between the 2 repairs.

In recent years, I have read a few reports on experimental studies on barbed sutures and wondered why these materials still attract the attention of investigators. This suture material has been in existence for 50 years and has already been studied extensively; it seems unnecessary to continue to study this well-tested material.

I use common and basic suture materials, such as looped nylon suture or coated nylon (eg, Ethilon), in repairing zone 2 flexor tendons. By creating proper configurations of suture passage in the tendon and ensuring a sufficient number of core suture strands across the repair site, the outcomes of repair have been quite good. I do not feel a particular need to search for better materials. Of course, if much stronger and easily usable suture materials become available, I will certainly use them. However, I do not think I will adopt new materials that offer no significant (or only slight) improvement in repair strength. The data reported thus far show that barbed materials do not substantially enhance the strength of tendon repair. Therefore, I feel that it is not a good use of our hand surgeons' time and efforts to continue testing barbed sutures.

I believe that any basic science investigations should be directed to difficult problems currently lacking good solutions. A study may result in publication of a paper, but sometimes it may not be worth the effort and time because there are many other more pressing or important topics to be investigated. I applaud the authors of this article and other 3 papers[1,2] in 2015 for publishing their studies with negative findings, which may avoid spending time in the search for ideal repair materials in the direction of a barbed suture.

J. B. Tang, MD, PhD

References

1. Ben-Amotz O, Kargel J, Mailey B, Sammer DM. The effect of barbed suture tendon repair on work of flexion. *J Hand Surg Am*. 2015;40:969-974.
2. Maddox GE, Ludwig J, Craig ER, et al. Flexor tendon repair with a knotless, bidirectional barbed suture: an in vivo biomechanical analysis. *J Hand Surg Am*. 2015; 40:963-968.

Single-Stage Flexor Tendon Grafting: Refining the Steps
Fletcher DR, McClinton MA (MedStar Union Memorial Hosp, Baltimore, MD)
J Hand Surg Am 40:1452-1460, 2015

Single-stage tendon grafting for reconstruction of zone I and II flexor tendon injuries is a challenging procedure in hand surgery. Careful patient selection, strict indications, and adherence to sound surgical principles are mandatory for return of digital motion.

▶ Single-stage tendon grafting is commonly called "tendon grafting." If tendon reconstruction requires multiple surgical procedures in 2 or more stages, the surgery is called "staged tendon reconstruction." It is not common to add "single-stage" before conventional tendon grafting. This review article describes the indications, procedures, pearls, and pitfalls of the well-described surgical procedure of secondary tendon grafting. I find the contents of this review quite standard with few controversies because this procedure is a classical method.

I use tendon grafting in cases with the same indications the authors describe, and my surgical methods are similar as well. The pulleys and sheath should be preserved as much as possible, and tension should be set to the grafted tendon to maintain partial digital flexion after making the proximal junction with an interweaving repair. I urge patients to perform partial early active motion after surgery, which helps reduce the risk of interphalangeal joint stiffness and improves tendon gliding. The palmaris longus tendon is used in almost all my cases.

I feel it is worth mentioning here a controversial procedure, primary tendon grafting, which is largely not used outside of Russia. In a few recent meetings in Europe, however, Russian surgeons reported its outcomes and proposed this unusual method in zone 2 primary flexor tendon repairs. They suggested its use in cases that would be repairable with direct end-to-end tendon repair. I think they are wrong. Primary tendon repair in the digital area has demonstrated far better outcomes than secondary tendon grafting. The reported outcomes of primary tendon grafting are generally worse than primary end-to-end repair. I am against the use of primary tendon grafting in zone 2 tendon repair.

J. B. Tang, MD, PhD

Comparison of Flexor Tendon Suture Techniques Including 1 Using 10 Strands

Lee HI, Lee JS, Kim TH, et al (Univ of Ulsan College of Medicine, Gangneung, Korea; Chung-Ang Univ, Seoul, Korea; et al)

J Hand Surg Am 40:1369-1376, 2015

Purpose.—To compare mechanical properties of a multistrand suture technique for flexor tendon repair with those of conventional suture methods through biomechanical and clinical studies.

Methods.—We describe a multistrand suture technique that is readily expandable from 6 to 10 strands of core suture. For biomechanical evaluation, 60 porcine flexor tendons were repaired using 1 of the following 6 suture techniques: Kessler (2-strand), locking cruciate (4-strand), Lim/Tsai's 6-strand, and our modified techniques (6-, 8-, or 10-strand). Structural properties of each tenorrhaphy were determined through tensile testing (ultimate failure load and force at 2-mm gap formation). Clinically we repaired 25 flexor tendons using the described 10-strand technique in zones I and II. Final follow-up results were evaluated according to the criteria of Strickland and Glogovac.

Results.—In the biomechanical study, tensile properties were strongly affected by repair technique; tendons in the 10-strand group had approximately 106%, 66%, and 39% increased ultimate load to failure (average, 87 N) compared with those in the 4-, 6-, and 8-strand groups, respectively. Tendons in the 10-strand group withstood higher 2-mm gap formation forces (average, 41 N) than those with other suture methods (4-strand, 26 N; 6-strand, 27 N; and 8-strand, 33 N). Clinically, we obtained 21 excellent, 2 good, and 2 fair outcomes after a mean of 16 months (range, 6—53 mo) of follow-up. No patients experienced poor results or rupture.

Conclusions.—The 10-strand suture repair technique not only increased ultimate strength and force at the 2-mm gap formation compared with conventional suture methods, it also showed good clinical outcomes. This multistrand suture technique can greatly increase the gap resistance of surgical repair, facilitating early mobilization of the affected digit.

Type of Study/Level of Evidence.—Therapeutic IV.

▶ From the early description of flexor tendon repair in zone II, researchers have sought to determine the technique that is strong enough for early active motion and can consistently produce excellent outcomes. Previous research has demonstrated that increasing core strand size and increasing the number of strands across the repair site produce stronger time 0 repair strength in a porcine model. The authors have demonstrated that their technique using up to 10 strands with a single knot within the tendon is relatively straightforward to perform and had the greatest 2-mm gap formation at time 0 and ultimate failure. They also resport good clinical outcomes in their series of 25 zone II flexor tendon repairs. They used a looped suture, which places each "pair" of sutures in the same area with in the suture, which is likely not the same as 2 separate sites within the tendon but may effectively increase the size of the tendon.

They tested the load for 2-mm gap formation and the ultimate failure. They did not describe the method of failure: suture pull out, suture rupture, knot unraveling. They did not evaluate the effect of increased number of sutures on the bulk of the repair or the extent to which the increased number of repairs has on gliding coefficient in a cadaver model. Although this repair is stronger than many others, we are still unable to accelerate the accrual of strength following flexor tendon repair, so therapy programs will continue to play a vital role in achieving the best outcomes. Clinically there are numerous factors beyond control of the surgeon that can affect outcomes (eg, patient compliance, edema, adhesion formation, pain limiting participation in rehabilitation, decreased gliding through pulleys).

Although we may be close to the limits of what we can study to the increase the strength of flexor tendon repairs, this new technique is worth considering because it increases the time 0 strength of the repair and appears straightforward to perform clinically.

W. C. Hammert, MD

Risk Assessment of Tendon Attrition Following Treatment of Distal Radius Fractures With Volar Locking Plates Using Audible Crepitus and Placement of the Plate: A Prospective Clinical Cohort Study
Yamazaki H, Uchiyama S, Komatsu M, et al (Aizawa Hosp, Matsumoto, Japan; Shinshu Univ School of Medicine, Matsumoto, Japan)
J Hand Surg Am 40:1571-1581, 2015

Purpose.—To identify risk factors for tendon attrition after volar locking plate fixation of distal radius fractures.

Methods.—We prospectively assessed attrition of the flexor pollicis longus tendon at volar plate removal in 127 hands in 126 patients. We also evaluated preoperative lateral wrist radiographs, sonographs, and crepitus with flexor pollicis longus tendon motion and compared the demographic and radiographic characteristics of patients with and without tendon attrition. Multivariate logistic regression analysis was employed to identify the factors independently associated with tendon attrition.

Results.—We found 12 cases of tendon attrition (10%) and 1 that presented with tendon rupture in our cohort. Crepitus was recognized in 14 patients (11%): 6 cases (50%) were among the 12 hands in 12 patients with tendon attrition whereas 8 (7%) were detected in the remaining 114 hands in 113 patients. Logistic regression examination revealed that audible crepitus and volar placement of the plate in lateral radiographs were independent predictors of tendon attrition.

Conclusions.—Crepitus and volar placement of hardware in lateral radiographs were independent risk factors for flexor tendon attrition after volar plating for distal radius fracture. These results may facilitate surgical decisions regarding early plate removal to prevent possible tendon rupture.

Type of Study/Level of Evidence.—Diagnostic II.

▶ The authors present a prospective study analyzing risk factors for tendon attrition after volar plating for distal radius fracture. Their hypothesis was that by identifying patients with crepitus during flexor pollicis longus motion, tendon rupture could be avoided by early hardware removal. Crepitus was identified by placing an electronic stethoscope 4 cm proximal to the patient's distal wrist crease and evaluating sounds (grinding, scraping, crackling, snapping, or gravel-like sounds) during thumb movement. The contralateral (nonfractured) wrists were evaluated as controls and were found to have "brushing or rustling" sounds during thumb movement. Crepitus was absent if the sounds were similar between sides. Ultrasounds were performed to evaluate the flexor pollicis longus during thumb motion and to evaluate for synovial thickening of the tendon. The authors found significantly more patients exhibiting crepitus with thumb motion in tendons with attritional findings compared with those without attrition. In addition, the interobserver reliability was 0.73. On ultrasound, patients with attrition had a significantly higher frequency of synovial thickening compared with tendons without attrition. Currently in my practice, at the final follow-up visit, I educate my patients as to the risks of tendon attrition and rupture, both on the flexor and extensor sides. When performing the surgery, I pay close attention to plate placement and make sure the plate does not lie distal to the watershed line. If a patient does present with crepitus, I evaluate his or her tendon with a dynamic ultrasound. At this time, I do not incorporate auditory evaluation of crepitance in my practice, but if future studies confirm these findings, this may provide cost savings for diagnosis of a preventable problem.

M. W. Kessler, MD, MPH

The Effect of the Epitendinous Suture on Gliding in a Cadaveric Model of Zone II Flexor Tendon Repair
Yaseen Z, English C, Stanbury SJ, et al (Univ of Rochester, NY)
J Hand Surg Am 40:1363-1368, 2015

Purpose.—We hypothesized that increasing core sutures (4–6) may be preferable in terms of gliding coefficient (GC) measurements when compared with adding an epitendinous suture to zone II flexor tendon repairs. We hypothesized that the inclusion of epitendinous suture in 2 standard repairs would contribute negatively to the GC of the repaired tendon.

Methods.—Nineteen fresh-frozen cadaveric fingers were used for testing. We compared a control group (dissected digits without repair) and 4-strand or 6-strand core tendon repairs with and without epitendinous suture. Arc of motion was driven by direct loading, and digital images were acquired and analyzed. Outcomes were defined as the difference in

GC between the native uninjured and the repaired state at each load. A linear mixed-model analysis was performed with comparisons between repairs to evaluate the statistically relevant differences between groups.

Results.—The test of fixed effects in the linear model revealed that repair type and the use of epitendinous suture significantly affected the change in GC. The addition of an epitendinous suture produced a significant decrement in gliding regardless of repair type.

Conclusions.—There was significant improvement in GC with the omission of the epitendinous suture in both repair types (4- or 6-strand).

Clinical Relevance.—The epitendinous suture used in this model resulted in poorer gliding of the repair, which may correspond with an expected increase in catching or triggering.

▶ This article discusses a perhaps important future topic: whether a strong core suture should be complemented by additional peripheral sutures. The present study was well designed and well performed, with clear clinical implications. I know some surgeons in Asia and Europe do not use peripheral sutures when they have placed a 6-strand core suture in the tendon, and their clinical outcomes are excellent. In fact, the present study shows that gliding resistance is increased significantly when peripheral sutures are added after a 4- or 6-strand core suture, and the addition of peripheral suture over a tendon with 4- or 6-strand repair might not be beneficial.

In vitro mechanical test data indicate that neither 4- nor 6-strand core sutures need peripheral sutures. However, I feel that for a 4-strand repair, a peripheral suture is still necessary, as I observed in patients that the tendon junction site is still rather easily movable when performing digital extension-flexion test. It is risky (even unacceptable in my view) to use only a 4-strand core suture without a peripheral suture. However, when 6-strand core sutures are used, adding a peripheral suture may not be necessary. A few of my colleagues do not use peripheral sutures with a 6-strand suture repair. In my practice, I tend to use a more secure approach; after I place a 6-strand core suture, I add 3 to 5 stitches of peripheral sutures to ensure that the 2 tendon cut surfaces approximate more smoothly. When a 6-strand core suture is used, I do not use complex peripheral sutures, and do not try to have many runs (eg, 7-8) of running peripheral sutures. Seven or eight runs are added only when the tendon ends are tidy and I can easily do so.

The simple running peripheral sutures described in textbooks are typical, but in practice, when a 6-strand repair is used, peripheral suture become less important; fewer runs can be used instead. Currently, only 1 or 2 reports have presented the outcomes of repair of zone 2 tendons with multistrand core sutures, without a peripheral suture. I look forward to more clinical reports on this subject. In addition, I found description of peripheral sutures in clinical reports generally lack sufficient details. Future clinical reports should give details of peripheral sutures, such as the number of runs, tensional status, and purchase length, because all of these would affect the efficacy of this repair component.

J. B. Tang, MD, PhD

Ultrasound-Guided Hyaluronic Acid Injections for Trigger Finger: A Double-Blinded, Randomized Controlled Trial

Liu D-H, Tsai M-W, Lin S-H, et al (Taipei Veterans General Hosp, Yilan, Taiwan; Natl Yang-Ming Univ, Taipei, Taiwan; et al)
Arch Phys Med Rehabil 96:2120-2127, 2015

Objectives.—To investigate the effects of ultrasound-guided injections of hyaluronic acid (HA) versus steroid for trigger fingers in adults.

Design.—Prospective, double-blinded, randomized controlled study.

Setting.—Tertiary care center.

Participants.—Subjects with a diagnosis of trigger finger (N = 36; 39 affected digits) received treatment and were evaluated.

Interventions.—Subjects were randomly assigned to HA and steroid injection groups. Both study medications were injected separately via ultrasound guidance with 1 injection.

Main Outcome Measures.—The classification of trigger grading, pain, functional disability, and patient satisfaction were evaluated before the injection and 3 weeks and 3 months after the injection.

Results.—At 3 months, 12 patients (66.7%) in the HA group and 17 patients (89.5%) in the steroid group exhibited no triggering of the affected fingers ($P = .124$). The treatment results at 3 weeks and 3 months showed similar changes in the Quinnell scale ($P = .057$ and .931, respectively). A statistically significant interaction effect between group and time was found for visual analog scale (VAS) and Michigan Hand Outcome Questionnaire (MHQ) evaluation ($P < .05$). The steroid group had a lower VAS at 3 months after injection (steroid 0.5 ± 1.1 vs HA 2.7 ± 2.4; $P < .001$). The HA group demonstrated continuing significant improvement in MHQ at 3 months (change from 3 wk: steroid -2.6 ± 14.1 vs HA 19.1 ± 37.0; $P = .023$; $d = .78$).

Conclusions.—Ultrasound-guided injection of HA demonstrated promising results for the treatment of trigger fingers. The optimal frequency, dosage, and molecular weight of HA injections for trigger fingers deserve further investigation for future clinical applications.

▶ This is a nice randomized study comparing 2 types of flexor tendon sheath injections for trigger fingers. The authors compare the standard steroid (triamcinolone) injection with hyaluronic acid (HA). Both are done under ultrasound guidance for accuracy, and follow-up is at 3 weeks and 3 months. Unfortunately, the authors try really hard to spine the data to indicate that the substances have relatively equal efficacy. They even try to say that HA gradually improves function over time.

However, patients are mainly concerned about whether they have relief of actual triggering. Using that measure alone, 90% of those getting steroid injections had relief at 3 months compared with only 67% of those receiving HA.

K. Bengston, MD

Self-regulated frequent power pinch exercises: A non-orthotic technique for the treatment of old mallet deformity

Macionis V (Vilnius Univ Hosp "Santariskiu Klinikos", Lithuania)
J Hand Ther 28:433-436, 2015

The utilization of an orthotic device to treat a mallet finger injury is common practice. This author describes a different approach to treating patients with an old mallet finger injury. The incorporation of frequent, self-regulated exercises without the use of an orthosis is described. — Victoria Priganc, PhD, OTR, CHT, CLT, Practice Forum Editor.

▶ This article introduces a novel approach to treating a mallet finger injury. Common and standard treatment of mallet deformities has been to use of orthotics to immobilize the distal interphalangeal (DIP) joint in extension. The author describes a technique to help avoid joint stiffness and other potential problems with standard orthotic treatment by using a self-directed power pinch throughout the day. The treatment is positioning the involved DIP joint in a power pinch or resting the digit on the table surface at frequent intervals during the day and nighttime as able. Limits of the clinical cases were in numbers of patients (6) in the trial and then only half of the patients available for follow-up, lack of control over exercise protocol, and probable results related to the effect of the central slip elongation. This elongation is caused by prolong flexion of the metacarpal and proximal interphalangeal joint and elongation of the central slip, thus, proximal slide of the terminal extensor. However, the study did have 1 case study with favorable results of a delayed or 3-week untreated mallet injury. It is my opinion that this may have some favorable exploration in the future with patients who refuse to comply with standard treatment with orthosis.

S. Kranz, OTR/L, CHT

Conservative treatment of mallet finger: A systematic review

Valdes K, Naughton N, Algar L (Drexel Univ, Philadelphia; Professional Orthopedics Associates, Scranton, PA; Northeast Orthopaedic and Hand Surgery, Waterbury, CT; et al)
J Hand Ther 28:237-246, 2015

Purpose.—To determine if there is a superior orthosis and wearing regimen for the conservative treatment of mallet finger injuries. The secondary purpose is to examine the current evidence to evaluate if a night orthosis is necessary following the initial immobilization phase.

Methods.—A comprehensive literature search was conducted using the search terms mallet finger, splint, orthosis, and conservative treatment.

Results.—Four randomized controlled trials (RCTs) were included in the systematic review. In all 4 RCTs mallet fingers were immobilized continuously for 6 weeks in acute injuries and 8 weeks for chronic injuries.

Conclusions.—Two of the three studies found a large effect size for orthotic intervention ranging from 2.17 to 12.12. Increased edema and age and decreased patient adherence seem to negatively influence DIP extension gains. Recommended immobilization duration is between 6 to 8 weeks and with additional weeks of immobilization in cases of persistent lags.

Level of Evidence.—1a.

▶ The authors present a systematic review of the conservative management of mallet finger injury in a literature search comparing 4 randomized, control trials. It had been more than 10 years since a similar systematic review took place. Disruption of the terminal extensor tendon at the distal interphalangeal joint is commonly known as a *mallet finger*. From the authors' comprehensive literature search, only 4 studies could be used for comparison value of conservative treatment. Systematic review of articles was confined to conservative measures, studies within the last 10 years, and in the English language. A portion of the article rationalized the exclusion criteria, in which, of 301 articles, only 4 could be used or were appropriate for the inclusion criteria. The review then went on to investigate the effectiveness of various orthoses and prescribed wearing schedules among the 4 studies. The review did discuss the study limitations, including small sample size in 3 of the 4 studies, patient compliance, and absence or lack of involvement of the hand therapist in the treatment. This review certainly gives the reader interest in a study to determine what the best practice for orthoses compliance is, and whether direct referral to hand therapy from the emergency room would improve the optimal care or outcomes.

S. Kranz, OTR/L, CHT

Stenosing flexor tenosynovitis: Validity of standard assessment tools of daily functioning and quality of life
Langer D, Luria S, Bar-Haim Erez A, et al (Hadassah and Hebrew Univ, Jerusalem, Israel; Hadassah-Hebrew Univ Med Ctr, Jerusalem, Israel; Ono Academic College, Kiryat-Ono, Israel; et al)
J Hand Ther 28:384-388, 2015

Study Design.—Cross-sectional.

Introduction.—Stenosing flexor tenosynovitis (SFT) is a common hand disease, yet there is a lack of valid standard assessments for this population.

Purpose of the Study.—Validation of assessment for the evaluation of disability and quality of life related to SFT clinical severity.

Methods.—Sixty five participants with SFT were matched to 71 controls. Participant's symptoms were graded using the Quinnell classification. Disability and quality of life were evaluated using the DASH and WHOQOL-BREF questionnaires.

Results.—Small to moderate correlations were found between SFT grade and the DASH and WHOQOLBREF. Both questionnaires differentiated between the first and third clinical grades and between SFT and healthy groups.

Discussion.—Both questionnaires are useful tools to distinguish between participants with SFT and controls and between mild and severe clinical grades.

Conclusion.—The DASH and WHOQOL-BREF may be implemented in the clinical management and research of SFT.

Level of Evidence.—Diagnostic III

▶ Stenosing flexor tenosynovitis (SFT) may affect quality of life, depending on the severity of the disease. To better understand SFT as it relates to function, the authors used the DASH and World Health Organization Quality of Life—BREF (WHOQOL-BREF) with 65 participants with SFT (Quinnell grades 1-3) and 71 healthy participants matched for age and gender. They found that participants with SFT had significantly higher DASH scores as well as a reduction in QoL scores that correlated with the severity of the disease. The DASH was able to differentiate between mild and severe forms of SFT and less between mild and moderate forms of SFT. The QoL was found to be the better measure for those with SFT unless they were in the severe (grade 3) category. Both of the outcome measures used were able to discriminate between the participants with SFT and the controls.

These findings are not unexpected considering the effect on quality of life that pain, swelling, and clicking of 1 or more digits in the hand have. The importance of this study is that the authors were able to determine that the DASH and WHOQOL-BREF are valid instruments to use when carrying out research on SFT. They are now in the position to continue their research using these outcome measures that accurately reflect the disability caused by SFT.

S. J. Clark, OTR/L, CHT

The Dorsal Triangular Fibrocartilage of the Metacarpophalangeal Joint: A Cadaveric Study

Hunter-Smith DJ, Slattery PG, Rizzitelli A, et al (Frankston Hosp, Victoria, Australia; et al)
J Hand Surg Am 40:1410-1415, 2015

Purpose.—To describe a fibrocartilaginous structure on the dorsal surface of the metacarpophalangeal (MCP) joint.

Methods.—A combination of anatomical dissection, histology, ultrasound, and magnetic resonance imaging was undertaken to explore the anatomical structure described, with clinical correlation undertaken by surgical exploration of MCP joints.

Results.—A dorsal structure of the MCP joint was identified as fibrocartilagenous in composition, triangular in shape, and—together with the volar plate and collateral and accessory collateral ligaments—forming a deepened dorsal fossa in which the metacarpal head invaginated. It was attached to the extensor tendon by loose connective tissue and formed part of the joint capsule.

Conclusions.—The dorsal fibrocartilage of the MCP joint is a constant anatomical structure that appears to complement the structural support for the metacarpal head and extensor tendon. Possible functions include stabilization of the extensor tendon, formation of a dorsal fossa, prevention of extensor tendon attrition, and synovial fluid production. Its structure and function may have implications in future development of joint replacement devices.

Clinical Relevance.—This study adds to the collective knowledge about the precise anatomy of the MCP joint. Reconstructive surgery and, in particular, joint replacement surgery should consider the potential function and importance of this structure when designing interventions on the joint.

▶ The authors report on a study using anatomic dissection, histology, ultrasound, MRI, and clinical correlation to define a known but not well-described fibrocartilaginous dorsal structure at the metacarpal-phalangeal joint. This triangular-shaped and meniscal-type structure interacts with the metacarpophalangeal (MCP) joint capsule and extensor tendon but is defined and separate from both. The authors suggest that this structure forms a deepened dorsal fossa that expands the contact area for the metacarpal head, and they hypothesize that this structure may function to stabilize the extensor tendon, improve the extensor moment at the MCP joint, prevent extensor tendon attrition, and assist in the production of synovial fluid.

This study contributes in a meaningful way to our understanding of the anatomy of the MCP joint and its supportive and surrounding structures. In my practice, this improved understanding of this dorsal triangular fibrocartilaginous structure will assist with the traumatic reconstruction of the extensor mechanism, dorsal capsule, and MCP joint. Knowledge of this anatomy may prove useful in my capsular reconstruction following MCP joint replacements and may also assist in the future development of a more anatomic MCP joint prosthesis.

J. L. Tueting, MD

10 Trauma

Reduction of Fifth Metacarpal Neck Fractures With a Kirschner Wire
Zhang X, Huang X, Shao X (Second Hosp of Qinhuangdao, Changli, Shangdong, China; Hebei Med Univ Third Hosp, Shijiazhuang, Shangdong, China; People's Hosp of Zhangqiu, Shangdong, China)
J Hand Surg Am 40:1225-1230, 2015

This article reports on a percutaneous joystick technique for reduction of fifth metacarpal neck fractures. The technique was performed in 76 hands. Reduction was achieved in all cases. The technique is a useful reduction maneuver in the treatment of fifth metacarpal neck fractures.

▶ In this level 4 report, the authors present a novel technique to reduce fifth metacarpal head fractures. Although as hand surgeons we are all familiar with transverse percutaneous pinning, the authors describe a Kapandji style reduction of the fifth metacarpal head. The authors present what seems to be a simple approach to the management of these common fractures. Their report on 76 fractures, over a 2-year period, showed successful healing of all fractures at an average of 7 weeks.

At the beginning of the report the authors cite the work of King and Beckenbaugh but dismiss their method as being "even more complex.[1] "However, the technique described in the report may not be so simple.

First, the procedure is invasive requiring pin care and dressing changes every 3 to 5 days. Also, as described, one needs to have power equipment available and maybe even an assistant to help transfix the fracture while the surgeon holds the reduction. These needs are drawbacks compared with the technique described by King and Beckenbaugh. Additionally the authors themselves make mention that this technique may have a learning curve. We must keep in mind "primum non nocere." In my practice I keep to the KISS principle.

The technique described does have some merit in obtaining a reduction. However, I do not appreciate the value over the King and Beckenbaugh noninvasive technique. As I have been reminded by my mentors, "just because we can, does not mean we have to—or we should."[1]

J. A. Ortiz, Jr, MD

Reference

1. King JC, Nettrour JF, Beckenbaugh RD. Traction reduction and cast immobilization for the treatment of boxer's fractures. *Tech Hand Up Extrem Surg.* 1999;3: 174-180.

Distal Oblique Bundle Reinforcement for Treatment of DRUJ Instability
Brink PRG, Hannemann PFW (Maastricht Univ Med Ctr, The Netherlands)
J Wrist Surg 4:221-228, 2015

Background.—Chronic, dynamic bidirectional instability in the distal radioulnar joint (DRUJ) is diagnosed clinically, based on the patient's complaints and the finding of abnormal laxity in the vicinity of the distal ulna. In cases where malunion is ruled out or treated and there are no signs of osteoarthritis, stabilization of the DRUJ may offer relief. To this end, several different techniques have been investigated over the past 90 years.

Materials and Methods.—In this article we outline the procedure for a new technique using a tendon graft to reinforce the distal edge of the interosseous membrane.

Description of Technique.—A percutaneous technique is used to harvest the palmaris longus tendon and to create a tunnel, just proximal to the sigmoid notch, through the ulna and radius in an oblique direction. By overdrilling the radial cortex, the knotted tendon can be pulled through the radius and ulna and the knot blocked at the second radial cortex, creating a strong connection between the radius and ulna at the site of the distal oblique bundle (DOB). The tendon is fixed in the ulna with a small interference screw in full supination, preventing subluxation of the ulna out of the sigmoid notch during rotation.

Results.—Fourteen patients were treated with this novel technique between 2011 and October 2013. The QuickDASH score at 25 months postoperatively (range 16—38 months) showed an improvement of 32 points. Similarly, an improvement of 33 points (67—34 months) was found on the PRWHE. Only one recurrence of chronic, dynamic bidirectional instability in the DRUJ was observed.

Conclusion.—This simple percutaneous tenodesis technique between radius and ulna at the position of the distal edge of the interosseous membrane shows promise in terms of both restoring stability and relieving complaints related to chronic subluxation in the DRUJ.

▶ This study describes a novel technique for restoring distal radioulnar joint (DRUJ) stability, focusing on reinforcement of the distal aspect of the interosseous membrane, the distal oblique bundle. The authors use a tendon graft to reinforce the distal edge of the interosseous membrane to restore stability and relieve complaints of laxity in the DRUJ. They have reported convincing clinical outcomes, as 13 of 14 patients were no longer experiencing the acute, sharp pain of subluxation postoperatively. Strengths of this study include a minimum

16-month follow-up in all subjects with a mean follow-up of 25 months and the use of validated patient-reported outcome scores both pre- and postoperatively. Randomized prospective studies or comparative studies of other stabilizing procedures will help strengthen evidence supporting the clinical use of this technique. Provided that patients are carefully selected, this simple percutaneous technique offers promising means of treating chronic instability in the DRUJ. It is important to emphasize that any underlying bony malunion must be corrected before consideration of this or any other soft tissue procedure to successfully stabilize the DRUJ.

Paul Kooner, BSc contributed to the writing of this review under the direction of Ruby Grewal, MD, MSc, FRCSC.

R. Grewal, MD, MSc, FRCSC

Impact of Joint Position and Joint Morphology on Assessment of Thumb Metacarpophalangeal Joint Radial Collateral Ligament Integrity

Shaftel ND, Ayalon O, Liu S, et al (New York Univ Hosp for Joint Diseases)
J Hand Surg Am 40:1838-1843, 2015

Purpose.—A 2-part biomechanical study was constructed to test the hypothesis that coronal morphology of the thumb metacarpophalangeal joint impacts the assessment of instability in the context of radial collateral ligament (RCL) injury.

Methods.—Fourteen cadaveric thumbs were disarticulated at the carpometacarpal joint. Four observers measured the radius of curvature of the metacarpal (MC) heads. In a custom jig, a micrometer was used to measure the RCL length as each thumb was put through a flexion and/or extension arc under a 200 g ulnar deviation load. Strain was calculated at maximal hyperextension, 0°, 15°, 30°, 45°, and maximal flexion. Radial instability was measured with a goniometer under 45 N stress. The RCL was then divided and measurements were repeated. Analysis of variance and Pearson correlation metrics were used.

Results.—The RCL strain notably increased from 0° to 30° and 45° of flexion. With an intact RCL, the radial deviation was 15° at 0° of flexion, 18° at 15°, 17° at 30°, 16° at 45°, and 14° at maximal flexion. With a divided RCL, instability was greatest at 30° of flexion with 31° of deviation. The mean radius of curvature of the MC head was 19 ± 4 mm. Radial instability was inversely correlated with the radius of curvature to a considerable degree only in divided RCL specimens, and only at 0° and 15° of flexion.

Conclusions.—The RCL contributes most to the radial stability of the joint at flexion positions greater than 30°. The results suggest that flatter MC heads contribute to stability when the RCL is ruptured and the joint is tested at 0° to 15° of metacarpophalangeal flexion.

Clinical Relevance.—The thumb MC joint should be examined for RCL instability in at least 30° of flexion.

▶ This interesting cadaveric biomechanical study adds knowledge to our understanding of radial collateral ligament injuries of the thumb metacarpophalangeal joint (MPJ). Many of our previous assumptions have been based on work performed on the more commonly injured ulnar collateral ligament. They conclude that the radial collateral ligament of the thumb MPJ is most taught between 30 and 45 degrees of flexion. Interestingly they also conclude that patients with a flat metacarpal head have increased stability over those with a more convex articulation. This study does not, however, look at the often troublesome volar subluxation of the base of the proximal phalanx in the presence of an incompetent radial collateral ligament of the thumb MPJ and may be an area for further work.

M. Hayton, MD

A Comparison of K-Wire Versus Screw Fixation on the Outcomes of Distal Phalanx Fractures

Hay RA, Tay SC (Duke-NUS Graduate Med School, Singapore; Singapore General Hosp)
J Hand Surg Am 40:2160-2167, 2015

Purpose.—To compare K-wire and screw fixation of distal phalanx (DP) fractures with respect to union and functional outcome.

Methods.—This retrospective study identified patients with DP fractures from a clinic registry taken from 2007 to 2013. Clinical data collected included patient demographics, range of motion (ROM), removal of implant (ROI), and complications. Radiographic data collected included fracture type, location, configuration, fracture displacement, and radiographic union. Statistical analysis was done using a chi-squared test for categorical variables and paired Student's t test for continuous variables.

Results.—A total of 172 patients with DP fractures were seen in our clinic between 2007 and 2013. Of these, 141 patients were managed conservatively and 31 patients had surgery for 33 DP fractures, of which 12 had K-wire and 21 had screw fixation. Mean union incidence for screw was 100% compared with 83% for K-wire. Time to union was 2.4 months for screw fixation compared with 4.1 months for K-wire fixation. ROM for screw fixation was significantly better (60°) compared with K-wire fixation (45°). ROM for non-transarticular K-wire (46°) was similar to transarticular K-wire (44°). ROI was performed in 52% of patients with screw fixation. Other than fingertip tenderness, which resolved after ROI, no other complications were noted.

Conclusions.—Our study showed that the union incidence and time to union for screw fixation were comparable to those for K-wire fixation. Screw fixation of DP fractures resulted in greater distal interphalangeal joint motion compared with K-wire fixation but required removal in half of cases.

Type of Study/Level of Evidence.—Therapeutic III.

▶ This retrospective study evaluated 172 patients with distal phalanx fractures. Thirty-one fractures in 33 fingers were indicated for surgery. Twenty-one were fixed with screws and 12 with k-wires. Based on the authors observations, K-wire fixation versus screw fixation demonstrated no significant difference in time to radiographic union. However, clinical union, defined as absence of pain, was noted much sooner in the screw fixation group (1 month for screw fixation and 2.4 months for K-wire fixation). Final DIP range of motion was significantly better in the patients who underwent screw fixation, although the clinical significance of less DIP motion may be minimal.

Additionally, patients undergoing screw fixation had a high incidence of hardware removal (50%) requiring return to the operating room. This was primarily due to tenderness at the fingertip.

The impact on current surgical practices may be minimal because the study was not randomized and the sample size was too small to support an evidence-based change in practice. This use of screw fixation does provide an alternative for patients who may have difficulty with pin care or in whom perhaps range of motion of the DIP joint is more critical. As a counterpoint, however, the increased return rate to OR in the setting of screw fixation is an increased burden on rising health care costs and should be a factor in decision making.

E. Lawler, MD

A Comparative Study of Attitudes Regarding Digit Replantation in the United States and Japan

Nishizuka T, Shauver MJ, Zhong L, et al (Nagoya Univ Graduate School of Medicine, Japan; Univ of Michigan, Ann Arbor)
J Hand Surg Am 40:1646-1656, 2015

Purpose.—To compare the societal preferences for finger replantation between the United States (US) and Japan and to investigate factors influencing the preferences.

Methods.—A sample of the general population without current hand disease or condition was recruited via flyers posted in public areas of 2 major academic centers in the US and Japan. The recruited subjects completed a survey presenting finger amputation scenarios and various factors that may affect treatment decisions. We performed univariate analysis using treatment preference as the outcome and all other factors as possible predictors using the chi-square test.

Results.—Most respondents in both countries preferred replantation and there was no significant difference between the US and Japan. Treatment preference was significantly associated with the importance of appearance, recovery time, and the chance of survival of the replanted digit. There was no association between treatment preference and attitudes regarding body

integrity or estimate of stigma toward finger amputees. Japanese participants agreed more with statements of body integrity, and Japanese respondents rated appearance, sensation, and chance of survival of the replant as
more important than did American participants.

Conclusions.—Patient preference is not driving the decrease in finger
replantations in the US. The general public in both countries prefer replantation over wound closure for digit amputations.

Type of Study/Level of Evidence.—Economic and decision analysis III.

▶ It has been reported that digital replant rates are significantly less in the
United States than in Japan. This report's self-reported purpose is to investigate
societal preferences for finger replantation and to investigate factors influencing
these preferences.

Forty-nine American and 81 Japanese volunteers were recruited from a major
academic medical center in each country. These volunteers were given surveys
exploring the individual's thoughts on sustaining a dominant index finger proximal interphalangeal amputation. The results were statistically evaluated specifically looking for differing trends within the 2 groups.

The authors' conclusion was that both countries' populations preferred digit
replantation over completion amputation.

This is an interesting report. In the United States, we seem to hear that Asian
societies push their hand surgeons to perform more frequent and more difficult
replant operations. The religious ideas of body integrity and the connotations of
Yakuza seem to lead the charge. This report refutes those ideas and replaces
them with the fact that both societies embrace the idea of digital replantation
after traumatic amputation.

Although it is an interesting report, one has to extrapolate that 49 people
(70% women) in one major academic medical center represent the views of
320,000,000 Americans. I also found some issue with the questions included
on the survey. The authors readily admit that there is no accepted measurement
tool for societal feelings toward digital amputation, but including survey items
such as "One's body is received from one's parents and therefore must be safe-
guarded" seems to be prebiased toward a single societal or religious viewpoint.

Overall, I found this report worth reading. As we become a more global medical community, we all should be critical of practice variations between geographic, social, political, or religious groups.

N. A. Hoekzema, MD

The Epidemiology of Upper Extremity Fractures in the United States, 2009
Karl JW, Olson PR, Rosenwasser MP (Columbia Univ Med Ctr, NY; Rosenberg
Cooley Metcalf Clinic, Park City, UT)
J Orthop Trauma 29:e242-e244, 2015

Background.—No single epidemiological study of upper extremity fractures in the United States exists using data from all payers. Current

epidemiological estimates are based on case series, foreign databases, or Medicare data, which are not representative of the entire US population. The objective of this project was to accurately describe the incidence of fractures of the upper extremity in a representative sample of the US population.

Methods.—Using *International Classification of Disease, Ninth Edition* codes for patient visits reported in the 2009 State Emergency Department Database and the State Inpatient Database, available from the Healthcare Cost and Utilization Project, and 2010 US Census data, we calculated the annual incidence rates per 10,000 persons of upper extremity fractures of all patients, regardless of age or payer type. This was done using a representative national sample from 8 states: Arizona, California, Iowa, Maryland, Massachusetts, New Jersey, and Vermont.

Results.—Overall, in this population of over 87 million Americans, there were 590,193 fractures of the upper extremity, yielding an annual incidence of 67.6 fractures per 10,000 persons. Distal radius and ulna fractures were the most common upper extremity fractures (16.2 fractures per 10,000 persons), followed by hand fractures (phalangeal and metacarpal fractures; 12.5 and 8.4 per 10,000, respectively), proximal humerus fractures (6.0 per 10,000), and clavicle fractures (5.8 per 10,000). The most common type of fracture for all age groups was distal radius fractures, except in the 18- to 34-year-old group, in which metacarpal and phalangeal fractures were more common (16.1 and 12.5 per 10,000, respectively) and the 35- to 49-year-old group, in which phalangeal fractures were most common (11.5 per 10,000). The incidence of distal radius fractures was bimodal, with the highest rates in the under 18 and over 65 age groups (30.18 and 25.42 per 10,000, respectively) with lower rates in the middle age groups. The most common type of fracture for males was phalangeal fractures (11.5 per 10,000), and distal radius and ulna fractures were the most common type for females (11.8 per 10,000). Interestingly, phalangeal and metacarpal fractures varied by socioeconomic status (SES), which decreased with increasing SES. No other fracture type varied by SES.

Conclusions.—Epidemiological studies are necessary for research, clinical applications, and public health and health policy initiatives. This study reports national estimates of upper extremity fractures with subgroup analysis.

▶ This study reports on the incidence of upper extremity fractures in Arizona, California, Iowa, Maryland, Massachusetts, New Jersey, and Vermont. The authors propose that these states (28% of the United States population) serve as a representative sample for the country. The geographic, economic, and cultural diversity of these states make this a reasonable claim.

The use of state inpatient and emergency department databases, which capture patients regardless of insurance status or payer type, allows for stratification by socioeconomic status. However, patients who receive care in outpatient clinic settings are not captured in this study. Therefore, the actual incidence of upper extremity fractures may be higher than reported in this study. This finding is particularly true for metacarpal and phalangeal fractures, which are the most common types of fractures in the 18- to 34-year-old and the 35- to 49-year-old groups.

Overall, this is an informative report on the epidemiology of upper extremity fractures in the United States, highlighting the differences in fracture type by age, sex, and socioeconomic status.

E. Kinnucan, MD

Early Versus Delayed Fourth Ray Amputation With Fifth Ray Transposition for Management of Mutilating Ring Finger Injuries
Sadek AF, Fouly EH, Hassan MY (Minia Univ Hosp, El-Minia, Egypt)
J Hand Surg 40:1389-1396, 2015

Purpose.—To compare hand function after early versus delayed fourth ray amputation and transposition of the fifth ray in mutilating ring finger injuries.

Methods.—We prospectively compared 2 groups of patients who sustained either isolated mutilating ring finger or complex hand injuries between January 2008 and December 2013. The first group (12 patients; 10 male and 2 female) was managed by early (within 14 d) fourth ray amputation with fifth ray transposition, and the second group (13 patients; 9 male and 4 female) was managed similarly but on a delayed basis (after 20 d). The postoperative fifth metacarpophalangeal joint active range of motion was recorded and compared with the preoperative value. Function was evaluated by measuring grip and key pinch strengths, supination and pronation strengths, and hand breadth. All parameters were evaluated by comparing the injured and the noninjured hands.

Results.—Group 1 patients exhibited superior results to group 2 patients regarding the postoperative grip and key pinch strength and pronation and supination strength in addition to the mean postoperative active range of motion of the transposed ray metacarpophalangeal joint. However, the results were statistically significant regarding only grip and pronation strengths. Postoperative active range of motion of the transposed ray metacarpophalangeal joint was significantly reduced in the cases having preoperative compromise of the transposed digit in group 1. The final subjective cosmetic satisfaction was better in group 1.

Conclusions.—Our results support early fourth ray amputation with fifth ray transposition for mutilating ring finger injuries.

Type of Study/Level of Evidence.—Therapeutic II.

▶ This is a very good article that provides useful information for the hand surgeon treating devastating injuries. The authors explain in great detail their surgical technique and postoperative protocol, which is often lacking from studies, and is very beneficial. Additionally, the article provides a nice review of the current literature regarding fourth ray amputation. The authors conclude that superior results are obtained with earlier intervention and aggressive therapy, which intuitively makes sense; however, by sharing their experience they have armed hand surgeons with information that can easily be discussed with patients to help determine optimal care with improved functional recovery.

P. Kane

Two Versus 3 Lag Screws for Fixation of Long Oblique Proximal Phalanx Fractures of the Fingers: A Cadaver Study
Zelken JA, Hayes AG, Parks BG, et al (MedStar Union Memorial Hosp, Baltimore, MD)
J Hand Surg Am 40:1124-1129, 2015

Purpose.—To compare 2- versus 3-screw fixation for oblique fractures of the proximal phalanx in a cadaver model that simulates active finger motion.

Methods.—We experimentally cut the proximal phalanges of the index, middle, and ring fingers of 9 cadaveric hands. Five fingers were assigned to a control group with no fixation, and 22 were fixed with either 2 or 3 lag screws. One digit was excluded because of iatrogenic fracture during preparation. The fingers were fitted with a differential variable reluctance transducer that measured maximum interfragment displacement while the fingers were subjected to 2,000 full flexion and extension cycles to simulate a 6-week active motion protocol.

Results.—Analysis of variance revealed a significant difference between the control group and both the 2- and the 3-screw group. The 2- and 3-screw group average displacements were not significantly different. Both of these groups were equivalent with a power of 90%.

Conclusions.—Biomechanical stability during simulated active motion protocol did not differ in simulated proximal phalanx fractures treated with 2 lag screws or 3.

Clinical Relevance.—Fracture fixation using 2 screws may be more cost and time effective and, therefore, more attractive to the surgeon, even when 3 screws can be placed. Furthermore, surgeons may consider using 2 screws rather than resorting to plate fixation when 3-screw fixation is not possible for these types of fractures.

▶ This study documents the biomechanic adequacy of 2 lag screws (vs 3) in the treatment of oblique proximal phalanx fractures. The study is well done, and the discussion adequately and appropriately addresses the limitations of the study. Most hand surgeons should know that 2 lag screws are all that are needed to control rotational stability while holding reduction. The authors argue that the third screw is often used for "peace of mind." Although this may be partially true, I contend that this is subtle and nuanced. Perhaps one of the screws did not have good purchase due to inadequate bone stock. Or, perhaps there is some "greenstick" or actual comminution that makes the surgeon uneasy about just 2 lag screws. This art of hand surgery will be difficult to overcome with even the most well-done biomechanical study. Of course, this third screw also comes with a potential price (both actual and figurative) with regard to the potential tendon irritation: bone comminution with insertion of the screw. That said, as a hand surgeon, I am sure I will be in this situation soon, and I very well may choose a third screw despite the study and perhaps despite myself.

B. T. Carlsen, MD

A review of phalangeal neck fractures in children

Al-Qattan MM, Al-Qattan AM (King Saud Univ, Riyadh, Saudi Arabia)
Injury 46:935-944, 2015

Phalangeal neck fractures are uncommon and are almost exclusively seen in children. Most paediatric hand fractures are treated conservatively and an excellent outcome is expected in almost all cases. Paediatric phalangeal neck fractures are different mainly because they are unstable and have a high risk of complications. Even minimally displaced phalangeal neck fractures are known to be unstable following reduction and hence k-wire fixation is required. Furthermore, complications such as persistent deformity, nonunion, and avascular necrosis are commonly seen following management of phalangeal neck fractures; such complications are extremely rare in other paediatric hand fractures. The current paper aims to review the diagnosis, classification, management and complications of these fractures in children. The paper also aims to introduce an extended classification of phalangeal neck fractures and to explain the clinical relevance of the extended classification.

▶ This report is based on a literature review of pediatric phalangeal neck fractures and the author's extensive personal experience. It discusses all facets of the subject including etiology of the injury in different age groups, the author's own expanded classification system, risk factors for poor outcome, various surgical techniques, and potential for remodeling of malunions.

The Al-Qattan classification system of nondisplaced (grade 1), displaced with bony contact at the fracture site (grade 2), and widely displaced (grade 3) fractures is further divided into fracture pattern (transverse, oblique, long oblique, and far distal) for grade 2 and direction of and type of displacement for the badly displaced grade 3 fractures. The grade 2 subdivisions are predictive of which type of pinning may be used. The grade 3 subdivisions may be predictive of mechanism but all generally need to be reduced open.

The Al-Qattan outcome criteria are based on clinical appearance and range of motion and are fairly stringent. Excellent results are defined as normal range of motion and normal alignment, good results have no residual malalignment and at least 90° of proximal interphalangeal joint (PIPJ) motion (or 50° of distal interphalangeal joint [DIPJ] motion), and fair results have only 50° to 90° of motion at the PIPJ or mild residual deformity. Poor results have nonunion, osteonecrosis, or motion less than 50° at the PIPJ. Based on this classification system, outcomes of these fractures are best in grade 1 fractures in which most results are excellent, moderate in grade 2 in which most results are good or excellent, and worst in grade 3 fractures in which there is frequently stiffness, nonunion, or osteonecrosis yielding a fair or poor result.

The author also details multiple techniques for pinning these fractures based on their pattern, age of the patient, or surgeon preference. These techniques include one clever method that leaves both PIPJ and DIPJ free of flexion deformity during immobilization but uses only one pin, rendering the fracture potentially rotationally unstable during healing. Other techniques such as an intrafocal pinning and osteoclasis are also detailed.

Finally, recommendations for treatment of nascent malunions and healed malunions are reviewed. Nascent malunions are safest, treated with osteoclasis (percutaneous breakup of healing) and closed pinning because open reduction has a high rate of osteonecrosis. Healed and malunited fractures are best treated by allowing the fracture to heal, remodel, and then later osteotomy or subcondylar fossa debridement if needed.

D. Bohn, MD

A Systematic Review of Outcomes after Revision Amputation for Treatment of Traumatic Finger Amputation

Yuan F, McGlinn EP, Giladi AM, et al (Univ of Michigan Health System, Ann Arbor)
Plast Reconstr Surg 136:99-113, 2015

Background.—Revision amputation is often the treatment for traumatic finger amputation injuries. However, patient outcomes are inadequately reported, and their impact is poorly understood. The authors performed a systematic review to evaluate outcomes of revision amputation and amputation wound coverage techniques.

Methods.—The authors searched all available English literature in the PubMed and Embase databases for articles reporting outcomes of nonreplantation treatments for traumatic finger amputation injuries, including revision amputation, local digital flaps, skin grafting, and conservative treatment. Data extracted were study characteristics, patient demographic data, sensory and functional outcomes, patient-reported outcomes, and complications.

Results.—A total of 1659 articles were screened, yielding 43 studies for review. Mean static two-point discrimination was 5.0 ± 1.5 mm ($n = 23$ studies) overall, 6.1 ± 2.4 mm after local flap procedures, and 3.8 ± 0.4 mm after revision amputation. Mean total active motion was 93 ± 8 percent of normal ($n = 6$ studies) overall. It was 90 ± 9 percent of normal after local flap procedures and 95 percent of normal after revision amputation. Seventy-seven percent of patients reported cold intolerance after revision amputation. Ninety-one percent of patients (217 of 238) reported "satisfactory" or "good/excellent" ratings regardless of treatment.

Conclusions.—Revision amputation and conservative treatments result in better static two-point discrimination outcomes compared with local flaps. All techniques preserve total active motion, although arc of motion is slightly better with revision amputation. Revision amputation procedures are frequently associated with cold intolerance. Patients report "satisfactory," "good," or "excellent" ratings in appearance and quality of life with all nonreplantation techniques.

▶ The current article is a meta-analysis aimed at clarifying the outcomes of treatments of finger amputations other than replantation. This includes diverse treatment modalities including revision amputation, local flaps, skin grafting, and conservative treatment. Total active motion is well preserved independent of the methods used. An interesting finding is that revision amputations were most frequently associated with cold intolerance. One would expect that local flap surgery would lead to a higher percentage of cold intolerance because these procedures are the most invasive. Unexpectedly, revision amputation, a far less invasive treatment modality, displayed the most frequent cold intolerance complications. The authors explain this by the fact that cold intolerance depends more on the vascular damage and nerve injuries sustained during the original trauma and not the trauma suffered during surgery.

Because the data collected for this meta-analysis is inhomogeneous and information on the patients' perception is lacking, the authors hope to bring more light on this topic through future studies.

M. Choi, MD

A Comparison of K-Wire Versus Screw Fixation on the Outcomes of Distal Phalanx Fractures

Hay RAS, Tay SC (Duke-NUS Graduate Med School, Singapore; Singapore General Hosp)
J Hand Surg Am 40:2160-2167, 2015

Purpose.—To compare K-wire and screw fixation of distal phalanx (DP) fractures with respect to union and functional outcome.

Methods.—This retrospective study identified patients with DP fractures from a clinic registry taken from 2007 to 2013. Clinical data collected included patient demographics, range of motion (ROM), removal of implant (ROI), and complications. Radiographic data collected included fracture type, location, configuration, fracture displacement, and radiographic union. Statistical analysis was done using a chi-squared test for categorical variables and paired Student's *t* test for continuous variables.

Results.—A total of 172 patients with DP fractures were seen in our clinic between 2007 and 2013. Of these, 141 patients were managed conservatively and 31 patients had surgery for 33 DP fractures, of which 12 had K-wire and 21 had screw fixation. Mean union incidence for screw was 100% compared with 83% for K-wire. Time to union was 2.4 months for screw fixation compared with 4.1 months for K-wire fixation. ROM for screw fixation was significantly better (60°) compared with K-wire fixation (45°). ROM for non-transarticular K-wire (46°) was similar to transarticular K-wire (44°). ROI was performed in 52% of patients with screw fixation. Other than fingertip tenderness, which resolved after ROI, no other complications were noted.

Conclusions.—Our study showed that the union incidence and time to union for screw fixation were comparable to those for K-wire fixation. Screw fixation of DP fractures resulted in greater distal interphalangeal joint motion compared with K-wire fixation but required removal in half of cases.

Type of Study/Level of Evidence.—Therapeutic III.

▶ The authors describe screw fixation of distal phalanx fractures, which is not a frequently used technique compared with K-wires in cases that require surgery for stabilization. The indications and surgical technique were nicely described. Screw fixation was introduced in response to the relatively high frequency of distal phalanx nonunions to provide better compression at the fracture site. The main differences in the results were in higher distal phalanx range of motion (60 compared with 45 degrees) in the screw fixation group and slightly higher union rate. In half of the cases, the screws required removal, but from my perspective, this is superior compared with the second group in which all K-wires were removed. Additional important information gained from this study is that a transarticular K-wire does not produce inferior results, which is helpful when there are some doubts of stability in some more complicated situations.

This research is retrospective and provides support for another option of phalangeal fixation with some pros and cons that appear reasonable. It can also be a good technique for secondary procedures in cases with complications, such as nonunions.

From my perspective, the indications for distal phalanx fracture fixation are rare in isolated injuries (similarly to these authors at 18%), mostly in cases with "big enough" comminuted fragments. Unfortunately, these fractures are often only part of more complicated injury (multiple injury, crush, amputation, etc) when the simple and fast K-wire technique is just enough to stabilize the bone and will allow work on the other injuries.

P. Czarnecki, MD

The Effect of Timing on the Treatment and Outcome of Combined Fourth and Fifth Carpometacarpal Fracture Dislocations

Zhang C, Wang H, Liang C, et al (Guangzhou Orthopedic Hosp, China; Sun Yat-sen Univ, Guangzhou, China)
J Hand Surg Am 40:2169-2175, 2015

Purpose.—In this study, we designed a prospective project to test the hypothesis that acute fourth and fifth carpometacarpal (CMC) fracture dislocations can be treated conservatively with good restoration of strength, range of motion (ROM), and function, whereas patients with delayed treatment of fourth and fifth CMC fracture dislocations should be treated with open reduction and internal fixation (ORIF).

Methods.—We evaluated the results of 20 patients with acute and 6 patients with subacute fourth and fifth CMC fracture dislocations. All 20 acute CMC fracture dislocations were treated conservatively, whereas 3 of the 6 patients with subacute injuries underwent operative intervention. The sensibility, ROM, and grip strength of the hands were tested during 1-year follow-up. The Michigan Hand Outcomes Questionnaire and control radiographs were also taken.

Results.—All 20 patients with acute CMC fracture dislocations showed good restoration of grip strength, ROM, and function, with an average Michigan Hand Outcomes Questionnaire score of 98 ± 2 at 1-year follow-up. Patients with delayed diagnosis who underwent conservative treatment had noticeable deformity of their injured hands, pain complaints, limited ROM at the fourth and fifth CMC joints, and decreased grip strength. The 3 patients with delayed diagnosis treated with ORIF showed good restoration of grip strength, ROM, and function.

Conclusions.—Patients with acute CMC fracture dislocations can be treated by closed reduction with good restoration of grip strength, ROM, and function. In patients with delayed presentation of CMC fracture dislocations, we recommend ORIF.

Type of Study/Level of Evidence.—Therapeutic IV.

▶ This retrospective study provides commentary on the already well-described behavior and management principles for acute and chronic ulnar carpometacarpal (CMC) fractures and dislocations. The authors review the management 20 acute and 6 dorsal CMC fracture-dislocations and seem to suggest that all acute injuries can be treated conservatively, whereas chronic injuries should be treated with open reduction and internal fixation.

For me, the treatment of these injuries is not so binary. In my practice, acute injuries that are stable, have joint congruity, and have soft tissues that will allow for meaningful splinting can be treated conservatively with closed reduction, splints or casts, and close follow-up. Acute injuries that are unstable, have joint incongruity, or have soft tissues that preclude splints or casts are best treated with closed reduction and percutaneous pinning or open reduction and internal fixation. Chronic presentations that have subluxation, dislocation or joint incongruity are usually treated with open reduction and internal fixation or CMC fusion. I have found CT scans helpful for the evaluation of subtle sub-luxation and for the evaluation of the CMC articular surface.

J. L. Tueting, MD

Dorsal Screw Penetration With the Use of Volar Plating of Distal Radius Fractures: How Can You Best Detect?
Hill BW, Shakir I, Cannada LK (Saint Louis Univ, MO)
J Orthop Trauma 29:e408-e413, 2015

Objectives.—To evaluate the most vulnerable position at which volar plate screws may penetrate the dorsal cortex of the radius and to determine which specific intraoperative fluoroscopic images (lateral, 45 degrees supination, 45 degrees pronation, and dorsal tangential) are most useful to detect dorsal cortex penetration.

Methods.—Four 2.5-mm locking screws were inserted distally using 18-, 20-, or 22-mm screws in 7 cadaveric specimens apiece. The specimens were then evaluated to count the number of screws breaching the dorsal cortex and the amount of penetration. Lateral, 45 degrees supination, 45 degrees pronation, and dorsal tangential fluoroscopic views were taken of each wrist. Sixty-three orthopaedic surgeons of varying experience were then asked to evaluate whether the screws penetrated the dorsal cortex after viewing each image.

Results.—Dorsal cortex screw penetration of at least 1 screw occurred in 3.6% of specimens with 18-mm screws, 25% of specimens with 20-mm screws, and 57% specimens with 22-mm screws. Radial-sided screws more commonly breached the dorsal cortex. The sensitivity was 58% on the lateral view, 88% on the 45 degrees supination view, 53% on the 45 degrees pronation view, and 67% on the dorsal tangential view. Additionally, surgeons with more experience were less accurate in detecting prominent screws.

Conclusions.—Clinicians should consider use of these views to evaluate dorsal screw penetration after volar plating but may opt to subtract a few millimeters from their measured screw lengths to avoid over penetration past the dorsal cortex.

▶ Over the past decade, the volar fixation of distal radius fractures has taken the orthopedic community by storm. This has led to an enormous amount of literature surrounding the advantages and pitfalls of this operative technique. The study by Hill et al is a high-quality cadaveric study evaluating the various radiographic views that can be useful to assess penetration of the dorsal cortex when plating these fractures.

Although it useful to know that the 45-degree supination view was the most sensitive at detecting screw penetration, it is important to remember that all of these views should be performed to minimize the risk of undetected dorsal tendon irritation by the screw tips. It would have been useful had the authors to determine the sensitivity of at least 1 view detecting a prominent screw.

To minimize dorsal tendon problems, I have continued to use smooth pegs to fixate the majority of my distal radius fractures. Although studies show better mechanical pullout strength with screws over pegs, pullout is not the typical mode of failure for this fracture. As the theory of volar plating is that the subchondral bone is supported by the fixed angle device distally, the presence of threads (and the sharp tip) has never seemed important to me.

Finally, I do not think that much can be made of the actual screw lengths and which length is more likely to penetrate at each position. There are too many variables to reliably say "the most radial screw should never be over an 18 mm." These variables include bone morphology, plate placement, screw trajectory, and measurement standards for individual manufacturers. Therefore, to avoid complications, it is critical to be aggressive in the imaging of the distal screws to look for dorsal penetration.

T. Hughes, MD

The Effect of Closed Reduction of Small Finger Metacarpal Neck Fractures on the Ultimate Angular Deformity

Pace GI, Gendelberg D, Taylor KF (Milton S. Hershey Med Ctr, PA)
J Hand Surg Am 40:1582-1585, 2015

Purpose.—To assess whether or not attempted closed reduction of fifth metacarpal neck fractures results in decreased fracture angulation at final follow-up.

Methods.—Retrospective chart review of all patients aged 18 and older managed for isolated fifth metacarpal neck fractures between 2004 and 2014.

Results.—Sixty-six patients managed for an isolated boxer fracture met inclusion criteria. Twenty-three patients underwent attempted reduction and 43 patients did not. Patients undergoing attempted reduction had a statistically significant improvement in fracture angulation following reduction compared with patients not undergoing attempted reduction. At final follow-up, there was no difference in fracture angle between the 2 groups.

Conclusions.—Closed reduction and splint immobilization of fifth metacarpal neck fractures was not an effective means of maintaining a significant improvement in fracture alignment upon healing. Other means, such as closed reduction with pin fixation or open reduction internal fixation, should be considered when maintenance of reduction is desired.

Type of Study/Level of Evidence.—Therapeutic III.

▶ Although there has been a relative paucity of literature addressing the natural history of conditions in hand surgery, this well thought through article bucks this trend by providing readers with an insight into the behavior of conservatively treated metacarpal neck fractures. In essence, they have found that attempted reduction of metacarpal neck fractures did not seem to affect the final fracture angulation after approximately 2.5 years of follow-up.

Together with an article on unoperated spiral metacarpal fractures, which showed that grip strength did not differ significantly from the uninjured side on long-term follow-up,[1] this article helps support the fact that in certain circumstances, accepting malunion in metacarpal fractures does not inevitably lead to poor outcomes. Thus, as they have alluded to in this article, the extra resources spent on reduction of this fracture may be better deployed elsewhere. It would also have been even more enlightening if both physician- and patient-rated outcomes were reported to further strengthen the case.

This study also prompts us to pursue several other research questions that may help us in our daily practice. First, in the setting of metacarpal fractures with rotational deformity, would reduction and conservative management be enough to deliver acceptable radiographic and functional outcomes? Second, do splints make a difference to final outcome when it comes to conservative treatment of small finger metacarpal neck fractures as well as isolated spiral metacarpal fractures? Last, what are the attitudes of hand surgeons with regard to conservative management of these fractures, especially in the light of this recent evidence?

For my patients with this injury, I usually highlight the "lost knuckle": prominent metacarpal head in the palm as well as any rotational deformity present to the patient. If patients feel that either of these are unacceptable in the long run, I offer them reduction and surgical fixation, usually in the form of bouquet or tension band wiring. If they accept these outcomes, I place them in a splint without attempting a reduction. This article has confirmed previous anecdotal evidence that attempted reduction usually does not change the final angular deformity.

A. Cheah, MD

Reference

1. Macdonald BB, Higgins A, Kean S, Smith C, Lalonde DH. Long-term follow-up of unoperated, non scissoring spiral metacarpal fractures. *Plast Surg (Oakv).* 2014; 22:254-258.

What Middle Phalanx Base Fracture Characteristics are Most Reliable and Useful for Surgical Decision-making?

Janssen SJ, on behalf of the Science Of Variation Group (Massachusetts General Hosp, Boston; et al)
Clin Orthop Relat Res 473:3943-3950, 2015

Background.—Fracture-dislocations of the proximal interphalangeal joint are vexing because subluxation and articular damage can lead to arthrosis and the treatments are imperfect. Ideally, a surgeon could advise a patient, based on radiographs, when the risk of problems merits operative intervention, but it is unclear if middle phalanx base fracture characteristics are sufficiently reliable to be useful for surgical decision making.

Questions/Purposes.—We evaluated (1) the degree of interobserver agreement as a function of fracture characteristics, (2) the differences in interobserver agreement between experienced and less-experienced hand surgeons, and (3) what fracture characteristics and surgeon characteristics were associated with the decision for operative treatment.

Methods.—Ninety-nine (33%) of 296 hand surgeons evaluated 21 intra-articular middle phalanx base fractures on lateral radiographs. Eighty-one surgeons (82%) were in academic practice and 57 (58%) had less than 10 years experience. Participants assessed six fracture characteristics and recommended treatment (nonoperative or operative: extension block pinning, external fixation, open reduction and internal fixation, volar plate arthroplasty, or hemihamate autograft arthroplasty) for all cases.

Results.—With all surgeons pooled together, the interobserver agreement for fracture characteristics was substantial for assessment of a 2-mm articular step or gap (kappa, 0.73; 95% CI, 0.60−0.86; $p < 0.001$), subluxation or dislocation (kappa, 0.72; 95% CI, 0.58−0.86; $p < 0.001$), and percentage of articular surface involved (intraclass correlation coefficient [ICC], 0.67; 95% CI, 0.54−0.81; $p < 0.001$); moderate for comminution (kappa, 0.55; 95% CI, 0.39−0.70; $p < 0.001$) and stability (kappa, 0.54; 95% CI, 0.39−0.69; $p < 0.001$); and fair for the number of fracture fragments (ICC, 0.39; 95% CI, 0.27−0.57; $p < 0.001$). When recommending treatment, interobserver agreement was substantial (kappa, 0.69; 95% CI, 0.50−0.88; $p < 0.001$) for the recommendation to operate or not to operate, but only fair (kappa, 0.34; 95% CI, 0.21−0.47; $p < 0.001$) for the specific type of treatment, indicating variation in operative techniques. There were no differences in agreement for any of the fracture characteristics or treatment preference between less-experienced and more-experienced surgeons, although statistical power on this comparison was low. None of the surgeon characteristics was associated with the decision for operative treatment, whereas all fracture characteristics were, except for stable and uncertain joint stability. Articular step or gap (β, 0.90; R-squared, 0.89; 95% CI, 0.75−1.05; $p < 0.001$), likelihood of subluxation or dislocation (β, 0.80; R-squared, 0.76; 95% CI, 0.59−1.02; $p < 0.001$), and unstable fractures (β, 0.88; R-squared, 0.81; 95% CI, 0.67−1.1; $p < 0.001$), are most strongly associated with the decision for operative treatment.

Conclusions.—We found that assessment of a step or gap and likelihood of subluxation were most reliable and are strongly associated with the decision for operative treatment. Surgeons largely agree on which fractures might benefit from surgery, and the variation seems to be with the operative technique. Efforts at improving the care of these fractures should focus on the comparative effectiveness of the various operative treatment options.

Level of Evidence.—Level III, diagnostic study.

▶ This study explores which fracture characteristics are most reliable in guiding surgical decision making for intraarticular middle phalanx fractures. The authors surveyed 91 hand surgeons and demonstrated strong interobserver agreement among surgeons in their interpretation of fracture characteristics and their reliability in recommending operative versus nonoperative treatment. The study design accounts for surgeon demographics, illustrating that both experienced and less experienced hand surgeons are equally proficient at assessing morphologic features of middle phalanx fractures. The authors successfully outline the importance of a 2-mm articular step or gap, likelihood of subluxation or dislocation, and percentage articular surface involvement as the most reliable factors in the decision for operative treatment. Although there was substantial agreement around the decision to operate, there was only fair agreement as to the type of surgery to offer. With a lack of clinical outcomes data, the treatment modality with the greatest clinical success remains uncertain. Given the difficult nature of this problem and potential complications associated with both treatment and lack of treatment, this study is an important first step in the development of guidelines that clinicians can use to best determine how to treat these injuries.

Paul Kooner, BSc contributed to the writing of this review under the direction of Ruby Grewal, MD, MSc, FRCSC.

R. Grewal, MD, MSc, FRCSC

Extension Block Pinning Versus Hook Plate Fixation for Treatment of Mallet Fractures

Toker S, Türkmen F, Pekince O, et al (Necmettin Erbakan Univ, Konya, Turkey)
J Hand Surg Am 40:1591-1596, 2015

Purpose.—To compare the outcomes and associated costs of the treatment of mallet fractures with either extension block pinning or open reduction and hook plate fixation.

Methods.—We treated 22 patients for a mallet fracture that involved at least 25% of the distal phalanx articular surface. Three joints demonstrated concomitant volar subluxation. Extension block pinning was used to treat 16 fractures (group 1) and 6 were treated with open reduction and hook plate fixation (group 2). All patients were evaluated at the second, fourth, and sixth weeks after surgery. Collected data included range of motion, extensor lag, and pain status. Patients were asked to grade preoperative and postoperative pain levels on a visual analog scale. Functional outcomes were determined by Crawford criteria. We retrospectively performed a cost analysis using our institutional records.

Results.—Mean follow-up was 12.7 months. Visual analog scale pain scores improved by a similar amount for both groups. Preoperative pain scores were 7.0 for group 1 and 7.5 for group 2. Postoperative levels were 2.0 and 2.0, respectively. Mean extensor lag was identical for both groups, 5°. Mean flexion was 70° for group 1 and 80° for group 2. Based on the Crawford criteria, group 1 had 5 patients rated as excellent, 6 as good, 3 as fair, and 2 as poor. Group 2 outcomes were 2 excellent, 2 good, and 2 fair. Five complications occurred in group 1, and 1 in group 2.

Differences noted between groups were not statistically significant. Extension block pinning was more cost-effective than hook plate fixation.

Conclusions.—We find extension block pinning to be an equally effective but more cost-efficient treatment than open reduction and hook plate fixation.

Type of Study/Level of Evidence.—Therapeutic III.

▶ The authors present a well-designed retrospective analysis comparing extension block pinning to open reduction internal fixation for mallet fractures. All fractures treated operatively involved greater than one-third of the articular surface of the distal interphalangeal joint. The authors acknowledge that there is no gold standard for operative fixation of mallet fractures; however, their goal was to determine whether there were any differences in outcomes or cost with either extension block pinning or plate fixation. The patients were randomly assigned to either a pinning or open reduction internal fixation group. Both groups of patients were protected in a mallet orthosis and were provided a program of protected mobilization for 6 weeks. Once bony union was achieved radiographically, the digits were assessed for residual pain, distal interphalangeal (DIP) joint flexion and extensor lag. Results indicated that there was no difference between groups in preoperative or postoperative pain scores, DIP joint flexion, extensor lag, nor complication rate. The total cost was 7 times higher for the plating procedure versus the pinning. In my practice, I have found the Ishiguro technique to be quite reliable for treating displaced mallet fractures, with volar joint subluxation. I do not typically fix these fractures unless the distal phalanx is volarly subluxated on the head of the middle phalanx. In this study, all fractures that involved greater than a third of the articular surface of the distal interphalangeal joint were indicated for surgery. I have found that many of these fractures can heal with nonoperative management with painless, functional digits.

M. W. Kessler, MD, MPH

Management of the Acutely Burned Hand

Pan BS, Vu AT, Yakuboff KP (Cincinnati Children's Hosp Med Ctr, OH; Univ of Cincinnati College of Medicine, OH)
J Hand Surg Am 40:1477-1484, 2015

Despite contributing a small percentage to the total body surface area, hands are the most commonly burned body part and are involved in over 90% of severe burns. Although the mortality of isolated hand burns is negligible, morbidity can be substantial given our need for functioning hands when performing activities of daily living. The greatest challenges of treating hand burns are 2-fold. First, determining the depth of injury can be difficult even for the most experienced surgeon, but despite many diagnostic options, clinical examination remains the gold standard. Second, appropriate postoperative hand therapy is crucial and requires a multidisciplinary approach with an experienced burn surgeon, hand surgeon, and hand therapist. Ultimately, the goals of treatment should include preservation of function and aesthetics. In this review, we present an approach to the management of the acutely burned hand with discussion of both conservative and surgical options. Regardless of the initial treatment decision, subsequent care for this subset of patients should be aimed at preventing debilitating postburn scar contractures that can severely limit hand function and ultimately require reconstructive surgery.

▶ This is a continuing medical education article dealing with the management of acutely burned hand. Written in a concise manner, it is helpful for hand surgeons who seek to become informed about the topic in a short time. Given this format, the article is focused on the basics of burn wound therapy. The authors point out that accurate diagnosis of burn wound depth can be a difficult task even for an experienced clinician. This is an important statement because misdiagnosis of burn wound depth can lead to significant treatment failure, resulting not only to prolonged therapy with an additional economic burden but also in unnecessary operations and unfavorable treatment results. Thus, accurate diagnosis needs to be verified by punch biopsy, if necessary.

I do not agree with the authors on the usefulness of silver-impregnated foam as a dressing in noninfected burn wounds. Even though dressings containing silver in either crystalline form or as sulphates are known to be antimicrobial, they may either lead to toxicity due to systemic absorption[1] or be less effective in reepithelialization of second-degree burns compared with antibiotic ointments.[2] For this reason, I do not routinely use silver-containing dressing materials for noninfected wounds or wounds that I do not consider prone to infection.

M. Choi, MD

References

1. Trop M, Novak M, Rodl S, Kroell W, Goessler W. Silver-coated dressing acticoat caused raised liver enzymes and argyria-like symptoms in burn patient. *J Trauma.* 2006;60:648-652.
2. Toussaint J, Chung WT, Osman N, McClain SA, Raut V, Singer AJ. Topical antibiotic ointment versus silver-containing foam dressing for second-degree burns in swine. *Acad Emerg Med.* 2015;22:927-933.

Early Versus Delayed Fourth Ray Amputation With Fifth Ray Transposition for Management of Mutilating Ring Finger Injuries

Sadek AF, Fouly EH, Hassan MY (Minia Univ Hosp, El-Minia, Egypt)
J Hand Surg Am 40:1389-1396, 2015

Purpose.—To compare hand function after early versus delayed fourth ray amputation and transposition of the fifth ray in mutilating ring finger injuries.

Methods.—We prospectively compared 2 groups of patients who sustained either isolated mutilating ring finger or complex hand injuries between January 2008 and December 2013. The first group (12 patients; 10 male and 2 female) was managed by early (within 14 d) fourth ray amputation with fifth ray transposition, and the second group (13 patients; 9 male and 4 female) was managed similarly but on a delayed basis (after 20 d). The postoperative fifth metacarpophalangeal joint active range of motion was recorded and compared with the preoperative value. Function was evaluated by measuring grip and key pinch strengths, supination and pronation strengths, and hand breadth. All parameters were evaluated by comparing the injured and the noninjured hands.

Results.—Group 1 patients exhibited superior results to group 2 patients regarding the postoperative grip and key pinch strength and pronation and supination strength in addition to the mean postoperative active range of motion of the transposed ray metacarpophalangeal joint. However, the results were statistically significant regarding only grip and pronation strengths. Postoperative active range of motion of the transposed ray metacarpophalangeal joint was significantly reduced in the cases having preoperative compromise of the transposed digit in group 1. The final subjective cosmetic satisfaction was better in group 1.

Conclusions.—Our results support early fourth ray amputation with fifth ray transposition for mutilating ring finger injuries.

Type of Study/Level of Evidence.—Therapeutic II.

▶ The authors compare early and delayed fifth ray transposition for mutilating injuries of the ring finger. They found early surgery to be superior to late intervention regarding grip and key pinch strength, pro- and supination strength, active range of motion, and cosmetic satisfaction. These results are not surprising because reconstruction at a later time is associated with more joint stiffness as early intervention. This is especially true for the setting of the present study, where early cases were operated on after a mean interval of only 3.7 ± 3.9 days, whereas late cases were reconstructed after 43 ± 24 days. When the mean interval is compared, late cases were cared for at least 11 times later than the early ones.

The article would have been even more informative if the authors would have reported and compared complications in both groups, especially on persistent pain.

M. Choi

Biomechanical Comparison of 2 Methods of Intramedullary K-Wire Fixation of Transverse Metacarpal Shaft Fractures
Hiatt SV, Begonia MT, Thiagarajan G, et al (Univ of Missouri—Kansas City; et al)
J Hand Surg Am 40:1586-1590, 2015

Purpose.—To determine the relative importance of intramedullary wire (IMW) diameter and IMW number in conferring stability to a metacarpal fracture fixation construct. Our research hypothesis was that the stiffness of IMW fixation for metacarpal shaft fractures using a single 1.6-mm-diameter (0.062-in) wire would be greater than three 0.8-mm-diameter (0.031-in) wires.

Methods.—Our study compared the biomechanical stiffness between one 1.6-mm K-wire and three 0.8-mm K-wires in a composite, fourth-generation, biomechanical metacarpal construct under cantilever testing to treat transverse metacarpal shaft fractures. Six composite bone-wire constructs were tested in each group using constant-rate, nondestructive testing. Stiffness (load/displacement) was measured for each construct.

Results.—All constructs demonstrated a linear load-displacement relationship. Wires were all tested in their elastic zone. The mean stiffness of the 1-wire construct was 3.20 N/mm and the mean stiffness of the 3-wire construct was 0.76 N/mm. These differences were statistically significant with a large effect size.

Conclusions.—The stiffness of IMW fixation for metacarpal shaft fractures using a single 1.6-mm-diameter wire was significantly greater than using three 0.8-mm-diameter wires.

Clinical Relevance.—When IMW fixation is clinically indicated for the treatment of metacarpal fractures, the increased stiffness of a single large-diameter construct provides more stability in the plane of finger flexion-extension.

▶ This well-designed study helps answer a question many hand surgeons ask themselves when performing procedures that require implants to be inserted: how many are necessary? We may ask this in the interest of operative efficiency and avoidance of extra costs. Another question related to the number of implants is the size that is required. In general, for hand fracture fixation, the higher the number of wires or screws used, the smaller the size used. This is because of the limited space that small hand bones afford to the treating surgeon.

The results seem to support the use of a single 1.6-mm wire over multiple smaller wires for intramedullary fixation of a transverse metacarpal fracture, especially if stiffness in the flexion-extension plane is the primary aim. It is of note that during placement of the wires, they were not "prebent"; the entry point was at the articular surface of the metacarpal base, and the fracture was incomplete with 3 mm of volar cortex spared to maintain fracture reduction. It may be that all these factors favor the ease of insertion of a single wire, whereas if one were to face the usual intraoperative situation in which the wires have to be prebent because of the eccentric entry point, insertion of the large 1.6-mm wire may prove challenging, particularly if perfect reduction of the fracture is not achieved.

This study also encourages investigators to answer other questions that follow the hypothesis tested here. It would be interesting to compare the rotational stability between these 2 constructs, especially because malrotation at the metacarpal shaft is amplified at the fingertips. In addition, it would be good to know the minimum stiffness needed for clinically stable fixation of a transverse metacarpal fracture in vivo as well as to identify the least invasive fixation method that can achieve this.

A. Cheah, MD

Anatomic Considerations for Plating of the Distal Ulna

Hazel A, Nemeth N, Bindra R (Loyola Univ Med Ctr, Maywood, IL)
J Wrist Surg 4:188-193, 2015

Purpose.—The purpose of our study was to examine the anatomy of the distal ulna and identify an interval that would be amenable to plating and would not cause impingement during wrist rotation nor irritation to the extensor carpi ulnaris (ECU) tendon.

Methods.—Six cadaveric forearms were dissected and the arc of the articular surface of the distal ulna was measured. The distal ulna was divided up as a clock face, with the ulnar styloid being assigned the 12 o'clock position, and the location of the ECU was identified accordingly. The distance from the ulnar styloid to where the dorsal sensory ulnar nerve crosses from volar to dorsal was also measured. Based on these measurements a safe zone was defined.

Results.—A safe zone was identified between the 12 and 2 o'clock position on the right wrist, and between the 10 and 12 o'clock on the left wrist. The dorsal sensory branch of the ulnar nerve crossed from volar to dorsal position at a variable location near the ulnar styloid. Two commercially available plates were utilized and could be placed in our designated interval and did not cause impingement when the forearm was rotated fully.

Conclusion.—Our study demonstrates a location for plating of the distal ulna that avoids impingement during forearm rotation and that is outside of the footprint of the ECU subsheath.

Clinical Relevance.—Plating of the distal ulna may be necessary with distal ulna fracture, and although plate placement may be dictated by the fracture pattern, it is important to understand the implications of plate placement. Although the ideal plate may not be possible because of comminution, the patient can be educated in regards to potential for tendon irritation, loss of motion, or need for hardware removal.

▶ The goal of this report was 2-fold. The first goal was to describe an anatomic safe zone for plating of the distal ulnar head, similar to placing a plate on a proximal radius. The second goal was to evaluate 2 commercially available plates designed for distal ulna fixation.

The authors dissected 6 cadaveric wrists and identified a 60° arc immediately volar to the extensor carpi ulnaris (ECU) tendon where the plate will be the least intrusive to the ECU and distal radioulnar joint (DRUJ). They do a nice job with the anatomic investigation; unfortunately, the authors cloud the description of the safe zone by using the concept of a clock face. The placement of the clock markers is side dependent and also depends on if one's point of view is from the fingers or from the elbow.

In the second part of the study, the investigators implanted Synthes and Accumed distal ulna-specific plates to determine how well they fit their newly defined safe zone. The authors admit that the Accumed plate is designed to be place volarly and proximal to the DRUJ and that the Synthes plate is designed to engage the ulnar styloid distally. They felt the plates could be utilized safely.

I feel this article is helpful to anyone having to surgically stabilize a distal ulna. There is a significant amount of anatomy and joint surfaces that must be accounted for during exposure and plate placement. I feel that the description of the safe zone was impeded by the clock face analogy, and simply stating that the safe zone is 60° volar to the ECU would have been more helpful.

N. A. Hoekzema, MD

11 Distal Radius Fractures

In Vivo Contact Characteristics of Distal Radioulnar Joint With Malunited Distal Radius During Wrist Motion
Xing SG, Chen YR, Xie RG, et al (Affiliated Hosp of Nantong Univ, Nantong, Jiangsu, China; Affiliated Hosp of Shandong Univ of Traditional Chinese Medicine, Jinan, China)
J Hand Surg Am 40:2243-2248, 2015

Purpose.—To determine whether distal radioulnar joint (DRUJ) contact characteristics were altered in patients with malunited distal radius fractures.

Methods.—We obtained computed tomography scans at 5 positions of both wrists of 6 patients who had unilateral malunited distal radius fractures with dorsal angulation from 10° to 20° and ulnar variance less than 3 mm. We reconstructed 3-dimensional images and mapped contact regions of DRUJ by calculating the shortest distance between the 2 opposing bones. The contact areas of the DRUJ were measured and the contact region centers were calculated and analyzed. The values of the malunited side were compared with those of the contralateral uninjured side.

Results.—In the uninjured wrist, the contact areas of the DRUJ increased slightly from wrist flexion to extension and ulnar deviation. In the malunited wrist, we found the contact areas of DRUJ to be progressively reduced from 20° flexion to neutral, 40° extension, and 20° extension, to ulnar deviation. The centroid of this area on the sigmoid notch moved to distal from flexion to extension. Compared with the contralateral uninjured wrist, the contact area significantly decreased during wrist extension and ulnar deviation, and significantly increased during wrist flexion. The centroids of this area on sigmoid notch all moved volarly in all selected wrist positions.

Conclusions.—The contact areas of the DRUJ and the centroid of contact area on sigmoid notch are altered in patients with malunited distal radius fractures. The contact area of the DRUJ increases during wrist flexion and decreases during wrist extension and ulnar deviation. The centroids of the contact area on sigmoid notch move volarly during wrist flexion-extension and ulnar deviation.

Clinical Relevance.—The *in vivo* findings suggest that alterations in joint mechanics may have an important role in the dysfunction associated with these injuries.

▶ This is a useful study that validated and expanded our current understanding of the distal radioulnar joint (DRUJ). It is certainly logical that the kinematics of the DRUJ will be altered by malunited distal radius fractures. This study provides specific information of exactly how this articulation is altered. The authors show that the contact area of the DRUJ increases during wrist flexion and decreases during wrist extension and ulnar deviation. Additionally, they illustrated how the contact area on the sigmoid notch moves volar during wrist flexion-extension and ulnar deviation. However the exact clinical significance of these findings is debatable. As the authors point out, altered contact stresses may lead to abnormal loading and the development of arthritis; however, further studies are needed to fully understand this relationship (Fig 4).

Only 6 patients were included in the study, and just as all fractures have unique characteristics, so will all malunited fractures. Consequently, although

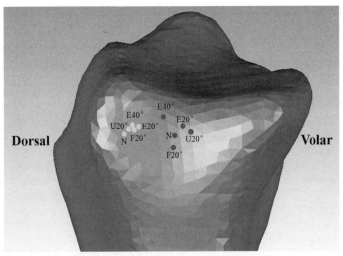

FIGURE 4.—Location of contact area center of the ulnar head in the sigmoid notch on both injured and uninjured sides. Red dots represent the center of contact area at different wrist positions on the injured side; yellow dots represent the center of contact area at different wrist positions on the uninjured side. For interpretation of the references to color in this figure legend, the reader is referred to web version of this article. (Reprinted from Xing SG, Chen YR, Xie RG, et al. *In vivo* contact characteristics of distal radioulnar joint with malunited distal radius during wrist motion. *J Hand Surg Am.* 2015;40:2243-2248, with permission from ASSH.)

the information is interesting, the universal application of these results to a patient with a malunited fracture is debatable.

P. Kane, MD

Volar, Intramedullary, and Percutaneous Fixation of Distal Radius Fractures
Alluri R, Longacre M, Pannell W, et al (Univ of Southern California, Los Angeles)
J Wrist Surg 4:292-300, 2015

Background.—The management of extra-articular distal radius fractures is highly variable, with no clear consensus regarding their optimal management.

Purpose.—To assess comparatively the biomechanical stability of Kirschner wire (K-wire) fixation, volar plating, and intramedullary nailing for unstable, extra-articular distal radius fractures with both (1) constant and (2) cyclical axial compression, simulating forces experienced during early postoperative rehabilitation.

Methods.—Twenty-six volar locking plate, intramedullary nail, and K-wire bone-implant constructs were biomechanically assessed using an unstable extra-articular distal radius bone model. Bone implant models were created for each type of construct. Three samples from each construct underwent compressive axial loading until fixation failure. The remaining samples from each construct underwent fatigue testing with a 50-N force for 2,000 cycles followed by repeat compressive axial loading until fixation failure.

Results.—Axial loading revealed the volar plate was significantly stiffer than the intramedullary nail and K-wire constructs. Both the volar plate and intramedullary nail required greater than 300 N of force for fixation failure, while the K-wire construct failed at less than 150 N. Both the volar plate and intramedullary nail demonstrated less than 1 mm of displacement during cyclic loading, while the K-wire construct displaced greater than 3 mm. Postfatigue testing demonstrated the volar plate was stiffer than the intramedullary nail and K-wire constructs, and both the volar plate and intramedullary nail required greater than 300 N of force for fixation failure while the K-wire construct failed at less than 150 N.

Conclusions.—Volar plating of unstable extra-articular distal radius fractures is biomechanically stiffer than K-wire and intramedullary fixation. Both the volar plate and intramedullary nail demonstrated the necessary stability and stiffness to maintain anatomic reduction during the postoperative rehabilitation period.

Clinical Relevance.—Both the volar plate and intramedullary nail demonstrated the necessary biomechanical stability to maintain postoperative reduction in extra-articular distal radius fractures, warranting further clinical comparison.

▶ This creative biomechanical study assessed mechanical stability of unstable extra-articular distal radius fractures treated by volar plating, Kirschner (K-wire) fixation and intramedullary nailing. As the authors indicate, numerous studies have found equivalent long-term functional outcomes regardless of fixation modality. In an effort to duplicate in vivo mechanics, bone implant models were created for each type of construct and underwent compressive axial loading and fatigue testing until fixation failure. Axial loading revealed that both volar plating and intramedullary fixation withstood forces of 300 N before failure, whereas K-wire fixation failed at less than 150 N. It should be noted that testing also revealed that both volar plating and intramedullary fixation demonstrated the necessary stiffness and stability to withstand typical stresses associated with postoperative rehabilitation.

The authors correctly note the inherent limitations of synthetic bone models, particularly the lack of a soft tissue envelope, which precludes true assessment of intramedullary fixation and K-wire fixation as these techniques avoid violation of soft tissues during surgical implantation, thereby imparting additional stability. Furthermore, torsional or rotational forces were not tested in this study model and may impart additional stressors to each of the implants tested. Nonetheless, this study indicates that both volar plating and intramedullary fixation withstand forces typically imparted to the distal radius in the early postoperative period. In the setting of extra-articular distal radius fractures, this model adds additional evidence that intramedullary implants offer adequate stabilization with less invasive insertion. Ultimately, in the setting of extra-articular distal radius fractures, surgeon preference and comfort will dictate use of either effective treatment option. Finally, K-wire fixation remains a reasonable alternative in the functionally low-demand patient or in patients who require expeditious operative time due to associated comorbidities.

S. M. Jacoby, MD

The Unstable Distal Radius Fracture—How Do We Define It? A Systematic Review
Walenkamp MMJ, Vos LM, Strackee SD, et al (Univ of Amsterdam, The Netherlands; et al)
J Wrist Surg 4:307-316, 2015

Background.—Unstable distal radius fractures are a popular research subject. However, to appreciate the findings of studies that enrolled patients with unstable distal radius fractures, it should be clear how the authors defined an *unstable distal radius fracture*.

Questions.—In what percentage of studies involving patients with unstable distal radius fractures did the authors define *unstable distal radius fracture*? What are the most common descriptions of an unstable distal radius fracture? And is there one preferred evidence-based definition for future authors?

Methods.—A systematic search of literature was performed to identify any type of study with the term *unstable distal radius fracture*. We assessed whether a definition was provided and determined the level of evidence for the most common definitions.

Results.—The search yielded 2,489 citations, of which 479 were included. In 149 studies, it was explicitly stated that patients with unstable distal radius fractures were enrolled. In 54% (81/149) of these studies, the authors defined an unstable distal radius fracture. Overall, we found 143 different definitions. The seven most common definitions were: displacement following adequate reduction; Lafontaine's definition; irreducibility; an AO type C2 fracture; a volarly displaced fracture; Poigenfürst's criteria; and Cooney's criteria. Only Lafontaine's definition originated from a clinical study (level IIIb).

Conclusion.—In only half of the studies involving patients with an unstable distal radius fracture did the authors defined what they considered an *unstable distal radius fracture*. None of the definitions stood out as the preferred choice. A general consensus definition could help to standardize future research.

▶ An unstable distal radius fracture is unable to resist displacement after attempted anatomic reduction. Interestingly, the diagnostic criteria available to us that define those parameters that constitute instability, and thereby dictate treatment intervention, are rather undefined and heterogeneous. The authors aim to eliminate variability of this definition and find an ideal definition to guide the study and management of distal radius fractures. It seems astounding that only half of the 254 clinical studies reviewed actually defined an unstable distal radius fracture and of the 479 total studies reviewed they found 143 descriptions of what constitutes an unstable distal radius fracture. The 7 most common definitions presented in the figure. Moreover, the majority of these diverse definitions, which are perpetuated by surgical training worldwide and our literature, are actually based on decades-old expert opinion classified as Level V by the Oxford Center for Evidence-based Medicine Levels of Evidence. It seems we should strive for a universally accepted definition based on clinically and biomechanically reviewed parameters to guide our discussions, management, and studies of unstable distal radius fractures.

A. Strohl, MD

Catastrophic Thinking Is Associated With Finger Stiffness After Distal Radius Fracture Surgery
Teunis T, Bot AGJ, Thornton ER, et al (Harvard Med School, Boston, MA; Univ of Amsterdam, the Netherlands)
J Orthop Trauma 29:e414-e420, 2015

Objectives.—To identify demographic, injury-related, or psychologic factors associated with finger stiffness at suture removal and 6 weeks after distal radius fracture surgery. We hypothesize that there are no factors associated with distance to palmar crease at suture removal.

Design.—Prospective cohort study.

Setting.—Level I Academic Urban Trauma Center.

Patients.—One hundred sixteen adult patients underwent open reduction and internal fixation of their distal radius fractures; 96 of whom were also available 6 weeks after surgery.

Intervention.—None.

Main Outcome Measurements.—At suture removal, we recorded patients' demographics, AO fracture type, carpal tunnel release at the time of surgery, pain catastrophizing scale, Whiteley Index, Patient Health Questionnaire-9, and disabilities of the arm, shoulder, and hand questionnaire, 11-point ordinal measure of pain intensity, distance to palmar crease, and active flexion of the thumb through the small finger. At 6 weeks after surgery, we measured motion, disabilities of the arm, shoulder, and hand, and pain intensity. Prereduction and postsurgery radiographic fracture characteristics were assessed.

Results.—Female sex, being married, specific surgeons, carpal tunnel release, AO type C fractures, and greater catastrophic thinking were associated with increased distance to palmar crease at suture removal. At 6 weeks, greater catastrophic thinking was the only factor associated with increased distance to palmar crease.

Conclusions.—Catastrophic thinking was a consistent and major determinant of finger stiffness at suture removal and 6 weeks after injury. Future research should assess if treatments that ameliorate catastrophic thinking can facilitate recovery of finger motion after operative treatment of a distal radius fracture.

▶ This prospective cohort study aimed to test the null hypothesis that there are no demographic, injury-related or psychology factors associated with finger stiffness after distal radius fracture fixation with volar plate. One hundred sixteen adult patients were prospectively enrolled at their office visit for suture removal. For each patient, demographic information was collected, radiographic fracture parameters were measured prereduction and after surgery, and each patient completed the pain catastrophizing scale, Whiteley Index, Patient Health Questionnaire-9, and DASH questionnaire. A single investigator measured finger motion. Distance to palmar crease was recorded as well as active flexion of the index through small finger and active thumb motion. Patients were evaluated at suture removal (average 11 days postoperatively) and 6 weeks postoperatively.

Although there were various factors associated with increased stiffness at the different time points, greater catastrophic thinking was the only consistent variable. Interestingly, thumb range of motion 6 weeks postoperatively was the only variable seemingly not affected by increased catastrophic thinking. Catastrophic thinking is defined as negative beliefs about pain, which leads to an overprotective response and then avoidance of activities that may cause pain. This response then leads to stiffness associated with disuse. Previous studies evaluated the effect of catastrophic thinking in patients with chronic low back pain, showing that a reduction in this thinking pattern was able to produce a reduction in symptoms and disability. As a provider, this finding will change my approach when counseling patients who exhibit signs of excessive stiffness or catastrophic thinking at their first appointment. Important future studies could be aimed at predicting which patients are more likely to have catastrophic thinking patterns as well as interventions aimed to minimize this response to determine if it will result in improved clinical outcomes.

E. J. Gauger, MD

Is Bone Grafting Necessary in the Treatment of Malunited Distal Radius Fractures?

Disseldorp DJG, Poeze M, Hannemann PFW, et al (Maastricht Univ Med Centre, The Netherlands)
J Wrist Surg 4:207-213, 2015

Background.—Open wedge osteotomy with bone grafting and plate fixation is the standard procedure for the correction of malunited distal radius fractures. Bone grafts are used to increase structural stability and to enhance new bone formation. However, bone grafts are also associated with donor site morbidity, delayed union at bone—graft interfaces, size mismatch between graft and osteotomy defect, and additional operation time.

Purpose.—The goal of this study was to assess bone healing and secondary fracture displacement in the treatment of malunited distal radius fractures without the use of bone grafting.

Methods.—Between January 1993 and December 2013, 132 corrective osteotomies and plate fixations without bone grafting were performed for malunited distal radius fractures. The minimum follow-up time was 12 months. Primary study outcomes were time to complete bone healing and secondary fracture displacement. Preoperative and postoperative radiographs during follow-up were compared with each other, as well as with radiographs of the uninjured side.

Results.—All 132 osteotomies healed. In two cases (1.5%), healing took more than 4 months, but reinterventions were not necessary. No cases of secondary fracture displacement or hardware failure were observed. Significant improvements in all radiographic parameters were shown after corrective osteotomy and plate fixation.

Conclusion.—This study shows that bone grafts are not required for bone healing and prevention of secondary fracture displacement after corrective osteotomy and plate fixation of malunited distal radius fractures.

Level of Evidence.—Therapeutic, level IV, case series with no comparison group

▶ In this article, the authors add one more piece to the puzzle in answering the question of whether bone grafting is necessary in corrective osteotomies of distal radius malunions.

The authors present a 20-year history during which 132 corrective osteotomies were performed. Of these cases, 128 of them were performed by the same surgeon. In the end, they conclude that bone grafting is not necessary in the treatment of distal radius malunions managed with opening wedge osteotomy. The results showed successful healing in all cases without the use of bone grafting. Of interest is the large number of malunions during this 20-year history. This was occurring during a time in which there was a significant change in the management of distal radius fractures.

The conclusion reached by the authors seems to be counterintuitive. I believe that many, if not most of us, have been trained to use bone graft to fill the void created by the osteotomy. In many cases, I have used the sculpted bone to facilitate correcting the malunion and then plate it once anatomic alignment has been obtained. With newer instrumentation, I have used the plate itself to help obtain and maintain the alignment. I have then used cancellous graft or allograft to fill the void. I have been comfortable doing so given that our newer plating systems are strong enough to hold the alignment without a structural component. However, I have yet to take the leap to treating these conditions with no bone graft—something I must consider the next time I am faced with this condition.

As an aside, I have gone to treating scaphoid nonunions with no structural graft. I rely on a screw to obtain and hold the alignment of the scaphoid, and I then fill the void with autograft from the distal radius. One wonders if the grafting is even needed in these cases as well.

J. A. Ortiz, Jr, MD

The Effect of Elbow Extension on the Biomechanics of the Osseoligamentous Structures of the Forearm

Malone PSC, Cooley J, Terenghi G, et al (Univ of Manchester, United Kingdom)
J Hand Surg Am 40:1776-1784, 2015

Purpose.—To investigate the hypothesis that elbow extension alters the biomechanics of forearm rotation including force transmission in the distal and proximal radioulnar joints (DRUJ and PRUJ) and the interosseous ligament (IOL).

Methods.—A cadaver model with a custom-designed jig was used to measure forearm pronosupination ranges, transmitted forces and contact areas across the PRUJ and DRUJ, and tension in the 3 main components of the IOL's central band. Testing with applied loads was undertaken throughout pronosupination with the elbow fully flexed (n = 15) and fully extended (n = 11).

Results.—Elbow extension-flexion affected the range of forearm pronosupination, shifting the arc of rotation such that the forearm supinated maximally with the elbow flexed and pronated maximally with the elbow extended. Elbow extension also increased transmitted forces across the DRUJ and PRUJ while also increasing contact areas within the DRUJ and PRUJ. Elbow extension significantly increased tension in the central band of the IOL when the forearm was maximally pronated.

Conclusions.—Maximum supination occurred with the elbow flexed. Maximum pronation occurred with it extended. Elbow position altered forearm biomechanics, including force transmission across the PRUJ and DRUJ and transmitted tension in the IOL.

Clinical Relevance.—The interplay of osseoligamentous forearm structures is such that we would anticipate surgical alteration of any one of them to have effects upon function of the others.

▶ There is ever-growing interest in understanding the effects of the interosseous ligament (IOL), and this important biomechanical article helps make an important stride forward in that understanding. The importance of the IOL in forearm biomechanics is well noted, but the secondary role of the position of the elbow in tensioning the forearm is not as well understood. This article sets an important foundation as we strive to understand the impact of the IOL on forearm rotation so that next step surgical interventions can be more accurately designed. This is a must read for anyone delving into the world of IOL surgery.

J. Froelich, MD

Arthroscopic assistance does not improve the functional or radiographic outcome of unstable intra-articular distal radial fractures treated with a volar locking plate: a randomised controlled trial
Yamazaki H, Uchiyama S, Komatsu M, et al (Aizawa Hosp, Matsumoto, Japan; et al)
Bone Joint J 97-B:957-962, 2015

There is no consensus on the benefit of arthroscopically assisted reduction of the articular surface combined with fixation using a volar locking plate for the treatment of intra-articular distal radial fractures. In this study we compared the functional and radiographic outcomes of fluoroscopically and arthroscopically guided reduction of these fractures.

Between February 2009 and May 2013, 74 patients with unilateral unstable intra-articular distal radial fractures were randomised equally into the two groups for treatment. The mean age of these 74 patients was 64 years (24 to 92). We compared functional outcomes including active range of movement of the wrist, grip strength and Disabilities of the Arm, Shoulder, and Hand scores at six and 48 weeks; and radiographic outcomes that included gap, step, radial inclination, volar angulation and ulnar variance.

There were no significant differences between the techniques with regard to functional outcomes or radiographic parameters. The mean gap and step in the fluoroscopic and arthroscopic groups were comparable at 0.9 mm (standard deviation (SD) 0.7) and 0.7 mm (SD 0.7) and 0.6 mm (SD 0.6) and 0.4 mm (SD 0.5), respectively; $p = 0.18$ and $p = 0.35$.

Arthroscopic reduction conferred no advantage over conventional fluoroscopic guidance in achieving anatomical reduction of intra-articular distal radial fractures when using a volar locking plate.

▶ This study compares functional and radiographic outcomes between distal radius fractures (DRF) fixed with volar plating with fluoroscopic guidance alone and DRF fixed with volar plating and arthroscopic-assisted reduction. Previous studies examining the role of arthroscopy in distal radius fixation suggested that fluoroscopy underestimated the articular gap and sometimes underestimated articular stepoff compared with measurements made arthroscopically.[1,2] These results might lead one to believe that the addition of arthroscopic reduction techniques would benefit patients, but neither of these studies included functional outcomes or CT evaluation.

In this study, the authors randomly assigned patients with intra-articular fractures to either volar plate fixation with fluoroscopic guidance alone or volar plate fixation with fluoroscopic guidance and arthroscopic reduction. They examined patients at 6, 12, 24, and 48 weeks and found no difference in range of motion or Disabilities of the Arm, Shoulder, and Hand score between the 2 groups. Perhaps most striking, they found no difference in gap, stepoff, radial inclination, volar angulation, or ulnar variance between the 2 groups as measured on CT 12 weeks postoperatively. Because all patients were treated by a single attending surgeon, that surgeon's bias could influence the study results (eg, accepting poor arthroscopic or fluoroscopic reductions). However the virtually equal radiographic findings on CT suggest that the intra-articular reduction is truly equivalent whether using just fluoroscopy or fluoroscopy and arthroscopy.

These results may represent the supreme skill of the author in interpreting fluoroscopic imaging of distal radius fractures and may not be widely generalizable. However, they suggest that the routine use of arthroscopy for treatment of distal radius fracture likely provides no benefit over modern volar plating techniques with fluoroscopic guidance.

C. M. Ward, MD

References

1. Edwards CC, Haraszti CJ, McGillivary GR, Gutow AP. Intra-articular distal radius fractures: arthroscopic assessment of radiographically assisted reduction. *J Hand Surg Am.* 2001;26:1036-1041.
2. Lutsky K, Boyer MI, Steffen JA, Goldfarb CA. Arthroscopic assessment of intra-articular distal radius fractures after open reduction and internal fixation from a polar approach. *J Hand Surg Am.* 2008;33:476-484.

Vitamin C to Prevent Complex Regional Pain Syndrome in Patients With Distal Radius Fractures: A Meta-Analysis of Randomized Controlled Trials
Evaniew N, McCarthy C, Kleinlugtenbelt YV, et al (McMaster Univ, Hamilton, Ontario, Canada)
J Orthop Trauma 29:e235-e241, 2015

Objective.—To determine whether vitamin C is effective in preventing complex regional pain syndrome (CRPS) in patients with distal radius fractures.

Data Sources.—MEDLINE (1946 to present), EMBASE (1974 to present), and The Cochrane Library (no date limit) were systematically searched up to September 6, 2014, using MeSH and EMTREE headings with free text combinations.

Study Selection.—Randomized trials comparing vitamin C against placebo were included. No exclusions were made during the selection of eligible trials on the basis of patient age, sex, fracture severity, or fracture treatment.

Data Extraction.—Two reviewers independently screened articles, extracted data, and applied the Cochrane Risk of Bias tool. Evidence was graded using the Grading of Recommendations Assessment, Development, and Evaluation approach.

Data Synthesis.—Heterogeneity was quantified using the χ^2 test and the I^2 statistic. Outcome data were combined with a random effects model.

Results.—Across 3 trials (n = 890) of patients with distal radius fractures, vitamin C did not reduce the risk for CRPS (risk ratio = 0.45; 95% confidence interval, 0.18–1.13; I^2 = 70%). This result was confirmed in sensitivity analyses to test the importance of missing data because of losses to follow-up under varying assumptions. Heterogeneity was explained by diagnostic criteria, but not regimen of vitamin C or fracture treatment.

Conclusions.—The evidence for vitamin C to prevent CRPS in patients with distal radius fractures fails to demonstrate a significant benefit. The overall quality of the evidence is low, and these results should be interpreted in the context of clinical expertise and patient preferences.

▶ This systematic review and meta-analysis was intended to determine the efficacy of vitamin C in preventing complex regional pain syndrome (CRPS) in patients with distal radius fractures within 1 year of follow-up based on evidence from randomized, controlled studies. This is a rather timely study, as there has been much debate on the utility of vitamin C following the 2010 American Academy of Orthopaedic Surgeons Clinical Practice Guideline that espoused a moderate strength recommendation that the treatment of distal radius fractures should include pre-emptive vitamin C for the prevention of disproportionate pain.

Two reviewers independently screened articles and extracted data from more than 127 articles and settled on 3 articles in the final meta-analysis. The authors excluded observational studies to minimize bias. In addition, the authors point out that of the 3 studies chosen, only one trial included results within the first 6 weeks of injury, whereas the remaining 2 focused on 1-year follow-up data. This finding indicates the possibility of early, mild CRPS that resolved by the 1-year follow-up check point. Nonetheless, the authors conclude that vitamin C administered in the early postinjury period did not reduce the risk of CRPS. The quality of evidence remains low, and the authors espouse additional studies aimed at evaluating the utility in patients who present with CRPS-type symptoms to augment the current data on patients treated proactively in the absence of CRPS symptoms. I do not routinely recommend vitamin C as an adjuvant in either nonoperative or operative distal radius fractures. However, I routinely recommend vitamin C in patients who I suspect have the slightest evidence of atypical findings, which include neuropathic pain, vasomotor or sudomotor instability, abnormal sweating, and swelling and joint/soft tissue stiffness. I find the antioxidant properties of vitamin C to be helpful as part of an aggressive approach to patients with CRPS that includes neuroleptic medication, occupational hand therapy, and often referral to a qualified pain management specialist to manage additional oral medication and consideration of sympathetic nerve blocks.

S. M. Jacoby, MD

Functional Outcomes Following Bridge Plate Fixation for Distal Radius Fractures

Lauder A, Agnew S, Bakri K, et al (Univ of Washington, Seattle; Northwestern Univ, Chicago, IL; Mayo Clinic, Rochester, MN)
J Hand Surg Am 40:1554-1562, 2015

Purpose.—To determine the functional outcomes of patients treated with dorsal spanning distraction bridge plate fixation for distal radius fractures.

Methods.—All adult patients at our institution who underwent treatment of a unilateral distal radius fracture using a dorsal bridge plate from 2008 to 2012 were identified retrospectively. Patients were enrolled in clinical follow-up to assess function. Wrist range of motion, grip strength, and extension torque were measured systematically and compared with the contralateral, uninjured wrist. Patients also completed *Quick*-Disabilities of the Arm, Shoulder, and Hand and Patient-Rated Wrist Evaluation outcomes questionnaires.

Results.—Eighteen of 100 eligible patients, with a minimum of 1 year from the time of implant removal, were available for follow-up (mean, 2.7 y). All fracture patterns were comminuted and intra-articular (AO 23.C3). There were significant decreases in wrist flexion (43° vs 58°), extension (46° vs 56°), and ulnar deviation (23° vs 29°) compared with the contralateral uninjured wrist. Grip strength was 86% and extension torque was 78% of the contralateral wrist. Comparison of dominant and nondominant wrist injuries identified nearly complete recovery of grip (95%) and extension (96%) strength of dominant-sided wrist injuries, compared with grip (79%) and extension (65%) strength in those with an injured nondominant wrist. Mean *Quick*-Disabilities of the Arm, Shoulder, and Hand and Patient-Rated Wrist Evaluation scores were 16 and 14, respectively. There were 2 cases of postoperative surgical site pain and no cases of infection, tendonitis, or tendon rupture.

Conclusions.—Distraction bridge plate fixation for distal radius fractures is safe with minimal complications. Functional outcomes are similar to those published for other treatment methods.

Type of Study/Level of Evidence.—Therapeutic IV.

▶ This study provides valuable retrospective evidence regarding dorsal bridge plating for distal radius fractures. Most importantly, the authors show distraction bridge plating to be safe with similar functional outcomes as other treatment options. The authors found decreased range of motion in the surgically treated wrist when compared with the contralateral uninjured wrist (flexion 43° vs 58°, extension 46° vs 56° and ulnar deviation 23° vs 29°). Obviously some loss of motion is to be expected given the injury. Additionally, the authors found good preservation of grip strength (87%) and extension torque (78%).

Slightly concerning is the limited percentage of patients treated with bridge plating that were able to participate (18 of 100); however, this is a frequently encountered problem with retrospective studies. The authors provide a succinct

TABLE 5.—Literature Review of Functional Outcomes Associated With Bridge Plate Fixation

Study	Level of Evidence	Size, Technique, Follow-Up	Functional Results (degrees)							Complications and DASH
			Flexion	Extension	Pronation	Supination	Radial Deviation	Ulnar Deviation	Grip Strength	
Ruch et al[27]	IV: prospective cohort	22 pts, avg age 55 y, 3rd metacarpal, 24.8 mo follow-up, avg 12 mo functional results	57	65	77	76			69% (contralateral)	3/22 infection 3/22 extensor lag DASH (24.8 mo): 11.5
Dodds et al[35]	IV: retrospective review	25 pts, avg age 54.6 y, second metacarpal, 6.6 mo follow-up and functional results	46	42	76	69	14	18		0/25 EPL entrapment 0/25 extensor tendon rupture 0/25 infection 0/25 radial sensory nerve injury 3/25 hardware failure DASH: N/A
Richard et al[26]	IV: retrospective review	33 pts, avg age 70 y, second metacarpal (12 pts), third metacarpal (21 pts), 11.8 mo follow-up and functional results	46	50	79	77				10/33 digital stiffness DASH (11.8 mo): 32
Mithani et al[36]	IV: case series	8 pts, avg age 68 y, third metacarpal ± volar plate, used for prior nonunion, final follow-up time not reported	36	40	79	72				1/8 persistent pain DASH (final): 27.6
Hanel et al[14]	IV: retrospective chart review	134 pts, second and third metacarpal, follow-up not obtained								2/134 wound healing 5/134 hardware failure 2/134 malunion 2/134 nonunion 2/134 deep infection 2/134 extensor tendon adhesions 1/134 EPL rupture DASH: N/A
Hanel et al[13]	IV: retrospective chart review	62 pts via chart review, second metacarpal								No CRPS, 1/62 ECRL rupture, 1/62 hardware failure, 0/62 postoperative digit stiffness DASH: N/A
Hanel et al[13]	IV: retrospective case report	1 pt case report via chart review, second metacarpal, 12 mo functional results	45	35	70	60	10	30		No complications DASH: N/A
Burke et al[4]	IV: case report	1 pt case report, third metacarpal, 4 y functional results	45	65	80	75				No complications DASH: N/A

Editor's Note: Please refer to original journal article for full references.

Pt, patient; avg, average; ECRL, extensor carpi radialis longus; EPL, extensor pollicus longus; N/A, not available; CRPS, complex regional pain syndrome.
Reprinted from Lauder A, Agnew S, Bakri K, et al. Functional outcomes following bridge plate fixation for distal radius fractures. *J Hand Surg Am.* 2015;40:1554-1562, with permission from American Society for Surgery of the Hand.

literature review of bridge plating in Table 5. Overall, the authors provide evidence to support the use of dorsal bridge plating illustrating the technique to be safe and effective.

P. Kane, MD

Are Volar Locking Plates Superior to Percutaneous K-wires for Distal Radius Fractures? A Meta-analysis
Chaudhry H, Kleinlugtenbelt YV, Mundi R, et al (McMaster Univ, Hamilton, Ontario, Canada; et al)
Clin Orthop Relat Res 473:3017-3027, 2015

Background.—Distal radius fractures are common, costly, and increasing in incidence. Percutaneous K-wire fixation and volar locking plates are two of the most commonly used surgical treatments for unstable dorsally displaced distal radius fractures. However, there is uncertainty regarding which of these treatments is superior.

Questions/Purposes.—We performed a meta-analysis of randomized controlled trials to determine whether patients treated with volar locking plates (1) achieved better function (2) attained better wrist motion, (3) had better radiographic outcomes, and (4) had fewer complications develop than did patients treated with K-wires for dorsally displaced distal radius fractures.

Methods.—We performed a comprehensive search of MEDLINE (inception to 2014, October Week 2), EMBASE (inception to 2014, Week 42), and the Cochrane Central Register of Controlled Trials to identify relevant randomized controlled trials; we supplemented these searches with manual searches. We included studies of extraarticular and intraarticular distal radius fractures. Adjunctive external fixation was acceptable as long as the intent was to use only K-wires where possible and external fixation was used in less than 25% of the procedures. We considered a difference in the DASH scores of 10 as the minimal clinically important difference. We performed quality assessment with the Cochrane Risk of Bias tool and evaluated the strength of recommendations using the Grades of Recommendation, Assessment, Development and Evaluation (GRADE) approach. Seven randomized trials with a total of 875 participants were included in the meta-analysis.

Results.—Patients treated with volar locking plates had slightly better function than did patients treated with K-wires as measured by their DASH scores at 3 months (mean difference [MD], 7.5; 95% CI, 4.4–10.6; $p < 0.001$) and 12 months (MD, 3.8; 95% CI, 1.2–6.3; $p = 0.004$). Neither of these differences exceeded the a priori-determined threshold for clinical importance (10 points). There was a small early advantage in flexion and supination in the volar locking plate group (3.7° [95% CI, 0.3°–7.1°; $p = 0.04$] and 4.1° [95% CI, 0.6°–7.6°; $p = 0.02$] greater, respectively) at 3 months, but not at later followups (6 or 12 months). There were no differences in radiographic outcomes (volar tilt, radial inclination, and radial height) between the two interventions. Superficial wound infection was more common in patients treated with K-wires (8.2% versus 3.2%; RR = 2.6; $p = 0.001$), but otherwise no difference in complication rates was found.

Conclusions.—Despite the small number of studies and the limitations inherent in a meta-analysis, we found that volar locking plates show better DASH scores at 3- and 12-month followups compared with K-wires for displaced distal radius fractures in adults; however, these differences were small and unlikely to be clinically important. Further research is required to better delineate if there are specific radiographic, injury, or patient characteristics that may benefit from volar locking plates in the short term and whether there are any differences in long-term outcomes and complications.

Level of Evidence.—Level I, therapeutic study.

▶ This meta-analysis examines the difference in outcomes between percutaneous pins and volar plating for treatment of distal radius fractures. Previous meta-analyses compared external fixation with volar plating. The authors included results from 7 randomized, controlled trials with a total of 875 patients. Patients ranged in age from 19 to 80 years. Although the authors did not report a mean age for the entire study group, the patient population skews older (mean ages, 50–80 years for individual studies). The authors reported a slightly better mean Disabilities of the Arm, Shoulder, and Hand (DASH) score at 3 months (7.5 points) in volar plate patients, although this did not meet their meaningful clinical difference criterion of a 10-point change. The difference in mean DASH score decreased to 3.8 points at final follow-up (6 or 12 months postoperatively). Similarly, the authors found no significant difference in range of motion or radiographic outcome between the 2 groups. The most notable difference was a higher incidence of infections in patients with percutaneous pins (8.2% vs 3.2%), whereas incidences of other complications were nearly equal.

Of note, although the authors included intra-articular and extra-articular fractures, they only included dorsally displaced fractures. Thus, this information can not necessarily be generalized to all patient populations. However, in my practice, these results reinforce my impression that percutaneous pinning is a reasonable option for extra-articular or simple intra-articular dorsally displaced distal radius fractures.

C. M. Ward, MD

Acute Median Nerve Problems in the Setting of a Distal Radius Fracture
Floyd WE IV, Earp BE, Blazar PE (Brigham and Women's Hosp, Boston, MA)
J Hand Surg 40:1669-1671, 2015

Background.—Patients who experience fracture of the distal radius may suffer median neuropathy. Often this resolves once the fracture is reduced, but if paresthesia persists after reduction, the clinician must consider whether the patient has median nerve contusion, acute carpal tunnel syndrome (ACTS), forearm compartment syndrome (FCS), or an exacerbation of underlying idiopathic CT syndrome. Operative intervention is generally not indicated for median nerve contusion or stretching, which will resolve with time. The characteristics of ACTS and FCS include worsening and disproportionate pain and pain on passive finger extension. ACTS is more likely among patients under age 40 years who suffer high-energy injuries, comminuted or displaced fractures, or polytrauma. Patients often do not seek treatment for several days after ACTS develops and the long-term prognosis is favorable after release. Surgeons often perform the release within 24 hours of diagnosis. A question was posed concerning the optimal management of median neuropathy for a patient with a distal radius fracture (DRF).

Current Evidence.—Six articles were reviewed for relevant information concerning the best course of treatment for median neuropathy associated with DRF. The findings were as follows: ACTS is more likely when the injury involves significant initial displacement, in male patients, with a higher energy injury, and with C-type fracture patterns. If ACTS is released within 32 hours from the time of injury, patients experience fewer residual symptoms. With respect to diagnosis, clinicians rely on changes in CT pressures. The postoperative volar plating CT pressure can range from 16 to 65 mm Hg. Lower pressures are more common with AO subtype A2 fractures than with A3 or C2 fractures. Prophylactic CT release may be indicated on the basis of monofilament sensory changes.

Analysis of the evidence notes that the relevant studies do not consistently distinguish among neurapraxia, ACTS, and preexisting idiopathic CT syndrome, with no widely accepted reference standard for their differentiation. In addition, the studies focusing on final median nerve function are shorter than those evaluating the potential for nerve recovery. No specific radiographic or clinical indicators have been identified that discern whether the patient suffered a high-energy injury. Studies monitoring CT pressure are promising but involve few patients and patients who may not represent either the typical or the high-risk individual.

Recommendations.—It is recommended that patients with nonprogressive numbness be observed, with release done only if the fracture is treated operatively. If numbness begins or progresses over the period after reduction, ACTS is diagnosed and urgent CT release done as soon as possible while addressing the fracture. Because peripheral nerve recovery requires an extended period of time, patients should be assessed at least 1 or 2 years after their injury to determine the prognosis for the median neuropathy. Future studies are needed to address the shortcomings of the current evidence.

▶ This is a review article published in the Evidence-based Medicine section of the *Journal of Hand Surgery*. It begins with a clinical vignette describing a patient with a distal radius fracture who had mild carpal tunnel syndrome exacerbated by his recent injury and subsequent fracture reduction.

The authors group distal radius fracture—related carpal tunnel symptoms into 4 categories:

1. Idiopathic, preexisting carpal tunnel syndrome (CTS)
2. Nerve contusion
3. Acute carpal tunnel syndrome (ACTS)
4. Forearm compartment syndrome

The literature is reviewed, including 6 applicable articles. In brief, the articles show (1) greater initial displacement correlates with ACTS; (2) ACTS is associated with male sex, higher energy injury, and C-type fracture pattern; (3) carpal tunnel pressure of 40 to 50 mm/Hg is suggested to be the threshold for ACTS; (4) patients tend to have fewer residual symptoms if ACTS is released less than 32 hours from the injury; (5) monofilament sensory changes are an indication for prophylactic CTR; (6) postoperative volar plating carpal tunnel pressures can range from 16 to 65 mm/Hg; and (7) AO subtype A2 fractures tend to have lower carpal tunnel pressures than A3 or C2.

The available published articles are criticized by these authors for having short follow-up and not differentiating between the types of fracture-related compression neuropathies at the wrist.

The authors summarize by outlining their current algorithm for management of fracture-related CTS. The authors propose observing patients with nonprogressive numbness and releasing the CT only if the fracture is treated operatively. If the patient has worsening numbness, the patient is considered to have ACTS, and the CT is released as soon as possible.

This article is both a concise summary of the few published articles and an expert opinion on a common topic. It is difficult to come up with a definitive consensus for treatment because of the wide variety of presentations, but I feel that the author's proposed management guidelines are very reasonable.

N. A. Hoekzema, MD

External Fixation and Adjuvant Pins Versus Volar Locking Plate Fixation in Unstable Distal Radius Fractures: A Randomized, Controlled Study With a 5-Year Follow-Up
Williksen JH, Husby T, Hellund JC, et al (Oslo Univ Hosp, Norway; et al)
J Hand Surg Am 40:1333-1340, 2015

Purpose.—To determine whether volar locking plates (VLP) are superior to external fixation (EF) with adjuvant pins in unstable distal radius fractures after 5 years of follow-up.

Methods.—We randomized 111 unstable distal radius fractures to treatment with either a VLP or EF using adjuvant pins. The patients' mean age was 54 years (range, 20—84 y). Twenty patients were lost to follow-up. At 5 years, 91 patients (82%) were assessed using the visual analog scale (VAS) pain score, Mayo wrist score, Quick Disabilities of the Arm, Shoulder and Hand (*Quick*DASH) questionnaire, range of motion, and

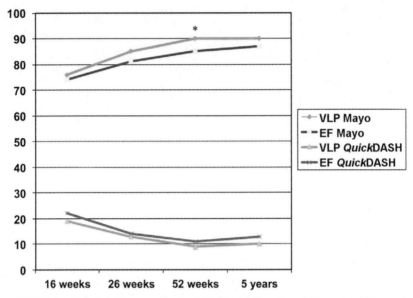

FIGURE 2.—All included fractures. Results at 16, 26, and 52 weeks and 66 months of Mayo wrist score (Mayo) and *Quick*DASH. The Mayo wrist score was statistically significant at 52 weeks (*P* =.02; SD, 10)* in favor of VLP over EF. At other time points and for the *Quick*DASH, there were no statistically significant differences. (Reprinted from Williksen JH, Husby T, Hellund JC, et al. External fixation and adjuvant pins versus volar locking plate fixation in unstable distal radius fractures: a randomized, controlled study with a 5-year follow-up. *J Hand Surg Am*. 2015;40:1333-1340, with permission from ASSH.)

radiological evaluation. The *Quick*DASH score at 5 years was the primary outcome measure.

Results.—The *Quick*DASH score was not statistically significantly different between the groups (VLP 10 vs EF 13) at 5 years. Patients with VLP had statistically significant better supination (85° vs 81°), better radial deviation (18° vs 16°), and less radial shortening (1 mm vs 2 mm). For AO/OTA type C2 fractures, the VLP had statistically significant better supination (84° vs 78°), flexion (64° vs 56°), grip strength (34 kg vs 28 kg), Mayo wrist score (92 vs 76), and less ulnar shortening (1 mm vs 3 mm). The *Quick*DASH score in the C2 subset analysis showed a difference of 10 (VLP 8 vs EF 18), but this was not statistically significant. In the VLP group, 11 patients (21%) had their plates removed owing to surgically related complications. In the EF group, 5 patients had proximal radial scar correction surgery owing to skin contracture.

Conclusions.—The findings were satisfactory for both groups at 5 years. The VLP provided statistically significantly better results for several clinical outcomes in the C2 subset analysis. However, 21% of the VLPs were removed because of surgical complications.

Type of Study/Level of Evidence.—Therapeutic I.

▶ This is a strong level-1 study that provides the treating physician with useful information regarding the treatment of distal radius fractures. The 5-year findings illustrated good outcomes in both treatment groups, external fixation versus volar locked plating, regarding the functional scores and wrist pain. Certain outcomes including ulnar variance, supination, and radial deviation favored the volar locked plating. However, the long-term follow-up with Mayo Wrist Score and QuickDASH was not statistically significant as the follow-up passed 1 year (Fig 2).

The authors do not provide a good description of their postoperative protocol for the groups, and although they acknowledge that 11 surgeons performed the surgeries, they do not discuss the training of theses surgeons or their particular familiarity with the implants, all factors that I feel are important in accurately interpreting their results.

The authors provide valid evidence that both external fixation and volar lock plating are acceptable treatment options. Given the recent trend toward volar plating, this article is useful to remind us that there are multiple ways of effectively treating patients with distal radius fractures. Additionally, from a training standpoint, this is important information, as we need to ensure residents and fellows are exposed to multiple methods of treatment.

P. Kane, MD

Utility and Cost Analysis of Radiographs Taken 2 Weeks Following Plate Fixation of Distal Radius Fractures

Stone JD, Vaccaro LM, Brabender RC, et al (Florida Orthopaedic Inst, Tampa; Foundation for Orthopaedic Res and Education, Tampa, FL)
J Hand Surg Am 40:1106-1109, 2015

Purpose.—To evaluate the utility of radiographs taken 2 weeks following plate fixation of distal radius fractures.

Methods.—A retrospective review of patients requiring operative fixation of distal radius fractures was performed with the objective of determining the utility of a 2-week postoperative radiograph in patient management.

Results.—Three out of 268 (1%) patients had loss of fixation noted radiographically at the 2-week visit that resulted in a reoperation. There was no statistically significant difference in radial inclination, radial height, or volar tilt measured at 2 weeks, 6 weeks, or final follow-up. The average cost of a series of wrist radiographs was $85 with no additional radiology reading fees.

Conclusions.—Routine 2-week postoperative radiographs of operatively treated distal radius fractures rarely resulted in a change in patient management; however, they may have added unnecessary cost to the patient and health care system.

Type of Study/Level of Evidence.—Economic and decision analysis IV.

▶ During an era in which health care costs continue to increase, this report offers a solution to help minimize cost in the postoperative management of surgically treated distal radius fractures.

The authors hypothesize that in the postoperative management of surgically treated distal radius fractures, elimination of the 2-week radiographs would have no impact on outcome. They report 268 distal radius fractures and found that in only 3 instances (~1%) did the 2-week radiograph result in an unexpected treatment of the patient. In all 3 cases, the patients sustained additional trauma after the initial surgery. Additionally, all 3 cases had initially sustained AO type C3 fractures.

Their data found that radiographic measurements such as radial inclination, radial height, and volar tilt showed no significant difference at 2 weeks compared with radiographs at 6 weeks.

Although retrospective in design, this study does show that not all distal radius fractures need to have routine radiographs at 2 weeks. Radiographs may be reserved for patients who initially have AO type C3 fractures or on those patients who sustain additional injury after surgery. This method would not only help to curtail costs but would also eliminate unnecessary radiation. In this study, there was no fee for reading the radiographs. Many institutions do have this added cost, the elimination of which results in even greater savings. Discontinuing routine radiography 2 weeks postoperatively would also have the added effect of improving clinical efficiency by decreasing demand on radiology departments, thus, improving patient throughput and impacting patient experience.

J. A. Ortiz, Jr, MD

Coronal Shift of Distal Radius Fractures: Influence of the Distal Interosseous Membrane on Distal Radioulnar Joint Instability
Trehan SK, Orbay JL, Wolfe SW (Hosp for Special Surgery, NY; Miami Hand and Upper Extremity Inst, FL)
J Hand Surg Am 40:159-162, 2015

Background.—Coronal shift of the distal radius, also termed radial translation, refers to the radial displacement of the articular fragment of a distal radius fracture in the coronal plane. It produces a narrowing of the radioulnar distance proximal to the site of the fracture, degreasing distal interosseous membrane (DIOM) tension and increasing laxity. Anatomic reduction of the coronal shift of distal radius fractures re-establishes tension in the DIOM, increases contact pressures, and seats the ulnar head within the sigmoid notch. Thus the coronal shift may be the most important predictor of distal radioulnar joint instability.

Anatomy.—Distal radius fractures are often accompanied by DRUJ injury, which can lead to pain of the ulnar side of the wrist, painful or

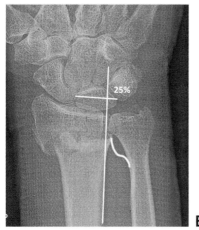 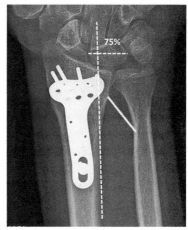

FIGURE 2.—**A** Posteroanterior radiograph of extra-articular distal radius fracture with associated coronal shift. Red line simulates DOB laxity. **B** Intra-operative radiograph after coronal shift reduction and fixation demonstrates restored DOB tension (red line) and restored alignment of the lunate. (For interpretation of the references to color in this figure legend, the reader is referred to web version of this article). (Reprinted from Trehan SK, Orbay JL, Wolfe SW. Coronal shift of distal radius fractures: influence of the distal interosseous membrane on distal radioulnar joint instability. *J Hand Surg Am.* 2015;40:159-162, with permission from ASSH.)

limited forearm rotation, weak grip strength, or degenerative arthritis. DRUJ stability is dependent on the triangular fibrocartilage complex (TFCC), bony articulation between the ulnar head and sigmoid notch of the radius, dorsal and palmar radioulnar ligaments, DIOM, and musculotendinous units of the extensor carpi ulnaris and pronator quadratus. The TFCC is the primary stabilizer of the DRUJ, with the DIOM serving a secondary role.

Clinical Evaluation.—Radial inclination, ulnar variance, volar tilt, and articular congruity are assessed, along with coronal plane reduction, to determine the need for distal radius fracture reduction. Coronal shift can occur in isolation but is more commonly seen with deformities such as dorsal tilt, dorsal comminution, and radial shortening. DRUJ instability has traditionally been attributed to avulsion of the distal radioulnar ligaments from the fovea or ligamentous detachment via a fracture of the basilar ulnar styloid when it is associated with distal radius fracture. Recent studies indicate the status of the basilar ulnar styloid fractures does not correlate with DRUJ instability and repair may not result in reestablishment of DRUJ stability. These indicate how important coronal plane reduction is to the maintenance of DRUJ stability.

Coronal shift is measured on standard posteroanterior (PA) radiographs. Extension of a line along the ulnar aspect of the radial diaphysis distally across the carpus reveals the percentage of lunate width remaining ulnar to the reference line and accurately demonstrates radial translation. Coronal shift may also be suspected if there is loss of the metaphyseal flare on the ulnar aspect of the distal radius proximal to the sigmoid notch or an overlap of the radial styloid on the radial metaphyseal flare.

Treatment.—A coronal shift as small as 2 mm should be reduced to restore DIOM tension and lessen the chance of DRUJ instability developing. A dorsal or volar approach is used for coronal shift reduction, with many techniques possible. The authors prefer to apply a radial reduction moment on a Hohmann retractor placed on the ulnar metaphyseal flare with counterpressure on the radial styloid.

Conclusions.—Coronal shift should be considered a classic measure of distal radius fracture requiring reduction based on its vital role in DRUJ stability.

▶ This review describes the importance of the distal interosseous membrane (DIOM) as a secondary stabilizer of the distal radioulnar joint (DRUJ). The DIOM originates palmar and proximal on the ulna and inserts distal and dorsal on the radius. Its anatomic location provides resting tension, therefore, making it an isometric stabilizer of the forearm. Coronal shift is defined as the radial displacement of the articular fragment of a distal radius fracture in the coronal plane, therefore, leading to narrowing of the radioulnar distance proximal to the fracture site. This narrowing decreases tension of the DIOM, resulting in increased laxity at the DRUJ. The authors reference a study by Fujitani et al that found that coronal shift was the most important predictor of DRUJ instability.[1] Coronal shift is measured on a posterior-anterior radiograph. A reference line is drawn along the ulnar border of the radial shaft and extended through the carpus; the percentage of lunate width remaining ulnar to this line is then calculated and serves as an accurate indicator of radial translation (see Fig 2). Mean percentage of lunate width ulnar to the reference line in normal individuals was 55%. The authors reference several surgical techniques that can be used intraoperatively to reduce coronal shift. A Gelpi retractor can be placed to spread apart the radius and ulna until tension is restored; an Army-Navy retractor can be placed into the interosseous space and turned 90° to provide tension, or a Hohmann retractor can be placed on the ulnar metaphyseal flare while counter pressure is applied at the radial styloid. The authors advocate for the evaluation of coronal shift to be included with the classic radiographic parameters (radial inclination, ulnar variance, volar tilt, and articular congruity) when assessing distal radius fracture reduction. This is a nice summary of the available literature and represents another tool that hand surgeons should use in the operating room to ensure appropriate restoration of anatomy while fixing distal radius fractures to minimize complications and improve patient outcomes.

E. J. Gauger, MD

Reference

1. Fujitani R, Omokawa S, Akahane M, Iida A, Ono H, Tanaka Y. Predictors of distal radioulnar joint instability in distal radius fractures. *J Hand Surg Am.* 2011; 36(12):1919-1925.

Volar Subluxation of the Ulnar Head in Dorsal Translation Deformities of Distal Radius Fractures: An In Vitro Biomechanical Study

Nishiwaki M, Welsh M, Gammon B, et al (Kawasaki Municipal Hosp, Japan; St Joseph's Health Care London, Ontario, Canada; Univ of Ottawa, Ontario, Canada)
J Orthop Trauma 29:295-300, 2015

Objectives.—To quantify the effects of dorsal translation deformities of the distal radius with and without dorsal angulation on volar displacement of the ulnar head during simulated active forearm rotation, both with the triangular fibrocartilage complex (TFCC) intact and sectioned conditions.

Methods.—Eight fresh-frozen cadaveric upper extremities were mounted in an active forearm motion simulator, and distal radial deformities of 0, 5, and 10 mm of dorsal translation with 0, 10, 20, and 30 degrees of dorsal angulation were simulated. Volar displacement of the ulnar head at the distal radioulnar joint as a result of each distal radial deformity was quantified during simulated active supination. The data were collected with the TFCC intact and after sectioning the TFCC at its ulnar insertion.

Results.—Increasing isolated dorsal translation deformities increased volar displacement of the ulnar head when the TFCC was intact ($P < 0.001$). Increasing dorsal translation combined with dorsal angulation increased volar displacement of the ulnar head compared with isolated dorsal angulation deformities ($P < 0.001$). Sectioning the TFCC increased the volar displacement of the ulnar head caused by each distal radial deformity ($P = 0.001$).

Conclusions.—These results emphasize the clinical importance of evaluating the magnitude of both dorsal translation and dorsal angulation when managing displaced distal radius fractures and malunions.

▶ Biomechanical studies are often overlooked by busy practitioners, but this one should be read everyone who treats distal radius fractures. The author's team developed a novel way of measuring the biomechanical effects of multiple plan deformities in distal radius fractures. Specifically, looking at dorsal angulation and dorsal displacement helps to create a more complete picture in evaluating these injuries. The finding that there is increased ulnar head volar translation with increased dorsal translation of the fracture opens the doors to rethink the parameters we consider when clinically treating distal radius fractures.

J. M. Froelich, MD

Distal Radioulnar Joint Reaction Force Following Ulnar Shortening: Diaphyseal Osteotomy Versus Wafer Resection

Canham CD, Schreck MJ, Maqsoodi N, et al (Univ of Rochester, NY; Univ of Rochester Orthopaedic Biomechanics Laboratory, NY; et al)
J Hand Surg Am 40:2206-2212, 2015

Purpose.—To compare how ulnar diaphyseal shortening and wafer resection affect distal radioulnar joint (DRUJ) joint reaction force (JRF) using a nondestructive method of measurement. Our hypothesis was that ulnar shortening osteotomy would increase DRUJ JRF more than wafer resection.

Methods.—Eight fresh-frozen human cadaveric upper limbs were obtained. Under fluoroscopic guidance, a threaded pin was inserted into the lateral radius orthogonal to the DRUJ and a second pin was placed in the medial ulna coaxial to the radial pin. Each limb was mounted onto a mechanical tensile testing machine and a distracting force was applied across the DRUJ while force and displacement were simultaneously measured. Data sets were entered into a computer and a polynomial was generated and solved to determine the JRF. This process was repeated after ulnar diaphyseal osteotomy, ulnar re-lengthening, and ulnar wafer resection. The JRF was compared among the 4 conditions.

Results.—Average baseline DRUJ JRF for the 8 arms increased significantly after diaphyseal ulnar shortening osteotomy (7.2 vs 10.3 N). Average JRF after re-lengthening the ulna and wafer resection was 6.9 and 6.7 N, respectively. There were no differences in JRF among baseline, relengthened, and wafer resection conditions.

Conclusions.—Distal radioulnar joint JRF increased significantly after ulnar diaphyseal shortening osteotomy and did not increase after ulnar wafer resection.

Clinical Relevance.—Diaphyseal ulnar shortening osteotomy increases DRUJ JRF, which may lead to DRUJ arthrosis.

▶ This cadaveric study on 8 fresh-frozen wrists found that a diaphyseal ulnar shortening of 3 mm increases the distal radioulnar joint (DRUJ) transverse articular forces by about 50%, whereas an open DRUJ wafer procedure of 3 mm does not. There are some weaknesses in this study, as the evaluation was only static in neutral forearm rotation, shortening was standardized as 3 mm in both groups, evaluation was done on ulnar neutral wrists, and the difference between Tolat 1 and 2 types of DRUJ was not addressed. Moreover, previous studies using pressure-sensitive devices already showed that ulnar shortening increases pressure at the DRUJ. However, the strength of the report was the use of an ingenious indirect mini-invasive evaluation of the articular pressure already in use in the knee research area. By simultaneously applying a joint distraction force and measuring joint displacement, a point was reached just before the joint surfaces separated when the compressive forces were overcome and the surfaces were no longer compressed but were not yet distracted. At this point, the distracting force applied was equal to the compressive forces acting across the joint (joint reaction force). This experimental study is the first one on the DRUJ using this concept, and despite the fact that a capsulotomy was necessary anyway to perform a wafer procedure, this method is appealing because it is by far less invasive than previous cadaveric studies using pressure-sensitive devices inserted into the joint. There is no doubt that other experiments using this concept will follow.

G. Herzberg, MD

In Vivo Contact Characteristics of Distal Radioulnar Joint With Malunited Distal Radius During Wrist Motion

Xing SG, Chen YR, Xie RG, et al (Affiliated Hosp of Nantong Univ, Nantong, Jiangsu; Affiliated Hosp of Shandong Univ of Traditional Chinese Medicine, Jinan, China)
J Hand Surg Am 40:2243-2248, 2015

Purpose.—To determine whether distal radioulnar joint (DRUJ) contact characteristics were altered in patients with malunited distal radius fractures.

Methods.—We obtained computed tomography scans at 5 positions of both wrists of 6 patients who had unilateral malunited distal radius fractures with dorsal angulation from 10° to 20° and ulnar variance less than 3 mm. We reconstructed 3-dimensional images and mapped contact regions of DRUJ by calculating the shortest distance between the 2 opposing bones. The contact areas of the DRUJ were measured and the contact region centers were calculated and analyzed. The values of the malunited side were compared with those of the contralateral uninjured side.

Results.—In the uninjured wrist, the contact areas of the DRUJ increased slightly from wrist flexion to extension and ulnar deviation. In the malunited wrist, we found the contact areas of DRUJ to be progressively reduced from 20° flexion to neutral, 40° extension, and 20° extension, to ulnar deviation. The centroid of this area on the sigmoid notch moved to distal from flexion to extension. Compared with the contralateral uninjured wrist, the contact area significantly decreased during wrist extension and ulnar deviation, and significantly increased during wrist flexion. The centroids of this area on sigmoid notch all moved volarly in all selected wrist positions.

Conclusions.—The contact areas of the DRUJ and the centroid of contact area on sigmoid notch are altered in patients with malunited distal radius fractures. The contact area of the DRUJ increases during wrist flexion and decreases during wrist extension and ulnar deviation. The centroids of the contact area on sigmoid notch move volarly during wrist flexion-extension and ulnar deviation.

Clinical Relevance.—The *in vivo* findings suggest that alterations in joint mechanics may have an important role in the dysfunction associated with these injuries.

▶ Although the detrimental effects of distal radius malunion on the radiocarpal and ulnocarpal joints have been extensively reported, the alterations to the mechanics of the distal radioulnar joint (DRUJ) have received less attention. The authors seek to describe the in vivo alterations of the kinematics of the DRUJ following distal radius malunions using 3-dimensional CT scans of the involved and contralateral uninvolved wrist.

Strengths include the contralateral control limb, multiple wrist positions tested, and apparent accuracy of centroid mapping of the sigmoid notch. Limitations include the inability to account for the influence of soft tissue injuries, a lack of active and dynamic in vivo assessment (all passive and static measurements), and the small and homogenous patient population (6 patients, 5 women, all 53-75 years old, and all 10°-20° of dorsal tilt).

The computerized mapping of the centroid representing load bearing on the sigmoid notch from a 3-dimensional CT scan was previously reported by these same authors and is reported to be accurate. This model cannot, however, account for individual patient differences in articular cartilage thickness of the sigmoid notch or ulnar head, and I am unsure how that affects the reported results.

The finding of a volar shift of the centroid in the sigmoid notch is logical given the dorsal displacement of the distal radius. The alteration of contact area particularly with wrist extension and ulnar deviation is noteworthy.

From a clinical application standpoint, I find the study enlightening in terms of highlighting the alterations in DRUJ kinematics; however, in the population they studied (middle aged to elderly women), I have not found late DRUJ arthritis to be a significant problem in my patients. This population has been found in numerous studies to clinically tolerate malunions very well, and I believe this includes DRUJ alterations. I do not plan on treating these fractures any differently given the current findings.

G. Gaston, MD

Reconstruction of the Distal Oblique Bundle of the Interosseous Membrane: A Technique to Restore Distal Radioulnar Joint Stability
Riggenbach MD, Wright TW, Dell PC (Univ of Florida, Gainesville)
J Hand Surg Am 40:2279-2282, 2015

The distal radioulnar ligament reconstruction is a technique that may be used for distal radioulnar joint instability without arthritis and failed nonsurgical management; clinical results demonstrate resolved or improved stability. Recent literature has focused on the distal oblique bundle of the interosseous membrane and its contributions to stability. This article describes a technically simple surgical technique to reconstruct the distal oblique bundle and restore distal radioulnar joint stability.

▶ This article describes a new surgical technique to reconstruct the distal oblique bundle of the interosseous membrane (IOM). The inconstant (40%) fibrous distal portion of the IOM (distal oblique band [DOB]) is found to play a significant role in distal radioulnar joint stability. The authors recommend using a palmaris longus or a split-hamstring graft through carefully positioned transosseous holes, one on the dorsal aspect of the distal one-sixth of the ulna and the other in the sagittal middle of the proximal aspect of the sigmoid notch. A postoperative position is 60° of supination is recommended. This technique is simple and well described in straightforward schematic drawings. Another strength is that it is based on a previous biomechanical study by the same authors. However, it is unclear from this report whether this DOB reconstruction should be used as an isolated procedure or combined with an Adams and Berger triangular fibrocartilage complex reconstruction. The bony bridges of the transosseous tunnels are small given the size of the tendon graft, and the surgical technique should be meticulous to avoid intraoperative problems. This technique should not be used in longitudinal forearm dissociation, as the obliquity of the DOB is opposite to the obliquity of the IOM central band. The authors acknowledge that "more studies are needed to determine the biomechanical and clinical efficacy of this reconstruction," but they should be commended for bringing up a simple technique that may be part of our armamentarium when treating the difficult problem of chronic distal radioulnar joint instability.

G. Herzberg, MD

The Unstable Distal Radius Fracture—How Do We Define It? A Systematic Review
Walenkamp MMJ, Vos LM, Strackee SD, et al (Univ of Amsterdam, The Netherlands; et al)
J Wrist Surg 4:307-316, 2015

Background.—Unstable distal radius fractures are a popular research subject. However, to appreciate the findings of studies that enrolled patients with unstable distal radius fractures, it should be clear how the authors defined an *unstable distal radius fracture*.

Questions.—In what percentage of studies involving patients with unstable distal radius fractures did the authors define *unstable distal radius fracture*? What are the most common descriptions of an unstable distal radius fracture? And is there one preferred evidence-based definition for future authors?

Methods.—A systematic search of literature was performed to identify any type of study with the term *unstable distal radius fracture*. We assessed whether a definition was provided and determined the level of evidence for the most common definitions.

Results.—The search yielded 2,489 citations, of which 479 were included. In 149 studies, it was explicitly stated that patients with unstable distal radius fractures were enrolled. In 54% (81/149) of these studies, the authors defined an unstable distal radius fracture. Overall, we found 143 different definitions. The seven most common definitions were: displacement following adequate reduction; Lafontaine's definition; irreducibility; an AO type C2 fracture; a volarly displaced fracture; Poigenfürst's criteria; and Cooney's criteria. Only Lafontaine's definition originated from a clinical study (level IIIb).

Conclusion.—In only half of the studies involving patients with an unstable distal radius fracture did the authors defined what they considered an *unstable distal radius fracture*. None of the definitions stood out as the preferred choice. A general consensus definition could help to standardize future research.

▶ The definition of an unstable distal radial fracture is often subjective. However, to interpret and compare the literature, a more objective definition of instability is required. In general, the term *"unstable"* is often used to describe a fracture that is highly likely to displace further from its original position. Of the articles reviewed that investigated "unstable" fractures, just more than half of them actually defined what they understand as unstable. Furthermore, the authors found 143 different descriptions of what an unstable fracture may be; however, the most common description was that of loss of reduction after initial manipulation and acceptable reduction. The authors suggest that future researchers in this area should clearly define what they understand to be an unstable distal radial fracture.

M. Hayton, MD

Effect of Volarly Angulated Distal Radius Fractures on Forearm Rotation and Distal Radioulnar Joint Kinematics

Nishiwaki M, Welsh MF, Gammon B, et al (Kawasaki Municipal Hosp, Japan; St. Joseph's Health Care London, Ontario, Canada; Univ of Ottawa, Ontario, Canada)
J Hand Surg Am 40:2236-2242, 2015

Purpose.—To examine the effect of volar angulation deformities of the distal radius with and without triangular fibrocartilage complex (TFCC) rupture on forearm range of motion and the kinematics of the ulnar head at the distal radioulnar joint (DRUJ) during simulated active forearm rotation.

Methods.—Volar angulation deformities of the distal radius with 10° and 20° angulation from the native orientation were created in 8 cadaveric specimens using an adjustable apparatus. Active supination and pronation were performed using a forearm motion simulator. Pronation and supination range of motion was quantified with each deformity. In addition, changes in the dorsovolar position of the ulnar head relative to the radius were calculated after simulating each distal radial deformity. Testing was performed with the TFCC intact and sectioned.

Results.—Volar angulation deformities of 20° decreased the supination range with preservation of pronation. There was no effect of TFCC status on the range of forearm rotation. With the TFCC intact, volar angulation deformities translated the ulna slightly dorsally in pronation and volarly in supination. After sectioning the TFCC, volar angulation deformities of 10° and 20° translated the ulna dorsally throughout forearm rotation.

Conclusions.—Volar angulation deformities reduce supination range and alter the DRUJ kinematics. The increased tension in the intact TFCC caused by volar angulation deformities likely prevented the expected dorsovolar displacement at the DRUJ and restricted supination. Dividing the TFCC released the constraining effect on the DRUJ and allowed the ulna to translate dorsally. However, supination remained limited, presumably because of impediment from the dorsally subluxated ulna.

Clinical Relevance.—This study demonstrated the importance of correcting volar angulation deformities of the distal radius to less than 20°

in order to maintain normal range of forearm rotation and to less than 10°
to maintain normal DRUJ kinematics when the TFCC is ruptured.

▶ This study examines the relationship between volarly angulated distal radius
fractures and forearm rotation. The authors evaluate the effects on the distal
radioulnar joint (DRUJ) with and without triangular fibrocartilage complex
(TFCC) rupture. The authors present an in vitro biomechanical model with
appropriate quantification of the volar angulation deformities using an active
motion simulator and previously described coordinate system. Their methodology and conclusions are sound, demonstrating the importance of correcting
distal radius deformities to less than 20° of volar angulation to maintain forearm
rotation and normal DRUJ kinematics. If the TFCC is ruptured, volar angulation
must be corrected to within 10°. Consideration must be given to the fact that
this is an in vitro model, and often volar angulation deformities are combined
with volar translation, radial translation, shortening, and pronation in the clinical setting. These additional factors may further influence range of motion or
DRUJ kinematics. This study takes an important step in quantifying volar angulation deformities and their significance in distal radius fracture malunion.

Paul Kooner, BSc, contributed to the writing of this review under the direction of Ruby Grewal, MD, MSc, FRCSC.

R. Grewal, MD, MSc, FRCSC

**No Difference in Adverse Events Between Surgically Treated Reduced and
Unreduced Distal Radius Fractures**
Teunis T, Mulder F, Nota SP, et al (Harvard Med School, Boston, MA)
J Orthop Trauma 29:521-525, 2015

Objectives.—To determine if closed reduction is worthwhile for the subset of patients who choose operative treatment before attempted reduction
of their distal radius fracture. We hypothesize that there are no differences
in (1) adverse events and (2) subsequent surgeries between patients treated
with manipulative reduction compared with those that were splinted without reduction.

Design.—Retrospective cohort study.

Setting.—Three affiliated urban hospitals in a single city in the United
States.

Patients/Participants.—One thousand five hundred eleven consecutive
adult patients who underwent open reduction and internal fixation of
their distal radius fracture between January 1, 2007, and December 31,
2012, of whom 102 (7%) were not reduced before surgery.

Intervention.—Manipulative reduction compared with splinting without reduction.

Main Outcome Measurements.—Adverse events were defined as any
infections, hematomas treated operatively, disproportionate finger stiffness,
(transient) neuropathology after surgery, delayed carpal tunnel release, malunion, reoperation for loss of alignment, hardware removal, and tendon

ruptures within 1 year after surgery. Outcome measures were grouped to determine the overall adverse event rate and subsequent surgery rate.

Results.—We found no difference in specific adverse events between unreduced and reduced fractures. After adjusting for possible confounding variables by logistic regression, we found no difference in overall rates of adverse events (adjusted odds ratio unreduced fractures 1.2, 95% confidence interval 0.67–2.0) and subsequent surgeries (adjusted odds ratio unreduced fractures 0.65, 95% confidence interval 0.23–1.8).

Conclusions.—Leaving the fracture unreduced before surgery was not associated with increased adverse events or subsequent surgeries. For patients who make an informed decision to undergo operative treatment for their closed neurovascular intact displaced distal radius fracture, manipulative reduction may not be helpful.

Level of Evidence.—Therapeutic Level III. See Instructions for Authors for a complete description of levels of evidence.

▶ Despite a busy title, this article addresses a practical aspect of the management of distal radius fractures (DRFs). The authors considered a group of 1511 consecutive patients over a 6-year period with acute, neurovascular uncomplicated DRF treated by 64 surgeons from 3 affiliated urban hospitals of a single US town. In all these patients, the decision of surgical treatment was taken before attempted reduction. Before surgery, 93.2% of this group had manipulative reduction, whereas 6.8% were splinted without reduction. Through chart review and statistical analysis, the authors demonstrated that leaving the fracture unreduced before surgery was not associated with increased adverse events or subsequent surgeries. The authors suggest that preoperative manipulative reduction and splinting may not be helpful when a decision of surgical treatment for acute neurovascularly uncomplicated DRF was made. It is worthwhile to be aware of this article when we are faced with this situation.

This article has several strengths: a large group of patients and sophisticated statistical analysis. It is also unique in a sense that in this group of patients the decision for surgery based on initial clinical and radiological presentation was made with the patient before any attempt at closed reduction. We all know that many authors recommend that DRFs are not considered for surgery until manipulative reduction is attempted.

There are also some weaknesses: the unreduced group is small compared with the reduced one, including hardware removal into the adverse effects is debatable, the study is based on retrospective chart analysis, and the age distribution is large (38-70 years) with no clear age stratification so that the conclusions may be different for different patients' profiles.

In our practice, given the high potential of redisplacement after closed reduction of acute displaced DRF and our large patient volume, we also make the decision for surgical treatment at the acute stage from a combined analysis of patient's profile, accident energy, and fracture displacement. We do not rely on the quality of a trial of closed reduction. Furthermore, we do not routinely use closed reduction and splinting for comfort before surgery unless the fracture was initially very displaced, especially in the sagittal plane. Actually, we noted on several occasions that the "closed reduction attempt" in the emergency department made the displacement worse!

G. Herzberg, MD

Wrist Fracture and Risk of Subsequent Fracture: Findings from the Women's Health Initiative Study
Crandall CJ, Hovey KM, Cauley JA, et al (Univ of California at Los Angeles; State Univ of New York at Buffalo; Univ of Pittsburgh, PA; et al)
J Bone Miner Res 30:2086-2095, 2015

Wrist fractures are common in postmenopausal women and are associated with functional decline. Fracture patterns after wrist fracture are unclear. The goal of this study was to determine the frequency and types of fractures that occur after a wrist fracture among postmenopausal women. We carried out a post hoc analysis of data from the Women's Health Initiative Observational Study and Clinical Trials (1993—2010) carried out at 40 US clinical centers. Participants were postmenopausal women aged 50 to 79 years at baseline. Mean follow-up duration was 11.8 years. Main measures included incident wrist, clinical spine, humerus, upper extremity, lower extremity, hip, and total non-wrist fractures and bone mineral density (BMD) in a subset. Among women who experienced wrist fracture, 15.5% subsequently experienced non-wrist fracture. The hazard for non-wrist fractures was higher among women who had experienced previous wrist fracture than among women who had not experienced wrist fracture: non-wrist fracture overall (hazard ratio [HR] = 1.40, 95% confidence interval [CI] 1.33—1.48), spine (HR = 1.48, 95% CI 1.32—1.66), humerus (HR = 1.78, 95% CI 1.57—2.02), upper extremity (non-wrist) (HR = 1.88, 95% CI 1.70—2.07), lower extremity (non-hip) (HR = 1.36, 95% CI 1.26—1.48), and hip (HR = 1.50, 95% CI 1.32—1.71) fracture. Associations persisted after adjustment for BMD, physical activity, and other risk factors. Risk of non-wrist fracture was higher in women who were younger when they experienced wrist fracture (interaction p value 0.02). Associations between incident wrist fracture and subsequent non-wrist fracture did not vary by baseline BMD category (normal, low bone density, osteoporosis). A wrist fracture is associated with increased risk of subsequent hip, vertebral, upper extremity, and lower extremity fractures. There may be substantial missed opportunity for intervention in the large number of women who present with wrist fractures.

▶ The study focuses on the association between wrist fractures and the risk of future fracture in postmenopausal women. The authors examined data from the Women's Health Initiative and reported an increased rate of secondary fractures (hip, spine, humerus, and other upper and lower extremity) in 160 930 women with wrist fractures. The hazard ratios for this ranged from 1.36 to 1.88 depending on the type of fracture.

Although previous literature database studies had already demonstrated a link between wrist fractures and subsequent fracture, this article is unique in that it provides more detail on the specific types of fractures sustained. The authors also demonstrated that the risk of second fracture was high after wrist fracture once age and bone mineral density are controlled for. The study strengths lie in the large sample size and standardized data collection, as well as the detail on specific types of fractures included. The weaknesses include the cross-sectional design and limited information on treatment and outcomes. The authors also classified radius fractures and carpal fractures as 1 group, although they have differing baseline characteristics. Finally, it would be interesting to know whether the wrist fracture cohort does indeed have an increase in mortality compared with the nonfracture cohort. In conclusion, this study highlights the importance of identifying patients with wrist fragility fractures and ensuring proper screening and treatment for osteoporosis in hopes of decreasing future fracture burden.

T. D. Rozental, MD

Catastrophic Thinking Is Associated With Finger Stiffness After Distal Radius Fracture Surgery
Teunis T, Bot AGJ, Thornton ER, et al (Massachusetts General Hosp, Boston; Univ of Amsterdam, the Netherlands)
J Orthop Trauma 29:e414-e420, 2015

Objectives.—To identify demographic, injury-related, or psychologic factors associated with finger stiffness at suture removal and 6 weeks after distal radius fracture surgery. We hypothesize that there are no factors associated with distance to palmar crease at suture removal.

Design.—Prospective cohort study.

Setting.—Level I Academic Urban Trauma Center.

Patients.—One hundred sixteen adult patients underwent open reduction and internal fixation of their distal radius fractures; 96 of whom were also available 6 weeks after surgery.

Intervention.—None.

Main Outcome Measurements.—At suture removal, we recorded patients' demographics, AO fracture type, carpal tunnel release at the time of surgery, pain catastrophizing scale, Whiteley Index, Patient Health Questionnaire-9, and disabilities of the arm, shoulder, and hand questionnaire, 11-point ordinal measure of pain intensity, distance to palmar crease, and active flexion of the thumb through the small finger. At 6 weeks after surgery, we measured motion, disabilities of the arm, shoulder, and hand, and pain intensity. Prereduction and postsurgery radiographic fracture characteristics were assessed.

Results.—Female sex, being married, specific surgeons, carpal tunnel release, AO type C fractures, and greater catastrophic thinking were associated with increased distance to palmar crease at suture removal. At 6 weeks, greater catastrophic thinking was the only factor associated with increased distance to palmar crease.

Conclusions.—Catastrophic thinking was a consistent and major determinant of finger stiffness at suture removal and 6 weeks after injury. Future research should assess if treatments that ameliorate catastrophic thinking can facilitate recovery of finger motion after operative treatment of a distal radius fracture.

Level of Evidence.—Prognostic Level I. See Instructions for Authors for a complete description of levels of evidence.

▶ This study by Ring et al prospectively evaluated a group of 116 adult patients with distal radius fractures treated with volar plate fixation over a 5-year period. The purpose of the study was to identify risk factors associated with finger stiffness at suture removal and 6 weeks after surgery. Of the 116 patients enrolled, 96 (83%) were available for examination at 6 weeks following surgery. The most significant finding of the study was that greater "catastrophic thinking" was a consistent and major determinant of finger stiffness at suture removal and 6 weeks after surgery. The authors point out that catastrophic thinking, or negative beliefs about pain leading to an overprotective response, is a critical risk factor that leads to digital stiffness following open reduction internal fixation (ORIF) of distal radius fractures.

Ring is once again to be commended for attempting to add science to a difficult and poorly understood subset of patients. Early recognition, supervised hand therapy, and early mobilization are all crucial to avoid permanent digital stiffness in this challenging population. In patients who do not exhibit full digital motion at the time of suture removal, I institute supervised hand therapy immediately. Permanent limitation in digital range of motion can severely compromise the result of an otherwise well-performed distal radius ORIF.

D. Zelouf, MD

Hemiarthroplasty for Complex Distal Radius Fractures in Elderly Patients
Vergnenègre G, Hardy J, Mabit C, et al (CHRU Limoges, France)
J Wrist Surg 4:169-173, 2015

Background.—In elderly patients, distal radius fractures frequently occur in osteoporotic bone and may be nonreconstructable. It is our hypothesis that a hemiarthroplasty replacment of the articular surface can provide satisfactory results in terms of range of motion, pain, and function for immediate salvage of a fracture that is not amenable to internal fixation.

Methods.—Between July 2009 and January 2012, eight elderly patients were treated with insertion of a Sophia distal radius implant (Biotech, Paris, France). Inclusion criteria consisted of an isolated AO type C2 distal radius fracture in patients over 70 years old. All patients were reviewed by an independent surgeon.

Results.—The mean follow-up was 25 months (range, 17—36 months). Mean wrist range of motion (ROM) was 45° (40—50°) of flexion, 44° (40—50°) of extension, and a mean pronation-supination arc of 160°. Mean grip force was 18 kgf. The mean QuickDASH (Disabilities of the

Arm, Shoulder and Hand) was 18.2/100 (6.82–29.55), and the mean visual analog scale (VAS) was 2.33 (0–4). X-ray images did not demonstrate implant loosening or ulnar translation of the carpus.

Conclusions.—The Sophia hemiarthroplasty provided rapid recovery of independence in elderly patients with a nonreconstructable comminuted distal radius fracture.

▶ Volar locking plate fixation for acute distal radius fractures is currently in vogue, but some authors have questioned its use in the elderly. In a prospective randomized study by Arora et al[1] comparing open reduction internal fixation with volar locking plate versus nonsurgical treatment in patients > 65 years of age, there were no differences in pain level, active range of motion, or DASH and Patient Rated Wrist Evaluation scores between the groups despite the malunions in the nonsurgical group. There were, however, more complications in the surgical group with 11 of 36 patients requiring revision surgery. The concept of inserting a wrist hemiarthroplasty (WHA) in elderly patients with acute distal radius fractures was proposed by Roux[2,3] using the Sophia prosthesis. This prosthesis is composed of a radial stem and an epiphyseal-metaphyseal block that articulates with both the carpus and the ulnar head. It replaces the distal carpal facet of the radius as well as the sigmoid notch. In Roux's series of 6 patients, the mean patient age was 73 years. At an mean follow-up of 27 months, the mean DASH score was 27.2. The mean arc of forearm rotation was 110 degrees, and the mean wrist flexion/extension arc was 90 degrees. Grip strength was 80% of the opposite side. There was 1 case of complex regional pain syndrome (CRPS).

In the current study, 8 patients underwent a primary WHA. The mean age of patients was 80 years old (range 74-85 years). All of the fractures were AO type C2 with metaphyseal and epiphyseal comminution. At a mean follow-up of 25 months (range 17-36 months), the mean visual analog scale (VAS) was 2 (range 0.5-3.5), and the QuickDash was 18 (SD 6.2). The mean arc of forearm rotation was 160 degrees, and the mean wrist flexion/extension arc was 89 degrees with an average wrist extension of 44 degrees. Grip strength was 92% of the opposite side. The patients were able to perform activities of daily living (ADLs) at an average of 3 weeks (range 0.5-5 weeks). There was 1 periprosthetic calcification.

Herzberg et al[4] reported similar results in 12 patients using the radial component of the Remotion total wrist arthroplasty (Small Bone Innovation, Morrisville PA) in 9 wrists, and a custom press-fit Cobra WHA implant (Groupe Lepine, Lyon, France) in 2 patients. The mean age was 76 years (range 65-88 years). At an average follow-up of 27 months, the average VAS was 1 (range 0-4), and the QuickDash was 32 (range 0-77). The mean arc of forearm pronation and supination was 151 degrees (range 120-170 degrees), and the mean wrist flexion/extension arc was 60 degrees (range 35-85 degrees), with a mean wrist extension of 34 degrees (range 15-50 degrees). Grip strength was 67% of the opposite side (range 36%-100%). Bone healing around the implants was satisfactory in all wrists. There were 3 patients with CRPS. One patient was reoperated at 20 months with significant finger stiffness due to tendon adhesions along with a tendency for ulnar deviation of the wrist. She underwent an extensor tenolysis combined with a tendon transfer on extensor carpi radialis longus to extensor carpi radialis brevis tendon transfer.

Study benefits:

Based on the experience of hemiarthroplasty for irreparable knee and shoulder fractures, a primary WHA leads to a rapid return to independent function and ADLs in elderly patients.

Study limitations:

Because the Sophia implant is bulky, the periosteum surrounding the distal radius in direct contact with the large metallic part of the implant. In addition, it would be difficult to reconstruct the large bony defect in case of implant removal. The use of this implant is contraindicated if there is an associated ulnar neck or head fracture. The long-term fate of the cartilage on the proximal carpal row due to direct metal on cartilage contact is uncertain. Erosion of the carpus due to prolonged contact with the cobalt chrome surface is likely. Longer-term follow-up and comparative studies with larger numbers of patients are needed to confirm the indications and safety of this approach in independently living elderly patients.

D. J. Slutsky, MD

References

1. Arora R, Gabl M. A prospective randomized trial comparing nonoperative treatment with volar locking plate fixation for displaced and unstable DRF in patients 65 years and older. *J Bone Joint Surg Am.* 2011;93A:2146-2153.
2. Roux JL. La prothèse de remplacement et resurfacage du radius distal: un nouveau concept thérapeutique. *Chirurgie de la Main.* 2009;28:10.
3. Roux JL. Treatment of intra-articular fractures of the distal radius by wrist prosthesis. *Orthop Traumatol Surg Res.* 2011;97S:S46-S53.
4. Herzberg G, Burnier M, Marc A, Izem Y. Primary wrist hemiarthroplasty for irreparable distal radius fracture in the independent elderly. *J Wrist Surg.* 2015;4:156-163.

Biomechanical Comparison of Volar Fixed-Angle Locking Plates for AO C3 Distal Radius Fractures: Titanium Versus Stainless Steel With Compression

Marshall T, Momaya A, Eberhardt A, et al (Univ of Alabama at Birmingham; et al)

J Hand Surg Am 40:2032-2038, 2015

Purpose.—To determine biomechanical differences between a fixed-angle locking volar titanium plate (VariAx; Stryker, Kalamazoo, MI) and a fixed-angle compression locking volar stainless steel plate (CoverLoc Volar Plate; Tornier, Amsterdam, Netherlands) in the fixation of simulated AO C3 distal radius fractures.

Methods.—Eighteen cadaveric upper extremities (9 matched pairs) with an average age of 54 years were tested. A 4-part AO C3 fracture pattern was created in each specimen. The fractures were reduced under direct vision and fixed with either the fixed-angle locking volar titanium plate or the fixed-angle compression locking volar stainless steel plate. Motion tracking analysis was then performed while the specimens underwent cyclic loading. Changes in displacement, rotation, load to failure, and mode of failure were recorded.

Results.—The fragments, when secured with the fixed-angle compression locking stainless steel construct, demonstrated less displacement and rotation than the fragments secured with the fixed-angle locking titanium plate under physiological loading conditions. In the fixed-angle compression locking stainless steel group, aggregate displacement and rotation of fracture fragments were 5 mm and 3° less, respectively, than those for the fixed-angle locking titanium group. The differences between axial loads at mechanical failure and stiffness were not statistically significant. The compression locking stainless steel group showed no trend in mode of failure, and the locking titanium plate group failed most often by articular fixation failure (5 of 9 specimens).

Conclusions.—The fixed-angle compression locking stainless steel volar plate may result in less displacement and rotation of fracture fragments in the fixation of AO C3 distal radius fractures than fixation by the fixed-angle locking volar titanium plate. However, there were no differences between the plates in mechanical load to failure and stiffness.

Clinical Relevance.—Fixation of distal radius AO C3 fracture patterns with the fixed-angle compression locking stainless steel plate may provide improved stability of fracture fragments.

▶ In this cadaveric study of 18 fresh-frozen specimens, the authors created reproducible intraarticular C3 type fractures and fixed them with 2 different volar plates that are available on the market (different concepts, materials—stainless steel vs titanium—and geometries). They applied physiological axial loading and demonstrated that load to failure was equivalent for the 2 plates. However, fragments displacements and rotation under cyclic loading were slightly superior ($P < .05$) when the titanium plate was used. The number and diameters of the epiphyseal screws were similar, but no information was provided about the length of the screws, which may have influenced the fragments displacement/rotation results. The strength of this study was a straightforward method of axial loading and fragments displacement/rotation recording. It was interesting to note that failures were most often due to loss of screw fixation. The reader should be aware that the funding of the study was provided by the company manufacturing one of the plates and that there was a conflict of interests for one of the authors. The authors conclude that "further research is necessary to determine if the results of this study are of clinical importance," and I agree with this statement.

G. Herzberg, MD

Volar Marginal Rim Fracture Fixation With Volar Fragment-Specific Hook Plate Fixation
O'Shaughnessy MA, Shin AY, Kakar S (Mayo Clinic, Rochester, MN)
J Hand Surg Am 40:1563-1570, 2015

Purpose.—To review the outcomes of patients treated with a volar hook plate specifically designed to capture volar marginal rim fractures.

Methods.—A retrospective study was performed over 18 months of patients treated with a volar hook plate in the management of AO type B or C distal radius fractures with a volar marginal rim fragment. Clinical and radiographic outcomes were evaluated.

Results.—The series included 26 wrists in 25 patients, average age 55 years. Average follow-up was 9 months (range, 3–30 mo). Twenty patients had AO type C fractures and 6 had AO type B fractures. All 6 AO type B were B3 fractures. Of the AO type C, 1 had C1, 7 had C2, and 12 had C3. No patients had loss of fixation of the critical volar ulnar corner and there was no evidence of carpal subluxation. Five patients required hardware removal. Four patients experienced hardware irritation requiring removal of all hardware including the volar hook plate. One patient required partial hardware removal that did not include the volar hook plate. All patients with volar hardware irritation had hook plates that were of second-generation design that had a prominent bend, which has since been modified. There were no cases of tendon rupture.

Conclusions.—Volar marginal rim fragments of intra-articular distal radius fractures are not amenable to standard volar plate fixation. Fragment-specific fixation using a volar hook plate designed specifically for these fragments allowed for stable fixation when combined with other fragment-specific fixation techniques. There was no loss of fixation of the critical corner in this series. Although hardware irritation can occur, fully seated hooks and subsequent modification of the design of the hook bend has diminished this complication.

Type of Study/Level of Evidence.—Therapeutic IV.

▶ This retrospective review highlights the importance of addressing the volar ulnar fragment in a case series of patients who have undergone fragment specific fixation of their comminuted distal radius fractures. The article focuses on the use of a specific type of implant, namely, a fixed angled hook plate, for the fixation on the volar ulnar corner. The authors have reported commendable outcomes and, importantly, no postoperative loss of reduction. It is also necessary to add that the average number of plates used per patient was 2.7 (range, 2-6 plates), implying that the volar hook plate was part of a more complex construct and the results described are best viewed in this context.

The volar ulnar corner may be stabilized with an array of implants, ranging from simple wires or screws to surgeon-bent plates originally meant for use for the phalanges and metacarpals. Wire forms are another good option for this purpose. In fact, in instances in which the volar ulnar fragment is large enough, biasing the placement of a conventional volar locking plate to the ulnar corner may also suffice. What must be emphasized in all these methods is that the implants have to be as flush as possible to the distal radius to avoid flexor tendon irritation. Although 4 of the 26 patients required removal of the hook plate placed at the volar ulnar corner for this exact complication, it is comforting to note that the new generation of this plate has been redesigned with a lower profile.

In essence, this report provides the evidence for use of another feasible option should the surgeon elect to fix the volar ulnar corner with a fixed angled device. A natural next step to gather higher levels of evidence would be to compare these different methods of fixation for the volar ulnar corner in a case-control or prospective comparative study.

A. Cheah, MD

Functional Outcomes of the Aptis-Scheker Distal Radioulnar Joint Replacement in Patients Under 40 Years Old

Rampazzo A, Gharb BB, Brock G, et al (Cleveland Clinic, OH; Univ of Louisville, KY; et al)
J Hand Surg Am 40:1397-1403, 2015

Purpose.—To study the functional results after Aptis-Scheker distal radioulnar joint (DRUJ) replacement in young patients.

Methods.—We performed a retrospective study selecting all patients under age 40 years, with a clinical and radiological follow-up longer than 2 years, who underwent DRUJ replacement. Patients' charts were reviewed and age at surgery, profession, hobbies, comorbidities, diagnosis, previous procedures, and complications were recorded. Preoperative and postoperative Disabilities of Arm, Shoulder, and Hand and Patient-Rated Wrist Evaluation scores, visual analog scale score, grip strength, lifting capacity, and wrist range of motion were recorded. Functional results and characteristics of the patients were correlated with linear regression. A Kaplan-Meier curve was plotted.

Results.—We performed 46 arthroplasties. Average patient age was 32 years. Forty-one arthroplasties were performed for pain and 5 for pain and instability. Average follow-up was 61 months. Thirty-seven patients underwent multiple procedures before DRUJ replacement (1.7 ± 1.2 procedures). Extensor carpi ulnaris release with implant coverage using a local adipofascial flap (5) or dermal-fat graft (4) was the most common procedure performed after implantation of the prosthesis. Thirty surgeries were undertaken to address complications after DRUJ replacement in 15 wrists. A total of 36 procedures not related to DRUJ replacement were performed in 15 wrists after the arthroplasty. Grip, lifting, Disabilities of Arm, Shoulder, and Hand and Patient-Rated Wrist Evaluation scores, visual analog scale score, and supination showed statistically significant improvement after surgery. Functional results were comparable in patients who received the implant with either a standard or extended stem. Patient age and number of the previous procedures did not correlate with functional results. The 5-year survival of the implant was 96%.

Conclusions.—In this group of young patients, the implant improved the functional status of the extremity. The most frequent complication was extensor carpi ulnaris tendonitis, which was addressed by interposition of an adipofascial flap.

Type of Study/Level of Evidence.—Therapeutic IV.

▶ Chronic distal radioulnar joint (DRUJ) pain, instability, and arthritis in young patients is one of the most challenging problems faced in hand surgery. Traditional management strategies of Sauve-Kapandji as well as partial/complete ulnar head resection with or without interposed materials are traditionally employed yet only occasionally leads to overly gratifying outcomes for the patient or physician. Concerns always exist for the use of this arthroplasty in young patients, particularly given the magnitude and size of the Aptis. An additional concern for this particular implant is the lack of unbiased published results because the majority of the publications are from the designer of the implant.

The strengths of this study include the relatively large number of patients, midterm follow-up, and inclusive reporting of any adverse subsequent event whether or not it was related to the index procedure. The 96% 5-year implant survival is certainly impressive, particularly in an active young patient cohort. Although half of the patients had a subsequent surgery, most of these were unrelated to the DRUJ arthroplasty. Of the complications related to the implant, most were tendonitis, which can be avoided with the addition of a retinacular sheath to protect the extensor carpi ulnaris (ECU; now recommended).

My personal experience with this implant, including patients under age 40, has far exceeded my expectations. The pain relief, range of motion, and patient satisfaction have far outperformed any other DRUJ salvage procedure in my hands. I believe the only thing lacking for the widespread adoption of this implant are longer term studies and nonbiased publications. A few technical pearls are critical for success including the ECU retinacular sling, the perpendicular bone cut and placement of the radial baseplate, and adequate exposure with release of the IOM.

This study further encouraged me to expand my comfort with this implant into a younger patient population, and I have been extremely happy with this decision. Although treatment must be individualized for patients with DRUJ chronic pain, instability, and arthritis, this procedure has become my personal "go-to" for a majority of patients.

G. Gaston, MD

Arthroscopic assistance does not improve the functional or radiographic outcome of unstable intra-articular distal radial fractures treated with a volar locking plate: a randomised controlled trial

Yamazaki H, Uchiyama S, Komatsu M, et al (Aizawa Hosp, Honjo, Matsumoto, Japan)

Bone Joint J 97-B:957-962, 2015

There is no consensus on the benefit of arthroscopically assisted reduction of the articular surface combined with fixation using a volar locking plate for the treatment of intra-articular distal radial fractures. In this study we compared the functional and radiographic outcomes of fluoroscopically and arthroscopically guided reduction of these fractures.

Between February 2009 and May 2013, 74 patients with unilateral unstable intra-articular distal radial fractures were randomised equally into the two groups for treatment. The mean age of these 74 patients was 64 years (24 to 92). We compared functional outcomes including active range of movement of the wrist, grip strength and Disabilities of the Arm, Shoulder, and Hand scores at six and 48 weeks; and radiographic outcomes that included gap, step, radial inclination, volar angulation and ulnar variance.

There were no significant differences between the techniques with regard to functional outcomes or radiographic parameters. The mean gap and step in the fluoroscopic and arthroscopic groups were comparable at 0.9 mm (standard deviation (SD) 0.7) and 0.7 mm (SD 0.7) and 0.6 mm (SD 0.6) and 0.4 mm (SD 0.5), respectively; $p = 0.18$ and $p = 0.35$.

Arthroscopic reduction conferred no advantage over conventional fluoroscopic guidance in achieving anatomical reduction of intra-articular distal radial fractures when using a volar locking plate.

▶ In modern orthopedics, arthroscopy is regarded as the gold standard in assessing intraarticular conditions. When facing a distal radius fracture with significant intraarticular involvement, the use of arthroscopy in evaluating the joint as well as in assisting reduction fixation becomes a natural desire or a logical choice for surgeons, especially for those who have acquired the skill. However, there is always a learning curve issue because arthroscopic intervention under such a situation can be one of the most challenging and technically demanding tasks in wrist arthroscopy. Additional cost is another concern, although from my point of view, for centers already equipped with standard wrist arthroscopic equipment and expertise, this should not be a hindrance. After all, the biggest drive for a surgeon to contemplate a more difficult or costly surgery is the difference in outcome. All arthroscopic surgeons would like to see their work being justified or rewarded by a better clinical result on the patients. They will probably be disappointed in reading this article, which shows no difference in arthroscopic treatment compared with treatment purely based on image intensifier. This study is a well-designed and well-conducted level I study of high quality. All surgeries were performed by a single experienced surgeon or under his supervision, CT imaging was used for evaluation both preoperatively and on follow-up instead of based on plain radiographs, assessors were blinded to the study, and there was a low default rate for follow-up. If they could produce a comparison on the costs, perhaps they could make an even stronger conclusion at the end. However, before their statements can become a testimonial, a few concerns must be addressed:

1. There was no report on the quality of reduction immediately after the operation for each method. Their technique also did not address the fixation of individual major articular fragments. We are uncertain whether the arthroscopic reduction was of the highest quality.

2. There were fewer complicated fractures in the fluoroscopic group (50% vs 61% C3 fractures), and this may be a bias in patient selection.

3. The average age of the patients in this study was approaching 65, which was much higher than in previous studies. Much evidence has shown that the clinical outcome on distal radius fractures in advanced aged patients did not vary with whatever treatment they received, and outcomes were generally good.

I look forward to seeing a similar study performed on the more challenging population of younger patients.

P. C. Ho, MD

Is it time to revisit the AO classification of fractures of the distal radius? Inter- and intra-observer reliability of the AO classification
Plant CE, Hickson C, Hedley H, et al (Univ of Warwick, Coventry, United Kingdom)
Bone Joint J 97-B:818-823, 2015

We conducted an observational radiographic study to determine the inter- and intraobserver reliability of the AO classification of fractures of the distal radius. Plain posteroanterior and lateral radiographs of 456 patients with an acute fracture of the distal radius were classified by a consultant orthopaedic hand specialist and two specialist trainees, and the k coefficient for the inter- and intra-observer reliability of the type, group and subgroup classification was calculated.

Only the type of fracture (A, B or C) was found to provide substantial intra-observer reliability (k_{type} 0.65). The inclusion of 'group' and 'subgroup' into the classification reduced the inter-observer reliability to fair (k_{group} 0.29, $k_{subgroup} = 0.28$) and the intra-observer reliability to moderate (k_{group} 0.53, $k_{subgroup}$ 0.49). Disagreement was found to arise between specific subgroups, which may be amenable to clarification.

▶ There are two types of classification philosophies. The "lumpers" approach is to simplify the concept into a system with few broad categories, easily recalled. The "splitters" approach is to divide and then further divide into more specific categories. The ideal result is a comprehensive descriptive intellectually appealing categorization that is impossible, except for the savant, to keep in mind. Ideally, classification systems should be the product of consensus committees of experts and nonexperts, perhaps using a consensus process such as the Delphi method. Perhaps the AO classification system would profit from a revision using a validated model for achieving consensus.

V. R. Hentz, MD

Functional Outcomes Following Bridge Plate Fixation for Distal Radius Fractures

Lauder A, Agnew S, Bakri K, et al (Univ of Washington, Seattle; Northwestern Univ, Chicago, IL; Mayo Clinic, Rochester, MN)
J Hand Surg Am 40:1554-1562, 2015

Purpose.—To determine the functional outcomes of patients treated with dorsal spanning distraction bridge plate fixation for distal radius fractures.

Methods.—All adult patients at our institution who underwent treatment of a unilateral distal radius fracture using a dorsal bridge plate from 2008 to 2012 were identified retrospectively. Patients were enrolled in clinical follow-up to assess function. Wrist range of motion, grip strength, and extension torque were measured systematically and compared with the contralateral, uninjured wrist. Patients also completed *Quick*-Disabilities of the Arm, Shoulder, and Hand and Patient-Rated Wrist Evaluation outcomes questionnaires.

Results.—Eighteen of 100 eligible patients, with a minimum of 1 year from the time of implant removal, were available for follow-up (mean, 2.7 y). All fracture patterns were comminuted and intra-articular (AO 23.C3). There were significant decreases in wrist flexion (43° vs 58°), extension (46° vs 56°), and ulnar deviation (23° vs 29°) compared with the contralateral uninjured wrist. Grip strength was 86% and extension torque was 78% of the contralateral wrist. Comparison of dominant and nondominant wrist injuries identified nearly complete recovery of grip (95%) and extension (96%) strength of dominant-sided wrist injuries, compared with grip (79%) and extension (65%) strength in those with an injured nondominant wrist. Mean *Quick*-Disabilities of the Arm, Shoulder, and Hand and Patient-Rated Wrist Evaluation scores were 16 and 14, respectively. There were 2 cases of postoperative surgical site pain and no cases of infection, tendonitis, or tendon rupture.

Conclusions.—Distraction bridge plate fixation for distal radius fractures is safe with minimal complications. Functional outcomes are similar to those published for other treatment methods.

Type of Study/Level of Evidence.—Therapeutic IV.

▶ Distal radius fractures are the most common fracture treated by hand surgeons. The use of bridge plates for the management of distal radius fractures has necessarily broadened the armamentarium of the treating surgeon. The authors of this article have a wealth of experience using this technique. They report on the functional outcome of patients treated with a unilateral bridge plate for distal radius fracture at their institution. The strengths of this article are that the authors had 100 patients who met the inclusion criteria. Selected outcome measures were reasonable and consistent with the literature for this injury. Although the duration of follow-up was nearly 3 years from injury for those included, a major limitation of the study is that only 18% of the patients were available for follow-up at 1 year after implant removal. This is in part related to the unique catchment area of the level 1 trauma center that services a large geographic area in the Pacific Northwest.

My clinical practice is consistent with that of the authors. I favor the use of bridge plates for distal radius fractures with metadiaphyseal extension with bone loss, polytrauma patients requiring early use of the limb for weight bearing or transfers, and unstable comminuted distal radius fractures not amenable to nonspanning fixation. My experience has been that these patients generally do well with this modality for these difficult fracture patterns. I have similarly experienced that wrist flexion seems to be the most difficult direction of range of motion to regain, but that patients overall rarely miss it. This article nicely demonstrates the expected functional outcomes after management with a bridge plate. This technique should be a skill of the proficient hand surgeon who cares for these injuries.

M. J. Richard

The Utility of the Fluoroscopic Skyline View During Volar Locking Plate Fixation of Distal Radius Fractures

Vaiss L, Ichihara S, Hendriks S, et al (Strasbourg Univ Hosp, Illkirch, France; et al)
J Wrist Surg 3:245-249, 2014

Background.—Open reduction and internal fixation (ORIF) using a volar locking plate is a common method for treating displaced distal radius fractures. There is, however, the risk of extensor tendon rupture due to protrusion of the screw tips past the dorsal cortex, which cannot always be adequately seen on a lateral fluoroscopic view. We therefore wished to compare the sensitivity of an intraoperative fluoroscopic skyline view to a lateral fluorosocopic view in detecting past pointing of these screws.

Material and Methods.—Our series included 75 patients with an average age of 59 years who underwent volar locked plate fixation of a displaced distal radius fracture. Intraoperative anteroposterior (AP), lateral, and skyline fluoroscopic views were performed in each case. The number of screws that were seen to protrude past the dorsal cortex of the distal fracture fragment were recorded for both the lateral and skyline views. The number of screws that required exchange was also documented.

Results.—No screws were seen to protrude past the dorsal cortical bone on the lateral fluroscopic views. 15 of 300 screws (5%) were seen to protrude past the dorsal cortex by an average of 0.8 mm (range, 0.5 to 2 mm) and were exchanged for shorter screws in 11/75 patients.

Conclusion.—Our results demonstrate that the skyline is more sensitive than a lateral fluoroscopic view at demonstrating protrusion of the screws in the distal fracture fragment following volar locked plate fixation.

Level of Evidence.—IV.

▶ Dorsal screw protrusion is a common problem during palmar plate fixation of the distal radius. The authors conclude that the fluoroscopic skyline view, previously also published as the dorsal horizon view, was superior to the standard lateral view in identifying protruding screws. The main methodological problem of this study is that there is no objective reference to screw protrusion. We do not know whether the screws, identified as too long, were actually protruding and how many protruding screws were missed even on the skyline view. Apart from that, the skyline view has been proven to be valuable in several previous experimental studies.

Personally, I think that the skyline view is difficult or even impossible to perform with smaller fluoroscopes. Rather than using cumbersome intraoperative views, my personal preference is to use screws that are 2 to 4 mm shorter than measured. There is solid biomechanical evidence that locking screws that are only 75% of the ideal length provide identical strength as bicortical fixation. In many fractures, true bicortical fixation is not possible anyway because of the lack of a stable dorsal cortex.

K. Megerle, MD

Are Volar Locking Plates Superior to Percutaneous K-wires for Distal Radius Fractures? A Meta-analysis

Chaudhry H, Kleinlugtenbelt YV, Mundi R, et al (McMaster Univ, Hamilton, Ontario, Canada; et al)
Clin Orthop Relat Res 473:3017-3027, 2015

Background.—Distal radius fractures are common, costly, and increasing in incidence. Percutaneous K-wire fixation and volar locking plates are two of the most commonly used surgical treatments for unstable dorsally displaced distal radius fractures. However, there is uncertainty regarding which of these treatments is superior.

Questions/Purposes.—We performed a meta-analysis of randomized controlled trials to determine whether patients treated with volar locking plates (1) achieved better function (2) attained better wrist motion, (3) had better radiographic outcomes, and (4) had fewer complications develop than did patients treated with K-wires for dorsally displaced distal radius fractures.

Methods.—We performed a comprehensive search of MEDLINE (inception to 2014, October Week 2), EMBASE (inception to 2014, Week 42), and the Cochrane Central Register of Controlled Trials to identify relevant randomized controlled trials; we supplemented these searches with manual searches. We included studies of extraarticular and intraarticular distal radius fractures. Adjunctive external fixation was acceptable as long as the intent was to use only K-wires where possible and external fixation was used in less than 25% of the procedures. We considered a difference in the DASH scores of 10 as the minimal clinically important difference. We performed quality assessment with the Cochrane Risk of Bias tool and evaluated the strength of recommendations using the Grades of Recommendation, Assessment, Development and Evaluation (GRADE) approach. Seven randomized trials with a total of 875 participants were included in the meta-analysis.

Results.—Patients treated with volar locking plates had slightly better function than did patients treated with K-wires as measured by their DASH scores at 3 months (mean difference [MD], 7.5; 95% CI, 4.4–10.6; $p < 0.001$) and 12 months (MD, 3.8; 95% CI, 1.2–6.3; $p = 0.004$). Neither of these differences exceeded the a priori-determined threshold for clinical importance (10 points). There was a small early advantage in flexion and supination in the volar locking plate group (3.7° [95% CI, 0.3°–7.1°; $p = 0.04$] and 4.1° [95% CI, 0.6°–7.6°; $p = 0.02$] greater, respectively) at 3 months, but not at later followups (6 or 12 months). There were no differences in radiographic outcomes (volar tilt, radial inclination, and radial height) between the two interventions. Superficial wound infection was more common in patients treated with K-wires (8.2% versus 3.2%; RR = 2.6; $p = 0.001$), but otherwise no difference in complication rates was found.

Conclusions.—Despite the small number of studies and the limitations inherent in a meta-analysis, we found that volar locking plates show better DASH scores at 3- and 12-month followups compared with K-wires for displaced distal radius fractures in adults; however, these differences were small and unlikely to be clinically important. Further research is required to better delineate if there are specific radiographic, injury, or patient characteristics that may benefit from volar locking plates in the short term and whether there are any differences in long-term outcomes and complications.

Level of Evidence.—Level I, therapeutic study.

▶ The study presents results from a meta-analysis of 7 randomized trials comparing outcomes for dorsally displaced distal radius fractures treated with volar locking plate (VLP) fixation versus K-wire fixation. The analysis demonstrated slightly better function in the VLP group, although differences between groups were less than 10 points on the DASH score, which is considered the minimum clinically significant difference. There were no differences in radiographic outcomes between groups. Complications were more common in the K-wire group, and most consisted of superficial pin infections.

The authors present an elegant pooled analysis of 875 patients from 7 randomized trials. Their results substantiate the existing literature and demonstrate that VLP and K-wire fixation result in similar outcomes at 1 year after surgery. VLP also appears to be more beneficial in the early-postoperative period (3 months). Despite a lack of consensus on reported outcomes after distal radius fracture fixation, all of the included trials included a minimum set of variables (DASH or quickDASH, range of motion, grip strength, radiographic data, and complications), which certainly adds to the strength of the meta-analysis. Study limitations include a relatively small number of included studies and, in some cases, a short duration of follow-up. It is also interesting to note that all but 1 study were performed in Europe, underlining the inherent difficulties of performing randomized surgical clinical trials in the United States. Lastly, it would have been interesting to analyze the cost for each treatment arm to determine which is most cost-effective in the treatment of these common injuries.

T. D. Rozental

The Minimum Clinically Important Difference of the Patient-rated Wrist Evaluation Score for Patients With Distal Radius Fractures
Walenkamp MMJ, de Muinck Keizer R-J, Goslings JC, et al (Univ of Amsterdam, The Netherlands; et al)
Clin Orthop Relat Res 473:3235-3241, 2015

Background.—The Patient-rated Wrist Evaluation (PRWE) is a commonly used instrument in upper extremity surgery and in research. However, to recognize a treatment effect expressed as a change in PRWE, it is important to be aware of the minimum clinically important difference (MCID) and the minimum detectable change (MDC). The MCID of an outcome tool like the PRWE is defined as the smallest change in a score that is likely to be appreciated by a patient as an important change, while the MDC is defined as the smallest amount of change that can be detected by an outcome measure. A numerical change in score that is less than the MCID, even when statistically significant, does not represent a true clinically relevant change. To our knowledge, the MCID and MDC of the PRWE have not been determined in patients with distal radius fractures.

Questions/Purposes.—We asked: (1) What is the MCID of the PRWE score for patients with distal radius fractures? (2) What is the MDC of the PRWE?

Methods.—Our prospective cohort study included 102 patients with a distal radius fracture and a median age of 59 years (interquartile range [IQR], 48–66 years). All patients completed the PRWE questionnaire during each of two separate visits. At the second visit, patients were asked to indicate the degree of clinical change they appreciated since the previous visit. Accordingly, patients were categorized in two groups: (1) minimally improved or (2) no change. The groups were used to anchor the changes observed in the PRWE score to patients' perspectives of what was clinically important. We determined the MCID using an anchor-based receiver operator characteristic method. In this context, the change in the PRWE score was considered a diagnostic test, and the anchor (minimally improved or no change as noted by the patients from visit to visit) was the gold standard. The optimal receiver operator characteristic cutoff point calculated with the Youden index reflected the value of the MCID.

Results.—In our study, the MCID of the PRWE was 11.5 points. The area under the curve was 0.54 (95% CI, 0.37–0.70) for the pain subscale and 0.71 (95% CI, 0.57–0.85) for the function subscale. We determined the MDC to be 11.0 points.

Conclusions.—We determined the MCID of the PRWE score for patients with distal radius fractures using the anchor-based approach and verified that the MDC of the PRWE was sufficiently small to detect our MCID.

Clinical Relevance.—We recommend using an improvement on the PRWE of more than 11.5 points as the smallest clinically relevant difference when evaluating the effects of treatments and when performing sample-size calculations on studies of distal radius fractures.

▶ Almost all of the clinical research conducted in hand surgery includes patient-reported outcome measures. For the wrist the Patient-Rated Wrist Evaluation (PRWE) is one of the standard measures used. This article attempts to identify the minimum clinically important difference (MCID) of the PRWE in patients with distal radius fractures. Essentially, the question they tried to answer was how large a change in PRWE in a group of patients with distal radius fractures likely to identify as making a clinically significant difference, rather than just a statistically important difference. For example, one could imagine a study on 2 types of distal radius fracture treatment that resulted in a statistically significant increase of 5 degrees of wrist radial deviation, but neither patients nor surgeons feel that such a difference is clinically significant.

The answer at which this article arrives is that the MCID for distal radius fractures is 11.5. Given the important characteristics and limitations of this study, this number is an important addition to the field, but further study is required before seeing it as generally applicable. First, the patients are drawn from 2 other studies and clinical practice, and the difference between the MCID of those in trials and the other patients is not presented. Some of the patients were treated surgically and others not. Second, these patients were all from the Netherlands, and the PRWE was administered in Dutch. There is an expectation that the MCID for many outcome measures in different conditions will vary among different populations and cultures. Third, significant recall bias was noted by the investigators.

Further study is needed to help us understand the MCID for these patients, but this is a starting point.

P. Blazar, MD

External Fixation and Adjuvant Pins Versus Volar Locking Plate Fixation in Unstable Distal Radius Fractures: A Randomized, Controlled Study With a 5-Year Follow-Up

Williksen JH, Husby T, Hellund JC, et al (Oslo Univ Hosp, Norway; et al)
J Hand Surg Am 40:1333-1340, 2015

Purpose.—To determine whether volar locking plates (VLP) are superior to external fixation (EF) with adjuvant pins in unstable distal radius fractures after 5 years of follow-up.

Methods.—We randomized 111 unstable distal radius fractures to treatment with either a VLP or EF using adjuvant pins. The patients' mean age was 54 years (range, 20–84 y). Twenty patients were lost to follow-up. At

5 years, 91 patients (82%) were assessed using the visual analog scale (VAS) pain score, Mayo wrist score, Quick Disabilities of the Arm, Shoulder and Hand (*Quick*DASH) questionnaire, range of motion, and radiological evaluation. The *Quick*DASH score at 5 years was the primary outcome measure.

Results.—The *Quick*DASH score was not statistically significantly different between the groups (VLP 10 vs EF 13) at 5 years. Patients with VLP had statistically significant better supination (85° vs 81°), better radial deviation (18° vs 16°), and less radial shortening (1 mm vs 2 mm). For AO/OTA type C2 fractures, the VLP had statistically significant better supination (84° vs 78°), flexion (64° vs 56°), grip strength (34 kg vs 28 kg), Mayo wrist score (92 vs 76), and less ulnar shortening (1 mm vs 3 mm). The *Quick*DASH score in the C2 subset analysis showed a difference of 10 (VLP 8 vs EF 18), but this was not statistically significant. In the VLP group, 11 patients (21%) had their plates removed owing to surgically related complications. In the EF group, 5 patients had proximal radial scar correction surgery owing to skin contracture.

Conclusions.—The findings were satisfactory for both groups at 5 years. The VLP provided statistically significantly better results for several clinical outcomes in the C2 subset analysis. However, 21% of the VLPs were removed because of surgical complications.

Type of Study/Level of Evidence.—Therapeutic I.

▶ The study presents results from a randomized trial comparing volar plate fixation (VLP) to external fixation (EF) and pinning for the treatment of unstable distal radius fractures in 95 patients at 5 years postsurgery. Using the quick-DASH score as a primary outcome, the authors demonstrated no significant differences between groups at final follow-up. There was a trend toward better outcomes for more complex intraarticular fracture patterns treated with VLP, but the VLP also had a higher rate of complications and reoperations.

The authors are to be commended for designing and executing a successful clinical trial. They were able to enroll a relatively large number of patients, had regular follow-up intervals, and had little crossover between treatment arms. Furthermore, the therapists who performed the final examination were blinded as to which treatment the patients had received. As noted by the authors, study limitations include an underpowered study for the primary outcome at 5-year follow-up, which also precluded meaningful subgroup analyses. The rate of plate removal was also higher than that typically reported after volar plate fixation yet the authors do not offer an explanation for this. Nonetheless, this study adds to the existing literature and substantiates that treatment outcomes after distal radius fracture are similar irrespective of the type of fixation used. In my practice, volar plating is still the preferred treatment method for displaced distal radius fractures, but EF and pinning are useful for more comminuted injuries or those with a shear component and significant instability.

T. D. Rozental, MD

A novel computational method for evaluating osteochondral autografts in distal radius reconstruction
Kollitz KM, Huang JI, Hsu JW, et al (Univ of Washington, Seattle)
Hand (N Y) 10:492-496, 2015

Background.—We describe a novel computational method for assessing the fit of an osteochondral graft. We applied our software to five normal wrist computed tomography (CT) scans to determine the fit of the scaphoid to the lunate fossa of the distal radius.

Methods.—CT scans of five wrists were digitally rendered. The capitate facet of the scaphoid was fit to the lunate fossa of the distal radius using custom software based on the iterative closest point (ICP) algorithm. This approach iteratively determines the optimal position of a model surface to minimize the sum of squares of distances from all points on a target surface. The fit of the two surfaces was reported by calculating the mean residual distance (MRD) between each point on one surface and its nearest neighbor on the other.

Results.—The MRD for the five subjects was found to be 0.25 mm, with 82.8–98.3% of the articular surfaces within 0.5 mm of each other.

Conclusions.—We have developed a software algorithm for comparing two articular surfaces to test fit for a proposed joint reconstruction. The software is versatile and may be applied to any bony surface to identify new graft donor sites. The fit assessment renders a richer, three-dimensional understanding of the fit of the graft as compared to traditional two-dimensional assessments.

Level of Evidence.—Decision analysis, Level V.

▶ The authors present a novel method for digitally assessing the congruency of 2 joint surfaces. They find that the capitate facet of the scaphoid provides a good match for the capitate head. The authors argue that the scaphoid therefore might be a suitable donor site for obtaining bone grafts that could replace a damaged lunate fossa. I cannot comment on the mathematical validity of the model, but I think the authors provide an interesting approach to simulate joint replacement by bone grafts in selected cases. However, I am not sure about the clinical applications of the graft investigated. I think the preferred motion-preserving procedure after destruction of the joint surface of the distal radius is radioscapholunate fusion with resection of the distal pole of the scaphoid. Usually, an acceptable range of wrist motion can be obtained, and I would argue that it is technically much less demanding than the procedure suggested by the authors. It will be interesting, however, to follow the authors' future publications on other grafts, such as the hemi-hamate arthroplasty used for replacing the proximal interphalangeal joint surfaces.

K. Megerle, MD

Wrist Fracture and Risk of Subsequent Fracture: Findings from the Women's Health Initiative Study

Crandall CJ, Hovey KM, Cauley JA, et al (David Geffen School of Medicine at the Univ of California at Los Angeles; State Univ of New York at Buffalo; Univ of Pittsburgh, PA; et al)
J Bone Miner Res 30:2086-2095, 2015

Wrist fractures are common in postmenopausal women and are associated with functional decline. Fracture patterns after wrist fracture are unclear. The goal of this study was to determine the frequency and types of fractures that occur after a wrist fracture among postmenopausal women. We carried out a post hoc analysis of data from the Women's Health Initiative Observational Study and Clinical Trials (1993–2010) carried out at 40 US clinical centers. Participants were postmenopausal women aged 50 to 79 years at baseline. Mean follow-up duration was 11.8 years. Main measures included incident wrist, clinical spine, humerus, upper extremity, lower extremity, hip, and total non-wrist fractures and bone mineral density (BMD) in a subset. Among women who experienced wrist fracture, 15.5% subsequently experienced non-wrist fracture. The hazard for non-wrist fractures was higher among women who had experienced previous wrist fracture than among women who had not experienced wrist fracture: non-wrist fracture overall (hazard ratio [HR] = 1.40, 95% confidence interval [CI] 1.33–1.48), spine (HR = 1.48, 95% CI 1.32–1.66), humerus (HR = 1.78, 95% CI 1.57–2.02), upper extremity (non-wrist) (HR = 1.88, 95% CI 1.70–2.07), lower extremity (non-hip) (HR = 1.36, 95% CI 1.26–1.48), and hip (HR = 1.50, 95% CI 1.32–1.71) fracture. Associations persisted after adjustment for BMD, physical activity, and other risk factors. Risk of non-wrist fracture was higher in women who were younger when they experienced wrist fracture (interaction p value 0.02). Associations between incident wrist fracture and subsequent non-wrist fracture did not vary by baseline BMD category (normal, low bone density, osteoporosis). A wrist fracture is associated with increased risk of subsequent hip, vertebral, upper extremity, and lower extremity fractures. There may be substantial missed opportunity for intervention in the large number of women who present with wrist fractures.

▶ This is an excellent and much-needed study. The large sample size, study design, and results highlight the prevalence and importance of bone health assessment in all persons with a fracture but especially in younger women presenting with a wrist fracture.

This research will have an impact on my practice (orthopedic nurse practitioner researching bone health) in the following ways: (1) I will initiate a bone health assessment on distal radius fractures with a focused intent to assess young postmenopausal initial fractures; (2) use my practice as an opportunity to educate referencing this research; and (3) reference this study in my community bone health presentations.

L. Fitton, CNP

12 Diagnostic Imaging

Efficacy of Magnetic Resonance Imaging and Clinical Tests in Diagnostics of Wrist Ligament Injuries: A Systematic Review
Andersson JK, Andernord D, Karlsson J, et al (Sahlgrenska Univ Hosp, Gothenburg, Sweden; Univ of Gothenburg, Sweden; et al)
Arthroscopy 31:2014-2020, 2015

Purpose.—To investigate the diagnostic performance of magnetic resonance imaging (MRI) and clinical provocative tests on injuries to the triangular fibrocartilage complex (TFCC), the scapholunate (SL) ligament, and the lunotriquetral (LT) ligament.

Methods.—An electronic literature search of articles published between January 1, 2000, and February 28, 2014, in PubMed, Embase, and the Cochrane Library was carried out in April 2014. Only studies of the diagnostic performance of MRI and clinical provocation tests using wrist arthroscopy as the gold standard were eligible for inclusion. The Preferred Reporting Items for Systematic Reviews and Meta-Analyses (PRISMA) checklist guided the extraction and reporting of data. The methodologic quality of the included articles was assessed with the revised Quality Assessment of Diagnostic Accuracy Studies (QUADAS-2) tool. The primary outcome measure was the negative predictive value (NPV) of wrist MRI and provocative wrist tests, which was defined as the probability of an intact wrist ligament given a negative investigation. The question was whether negative results of MRI or provocative tests were enough to safely discontinue further investigation with arthroscopy. A minimum NPV of 95% was considered a clinically relevant cutoff value. The secondary outcome measures were the positive predictive value (PPV), sensitivity, and specificity.

Results.—A total of 7 articles (327 patients with MRI and 105 patients with clinical tests) were included in this systematic review. The included articles displayed heterogeneity regarding participants, diagnostic methods, and study design. Seven articles investigated the diagnostic performance of MRI, whereas 1 article investigated clinical testing. The NPVs of MRI were as follows: TFCC, 37% to 90%; SL ligament, 72% to 94%; and LT ligament, 74% to 95%. The NPVs of clinical tests were 55%, 74%, and 94% for the TFCC, SL ligament, and LT ligament, respectively. Only 1 study reached the predetermined cutoff value for the primary outcome measure (NPV ≥95%) but only for MRI of the LT ligament; this study also reached a borderline-cutoff NPV of 94% for MRI of the SL ligament. Another study reached borderline-cutoff NPVs of 94% both for MRI and for clinical tests of the LT ligament.

Conclusions.—A negative result from MRI is unable to rule out the possibility of a clinically relevant injury to the TFCC, SL ligament, or LT ligament of the wrist. Clinical provocation wrist tests were of limited diagnostic value. The current gold standard—wrist arthroscopy—remains the preferred diagnostic technique with sufficient conclusive properties when it comes to wrist ligament injuries.

Level of Evidence.—Level II, systematic review of Level II diagnostic studies.

▶ This study searched the literature for articles that evaluate the negative predictive value (NPV) of MRI and provocative tests on the diagnosis of scapholunate (SL) ligament, lunotriquetral (LT) ligament, and triangular fibrocartilage complex (TFCC) injuries. As expected, the physical examination tests had a very low NPV. More surprising was that only 1 study demonstrated a >95% NPV for MRI, and that was only for LT tears. Most studies demonstrated that MRIs frequently miss these injuries as well.

The study points out that the gold standard test for intercarpal ligament injury remains arthroscopy. So in patients with "normal" MRIs, even in the presence of negative provocative maneuvers, surgical exploration with arthroscopy may frequently make the missed diagnosis. Obviously, with negative exam findings and MRI, a high index of suspicion is needed to proceed with surgery.

One important distinction this article does not make is the presence of a "ligament" injury versus the presence of a "destabilizing ligament injury." Just having a small foveal irregularity of the TFCC does not explain distal radioulna joint laxity. Having a tear of the membranous portion of the SL ligament that might be missed by MRI does not mean that every wrist should be scoped to identify these nonstructural tears. Therefore, a combination of exam findings, the chronicity of symptoms, the MRI findings, and the clinical scenario can all help guide the practitioner to wrist arthroscopy when needed to confirm and treat the diagnosis.

T. Hughes, MD

Approach to the Swollen Arm With Chronic Dialysis Access: It's Not Just Deep Vein Thrombosis
Reddy SN, Boros MC, Horrow MM (Einstein Med Ctr, Philadelphia, PA)
J Ultrasound Med 34:1901-1910, 2015

The purposes of this pictorial essay are as follows: (1) Review a systematic approach to using sonography in the initial evaluation of patients with acute arm swelling and permanent dialysis access. (2) Identify normal grayscale and Doppler findings in arteriovenous fistulas and grafts.

(3) Discuss a spectrum of vascular differential diagnoses for arm swelling in this setting, including stenosis of the access, draining vein complications, thrombosis, steal syndrome, and aneurysms, as well as several non-vascular causes. (4) Recognize findings that warrant further imaging evaluation or intervention.

▶ The authors of this article review important principles of vascular ultrasound findings and define a systematic clinical approach to differentiating both vascular and nonvascular etiologies of upper extremity swelling. In addition, they provide sound evidence, excellent pictorial examples, and a methodical approach that allow it to be adopted into clinical practice, benefiting the patient.

D. Barnes, MD

Calcific tendinopathy of the rotator cuff: the correlation between pain and imaging features in symptomatic and asymptomatic female shoulders
Sansone V, Consonni O, Maiorano E, et al (Università degli Studi di Milano, Italy; et al)
Skeletal Radiol 45:49-55, 2016

Objective.—To provide new epidemiological data regarding the prevalence, distribution and macroscopic features of shoulder rotator cuff calcific tendinopathy (calcific tendinopathy), and to identify the characteristics of calcific deposits associated with shoulder pain.

Materials and Methods.—Three hundred and two female volunteers (604 shoulders) who had been referred to a gynaecological clinic participated in the study. The subjects underwent a high-resolution ultrasonography of both shoulders, and those with a diagnosis of calcific tendinopathy compiled a standardized questionnaire relating to shoulder symptoms. We determined the prevalence of symptomatic and asymptomatic rotator cuff calcific tendinopathy, and compared differences in distribution and macroscopic features of the symptomatic and asymptomatic calcifications.

Results.—The prevalence of calcific tendinopathy was 17.8% (103 shoulders). Ninety-five shoulders (15.7%) were symptomatic; of these, calcific tendinopathy was found in 34 shoulders (33%) on imaging. Of the 509 asymptomatic (84.3%) shoulders, calcific tendinopathy was observed in 69 cases (67%). Among tendons, supraspinatus (53.4%) and infraspinatus (54.6%) were the most frequently involved. The majority of calcific deposits were of maximum diameter between 2 and 5 mm (77.9%), and were linear in form (69.9%). The involvement of multiple tendons and a location in the supraspinatus tendon were found to be significantly correlated with pain ($p = 0.023$, $p = 0.043$ respectively), as were age ($p = 0.041$) and an excessive body mass index ($p = 0.024$).

Conclusion.—In this sample from the general population of working age females, both intrinsic factors (location in supraspinatus, multiple tendon involvement) and extrinsic variables (age, abnormally high BMI) were correlated with pain in calcific tendinopathy.

Level of Evidence.—Level III, cross-sectional study, prevalence study.

▶ The authors present a cross-sectional study to identify the prevalence, distribution, and macroscopic features of rotator cuff (RTC) calcific tendinopathy using high-resolution ultrasonography (US) as well as characteristics of calcific deposits associated with shoulder pain. A total of 302 women (604 shoulders) who presented for routine gynecologic appointments volunteered to participate in the study with an unknown number of patients being excluded or declining to participate. A high-resolution US was performed by a single radiologist, and without being informed of the results, the patients completed a questionnaire regarding shoulder pain. Calcific tendinopathy was found in 103 (17.8%) shoulders (Table 2). Ninety-five shoulders (15.7%) were symptomatic with 34 of the 95 (33%) found to have calcific tendinopathy. The supraspinatus (53.4%) and infraspinatus (54.6%) were most frequently involved with 77.9% calcific deposits between 2 and 5 mm and 66.9% linear in shape.

The results were presented based on number of shoulders instead of patients, with no data on the prevalence in both shoulders of the same patient. Furthermore, previous studies found that calcific tendinopathy affects women more than men, so it is difficult to generalize the results of this study to a male population. Because a detailed physical examination of the shoulder was not performed and there was no US documentation of rotator cuff tears or other conditions and no further imaging modalities such as magnetic resonance imaging, it is incorrect to assume that RTC calcific tendinopathy was the cause of the symptoms in the patients who were positively identified has having pain on the questionnaire. Overall, the article provides good epidemiologic data, which is limited in utility for the above-mentioned reasons. In my clinic, symptomatic calcific tendinopathy is essentially a diagnosis of exclusion once all other causes of shoulder pain have been ruled out and typically responds to nonoperative management. If pain (particularly impingement type symptoms)

TABLE 2.—Results of US Examination and Pain Questionnaire

	Symptomatic Shoulders	Asymptomatic Shoulders	Total Shoulders
Calcific tendinopathy	33.0% ($n = 34$)	67.0% ($n = 69$)	100% ($n = 103$)
No calcific tendinopathy	12.2% ($n = 61$)	87.8% ($n = 440$)	100% ($n = 501$)
Total	15.7% ($n = 95$)	84.3% ($n = 509$)	100% ($n = 604$)
Odds ratio = 3.554 (95% CI: 2.177−5.803)*			

n number of shoulders.
*Statistically significant correlation between pain and calcific tendinopathy.
Reprinted from Sansone V, Consonni O, Maiorano E, et al. Calcific tendinopathy of the rotator cuff: the correlation between pain and imaging features in symptomatic and asymptomatic female shoulders. *Skeletal Radiol* 2016;45:49-55, with permission from ISS.

persists after a several-month trial of oral anti-inflammatories, physical therapy, and corticosteroid injections, I will consider other treatment modalities.

E. Gauger, MD

The Reliability of Ultrasound Measurements of the Median Nerve at the Carpal Tunnel Inlet

Fowler JR, Hirsch D, Kruse K (Univ of Pittsburgh, PA)
J Hand Surg Am 40:1992-1995, 2015

Purpose.—To determine the interrater and intra-rater reliability of ultrasound (US) measurement of the cross-sectional area (CSA) of the median nerve at the carpal tunnel inlet.

Methods.—Three examiners of varying levels of experience performed US measurements of the CSA of the median nerve at the carpal tunnel inlet of both wrists of 11 healthy volunteers. Each examiner was blinded to the measurements of the other examiners. The measurements were repeated 2 weeks later in random order to test intra-rater reliability. The Lin concordance correlation coefficient (LCCC) for interrater and intra-rater reliability was calculated.

Results.—The overall inter-rater LCCC was 0.59 (95% confidence interval [CI], 0.41–0.73). Intrarater LCCC varied based on examiner experience. The senior author had an intra-rater LCCC of 0.91 (95% CI, 0.80–0.96), the hand fellow had an intra-rater LCCC of 0.45 (95% CI, 0.17–0.66), and the first-year resident had an intra-rater LCCC of 0.78 (95% CI, 0.55–0.90).

Conclusions.—There is moderate agreement among examiners of varying levels of experience when measuring the CSA of the median nerve at the carpal tunnel inlet. Examiner experience affected intra-rater reliability of measurements; an experienced examiner had nearly perfect agreement compared with moderate agreement for less experienced examiners.

▶ This article by Fowler et al looked at interrater and intrarater reliability of ultrasound (US) measurement of the cross-sectional area (CSA) of the median nerve at the carpal tunnel inlet in 11 volunteers without CT scan (CTS). The methodology of using 3 examiners with varied US experience at varied levels of surgical training is sound and re-creates what might be seen in clinical practice. The study was strengthened by blinding each examiner to the others' measurements and separating repeat measurements by 2 weeks for intraobserver reliability. This article does not question the diagnostic reliability of US but rather the inter/intraobserver reliability specifically regarding measurements by 3 individuals with varying skill in diagnostic US. It did demonstrate that the most experienced examiner had nearly perfect agreement compared with moderate agreement for less experienced examiners. It was quite concerning that the first-year resident had greater interobserver reliability than the hand fellow. Given that a difference in CSA of 1 mm^2 could be the difference between a positive and negative test when using US to confirm a diagnosis of CTS, I find this worrisome.

A number of articles from this group and others have recently been published touting US as valuable in the evaluation of CTS. In a previous study, this same group of authors reported that US confirmed the diagnosis of CTS with better specificity and equal sensitivity compared with electrodiagnostic testing. It is certainly true that US is noninvasive, nonpainful, and can be performed in the office at the time of initial evaluation. Based on this article, it is clear, however, that there is definitely a learning curve, and experience is required before using it as the gold standard. Electrical studies, although "invasive" and uncomfortable at times, still provide useful diagnostic and prognostic information that I continue to utilize in my daily practice.[1]

D. Zelouf, MD

Reference

1. Fowler JR, Munsch M, Tosti R, Hagberg WC, Imbriglia JE. Comparison of ultrasound and electrodiagnostic testing for diagnosis of carpal tunnel syndrome: study using a validated clinical tool as the reference standard. *J Bone Joint Surg Am.* 2014;96:e148.

Routine Imaging after Operatively Repaired Distal Radius and Scaphoid Fractures: A Survey of Hand Surgeons

Bohl DD, Lese AB, Patterson JT, et al (Yale School of Medicine, New Haven, CT)
J Wrist Surg 3:239-244, 2013

Background.—There is currently no standard of care for imaging after hand and upper-extremity procedures, and current imaging practices have not been characterized.

Questions/Purposes.—To characterize current imaging practices and to compare those practices to the best available evidence.

Patients and Methods.—A survey was distributed to attending-level surgeons at a regional hand and upper-extremity surgery conference in the United States in 2013. 40 out of 75 surgeons completed the survey (53%).

Results.—All results are presented for distal radius and scaphoid fractures, respectively. There was a high degree of variability between respondents in the number of radiographic series routinely ordered during follow-up of asymptomatic patients, with the number of series ranging from 1—6 and 1—6. On average, respondents did not order an excessive number of follow-up radiographs for asymptomatic patients, with means (± standard deviations) of 2.6 ± 1.0 and 3.3 ± 1.2 radiographic series. Radiographic series were taken at only 74% and 81% of postoperative visits with asymptomatic patients. Only 10% and 8% of respondents felt it was acceptable medical practice to save costs by ordering postoperative radiographs only when patients are symptomatic.

Conclusions.—Among a sample of 40 fellowship-trained hand surgeons, these findings demonstrate a high degree of variability in number of radiographs obtained after operative repair of distal radius and scaphoid fractures. On average, respondents were relatively efficient with respect to total number of postoperative radiographs ordered.

Level of Evidence.—Diagnostic study, level IV.

▶ The authors used a survey to study current imaging practices among hand surgeons, specifically for distal radius fractures and scaphoid fractures. As they stated, "imaging contributes substantially to the rising cost of health care."

The authors are trying to shed light on a practice that may be partially responsible for the increased costs in health care. They look specifically at 2 common surgeries performed by hand surgeons and the number of postoperative radiographs that accompany them. The current studies in the literature have looked at postoperative radiographs in other orthopaedic specialties, for example, spine and total joint arthroplasty.

This survey was handed out to hand surgeons at a regional conference, with only 40 of 75 surgeons completing the survey (response rate of 53%). As the authors pointed out, these data were obtained from surgeon self-report, which is certainly not as reliable as data collected directly from the patients' records.

I am personally not a fan of surveys or the studies that are gleaned from their data. I do not believe that quality of the data can lead, in most cases, to any significant conclusions. That said, I was surprised by the number of surgeons who routinely order radiographs for asymptomatic patients at the first postoperative visit following distal radius and scaphoid repair (80% and 77%, respectively). I do not. Like the respondents in this survey, I probably obtain between 2 and 3 sets of postoperative radiographs following repair of distal radius and scaphoid fractures, but the actual number depends on the individual patient, the complexity of the fracture, and its potential for healing.

S. S. Shin, MD, MMSc

Advanced imaging of the scapholunate ligamentous complex
Shahabpour M, Staelens B, Van Overstraeten L, et al (Universitair Ziekenhuis Brussel (UZ Brussel), Belgium; Hand and Foot Surgery Unit (HFSU), Brussel, Belgium)
Skeletal Radiol 44:1709-1725, 2015

The scapholunate joint is one of the most involved in wrist injuries. Its stability depends on primary and secondary stabilisers forming together the scapholunate complex. This ligamentous complex is often evaluated by wrist arthroscopy. To avoid surgery as diagnostic procedure, optimization of MR imaging parameters as use of three-dimensional (3D) sequences with very thin slices and high spatial resolution, is needed to detect lesions of the intrinsic and extrinsic ligaments of the scapholunate complex. The paper reviews the literature on imaging of radial-sided carpal ligaments with advanced computed tomographic arthrography (CTA) and magnetic resonance arthrography (MRA) to evaluate the scapholunate complex. Anatomy and pathology of the ligamentous complex are described and illustrated with CTA, MRA and corresponding arthroscopy. Sprains, mid-substance tears, avulsions and fibrous infiltrations of carpal ligaments could be identified on CTA and MRA images using 3D fat-saturated PD and 3D DESS (dual echo with steady-state precession) sequences with 0.5-mm-thick slices. Imaging signs of scapholunate complex pathology include: discontinuity, nonvisualization, changes in signal intensity, contrast extravasation (MRA), contour irregularity and waviness and periligamentous infiltration by edema, granulation tissue or fibrosis. Based on this preliminary experience, we believe that 3 T MRA using 3D sequences with 0.5-mm-thick slices and multiplanar reconstructions is capable to evaluate the scapholunate complex and could help to reduce the number of diagnostic arthroscopies.

▶ The authors provide a comprehensive review of available radiographic studies available to evaluate for pathology related to the scapholunate ligament complex. Arthroscopy is considered the gold standard with respect to evaluating intra-articular structures in the wrist. The concern is that this is an invasive procedure used for diagnosis that carries with it an inherent risk of complications or trauma to undisturbed anatomy. Plain radiography can be useful when evaluating carpal instability if there has been a change in the scapholunate angle or scapholunate distance. CT arthrography is a useful test with an excellent sensitivity and specificity for evaluating scapholunate pathology, but it exposes the patient to radiation. Standard MRI can be useful for evaluating soft tissue injuries in the wrist, but this is significantly enhanced by the addition of arthrography. The authors show that a multitude of studies reveal the significant improvement in sensitivity and specificity when an magnetic resonance arthrogram is performed, compared with a standard MRI. The most accurate test was an MRA with 3-dimensional sequences with 0.5-mm-thick slices and multiplanar reconstructions on 3-T scanners. Currently, if I am concerned that a patient may have a scapholunate injury, I send the patient for a MRA on a 3-T scanner. It is clear that this study can provide more detailed information than a standard MRI and can save health care dollars if it is ordered initially, rather than ordering a standard MRI and not obtaining a high-quality study that then requires additional evaluation.

M. W. Kessler, MD, MPH

Cine MRI: a new approach to the diagnosis of scapholunate dissociation

Langner I, Fischer S, Eisenschenk A, et al (Univ Medicine Greifswald, Germany)
Skeletal Radiol 44:1103-1110, 2015

Objective.—To evaluate the feasibility of cine MRI for the detection of scapholunate dissociation (SLD) and to compare the sensitivity and specificity of cine MRI with those of cineradiography and arthroscopy.

Materials and Methods.—To evaluate feasibility, healthy subjects underwent cine MRI of the wrist. To evaluate sensitivity and specificity, patients with clinically suspected scapholunate ligament (SLL) injury after trauma to the wrist were prospectively included and underwent radiographic examination, cineradiography, and cine MRI. In 25 out of 38 patients, subsequent arthroscopy was performed. Results of cineradiography and cine MRI correlated with those of arthroscopy.

Results.—Cine MRI was of diagnostic quality in all healthy subjects and patients with good interrater agreement. There was excellent correlation between cineradiography and cine MRI. Scapholunate distance differed significantly between healthy subjects and patients with scapholunate dissociation ($p < 0.001$), but not between imaging modalities in the patient group. Cine MRI had 85% sensitivity and 90% specificity for the detection of SLD.

Conclusion.—Cine MRI of the wrist is a fast and reliable technique for the detection of SLD with diagnostic accuracy comparable to cineradiography. It can be easily implemented as a routine clinical MRI examination, facilitating diagnostic workup of patients with suspected SLD while avoiding radiation exposure.

▶ The diagnosis and treatment of scapholunate dissociation (SLD) is definitely one of the unsolved problems in hand surgery. We lack a consensus definition of the disorder and a noninvasive way to reliably diagnose the pathoanatomy, and treatment results from the large number of published repair techniques show limited success. This article adds an interesting potential diagnostic technique, cine MRI. Published MRI techniques in the past have focused almost exclusively on static images or a series of static images in different positions. Cine MRI actually acquires images on a moving joint, albeit one that is restrained, and the motion observed is limited to 1 plane by a support. Similar information can be gained by cineradiography, but that technique does not provide the same opportunity for 3-dimensional analysis and requires exposure to radiation.

The authors used scapholunate distance as the indicator of scapholunate injury in a group of patients who had sustained wrist trauma at least 1 month before the evaluation. The authors are clear on the limitations of their study: the specificity found is less than reported for cineradiography, the gold standard of arthroscopy was only used for patients with positive imaging, and other indicators of scapholunate injury were not investigated.

On the basis of this article, it is unclear whether cine MRI should be a modality of choice for diagnosis of SLD. It does not appear to equal cineradiography and, at least from this article, it is unclear that is equal or superior to a traditional MRI.

P. Blazar, MD

Elbow US: Anatomy, Variants, and Scanning Technique
Tagliafico AS, Bignotti B, Martinoli C (Univ of Genoa, Italy)
Radiology 275:636-650, 2015

As with other musculoskeletal joints, elbow ultrasonography (US) depends on the examination technique. Deep knowledge of the relevant anatomy, such as the bone surface anatomy, tendon orientation, nerves, and vessels, is crucial for diagnosis. It is important to be aware of the primary imaging pitfalls related to US technique (anisotropy) in the evaluation of deep tendons such as the distal biceps and peripheral nerves. In this article, US scanning technique for the elbow as well as the related anatomy, primary variants, and scanning pitfalls are described. In addition, an online video tutorial of elbow US describes a possible approach to elbow evaluation. Online supplemental material is available for this article.

▶ This article comprehensively reviews musculoskeletal ultrasound essential principles for clinical evaluation of the elbow. Musculoskeletal ultrasound scan has rapidly gained increased clinical adoption over the last several years in multiple specialties including orthopedics, physiatry, radiology, rheumatology, and sports medicine. This increased adoption is in part owing to the significant reduction in cost of sonographic equipment but is also secondary to a significant increase in the ability to produce high-resolution, high-quality static and dynamic images. Although this article focuses on scanning techniques to optimize the visualization of specific anatomic structures in the elbow for diagnostic purposes, including pitfalls to avoid when scanning the elbow, it is important to understand these techniques to properly perform interventional procedures that are becoming more widespread among many specialties. This article contains photographs of surface anatomy and anatomic dissections, schematic drawings, and sonographs. This article also uses multimedia, including online supplemental materials (eg, movie clips), truly making it a useful and comprehensive review article for the learner.

D. Barnes, MD

13 Elbow: Trauma

An Expedited Care Pathway with Ambulatory Brachial Plexus Analgesia Is a Cost-effective Alternative to Standard Inpatient Care after Complex Arthroscopic Elbow Surgery: A Randomized, Single-blinded Study

Cruz Eng H, Riazi S, Veillette C, et al (Univ of Toronto, Ontario, Canada)
Anesthesiology 123:1256-1266, 2015

Background.—Common standard practice after complex arthroscopic elbow surgery includes hospital admission for 72 h. The authors hypothesized that an expedited care pathway, with 24 h of hospital admission and ambulatory brachial plexus analgesia and continuous passive motion at home, results in equivalent elbow range of motion (ROM) 2 weeks after surgery compared with standard 72-h hospital admission.

Methods.—A randomized, single-blinded study was conducted after obtaining approval from the research ethics board. Forty patients were randomized in a 1:1 ratio using a computer-generated list of random numbers into an expedited care pathway group (24-h admission) and a control group (72-h admission). They were treated equally aside from the predetermined hospital length of stay.

Results.—Patients in the control (n = 19) and expedited care pathway (n = 19) groups achieved similar elbow ROM 2 weeks (119 ± 18 degrees and 121 ± 15 degrees, $P = 0.627$) and 3 months (130 ± 18 *vs.* 130 ± 11 degrees, $P = 0.897$) postoperatively. The mean difference in elbow ROM at 2 weeks was 2.6 degrees (95% CI, −8.3 to 13.5). There were no differences in analgesic outcomes, physical function scores, and patient satisfaction up to 3 months postoperatively. Total hospital cost of care was 15% lower in the expedited care pathway group.

Conclusion.—The results suggest that an expedited care pathway with early hospital discharge followed by ambulatory brachial plexus analgesia and continuous passive motion at home is a cost-effective alternative to 72 h of hospital admission after complex arthroscopic elbow surgery.

▶ This article details a carefully constructed, appropriately powered, and patiently executed randomized trial over 4 years. The anesthesia and postoperative therapy protocol were complexly detailed. There was a high rate of participation by eligible enrollees (90%). The authors should be commended for their diligent execution of this trial for a relatively rare condition.

The most important finding is that the clinical results were as good (if not better) for the group of patients discharged on postoperative day 1 rather than the standard postoperative day 3. Furthermore, both groups improved significantly (the primary goal of surgery) from their preoperative status in terms of range of motion and function. No patient in either group required unexpected readmission or significantly increased cost due to a complication, confirming that this is a relatively safe procedure (both with expedited or standard admission).

As expected, there was a significant reduction in costs for the group discharged early. Nevertheless, it was only a 15% savings per patient. The average cost for the 3-day stay was $6646 versus $5675 for the 1-day stay. This is an average savings of approximately $1000 (in Canadian dollars) per patient. This study was performed in the Canadian provincial health insurance system. Costs within the US health care system tend to be dramatically higher, so one would expect the per-patient savings to be even greater in the United States.

This study also begs the question, "Do patients need to be admitted at all?" The major complication in both groups was that the catheter dislodged intraoperatively and had to be replaced, but this was done in the recovery room.

D. Bohn, MD

A survey of current practices and preferences for internal fixation of displaced olecranon fractures

Wood T, Thomas K, Farrokhyar F, et al (McMaster Univ, Hamilton, ON; et al)
Can J Surg 58:250-256, 2015

Background.—Olecranon fractures represent 10% of upper extremity fractures. There is a growing body of literature to support the use of plate fixation for displaced olecranon fractures. The purpose of this survey was to gauge Canadian surgeons' practices and preferences for internal fixation methods for displaced olecranon fractures.

Methods.—Using an online survey tool, we administered a cross-sectional survey to examine current practice for fixation of displaced olecranon fractures.

Results.—We received 256 completed surveys for a response rate of 31% (95% confidence interval [CI] 30.5–37.5%). The preferred treatment was tension band wiring (78.5%, 95% CI 73–83%) for simple displaced olecranon fractures (Mayo IIA) and plating (81%, 95% CI 75.5–85%) for displaced comminuted olecranon fractures (Mayo IIB). Fracture morphology with a mean impact of 3.31 (95% CI 3.17–3.45) and comminution with a mean impact of 3.34 (95% CI 3.21–3.46) were the 2 factors influencing surgeons' choice of fixation method the most. The major deterrent to using tension band wiring for displaced comminuted fractures (Mayo IIB) was increased stability obtained with other methods described by 75% (95% CI 69–80%) of respondents. The major deterrent for using plating constructs for simple displaced fractures (Mayo

IIA) was better outcomes with other methods. Hardware prominence was the most commonly perceived complication using either method of fixation: 77% (95% CI 71.4–81.7%) and 76.2% (95% CI 70.6–81.0%) for tension band wiring and plating, respectively.

Conclusion.—Divergence exists with current literature and surgeon preference for fixation of displaced olecranon fractures.

▶ The authors suggest that plate fixation of olecranon fractures is the optimal method for fixation based on a randomized, controlled study from 1992.[1] comparing tension band wiring and plate fixation. That trial found that there was more hardware prominence requiring hardware removal and more frequent loss of fixation or settling with tension bands compared with plates.

This report then surveyed Canadian orthopedic surgeons regarding their practices and perceptions surrounding olecranon fracture fixation to see whether current practices match the best available information in the literature. Although most respondents (81%) believed that the best method for fixation of a comminuted displaced olecranon fracture is plate osteosynthesis, 78% still routinely use a tension band construct for uncomminuted fractures. Of note, respondents from academic institutions were more likely to recommended plate fixation for both noncomminuted and comminuted fractures (12% and 6%, respectively) than community orthopedists. This finding can potentially be attributed to academic surgeons being more familiar with current literature, but the information is more than 10 years old, and a very high rate of academic surgeons (77%) still use tension band wiring for simple fractures.

This article reports the difficulty in changing practice despite level 1 evidence that one method of treatment is better than another. It also reviews the findings of an important randomized, controlled trial of tension band versus plate fixation for olecranon fractures.

D. Bohn, MD

Reference

1. Hume MC, Wiss DA. Olecranon fractures: a clinical and radiographic comparison of tension band wiring and plate fixation. *Clin Orthop Relat Res.* 1992;285: 229-235.

What Factors are Associated With a Surgical Site Infection After Operative Treatment of an Elbow Fracture?
Claessen FMAP, Braun Y, van Leeuwen WF, et al (Massachusetts General Hosp, Boston; et al)
Clin Orthop Relat Res 474:562-570, 2016

Background.—Surgical site infections are one of the more common major complications of elbow fracture surgery and can contribute to other adverse outcomes, prolonged hospital stays, and increased healthcare costs.

Questions/Purposes.—We asked: (1) What are the factors associated with a surgical site infection after elbow fracture surgery? (2) When taking the subset of closed elbow fractures only, what are the factors associated with a surgical site infection? (3) What are the common organisms isolated from an elbow infection after open treatment?

Methods.—One thousand three hundred twenty adult patients underwent surgery for an elbow fracture between January 2002 and July 2014 and were included in our study. Forty-eight of 1320 patients (4%) had a surgical site infection develop. Thirty-four of 1113 patients with a closed fracture (3%) had a surgical site infection develop.

Results.—For all elbow fractures, use of plate and screw fixation (adjusted odds ratio [OR] = 2.2; 95% CI, 1.0–4.5; $p = 0.041$) and use of external fixation before surgery (adjusted OR = 4.7; 95% CI, 1.1–21; $p = 0.035$) were associated with higher infection rates. When subset analysis was performed for closed fractures, only smoking (adjusted OR = 2.2; 95% CI, 1.1–4.5; $p = 0.023$) was associated with higher infection rates. *Staphylococcus aureus* was the most common bacteria cultured (59%).

Conclusions.—The only modifiable risk factor for a surgical site infection after open reduction and internal fixation was cigarette smoking. Plate fixation and temporary external fixation are likely surrogates for more complex injuries, therefore no recommendations should be inferred from this association. Surgeons should counsel patients who smoke.

Level of Evidence.—Level IV, prognostic study.

▶ The authors investigate factors associated with and characteristics of surgical site infection in a series of 1320 patients who underwent elbow fracture surgery. In this series, a 4% incidence (n = 48) of infection was noted. *Staphylococcus aureus* was the most commonly implicated organism. Risk factors associated with an infection included cigarette smoking (odds ratio [OR], 2.2), use of plate and screw fixation (OR, 2.2) and external fixation (OR, 4.7). Male sex was also more likely to be associated with an infection. Although use of plate and screw and external fixation devices was associated with a higher risk of infection, these are also often used in association with more complex injuries, so this must be interpreted with caution. Thus, the modifiable risk factor of smoking should be the focus of efforts to decrease this potentially devastating complication.

J. E. Adams, MD

Distal Biceps Tendon Ruptures: An Epidemiological Analysis Using a Large Population Database
Kelly MP, Perkinson SG, Ablove RH, et al (Univ of Wisconsin, Madison; Mayo Clinic Health System, Owatonna, MN; State Univ of New York at Buffalo)
Am J Sports Med 43:2012-2017, 2015

Background.—The incidence of distal biceps tendon ruptures was studied more than 10 years ago in a small patient cohort. Recent diagnostic advancements have improved the ability to detect this rare injury.

Hypothesis.—The incidence of distal biceps tendon ruptures will be significantly greater than previously reported.

Study Design.—Descriptive epidemiologic study.

Methods.—A query of the PearlDiver Technologies national database containing public and private insurance patients was used to estimate the national incidence of distal biceps tendon ruptures in the United States. A retrospective chart review of our local population identified demographic groups and risk factors that increased likelihood of injury.

Results.—The estimated national incidence of distal biceps tendon rupture was 2.55 per 100,000 patient-years. The local incidence was 5.35 per 100,000 patient-years. The mean and median ages of patients in our regional cohort were 46.3 and 46 years, respectively. Males composed the majority of the injured population (national 95%, regional 96%). Smoking and elevated body mass index were found to be associated with increased likelihood of injury, while diabetes mellitus showed no association.

Conclusion.—The incidence of distal biceps tendon ruptures in this study was higher than previously reported.

▶ The authors use an interesting methodology to establish the recent incidence of distal biceps tendon ruptures. Based on their study population that includes approximately 20 million patients annually, a steady increase from 2.46 to 2.63 per 100 000 patient-years was observed nationally between 2006 and 2010. These data show a significant higher incidence than previously reported.[1] Although the authors argue that current diagnostic tools, including physical examination and advanced imaging, have improved our ability to diagnose distal biceps ruptures, their data are derived from operative databases. As such, an increase in surgical management for these injuries could also have played an important role. Although surgical repair is considered the standard treatment of distal biceps tendon ruptures, nonoperative management can yield satisfactory outcomes in subsets of older less-active patients. It is unclear what the baseline age distribution of the included population is. It is to be assumed that a considerable proportion of data originated from Medicare databases. As such, even though included, younger patients (those with the highest incidence and almost invariably undergoing surgery) may be underrepresented. Furthermore, nonoperatively treated ruptures in the elderly are not included. Both factors could have the potential of underestimating the true incidence of this injury. The discrepancy between the local incidence (5.35 per 100,000 years) and the national incidence (2.55 per 100,000 years) raises the question whether different patterns in the treatment exist throughout the country as seen for other orthopedic injuries.[2-4]

P. Streubel, MD

References

1. Weinstein JN, Birkmeyer JD, eds. The Dartmouth Atlas of Musculoskeletal Health Care. Chicago, IL: American Hospital Publishing; 2000.
2. Koval KJ, Lurie J, Zhou W, et al. Ankle fractures in the elderly: what you get depends on where you live and who you see. *J Orthop Trauma.* 2005;19:635-639.
3. Keller RB, Soule DN, Wennberg JE, Hanley DF. Dealing with geographic variations in the use of hospitals. The experience of the Maine Medical Assessment Foundation Orthopaedic Study Group. *J Bone Joint Surg Am.* 1990;72: 1286-1293.
4. Sporer SM, Weinstein JN, Koval KJ. The geographic incidence and treatment variation of common fractures of elderly patients. *J Am Acad Orthop Surg.* 2006;14: 246-255.

Revisiting the 'bag of bones': functional outcome after the conservative management of a fracture of the distal humerus
Aitken SA, Jenkins PJ, Rymaszewski L (Glasgow Royal Infirmary, United Kingdom)
Bone Joint J 97-B:1132-1138, 2015

The best method of managing a fracture of the distal humerus in a frail low-demand patient with osteoporotic bone remains controversial. Total elbow arthroplasty (TEA) has been recommended for patients in whom open reduction and internal fixation (ORIF) is not possible. Conservative methods of treatment, including the 'bag of bones' technique (acceptance of displacement of the bony fragments and early mobilisation), are now rarely considered as they are believed to give a poor functional result.

We reviewed 40 elderly and low-demand patients (aged 50 to 93 years, 72% women) with a fracture of the distal humerus who had been treated conservatively at our hospital between March 2008 and December 2013, and assessed their short- and medium-term functional outcome.

In the short-term, the mean Broberg and Morrey score improved from 42 points (poor; 23 to 80) at six weeks after injury to 67 points (fair; 40 to 88) by three months.

In the medium-term, surviving patients (n = 20) had a mean Oxford elbow score of 30 points (7 to 48) at four years and a mean Disabilities of the Arm, Shoulder and Hand score of 38 points (0 to 75): 95% reported a functional range of elbow flexion. The cumulative rate of fracture union at one year was 53%. The mortality at five years approached 40%.

Conservative management of a fracture of the distal humerus in a low-demand patient only gives a modest functional result, but avoids the substantial surgical risks associated with primary ORIF or TEA.

▶ The authors remind us that nonsurgical treatment of distal humerus fractures is a reasonable option in elderly, osteoporotic, and medically complicated patients. Open reduction and internal fixation can be challenging in this population, especially in comminuted and distal fracture patterns. Total elbow arthroplasty is recommended in these instances, but the risks and potential complications are high, even in healthy, middle-age patients.

The study has limitations similar to any retrospective case series. The number of subjects is small, with only 50% of patients at final follow-up. Additionally, the cohort was not truly nonoperative. Patients that underwent anesthesia for early excision of potentially impinging bony fragments were included in the study (n = 5). Of the remaining 34 patients, 5 underwent delayed surgical treatment of the fracture. It appears all patients were included in the short- and medium-term functional data.

Despite the recognized limitations, the study provides surgeons with functional outcome data that may assist during a discussion with patients on the various treatment options. In a low-demand patient with severe medical comorbidities, nonoperative management of a distal humerus fracture may be a reasonable and appropriate intervention and should remain in a surgeon's treatment armamentarium.

A. Moeller

Clinical and functional outcomes and treatment options for paediatric elbow dislocations: Experiences of three trauma centres
Subasi M, Isik M, Bulut M, et al (Univ of Gaziantep, Turkey; Univ of Dicle, Turkey; et al)
Injury 46:S14-S18, 2015

Although elbow dislocations are seen rarely in children, their management remains controversial. In this study, over a 7 years period, we evaluated retrospectively the clinical and functional results of paediatric elbow dislocations managed in three different trauma centres. Pure dislocations and dislocations with associated injuries were evaluated separately. In total 56 patients met the inclusion criteria. The number of patients without additional injury was 22 out of which according to the Robert's criteria, 15 children (68%) had an excellent, four (18%) a good, one (5%) a fair, and two (9%) a poor outcome. From the thirty-four patients that had associated injuries, two (6%) had an excellent, 6 (18%) a good, 10 (29%) a fair and 16 (47%) a poor result.

Overall, patients with pure dislocation were found to have a better range of motion compared to patients with dislocation and associated injuries. Prolonged follow ups, and effective rehabilitation programs are required in order to expect good outcomes.

▶ This study reports the authors' experience treating pediatric elbow dislocations at 3 trauma centers over 7 years. Only 56 cases were included, so 2 to 3 cases per year per institution. Thirty-nine percent of patients had a pure posterior elbow dislocation diagnosed and 61% had associated injuries. The most common associated injuries were medial epicondyle (20), lateral condyle (4) (Fig 4), and radial neck (4) fractures. Of the pure dislocations, 86% had good or excellent results, 5% had fair results, and 9% had poor results. In

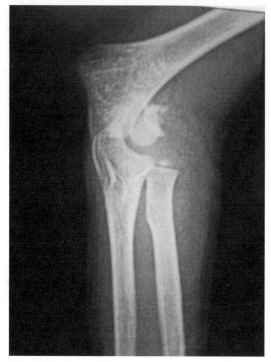

FIGURE 4.—Radiograph of posteromedial dislocation of elbow with olecranon fracture, and fracture of lateral condyle. (Reprinted from Subasi M, Isik M, Bulut M, et al. Clinical and functional outcomes and treatment options for paediatric elbow dislocations: experiences of three trauma centres. *Injury.* 2015;46:S14-S18, with permission from Elsevier.)

patients with associated injuries, results were good or excellent in only 24%, fair in 29%, and poor in 47%.

The treatment algorithm used is not entirely clear. They report that each child had a closed reduction under sedation followed by stressing of the joint. If it was easy to redislocate, the patient was treated surgically. However, they did not say if there were cases of ligament repair only or if those patients all had associated injuries requiring stabilization. Furthermore, patients with displaced fractures deemed to be unstable were taken to surgery for fixation of the fractures. Yet, 2 of the medial epicondyle fractures were deemed nondisplaced and treated with a cast. It is difficult to imagine a pediatric elbow dislocation with a fracture through the medial epicondyle that is nondisplaced.

The length of follow-up was not discussed, although "lost to follow-up" was their only exclusion criterion. In fact, it sounded like one of their patients with an ulnar neurapraxia had nerve function recovery at 8 weeks but was given a poor result because of interosseous atrophy and mild finger contractures that developed within that timeframe. A second patient with median neurapraxia "leading to severe loss of elbow movement" had nerve function recovery at 3 months. Hand atrophy and contractures contributed to that patient's poor result as well. The natural history for traumatic neurapraxia in children is full recovery over time, leading one to believe that the follow-up period may have been insufficient.

The most important contribution this report makes is to point out that vigilance in identifying associated injuries, appropriately treating them, and close monitoring are important for obtaining good and excellent results in pediatric elbow dislocations.[1]

D. Bohn, MD

Reference

1. Lieber J, Zundel SM, Luithle T, Fuchs J, Kirchner HJ. Acute traumatic posterior elbow dislocation in children. *J Pediatr Orthop B*. 2012;21:474-481.

The frequency and risk factors for subsequent surgery after a simple elbow dislocation
Modi CS, Wasserstein D, Mayne IP, et al (Toronto Western Hosp, ON, Canada; Sunnybrook Health Sciences Centre, Toronto, ON, Canada; et al)
Injury 46:1156-1160, 2015

Introduction.—Simple elbow dislocations treated by closed reduction are thought to result in a satisfactory return of function in most patients. Little, however, is known about how many patients ultimately proceed to subsequent surgical treatment due to the low patient numbers and significant loss to follow-up in the current literature. The purpose of this study was to establish the rate of and risk factors for subsequent surgical treatment after closed reduction of a simple elbow dislocation at a population level.

Patients and Methods.—All patients aged 16 years or older who underwent closed reduction of a simple elbow dislocation between 1994 and 2010 were identified using a population database. Subsequent procedures performed for joint contractures, instability or arthritis were recorded. Outcomes were modelled as a function of age, sex, income quintile, co-morbidity, urban/rural status, physician speciality performing the initial reduction and whether orthopaedic consultation and/or post-reduction radiograph was performed within 28 days of the injury, in a time-to-event analysis.

Results.—We identified 4878 elbow dislocations with a minimum 2-year follow-up: stabilisation surgery was performed in 112 (2.3%) at a median time of 1 month, contracture release in 59 (1.2%) at median 9 months and arthroplasty in seven (0.1%) at median 25 months. Admission to hospital for the initial reduction was associated with an increased risk of undergoing stabilisation (hazard ratio (HR), 2.50; 95% confidence interval (CI), 1.67–3.74) and contracture release (HR, 1.93; CI, 1.08–3.44). Multiple reduction attempts increased the risk of requiring contracture release (HR, 3.71; CI, 1.22−11.29). Survival analysis demonstrated that all subsequent procedures had taken place by 4−5 years.

Conclusion.—Few patients with simple elbow dislocations develop complications requiring surgery, but those that do most commonly undergo soft-tissue stabilisation or contracture release within 4 years of the injury. Contrary to current thinking, surgery for instability is performed more often than joint contracture release, albeit with slightly different time patterns.

▶ This study is helpful for counseling patients with simple elbow dislocations about the likelihood of needing surgical treatment for their injury (Tables 1 and 2). The authors investigated a large cohort (almost 5,000) of patients with simple elbow dislocations with a minimum follow-up of 2 years (median of 9.3 years), looking at whether surgical intervention was required for elbow stabilization, elbow contracture release, or to address posttraumatic arthritis in the elbow.

Based on the results of this study, a patient with a simple elbow dislocation should be advised that chances of needing surgery are low, approximately 3% to 4%. However, if surgery is required, it is twice as likely to be an elbow-stabilizing procedure as a contracture release. Furthermore, elbow-stabilizing procedures are more likely to be performed acutely. The treating physician should be aware that the risk of surgery increases if the patient is admitted to the hospital at the time of the initial reduction or if multiple reductions are attempted.

The sequelae of simple elbow dislocations that do not require surgical management are also of concern to the patient and physician. Anakwe et al[1] investigated 110 patients with simple elbow dislocations, more than half of whom reported subjective stiffness and residual pain after the injury. Given the apparent frequency of these concerns in patients with simple elbow dislocations,

TABLE 1.—Inclusion and exclusion criteria for the simple dislocation cohort

	No.
Inclusion criterion	
OHIP fee code #D009 (elbow dislocation − closed reduction)	14,736
Exclusion criteria	
Age <16 years	6886
Non-Ontario residents	11
Previous elbow dislocation	26
Previous elbow fracture	336
Concurrent elbow fracture	1913
Other concurrent fractures	644
Death at index date	2
Missing demographic data	40
Cohort size after exclusions	4878

OHIP, Ontario Health Insurance Plan.
Reprinted from Modi CS, Wasserstein D, Mayne IP, et al. The frequency and risk factors for subsequent surgery after a simple elbow dislocation. *Injury.* 2015;46:1156-1160, with permission from Elsevier.

TABLE 2.—Characteristics of simple elbow dislocation cohort

Variable	Stabilisation, no. (%)			Contracture Release with Ulnar Nerve, no. (%)			Arthroplasty, no. (%)		
	Had Surgery	No Surgery	p-Value	Had Surgery	No Surgery	p-Value	Had Surgery	No Surgery	p-Value
Age	46.08 ± 17.56	42.09 ± 17.79	0.042	39.47 ± 14.01	42.19 ± 17.83	0.24	51.00 ± 22.34	42.14 ± 17.78	0.22
Sex (female)	48 (57.8)	2559 (53.4)	0.42	31 (52.5)	2576 (53.5)	0.89	5 (83.3)	2602 (53.4)	0.14
Urban (versus Rural)	73 (88.0)	4201 (87.6)	0.93	54 (91.5)	4220 (87.6)	0.36	6 (100)	4268 (87.6)	0.36
Income quintile			0.10			0.20			0.40
1	23 (27.7)	956 (19.9)		12 (20.3)	967 (20.1)		0 (0)	979 (20.1)	
2	15 (18.1)	988 (20.6)		16 (27.1)	987 (20.5)		2 (33.3)	1001 (20.5)	
3	21 (25.3)	942 (19.6)		16 (27.1)	947 (19.7)		2 (33.3)	961 (19.7)	
4	15 (18.1)	940 (19.6)		8 (13.6)	947 (19.7)		2 (33.3)	953 (19.6)	
5	9 (10.8)	969 (20.2)		7 (11.9)	971 (20.1)		0 (0)	978 (20.1)	
Comorbidities			0.27			0.35			0.01
0–4	40 (48.2)	2731 (57.0)		38 (64.4)	2733 (56.7)		2 (33.3)	2769 (56.8)	
5–8	41 (49.4)	1984 (41.4)		21 (35.6)	2004 (41.6)		3 (50.0)	2022 (42.2)	
9+	2 (2.4)	80 (1.7)		0 (0)	82 (1.7)		1 (16.7)	81 (1.7)	
Admission to hospital for initial reduction	27 (32.5)	765 (16.0)	<0.001	17 (28.8)	775 (16.1)	0.008	0 (0)	792 (16.3)	0.28
Multiple reduction attempts (>1)	9 (10.8)	281 (5.9)	0.06	5 (8.5)	285 (5.9)	0.41	0 (0)	290 (6.0)	0.54
Initial reduction by orthopaedics	31 (37.3)	1174 (24.5)	0.007	24 (40.7)	1181 (24.5)	0.004	2 (33.3)	1203 (24.7)	0.62
Orthopaedic consult within 28 days	73 (88.0)	3795 (79.1)	0.05	51 (86.4)	3817 (79.2)	0.17	5 (83.3)	3863 (79.3)	0.81
Follow-up radiograph within 28 days	20 (24.1)	1051 (21.9)	0.64	18 (30.5)	1053 (21.9)	0.11	3 (50.0)	1068 (21.9)	0.48

Reprinted from Modi CS, Wasserstein D, Mayne IP, et al. The frequency and risk factors for subsequent surgery after a simple elbow dislocation. *Injury.* 2015;46:1156-1160, with permission from Elsevier.

additional research focusing on pain, stiffness, and function in this large cohort may yield useful information for the future care and counseling of patients with this injury.

E. Kinnucan, MD

Reference

1. Anakwe RE, Middleton SD, Jenkins PJ, McQueen MM, Court-Brown CM. Patient-reported outcomes after simple dislocation of the elbow. *J Bone Joint Surg Am.* 2011;93:1220-1226.

Current Treatment Concepts for "Terrible Triad" Injuries of the Elbow
Bohn K, Ipaktchi K, Livermore M, et al (Univ of Colorado School of Medicine, Aurora; Denver Health Med Ctr, CO; et al)
Orthopedics 37:831-837, 2014

Elbow fracture-dislocations destabilize the elbow, preventing functional rehabilitation. If left untreated, they commonly result in functional compromise and poor outcomes. The "terrible triad" injury is classically described as a combination of a coronoid process and radial head fractures, as well as a posterolateral elbow dislocation. Surgical treatment to restore stable elbow range of motion has evolved in the past few decades based on increased understanding of elbow biomechanics and the anatomy of these injuries. This article highlights current concepts in the treatment of these complicated injuries.

▶ Bohn et al provide an overview of terrible triad elbow injuries. The authors provide a review of the basic anatomy but not a detailed description of ligament attachments or surgical approaches. They also review basic treatment algorithms and common complications. This article provides a nice framework for understanding terrible triad injuries, but an inexperienced surgeon would be advised to seek out more in-depth articles before approaching one of these challenging injuries.

C. Ward, MD

Incarcerated Medial Epicondyle Fracture Following Pediatric Elbow Dislocation: 11 Cases
Dodds SD, Flanagin BA, Bohl DD, et al (Yale School of Medicine, New Haven, CT; Connecticut Orthopaedic Specialists, Hamden)
J Hand Surg 39:1739-1745, 2014

Purpose.—To describe outcomes after surgical management of pediatric elbow dislocation with incarceration of the medial epicondyle.

Methods.—We conducted a retrospective case review of 11 consecutive children and adolescents with an incarcerated medial epicondyle fracture after elbow dislocation. All patients underwent open reduction internal fixation using a similar technique. We characterized outcomes at final follow-up.

Results.—Average follow-up was 14 months (range, 4–56 mo). All patients had clinical and radiographic signs of healing at final follow-up. There was no radiographic evidence of loss of reduction at intervals or at final follow-up. There were no cases of residual deformity or valgus instability. Average final arc of elbow motion was 4° to 140°. All patients had forearm rotation from 90° supination to 90° pronation. Average Mayo elbow score was 99.5. Four of 11 patients had ulnar nerve symptoms postoperatively and 1 required a second operation for ulnar nerve symptoms. In addition, 1 required a second operation for flexion contracture release with excision of heterotopic ossification. Three patients had ulnar nerve symptoms at final follow-up. Two of these had mild paresthesia only and 1 had both mild paresthesia and weakness.

Conclusions.—Our results suggest that open reduction internal fixation of incarcerated medial epicondyle fractures after elbow dislocation leads to satisfactory motion and function; however, the injury carries a high risk for complications, particularly ulnar neuropathy.

▶ Dodds et al performed a retrospective review of 11 pediatric patients who suffered an incarcerated medial epicondyle fracture associated with an elbow dislocation. In all cases, patients were treated with open reduction internal fixation. Five of 6 patients with ulnar nerve symptoms preoperatively underwent ulnar nerve neurolysis, but the nerve was not transposed during the index procedure in any patients.

Surgeons noted some articular damage at the time of surgery in all cases. Most patients regained motion (average arc of motion: 4°-140°). More than half of the patients experienced ulnar nerve symptoms preoperatively, and 3 of 11 patients had continued ulnar nerve symptoms at final follow-up despite ulnar nerve neurolysis in 2 of those cases. Eighteen percent of patients underwent a second operation, which the authors noted was higher than previous reported reoperation rates for medial epicondyle fractures (with or without incarceration).

Although the authors report an average follow-up of 14 months, this time may not best represent this patient group, as 8 of 11 patients had less than 12 months of follow-up. The median follow-up was 7 months, and 3 patients had less than 6 months of follow-up. With that in mind, further follow-up may reveal changes in both ulnar nerve function and elbow range of motion. The included patients were skeletally immature, and growth disturbances or other issues related to the noted articular damage may not be evident so soon after the injury.

C. Ward, MD

Extension Test and Ossal Point Tenderness Cannot Accurately Exclude Significant Injury in Acute Elbow Trauma

Jie KE, van Dam LF, Verhagen TF, et al (Sint Antonius Ziekenhuis, Nieuwegein, the Netherlands)

Ann Emerg Med 64:74-78, 2014

Study Objective.—Elbow injury is a common presentation at the emergency department (ED). There are no guidelines indicating which of these patients require radiography, whereas clinical decision rules for other limb injuries are widely accepted and resulted in less radiography and reduced waiting times. We aim to identify clinical signs that can be used to predict the need for radiography in elbow injury.

Methods.—A prospective observational study at 2 ED locations in the Netherlands was performed. For every eligible patient with acute elbow injury, elbow extension and addition of point tenderness at the olecranon, epicondyles, and radial head were evaluated for predicting the need for radiography (primary endpoint). A subgroup of patients was assessed by a blinded second investigator to analyze interobserver variability (secondary endpoint). All patients received anterior-posterior and lateral elbow radiographs. Fractures were treated according to current guidelines and patients were followed at outpatient clinics.

Results.—In total, 587 patients were included. Normal extension was observed in 174 patients (30%). Normal extension predicted absence of a fracture or isolated fat pad with 88% sensitivity and 55% specificity. Five patients with normal extension had a fracture that required surgery. Absence of point tenderness in patients with normal extension was observed in only 24 patients, of whom 3 showed a fracture and 1 required surgery. Addition of point tenderness to the extension test to predict absence of a fracture or isolated fat pad resulted in 98% sensitivity and 11% specificity. Interobserver analysis for extension and palpation of olecranon, epicondyles, and radial head resulted in κ values between 0.6 and 0.7.

Conclusion.—In contrast with previous studies, ours shows that in acute elbow injury, the extension test alone or in combination with point tenderness assessment does not safely rule out clinically significant injury. Interobserver variability was substantial. We would not recommend the use of the extension test (+/− point tenderness assessment) as a clinical decision rule to guide radiologic diagnostics in acute elbow trauma.

▶ This study prospectively evaluated patients who presented to the emergency department with acute elbow injury to determine if specific clinical findings could be used to rule out fracture without requiring radiographs. Arundel et al had previously described the "East Riding Elbow Rules," which reported that radiographs were very unlikely to identify a clinically relevant elbow fracture if the patient had full active elbow extension, and there was no bony tenderness at the olecranon, epicondyles, and radial head and if the patient had full active elbow extension.[1] In essence, they attempted to create something similar to the Ottawa Ankle Rules for the elbow. The current study prospectively evaluated 587 emergency department patients (adults and children > 3 years old) using these physical examination tests as well as anterior-posterior and lateral elbow radiographs.

Most patients (77%) with normal elbow extension had no fracture, but 12% had a fracture and 3% required surgery for their fracture. The remaining 11% had an abnormal fat pad sign. Most patients (73%) with abnormal extension test also had abnormal radiographs. Authors calculated that abnormal extension alone had a sensitivity of 88% and a specificity of 55% for fracture.

Sensitivity increased to 98% when authors combined extension testing with bony tenderness, but this substantially decreased specificity. And even in the 24 patients with a normal extension test and no bony tenderness, radiographs identified fractures in 3 patients (13%). The authors conclude that the missed fracture rate when using East Riding Elbow Rules is likely higher in practice than in the original report. In short, physicians must continue to use their clinical judgment when determining whether to obtain radiographs in acute elbow injuries.

C. Ward, MD

Reference

1. Arundel D, Williams P, Townend W. Deriving the East Riding Elbow Rule (ER2): a maximally sensitive decision tool for elbow injury. *Emerg Med J*. 2014;31: 380-383.

14 Elbow: Miscellaneous

Total elbow joint replacement for fractures in the elderly—Functional and radiological outcomes
Pooley J, Salvador Carreno J (Queen Elizabeth Hosp, Gateshead, United Kingdom; Hosp Universitari Mutua Terassa, Barcelona, Spain)
Injury 46S:S37-S42, 2015

Aim.—The purpose of this paper was to review the literature on the treatment of intra-articular fractures of the distal humerus in the elderly in order to evaluate the place for total elbow replacement (TER) in the light of our experience over the past 15 years.

Methods.—A review of the records of 11 consecutive patients over the age of 60 years who underwent primary TER for comminuted fractures of the distal humerus between 1997 and 2011 were reviewed and the surviving patients were interviewed. The Scopus database was used to perform a pragmatic review of the literature published between the mid-1990s and the present-day.

Results.—At the time of the most recent follow-up 3.5 years following surgery (range: 2—6 years) 7 patients assessed with the Mayo elbow performance index were classified as excellent, 4 were classified as good. There were no complications requiring further procedures encountered. Five surviving patients remain satisfied with the function of their TER. The number of papers recommending TER for treatment of these fractures continues to increase with time.

Conclusions.—TER is now the treatment of choice for unreconstructable fractures of the distal humerus in the elderly. This option should therefore be available at the time of surgery for all distal humeral fractures in this patient population. A surgical approach other than olecranon osteotomy, which would preclude TER is therefore required.

▶ This enlightening article offers a review of the literature and the authors' personal experiences with total elbow replacement (TER) for acute intra-articular fractures of the distal humerus in an elderly population. The authors correctly note the paradigm shift in treatment philosophy for these relatively rare but highly disabling fractures in the upper extremity. Briefly restated, comminuted intra-articular distal humerus fractures in the elderly frequently have displaced fragments devoid of soft tissue attachment and inherently poor bone quality. Cleverly compared with Neer 4-part proximal humerus fractures, distal humerus fractures in the elderly are a biological equivalent to this more proximal injury pattern.

The authors cite numerous studies that indicate an evolution of thought and practicality of TER for distal humerus fractures in this patient population based on outcome data although admittedly often limited in size because of the relative infrequent occurrence of these devastating injuries. The authors' personal experiences of 11 consecutive patients treated with TER yielded good to excellent results in those patients available for follow-up, and none required additional surgery and were satisfied with their elbow function after TER.

Final summary points offered by this report are that the TER remains not only a viable option for comminuted distal humerus fractures in the elderly but is rapidly becoming the treatment of choice based on patient satisfaction and implant survivability with few medium- to long-term complications. It is also critical that the surgeon prepare for the possibility of TER in the acute setting, both with implant availability and a surgical approach that avoids olecranon osteotomy, which complicates implantation of the ulnar component.

S. M. Jacoby, MD

Corticosteroid and platelet-rich plasma injection therapy in tennis elbow (lateral epicondylalgia): a survey of current UK specialist practice and a call for clinical guidelines
Titchener AG, Booker SJ, Bhamber NS, et al (Royal Derby Hosp, UK)
Br J Sports Med 49:1410-1413, 2015

Background.—Tennis elbow is a common condition with a variety of treatment options, but little is known about which of these options specialists choose most commonly. Corticosteroid injections in tennis elbow may reduce pain in the short-term but delay long-term recovery. We have undertaken a UK-wide survey of upper limb specialists to assess current practice.

Methods.—Cross-sectional electronic survey of current members of the British Elbow and Shoulder Society (BESS) and the British Society for Surgery of the Hand (BSSH).

Results.—271 of 1047 eligible members responded (25.9%); consultant surgeons constituted the largest group (232/271, 85%). 131 respondents (48%) use corticosteroid injections as their first-line treatment for tennis elbow. 206 respondents (77%) believed that corticosteroid injections are not potentially harmful in the treatment of tennis elbow, while 31 (11%) did not use them in their current practice. In light of recent evidence of the potential harmful effects of corticosteroid therapy, 136 (50%) had not changed their practice while 108 (40.1%) had reduced or discontinued their use. 43 respondents (16%) reported having used platelet-rich plasma injections.

Conclusions.—Recent high-quality evidence that corticosteroids may delay recovery in tennis elbow appears to have had a limited effect on current practice. Treatment is not uniform among specialists and a proportion of them use platelet-rich plasma injections.

▶ Recent studies of corticosteroid injection for tennis elbow cast concern about the long-term benefit, complication rate, and efficacy of such injections. This study consisted of a survey sent to physicians practicing in the United Kingdom to assess practice patterns in light of these recent findings. The survey demonstrated a variety of practice patterns with respect to the management of tennis elbow with steroid injection that did not necessarily reflect incorporation of the recent literature. The authors rightly recommend the development of best practice guidelines for practitioners. Additionally, the authors suggest the development of patient information reflecting the current state of knowledge.

W. T. Payne, MD

Factors Associated With Failure of Nonoperative Treatment in Lateral Epicondylitis
Knutsen EJ, Calfee RP, Chen RE, et al (George Washington Univ School of Medicine and Health Sciences; Washington Univ School of Medicine, St Louis, MO; et al)
Am J Sports Med 43:2133-2137, 2015

Background.—Lateral epicondylitis is a common cause of elbow pain that is treated with a variety of nonoperative measures and often improves with time. Minimal research is available on patients in whom these nonoperative treatments fail.

Purpose.—To identify baseline patient and disease factors associated with the failure of nonoperative treatment of lateral epicondylitis, defined as surgery after a period of nonoperative treatment.

Study Design.—Case control study; Level of evidence, 3.

Methods.—A total of 580 patients treated for lateral epicondylitis at a tertiary center between 2007 and 2012 were analyzed. Disease-specific and patient demographic characteristics were compared between patient groups (nonoperative vs surgical treatment). A multivariable logistic regression model was created based on preliminary univariate testing to determine which characteristics were associated with failure of nonoperative treatment.

Results.—Of the 580 patients, 92 (16%) underwent surgical treatment at a mean of 6 months (range, 0-31 months) from their initial visit. Univariate analysis demonstrated a potential association ($P < .10$) between operative management and the following factors at initial diagnosis: increased age, body mass index, duration of symptoms, presence of radial tunnel syndrome, prior injection, physical therapy, splinting, smoking, workers' compensation, a labor occupation, use of narcotics, use of antidepressant medications, and previous orthopaedic surgery. In the final multivariable model, a workers' compensation claim (odds ratio [OR], 8.1), prior injection (OR, 5.6), the presence of radial tunnel syndrome (OR, 3.1), previous orthopaedic surgery (OR, 3.2), and duration of symptoms >12 months (OR, 2.5) remained significant independent predictors of surgical treatment.

Conclusion.—This study identifies risk factors for surgical treatment for lateral epicondylitis. While these findings do not provide information regarding causal factors associated with surgery, these patient and disease-specific considerations may be helpful when counseling patients regarding treatment options and the likelihood of the success of continued nonoperative treatment.

▶ The authors present an interesting plan in this article: to discover which patients with lateral epicondylitis are likely to progress to surgery. They have a large cohort of 580 patients retrospectively reviewed for their data set, which adds a nice robustness to the article, but the clinical impact is still wanting. The authors do a nice job in the discussion describing the limitations of the study, which should be read (not just the abstract), as the summary could be a bit misleading. One of the most interesting takeaways from the article is the increased risk to advance to surgical intervention in patients that received an injection. It should be noted that the endpoint or failure point of intervention is an arbitrary choice of proceeding to surgery, which is a soft decision that rarely is the same construct for each patient.

J. M. Froelich, MD

Plate and Screw Fixation of Bicolumnar Distal Humerus Fractures: Factors Associated With Loosening or Breakage of Implants or Nonunion
Claessen FMAP, Braun Y, Peters RM, et al (Massachusetts General Hosp, Boston)
J Hand Surg Am 40:2045-2051, 2015

Purpose.—To identify factors associated with reoperation for early loosening or breakage of implants or nonunion after operative treatment of AO type C distal humerus fractures.

Methods.—We retrospectively analyzed 129 adult patients who had operative treatment of an isolated AO type C distal humerus fracture at 1 of 5 hospitals to determine factors associated with reoperation for early loosening or breakage of implants or nonunion.

Results.—Within 6 months of original fixation, 16 of 129 fractures (12%) required reoperation for loosening or breakage of implants (n = 8) or nonunion (n = 8). In bivariate analyses, the Charlson comorbidity index, smoking, a coded diagnosis of obesity, diabetes mellitus, and radiographic osteoarthritis were significantly associated with reoperation for early loosening or breakage of implants or nonunion.

Conclusions.—With the numbers available, patient factors rather than technical factors were associated with reoperation for loosening or breakage of implants and nonunion. Because of the relative infrequency of fixation problems and nonunion, a much larger study is needed to address technical deficiencies.

Type of Study/Level of Evidence.—Therapeutic IV.

▶ Distal humerus fractures are a challenging problem in an upper extremity surgeon's practice. The authors did a nice job of creating a tight lens to evaluate the risk factors for nonunion/hardware failure by isolating specifically AO type C bicolumnar fracture patterns. They showed that obesity, increased comorbidities, diabetes, smoking, and, interestingly, osteoarthritis were associated with a higher reoperation rate. This article helps frame discussions with patients preoperatively and lay a foundation for understanding nonsurgical technique influences on the outcomes of these complex cases.

J. Froelich, MD

Subcutaneous Versus Submuscular Anterior Transposition of the Ulnar Nerve for Cubital Tunnel Syndrome: A Systematic Review and Meta-Analysis of Randomized Controlled Trials and Observational Studies

Liu C-H, Wu S-Q, Ke X-B, et al (Fujian Univ of Traditional Chinese Medicine, Fuzhou, China; Second Affiliated Hosp of Fujian Med Univ, Quanzhou, China; et al)
Medicine (Baltimore) 94:e1207, 2015

Subcutaneous and submuscular anterior ulnar nerve transposition have been widely used in patients with cubital tunnel syndrome. However, the reliable evidence in favor of 1 of 2 surgical options on clinical improvement remains controversial.

To maximize the value of the available literature, we performed a systematic review and meta-analysis to compare subcutaneous versus submuscular anterior ulnar nerve transposition in patients with ulnar neuropathy at the elbow.

PubMed, Cochrane Library, and EMBASE databases were searched for randomized and observational studies that compared subcutaneous transposition with submuscular transposition of ulnar nerve for cubital tunnel syndrome. The primary outcome was clinically relevant improvement in function compared to the baseline. Randomized and observational studies were separately analyzed with relative risks (RRs) and 95% confidence intervals (CIs).

Two randomized controlled trials (RCTs) and 7 observational studies, involving 605 patients, were included. Our meta-analysis suggested that no significant differences in the primary outcomes were observed between comparison groups, both in RCT (RR, 1.16; 95% CI 0.68−1.98; $P = 0.60$; $I^2 = 81\%$) and observational studies (RR, 1.01; 95% CI 0.95−1.08; $P = 0.69$; $I^2 = 0\%$). These findings were also consistent with all subgroup analyses for observational studies. In the secondary outcomes, the incidence of adverse events was significantly lower in subcutaneous group than in submuscular group (RR, 0.54; 95% CI 0.33–0.87; $P = 0.01$; $I^2 = 0\%$), whereas subcutaneous transposition failed to reveal more superiority than submuscular transposition in static two-point discrimination (MD, 0.04; 95% CI −0.18–0.25; $P = 0.74$; $I^2 = 0\%$).

The available evidence is not adequately powered to identify the best anterior ulnar nerve transposition technique for cubital tunnel syndrome on the basis of clinical outcomes, that is, suggests that subcutaneous and submuscular anterior transposition might be equally effective in terms of postoperative clinical improvement. However, differences in clinical outcomes metrics should be noted, and these findings largely rely on the outcomes data from observational studies that are potentially subject to a high risk of selection bias. Therefore, more high-quality and adequately powered RCTs with standardized clinical outcomes metrics are necessary for proper comparison of these techniques.

▶ The quest for evidence-based guidelines for treatment of cubital tunnel syndrome remains quite active as highlighted by the number of published articles on this topic in recent years. This meta-analysis consisted of 2 randomized control trials (RCT) and 7 observational studies comparing anterior subcutaneous and submuscular transposition. It is not clear whether these were primary or revision procedures or a combination. Of the total patients included, less than 2% were in the RCT studies. The potential bias is high when most collected data were from retrospective observational studies. Additionally, each of the 9 included studies had a different primary outcome; therefore, the authors converted the results to "improvement" or "no improvement." This method may limit the reliability of the results. The authors conclude that although no differences in the primary outcome were detected between the 2 operative procedures, the study was not adequately powered to detect a difference.

Our quest continues. This meta-analysis has not changed my clinical practice. In primary cubital tunnel decompression, in situ decompression is my treatment of choice unless ulnar nerve subluxation or osseous deformity is present. In revision surgery, I would consider submuscular transposition if previous subcutaneous transposition had been performed.

A. Moeller

Outcomes After Ulnar Nerve *In Situ* Release During Total Elbow Arthroplasty
Dachs RP, Vrettos BC, Chivers DA, et al (Univ of Cape Town, South Africa)
J Hand Surg Am 40:1832-1837, 2015

Purpose.—Ulnar nerve (UN) lesions are a significant complication after total elbow arthroplasty (TEA), with potentially debilitating consequences. Outcomes from a center, which routinely performs an *in situ* release of the nerve without transposition, were investigated.

Methods.—Eighty-three primary TEAs were retrospectively reviewed for the intraoperative management of the UN and presence of postoperative UN symptoms.

Results.—Three patients had documented preoperative UN symptoms. One patient had a prior UN transposition. The nerve was transposed at the time of TEA in 4 of the remaining 82 elbows (5%). The indication for transposition in all cases was abnormal tracking or increased tension on the nerve after insertion of the prosthesis. Of the 4 patients who underwent UN transposition, 2 had postoperative UN symptoms. Both were neuropraxias, which resolved in the early postoperative period. The remaining 78 TEAs received an *in situ* release of the nerve. The incidence of postoperative UN symptoms in the *in situ* release group was 5% (4 of 78). Two patients had resolution of symptoms, whereas 2 continued to experience significant UN symptoms requiring subsequent transposition. Seven patients had preoperative flexion of less than 100°. Of these, 2 had a UN transposition at the time of TEA. Of the remaining 5 elbows with preoperative flexion less than 100°, 2 had postoperative UN symptoms after *in situ* release, with 1 requiring subsequent UN transposition.

Conclusions.—A 3% incidence of significant UN complications after TEA compares favorably with systematic reviews. We do not believe that transposition, which adds to the handling of the nerve and increases surgical time, is routinely indicated and should rather be reserved for cases with marked limitation of preoperative elbow flexion or when intraoperative assessment by the surgeon deems it necessary.

Type of Study/Level of Evidence.—Therapeutic IV.

▶ Total elbow arthroplasty carries a high rate of complications and yet is still an important option in the treatment of end-stage arthritis of the elbow or post-traumatic conditions. As the procedure continues to evolve, investigators try to identify ways of decreasing the complications associated with the procedure. This retrospective study describes the results of a series of 78 patients who underwent ulnar nerve release without transposition during total elbow arthroplasty. Four of the 78 patients had documented ulnar nerve symptoms postoperatively, and 2 required reoperation to transpose the ulnar nerve. Optimal management of the ulnar nerve during total elbow arthroplasty is still unclear, and surgeons should strive to protect the ulnar nerve during the procedure.

W. T. Payne, MD

Elbow Positioning and Joint Insufflation Substantially Influence Median and Radial Nerve Locations
Hackl M, Lappen S, Burkhart KJ, et al (Univ Med Ctr of Cologne, Germany; Univ of Cologne, Germany; et al)
Clin Orthop Relat Res 473:3627-3634, 2015

Background.—The median and radial nerves are at risk of iatrogenic injury when performing arthroscopic arthrolysis with anterior capsulectomy.

Although prior anatomic studies have identified the position of these nerves, little is known about how elbow positioning and joint insufflation might influence nerve locations.

Questions/Purposes.—In a cadaver model, we sought to determine whether (1) the locations of the median and radial nerves change with variation of elbow positioning; and whether (2) flexion and joint insufflation increase the distance of the median and radial nerves to osseous landmarks after correcting for differences in size of the cadaveric specimens.

Methods.—The median and radial nerves were marked with a radiopaque thread in 11 fresh-frozen elbow specimens. Three-dimensional radiographic scans were performed in extension, in 90° flexion, and after joint insufflations in neutral rotation, pronation, and supination. Trochlear and capitellar widths were analyzed. The distances of the median nerve to the medial and anterior edge of the trochlea and to the coronoid were measured. The distances of the radial nerve to the lateral and anterior edge of the capitulum and to the anterior edge of the radial head were measured. We analyzed the mediolateral nerve locations as a percentage function of the trochlear and capitellar widths to control for differences regarding the size of the specimens.

Results.—The mean distance of the radial nerve to the lateral edge of the capitulum as a percentage function of the capitellar width increased from 68% ± 17% in extension to 91% ± 23% in flexion (mean difference = 23%; 95% confidence interval [CI], 5%−41%; $p = 0.01$). With the numbers available, no such difference was observed regarding the location of the median nerve in relation to the medial border of the trochlea (mean difference = 5%; 95% CI, −13% to 22%; $p = 0.309$). Flexion and joint insufflation increased the distance of the nerves to osseous landmarks. The mean distance of the median nerve to the coronoid tip was 5.4 ± 1.3 mm in extension, 9.1 ± 2.3 mm in flexion (mean difference = 3.7 mm; 95% CI, 2.04−5.36 mm; $p < 0.001$), and 12.6 ± 3.6 mm in flexion and insufflation (mean difference = 3.5 mm; 95% CI, 0.81−6.19 mm; $p = 0.008$). The mean distance of the radial nerve to the anterior edge of the radial head increased from 4.7 ± 1.8 mm in extension to 7.7 ± 2.7 mm in flexion (mean difference = 3.0 mm; 95% CI, 0.96−5.04 mm; $p = 0.005$) and to 11.9 ± 3.0 mm in flexion with additional joint insufflation (mean difference = 4.2 mm; 95% CI, 1.66−6.74 mm; $p = 0.002$).

Conclusions.—The radial nerve shifts medially during flexion from the lateral to the medial border of the inner third of the capitulum. The median nerve is located at the medial quarter of the joint. The distance of the median and radial nerves to osseous landmarks doubles from extension to 90° flexion and triples after joint insufflation.

Clinical Relevance.—Elbow arthroscopy with anterior capsulectomy should be performed cautiously at the medial aspect of the joint to avoid median nerve lesions. Performing arthroscopic anterior capsulectomy in flexion at the lateral aspect of the joint and in slight extension at the medial edge of the capitulum could enhance safety of this procedure.

▶ Latrogenic nerve injury is one of the most feared complications of elbow arthroscopy for capsular release. The findings of this cadaveric study serve to support the concepts of flexing the elbow to 90° and insufflating the joint to increase the distance of the nerves from the bone. Although these techniques are found to increase the distance of the median and radial nerves from anterior bony landmarks, it is unclear if this finding is reproducible in joints with capsular contracture; therefore, caution is still advised when performing anterior elbow joint capsular release arthroscopically.

W. T. Payne, MD

Trends in Medial Ulnar Collateral Ligament Reconstruction in the United States: A Retrospective Review of a Large Private-Payer Database From 2007 to 2011
Erickson BJ, Nwachukwu BU, Rosas S, et al (Rush Univ Med Ctr, Chicago, IL; Hosp for Special Surgery, NY; Holy Cross Hosp Orthopaedic Inst, Fort Lauderdale, FL)
Am J Sports Med 43:1770-1774, 2015

Background.—Overuse injuries to the elbow in the throwing athlete are common. Ulnar collateral ligament reconstruction (UCLR), commonly known as Tommy John surgery, is performed on both recreational and high-level athletes. There is no current literature regarding the incidence and demographic distribution of this surgical procedure in relation to patient age, location within the Unites States, and sex.

Purpose.—To determine the current demographic distribution of UCLR within the US population included in the PearlDiver database.

Study Design.—Descriptive epidemiology study.

Methods.—A retrospective analysis of the PearlDiver supercomputer database, a private-payer database, was performed to identify UCLR procedures performed between 2007 and 2011. The Current Procedural Terminology (CPT) code 24346 (reconstruction of the ulnar collateral ligament of the elbow with the use of a tendinous graft) was used.

Results.—Between 2007 and 2011, a total of 790 patients underwent UCLR. The average ($\pm$SD) annual incidence was 3.96 ± 0.38 per 100,000 patients for the overall population but was 22 ± 3.4 for patients aged 15 to 19 years. The overall average annual growth was 4.2%. There were 695 males and 95 females. The 15- to 19-year-old patients accounted for significantly more procedures than any other age group (56.8%; $P < .001$), followed by 20- to 24-year-olds (22.2%). The incidence of UCLR in the 15- to 19-year-old group increased at an average rate of 9.12% per year ($P = .009$). Significantly more UCLR procedures were performed in the southern United States than in any other region ($P < .001$). The number of procedures significantly increased over time ($P = .039$).

Conclusion.—According to this database of a privately insured population, UCLR was performed significantly more in patients aged 15 to 19 than any other age group. The average annual incidence of UCLR per 100,000 people for patients aged 15 to 19 was 22 ± 3.4. Further, this database showed that the number of UCLR procedures is increasing over time. Further work should address risk reduction efforts in this at-risk population.

▶ The findings of this retrospective database review are not surprising. The number of ulnar collateral ligament reconstructions performed is increasing, most significantly in patients aged 15 to 19 years. These surgeries tend to be performed at the beginning of the baseball season (April to June) when athletes are perhaps more prone to injury.

These findings may be a result of increasing demands on young athletes. Children are beginning sports at a younger age and are practicing more frequently for more prolonged periods. Alternatively, as mentioned by the authors, ulnar collateral ligament reconstruction may be a perceived panacea by athletes, their parents, and coaches. The cohort of patients in this study was from a private payer database. It is more likely that these families can afford surgical reconstruction of the ulnar collateral ligament with hopes that their child will be the next Major League Baseball pitcher!

Efforts should be focused on education of athletes, parents and coaches.

A. Moeller

Prognostic Factors of Arthroscopic Extensor Carpi Radialis Brevis Release for Lateral Epicondylitis

Yoon JP, Chung SW, Yi JH, et al (Kyungpook Natl Univ Hosp, Daegu, Republic of Korea; Asan Med Ctr, Seoul, Republic of Korea; et al)
Arthroscopy 31:1232-1237, 2015

Purpose. The purpose of this study was to analyze factors affecting the treatment outcomes and prognoses of arthroscopic debridement for refractory lateral epicondylitis.

Methods.—We included 45 patients who had undergone arthroscopic extensor carpi radialis brevis release for chronic refractory lateral epicondylitis between October 2008 and December 2012. Demographic data, magnetic resonance imaging studies, and arthroscopic findings were examined and analyzed.

Results.—The mean age of the enrolled patients (23 men and 22 women) was 45.9 ± 7.8 years, and the mean follow-up duration was 26.9 ± 9.0 months. All the patients showed significant clinical improvement on all parameters assessed using the visual analog scale (6.9

preoperatively to 0.9 postoperatively), the Upper Extremity Functional Scale (34.8 to 66.7), and the Mayo Elbow Score (63.5 to 92.3) ($P < .05$). There were no reports of serious surgical complications. At final follow-up, 37 patients (82.2%) were satisfied with their outcomes whereas 8 patients (17.8%) were dissatisfied. In terms of demographic factors, female sex was significantly different between the 2 groups. On preoperative magnetic resonance imaging, 7 patients in the satisfied group (18.9%) had a definite tendon lesion (grade III defect, ≥ 6 mm) whereas 6 patients in the dissatisfied group (75%) had a grade III defect ($P = .016$).

Conclusions.—Overall, clinical outcome scores showed improvement after arthroscopic extensor carpi radialis brevis release for refractory lateral epicondylitis. However, preoperative tendon status and sex were associated with dissatisfaction and poor postoperative outcomes after the arthroscopic release procedure.

Level of Evidence.—Level IV, therapeutic case series.

▶ The authors present a case series of arthroscopic release of the extensor carpi radialis brevis (ECRB) for lateral epicondylitis and try to identify risk factors for unsatisfactory outcomes from the surgery.

Forty-five patients were retrospectively reviewed, which included all arthroscopic treatment of lateral epicondylitis over a 4-year period. Patients must have not responded to conservative management with medication, activity modification, physical therapy, bracing, and at least 1 local injection with steroid. Patients with bilateral disease, prior surgery, concomitant arthritis, or lack of follow-up of at least 1 year with functional outcome evaluation were excluded.

Functional evaluations included a visual analog scale (VAS) for pain, the Mayo Elbow Score (MES), and the Upper Extremity Functional Scale (UEFS). Other clinical variables including smoking status, work status, sports activity, hand dominance, and history of trauma were recorded. MR images were assessed

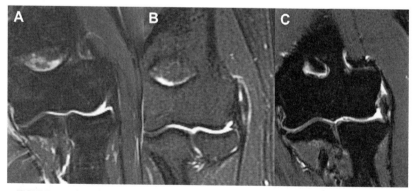

FIGURE 1.—The size of the extensor carpi radialis brevis tendon defect was examined on magnetic resonance imaging. (A) A grade I tendon defect has a normal shape, homogeneous low intensity, or mild focally increased tendon signals. (B) A 2- to 5-mm defect is classified as a grade II defect. (C) A defect of 6 mm or greater is classified as a grade III defect. (Reprinted from Yoon JP, Chung SW, Yi JH, et al. Prognostic factors of arthroscopic extensor carpi radialis brevis release for lateral epicondylitis. *Arthroscopy.* 2015;31:1232-1237, with permission from Arthroscopy Association of North America.)

TABLE 3.—Demographic and Clinical Differences Between Satisfied and Dissatisfied Groups

Variable	Satisfied Group (n = 37)	Dissatisfied Group (n = 8)	P Value
Age, yr	45.2 ± 7.9	48.8 ± 7.4	.248
Sex, male/female	22/15	1/7	.016
Dominant side, dominant/ nondominant	24/13	3/5	.152
Symptom duration, mo	15.2 ± 10.4	17.7 ± 6.0	.522
Symptom aggravation, mo	1.6 ± 0.8	1.6 ± 0.5	.783
Diabetes	2 (35 without diabetes)	2 (6 without diabetes)	.077
Hypertension	9 (28 without hypertension)	2 (6 without hypertension)	.968
Smoking	8 (29 nonsmokers)	1 (7 nonsmokers)	.559
No. of previous steroid injections	2.3 ± 1.1	2.6 ± 0.9	.478
Traumatic event, yes/no	4/33	2/6	.284
Level of sports activity, low/ medium/high	11/17/9	3/4/1	.493
Work level, low/medium/high	9/18/10	1/3/4	.223
Calcification, I/II/III	5/5/6	3/0/0	.208
Tendon defect grade, I/II/III	18/12/7	2/0/6	.016
Capsular tear, I/II/III	10/14/13	1/4/3	.663
Presence of plicae, yes/no	12/25	3/5	.783
Degree of synovitis, I/II/III	11/17/9	0/5/3	.08
Postoperative VAS	0.5 ± 0.5	2.5 ± 0.5	< .001
Postoperative UEFS	70.1 ± 5.8	51.2 ± 9.1	< .001
Postoperative MES	96.6 ± 4.8	72.5 ± 7.0	< .001
Postoperative grip strength, kg	33.5 ± 6.9	24.7 ± 4.4	.001

NOTE. Data are given as mean ± SD or number of patients, unless otherwise indicated.
MES, Mayo Elbow Score; UEFS, Upper Extremity Functional Scale; VAS, visual analog scale.
Reprinted from Yoon JP, Chung SW, Yi JH, et al. Prognostic factors of arthroscopic extensor carpi radialis brevis release for lateral epicondylitis. *Arthroscopy.* 2015;31:1232-1237, with permission from Arthroscopy Association of North America.

for calcification and tendon defects, which were graded (Fig 1). Arthroscopic findings of plicae, capsular tears, and synovitis were recorded. Finally, patient satisfaction was recorded at final follow-up. Patients who were "enthusiastic" or "satisfied" were categorized as satisfied, whereas those who responded "noncommittal" or "disappointed" were categorized as dissatisfied.

All patients reported improved pain on the VAS and better function as reported on UEFS and the MES. Overall, women had worse clinical outcomes compared with men on the VAS and MES. Thirty-seven patients (82.2%) were satisfied, whereas 8 patients (17.8%) were dissatisfied. Dissatisfied patients reported significantly worse scores on the VAS, UEFS, MES, and grip strength measurements.

Women were 10.2 times more likely to be dissatisfied with results than men, and patients with grade III tendon lesions were 12.8 times more likely to be dissatisfied compared with patients who had grade I or grade II lesions. The combination of women with grade III lesions had an odds ratio of 29.1 for dissatisfaction. No other variables were identified as correlated with satisfaction (Table 3).

The authors point out that their study is in agreement with other studies that show increased pain severity and duration in female patients than their male counterparts. They also recognize that women have a smaller extensor tendon, and they may not compensate as effectively after debridement. They also suggest that grade III tendon defects may benefit from tendon repair after debridement, as these larger defects did not do as well as smaller defects, a finding confirmed in the literature.

The study is limited by the small number of patients in the dissatisfied group (8 of 45); of note, there was only one man who reported dissatisfaction after surgery. The authors do not present a posthoc power analysis, and admit that a large number of patients were excluded from the study because they were lost to follow-up.

K. Kollitz, MD

Impact of Ulnar Collateral Ligament Tear on Posteromedial Elbow Biomechanics

Anand P, Parks BG, Hassan SE, et al (MedStar Union Memorial Hosp, Baltimore, MD; et al)
Orthopedics 38:e547-e551, 2015

Ulnar collateral ligament insufficiency has been shown to result in changes in contact pressure and contact area in the posteromedial elbow. This study used new digital technology to assess the effect of a complete ulnar collateral ligament tear on ulnohumeral contact area, contact pressure, and valgus laxity throughout the throwing motion. Nine elbow cadaveric specimens were tested at 90° and 30° of elbow flexion to simulate the late cocking/early acceleration and deceleration phases of throwing, respectively. A digital sensor was placed in the posteromedial elbow. Each specimen was tested with valgus torque of 2.5 Nm with the anterior band of the ulnar collateral ligament intact and transected. A camera-based motion analysis system was used to measure valgus inclination of the forearm with the applied torque. At 90° of elbow flexion, mean contact area decreased significantly (107.9 mm^2 intact vs 84.9 mm^2 transected, $P = .05$) and average maximum contact pressure increased significantly (457.6 kPa intact vs 548.6 kPa transected, $P < .001$). At 30° of elbow flexion, mean contact area decreased significantly (83.9 mm^2 intact vs 65.8 mm^2 transected, $P = .01$) and average maximum contact pressure increased nonsignificantly (365.9 kPa intact vs 450.7 kPa transected, $P = .08$). Valgus laxity increased significantly at elbow flexion of 90° ($1.1°$ intact vs $3.3°$ transected, $P = .01$) and 30° ($1.0°$ intact vs $1.7°$ transected, $P = .05$). Ulnar collateral ligament insufficiency was associated with significant changes in contact area, contact pressure, and valgus laxity during both relative flexion (late cocking/early acceleration phase) and relative extension (deceleration phase) moments during the throwing motion arc.

▶ Complete injuries to the ulnar collateral ligament in the overhead throwing athlete may be associated with overload syndromes of the elbow. This study used a digital sensor to measure the alteration in pressure that occurs with

TABLE 1.—Data Comparing Intact Versus Transected Ulnar Collateral Ligament

Comparison	Intact (n = 9)	Cut (n = 9)	P
30°, mean ± SD			
Contact pressure, kPa	365.9 ± 114.6	450.7 ± 176.5	.08
Contact area, mm²	83.9 ± 29.3	65.8 ± 29.1	.01
Valgus laxity	1.0° ± 0.4°	1.7° ± 1.0°	.05
90°, mean ± SD			
Contact pressure, kPa	457.6 ± 155.0	548.6 ± 147.9	<.001
Contact area, mm²	107.9 ± 23.6	84.9 ± 23.9	.05
Valgus laxity	1.1° ± 0.3°	3.3° ± 1.2°	.01

Reprinted from Anand P, Parks BG, Hassan SE, et al. Impact of ulnar collateral ligament tear on posteromedial elbow biomechanics. Orthopedics 2015;38:e547-e551, with permission from SLACK Incorporated.

valgus load in 30° and 90° of elbow flexion. Contact area was decreased in both positions of elbow flexion with load after section of the ulnar collateral ligament. Contact pressure was significantly increased at 90° but not at 30°. Valgus laxity was increased in both positions of elbow flexion with motion analysis.

The findings of this study (Table 1) support the findings of other studies using older techniques of measuring joint mechanical alteration with ulnar collateral ligament deficiency. Increased pressure over a smaller area of the joint may play a role in wear and chondromalacia that are seen clinically in these patients.

W. T. Payne, MD

Restoring Isometry in Lateral Ulnar Collateral Ligament Reconstruction

Alaia MJ, Shearin JW, Kremenic IJ, et al (NYU Hosp for Joint Diseases; Lenox Hill Hosp, NY)

J Hand Surg 40:1421-1427, 2015

Purpose.—To ascertain whether placing the humeral attachment of the lateral ulnar collateral ligament (LUCL) at the humeral center of rotation (hCOR) on the humerus would provide the most isometric reconstruction.

Methods.—We analyzed 13 cadaver limbs from mid-humerus to the hand. The morphology of the ligament complex was assessed. The hCOR was then found using radiographic parameters. We chose 7 points on the humerus located at and around the hCOR and 3 points paralleling the supinator crest of the ulna and then calculated distances from these points using a digital caliper at 0°, 30°, 60°, 90°, and 130° flexion. Differences in potential ligamentous lengths (termed graft elongation) were then calculated and statistical analysis was performed.

Results.—There was no perfectly isometric point along the humerus or ulna. However, in all specimens the hCOR was the most isometric point for the humeral reconstruction site, with an average graft elongation of 1.1 mm. Differences in humeral tunnel position dramatically affected graft elongation at all 3 ulnar insertions. Overall, ulnar position had a minimal effect on graft elongation.

Conclusions.—Although no perfectly isometric points were found, the humeral center of rotation consistently reproduced the most isometry when assessing graft elongation over range of motion. These data may assist surgeons in proper tunnel placement in LUCL reconstruction.

Clinical Relevance.—In LUCL reconstruction, the humeral tunnel should be placed as close as possible to the center of rotation, whereas placement on the ulna is less critical.

▶ When we perform surgery to repair the musculoskeletal system, whether it is bone, ligament, or tendon, our goal is to restore normal anatomy in an effort to obtain normal function. In the more chronic cases, we are then are required to reconstruct normal anatomy to obtain normal function. At times we do have to create abnormal anatomy with the goal of obtaining normal function. Likewise, when dealing with lateral ulnar collateral ligament reconstruction, our goal is to obtain normal function. The authors attempt to describe what the normal position of the ligament attachment points are.

This study confirms what most of us understand to be the ideal location for graft placement. It is interesting that the ulnar attachment isn't as crucial as the humeral attachment. This location allows for a greater degree of freedom during reconstruction.

In primary repairs of the lateral ulnar collateral ligament, one can see the footprint of the original attachment on the humerus and in many cases some residual fibers that remain. This visualization aides in facilitating attachment to the right location. With reconstruction, the attachment point it isn't as clear. One pearl I have adopted is to ensure that I fully expose the lateral epicondyle. I have found that failure to do so may result in erroneously choosing an attachment point that is not the true humeral center of rotation.

In many cases, the most difficult component of this procedure is in making the correct diagnosis to begin with. However, once diagnosed, placing the graft in the correct position is critical to obtaining the optimum outcome.

J. A. Ortiz, Jr, MD

Radial head dislocation due to gigantic solitary osteochondroma of the proximal ulna: case report and literature review

Hamada Y, Hibino N, Horii E (Tokushima Prefectural Central Hosp, Kuramoto-cho, Japan; Tokushima Naruto Hosp, Japan; Nagoya Daiichi Red Cross Hosp, Japan)
Hand 10:305-308, 2015

Developmental anterior dislocation of the radial head resulting from a congenital solitary osteochondroma of the proximal ulna is an extremely rare condition. We present a case of a 4-year-old girl with this condition affecting her right elbow, which was treated by a trapezoidal shortening osteotomy at the radial neck following an oblique ulnar osteotomy with angulation and elongation after a complete resection of the tumor mass. The child remained asymptomatic with symmetric carrying angles during 2.5 years of follow-up post-surgery. We discuss the nature of this condition and review the literature.

▶ The authors present a nicely formed review of a complicated situation. This article is a nice addition to the literature, as it provides thoughtful insight into the decision making and timing as well as preoperative planning when dealing with a complex case such as this. The excellent intraoperative images and clinical correlation images help create a clear picture of the process and aid its readers in understanding how to address this issue.

J. M. Froelich, MD

Cold Hyperalgesia Associated with Poorer Prognosis in Lateral Epicondylalgia: A 1-Year Prognostic Study of Physical and Psychological Factors
Coombes BK, Bisset L, Vicenzino B (The Univ of Queensland, St Lucia, Australia; Griffith Univ, Queensland, Australia; et al)
Clin J Pain 31:30-35, 2014

Background.—Predictors of outcome in lateral epicondylalgia, which is mainly characterized as a mechanical hyperalgesia, are largely limited to sociodemographic and symptomatic factors. Quantitative sensory testing is used to study altered pain processing in various chronic pain conditions and may be of prognostic relevance.

Methods.—The predictive capacity of early measures of physical and psychological impairment on pain and disability and mechanical hyperalgesia, were examined using data from 41 patients assigned to placebo in a prospective randomized controlled trial of unilateral lateral epicondylalgia. Quantitative sensory testing (pressure, cold pain thresholds), motor function (pain-free grip), and psychological factors (Tampa Scale of Kinesiophobia, Hospital Anxiety and Depression Scale) were measured at baseline. The outcome measures were the Patient-rated Tennis Elbow Evaluation (PRTEE) scale and pressure pain threshold (PPT) measured by digital algometry at the affected elbow. Backward stepwise linear regression was used to predict PRTEE and PPT scores at 2 and 12 months.

Results.—Cold pain threshold was the only consistent predictor for both PRTEE ($P < 0.034$) and PPT ($P < 0.048$). Initial PRTEE was the strongest single predictor of PRTEE at 2 months, whereas female sex was the strongest single predictor of PPT ($P < 0.002$). At 1 year, final models explained 9% to 52% of the variability in pain and disability and mechanical hyperalgesia, respectively.

Discussion.—Early assessment of cold pain threshold could be a useful clinical tool to help identify patients at risk of poorer outcomes and might provide direction for future research into mechanism-based treatment approaches for these patients.

▶ Despite the frequent occurrence of lateral epicondylitis (called *lateral epicondylalgia* in this study), this condition can be challenging to treat. The authors of this study examined the value of several sensory tests and psychological surveys to predict the level of symptoms 1 year from study initiation. The study included 41 patients that enrolled in the placebo arm (saline injection) of a randomized, controlled trial evaluating treatment of lateral epicondylitis. Patients completed the Patient-rated Tennis Elbow Evaluation (PRTEE) at baseline, 2 months, and 12 months after initiating the study. Patients also underwent a cold threshold test (applying a probe with gradually decreasing temperatures to the lateral elbow), pressure pain threshold test (applying a probe with gradually increasing pressure to the lateral elbow), and 2 psychological questionnaires (1 addressing depression and anxiety, and 1 assessing kinesiophobia). Researchers then performed a regression analysis to see which of these tests could predict the level of symptoms at 2 and 12 months after study initiation. As seen in many other lateral epicondylitis studies, most patients improved quite a bit at a year, with the mean PRTEE score decreasing from 41.6 to 5.2. At 2 months, initial symptoms level (PRTEE score) and cold pain threshold best predicted current PRTEE score, with initial PRTEE score being the best predictor of 2-month PRTEE score. At 12 months, cold pain threshold test proved the most predictive but accounted for only 9% of PRTEE score variance.

Although the authors identified a statistical relationship between cold pain threshold and lateral epicondylitis symptoms, cold pain threshold was a weak predictor of final clinical results. I doubt that cold pain threshold testing represents a meaningful contribution to lateral epicondylitis treatment given that this testing requires specialized equipment and does not offer any insight into particular treatment selection.

C. Ward, MD

Trends in Revision Elbow Ulnar Collateral Ligament Reconstruction in Professional Baseball Pitchers

Wilson AT, Pidgeon TS, Morrell NT, et al (Warren Alpert Med School of Brown Univ, Providence, RI)
J Hand Surg Am 40:2249-2254, 2015

Purpose.—To determine the frequency of revision elbow ulnar collateral ligament (UCL) reconstruction in professional baseball pitchers.

Methods.—Data were collected on 271 professional baseball pitchers who underwent primary UCL reconstruction. Each player was evaluated retrospectively for occurrence of revision UCL reconstructive surgery to treat failed primary reconstruction. Data on players who underwent revision UCL reconstruction were compiled to determine total surgical revision incidence and revision rate by year. The incidence of early revision was analyzed for trends. Average career length after primary UCL reconstruction was calculated and compared with that of players who underwent revision surgery. Logistic regression analysis was performed to assess risk factors for revision including handedness, pitching role, and age at the time of primary reconstruction.

Results.—Between 1974 and 2014, the annual incidence of primary UCL reconstructions among professional pitchers increased, while the proportion of cases being revised per year decreased. Of the 271 pitchers included in the study, 40 (15%) required at least 1 revision procedure during their playing career. Three cases required a second UCL revision reconstruction. The average time from primary surgery to revision was 5.2 ± 3.2 years (range, 1–13 years). The average length of career following primary reconstruction for all players was 4.9 ± 4.3 years (range, 0–22 years). The average length of career following revision UCL reconstruction was 2.5 ± 2.4 years (range, 0–8 years). No risk factors for needing revision UCL reconstruction were identified.

Conclusions.—The incidence of primary UCL reconstructions among professional pitchers is increasing; however, the rate of primary reconstructions requiring revision is decreasing. Explanations for the decreased revision rate may include improved surgical technique and improved rehabilitation protocols.

Type of Study/Level of Evidence.—Therapeutic IV.

▶ The rate of ulnar collateral ligament (UCL) reconstruction in professional baseball pitchers has steadily increased since Tommy John first underwent the procedure in 1974. With this increasing rate of primary reconstructions, there has evolved a need for revision UCL reconstruction. The authors appropriately reviewed the available data from Major League Baseball to create a database of professional pitchers undergoing UCL reconstruction. Two hundred and seventy-one UCL reconstructions were performed over 40 years with revision UCL reconstruction accounting for 40 surgeries and a second revision performed in 3 pitchers. What is most interesting is that despite the total number of revision UCL reconstructions progressively rising since 1989, the rate of revision surgery has decreased over time. This can be attributed to improvements in surgical technique, better rehabilitation protocols, and a better understanding of throwing mechanics.

In this study, no specific risk factors for requiring revision UCL reconstruction were identified. Future research should be directed at understanding the risks factors for UCL injury in baseball pitchers and focusing on preventive care. In professional baseball, this information is critical to teams in their evaluation of pitching talent. Because major league baseball contracts are guaranteed, the ability to predict the risk for UCL reconstruction would affect the size and duration of contracts offered by teams. UCL injury in baseball pitchers is not limited to professional baseball. There are significantly more UCL reconstructions being performed in youth baseball than in previous years. Adherence to safety measures directed at preventing UCL injury in youth baseball is critical. Furthermore, there exists a misperception among youth players, parents and coaches regarding the indications and outcomes of UCL reconstruction. The ultimate management of UCL injuries begins with education, proper throwing techniques, and adherence to pitching limitations in youth baseball.

M. J. Richard, MD

Elbow Positioning and Joint Insufflation Substantially Influence Median and Radial Nerve Locations
Hackl M, Lappen S, Burkhart KJ, et al (Univ Med Ctr of Cologne, Germany; et al)
Clin Orthop Relat Res 473:3627-3634, 2015

Background.—The median and radial nerves are at risk of iatrogenic injury when performing arthroscopic arthrolysis with anterior capsulectomy. Although prior anatomic studies have identified the position of these nerves, little is known about how elbow positioning and joint insufflation might influence nerve locations.

Questions/Purposes.—In a cadaver model, we sought to determine whether (1) the locations of the median and radial nerves change with variation of elbow positioning; and whether (2) flexion and joint insufflation increase the distance of the median and radial nerves to osseous landmarks after correcting for differences in size of the cadaveric specimens.

Methods.—The median and radial nerves were marked with a radiopaque thread in 11 fresh-frozen elbow specimens. Three-dimensional radiographic scans were performed in extension, in 90° flexion, and after joint insufflations in neutral rotation, pronation, and supination. Trochlear and capitellar widths were analyzed. The distances of the median nerve to the medial and anterior edge of the trochlea and to the coronoid were measured. The distances of the radial nerve to the lateral and anterior edge of the capitulum and to the anterior edge of the radial head were measured. We analyzed the mediolateral nerve locations as a percentage function of the trochlear and capitellar widths to control for differences regarding the size of the specimens.

Results.—The mean distance of the radial nerve to the lateral edge of the capitulum as a percentage function of the capitellar width increased from 68% ± 17% in extension to 91% ± 23% in flexion (mean difference = 23%; 95% confidence interval [CI], 5%−41%; $p = 0.01$). With the numbers available, no such difference was observed regarding the location of the median nerve in relation to the medial border of the trochlea (mean difference = 5%; 95% CI, −13% to 22%; $p = 0.309$). Flexion and joint insufflation increased the distance of the nerves to osseous landmarks. The mean distance of the median nerve to the coronoid tip was 5.4 ± 1.3 mm in extension, 9.1 ± 2.3 mm in flexion (mean difference = 3.7 mm; 95% CI, 2.04−5.36 mm; $p < 0.001$), and 12.6 ± 3.6 mm in flexion and insufflation (mean difference = 3.5 mm; 95% CI, 0.81−6.19 mm; $p = 0.008$). The mean distance of the radial nerve to the anterior edge of the radial head increased from 4.7 ± 1.8 mm in extension to 7.7 ± 2.7 mm in flexion (mean difference = 3.0 mm; 95% CI, 0.96−5.04 mm; $p = 0.005$) and to 11.9 ± 3.0 mm in flexion with additional joint insufflation (mean difference = 4.2 mm; 95% CI, 1.66−6.74 mm; $p = 0.002$).

Conclusions.—The radial nerve shifts medially during flexion from the lateral to the medial border of the inner third of the capitulum. The median nerve is located at the medial quarter of the joint. The distance of the median and radial nerves to osseous landmarks doubles from extension to 90° flexion and triples after joint insufflation.

Clinical Relevance.—Elbow arthroscopy with anterior capsulectomy should be performed cautiously at the medial aspect of the joint to avoid median nerve lesions. Performing arthroscopic anterior capsulectomy in flexion at the lateral aspect of the joint and in slight extension at the medial edge of the capitulum could enhance safety of this procedure.

▶ Detailed knowledge of the anatomic course of the radial and median nerves can be of help for elbow surgeons to minimize risk of neurologic complications when performing arthroscopic anterior capsulectomy, in the setting of arthrofibrosis. The purpose of the present study was to analyze the anatomic course of the median and radial nerves in relation to bony landmarks depending on elbow positioning and joint distension by means of an innovative investigational design. An anterior Henry approach was used. A fine, radiopaque thread was then placed and sutured onto each nerve at regular 2-cm intervals. The overlying subcutaneous and skin tissue was subsequently repaired. Immediately after specimen dissection, 3-dimensional (3D) x-ray imaging was performed to visualize the radiopaque threads imitating the course of the respective nerve. Scans were performed in pronation, supination, and neutral forearm rotation with the elbow (1) in full extension, (2) in 90 degrees of flexion, and (3) in 90 degrees of flexion with additional joint insufflation with 20 cc of 0.9% normal saline solution. Through the digital radiologic evaluation software, 3D reconstructions of the obtained imaging data were built, and measurements thus made. The results of this study show that 90 degrees of elbow flexion doubles the bone to nerve distance compared with full extension. Additional joint insufflation with 20 cc of normal saline solution approximately triples the distance of the median and radial nerves to osseous landmarks. Although joint insufflation increases the bone-to-nerve distance, it has been previously shown in other studies that capsule-to-nerve distance does not improve with joint distension but rather remains unchanged. These factors have to be carefully considered when performing arthroscopic anterior capsulectomy.

E. Cheung, MD

Restoring Isometry in Lateral Ulnar Collateral Ligament Reconstruction

Alaia MJ, Shearin JW, Kremenic IJ, et al (NYU Hosp for Joint Diseases, New York; Lenox Hill Hosp, New York)
J Hand Surg Am 40:1421-1427, 2015

Purpose.—To ascertain whether placing the humeral attachment of the lateral ulnar collateral ligament (LUCL) at the humeral center of rotation (hCOR) on the humerus would provide the most isometric reconstruction.

Methods.—We analyzed 13 cadaver limbs from mid-humerus to the hand. The morphology of the ligament complex was assessed. The hCOR was then found using radiographic parameters. We chose 7 points on the humerus located at and around the hCOR and 3 points paralleling the supinator crest of the ulna and then calculated distances from these points using a digital caliper at 0°, 30°, 60°, 90°, and 130° flexion. Differences in potential ligamentous lengths (termed graft elongation) were then calculated and statistical analysis was performed.

Results.—There was no perfectly isometric point along the humerus or ulna. However, in all specimens the hCOR was the most isometric point for the humeral reconstruction site, with an average graft elongation of 1.1 mm. Differences in humeral tunnel position dramatically affected graft elongation at all 3 ulnar insertions. Overall, ulnar position had a minimal effect on graft elongation.

Conclusions.—Although no perfectly isometric points were found, the humeral center of rotation consistently reproduced the most isometry when assessing graft elongation over range of motion. These data may assist surgeons in proper tunnel placement in LUCL reconstruction.

Clinical Relevance.—In LUCL reconstruction, the humeral tunnel should be placed as close as possible to the center of rotation, whereas placement on the ulna is less critical.

▶ This prospective anatomic study was developed to determine the most isometric placement of the humeral tunnel during elbow lateral ulnar collateral ligament reconstruction. Many previous studies have shown that the lateral ulnar collateral ligament is a widely variable anisometric ligament that is critical to maintaining elbow stability through the full arc of motion. The authors in this study developed a thoughtful approach to evaluate which humeral tunnel location provides the most isometric position by measuring graft elongation in 13 cadavers with various graft positions in both the humerus and the ulna. The authors found that the ulnar position had a minimal effect on graft elongation, whereas humeral tunnel position contributed significantly to graft isometry. A humeral tunnel placed directly in the center of rotation of the humerus provided the most isometry. A tunnel placed 3 mm posterior to this location provided the least isometry.

In my practice, establishing isometric tunnels for both ulnar collateral and lateral collateral elbow ligament reconstruction is critical to maintain adequate and appropriate ligament tension throughout the full arc of motion. Poorly placed tunnels clearly contribute to persistent instability, graft failure, elbow stiffness, and/or posttraumatic arthritis secondary to overconstraining the elbow joint. This study provides a concise, methodical, and detailed analysis of the ideal placement of both the humeral and ulnar tunnels for lateral collateral ligament reconstruction. This study clearly improves our understanding of lateral ulnar collateral ligament anatomy and will serve as an extremely useful guide for positioning my tunnels during future reconstructive procedures.

J. L. Tueting, MD

Repair of distal biceps brachii tendon assessed with 3-T magnetic resonance imaging and correlation with functional outcome
Alemann G, Dietsch E, Gallinet D, et al (Univ Hosp of Besancon, France; et al)
Skeletal Radiol 44:629-639, 2015

Objective.—Objectives were to study the MRI appearance of the repaired distal biceps tendon (DBT), anatomically reinserted, and to search for a correlation between tendon measurements and functional results.

Materials and Methods.—Twenty-five patients (mean age, 49 ± 4.9 years old) who benefited from 3-T MRI follow-up of the elbow after surgical reinsertion of the DBT were retrospectively included and compared to a control group ($n = 25$ mean age, 48 ± 10 years old). MRI was performed during the month of clinical follow-up and on average 22 months after surgery. Delayed complications (secondary avulsion, new rupture), intratendinous osteoma, tendinous signal on T1-weighted ($T1_w$) and fat-suppressed proton density-weighted ($FS-PD_w$) images as well as DBT measurements were recorded. The maximum isometric elbow flexion strength (MEFS) and range of motion of the elbow were assessed.

Results.—Repaired DBT demonstrated a heterogeneous but normally fibrillar structure. Its low $T1_w$ signal was less pronounced than that of normal tendons, and the $FS-PD_w$ image signal was similar to that of $T1_w$ images. MRI detected seven osteomas ($Se = 53\%$ vs. plain radiography), one textiloma and one secondary avulsion. Repaired DBT measurements were significantly correlated with MEFS (dominant arm R2: 0.38 nondominant arm R2: 0.54) this correlation involved the insertion surface ($\Delta = -75.7$ mm^2, $p = 0.046$), transverse diameter ($\Delta = -2.6$ mm, $p = 0.018$), anteroposterior diameter at the level of the radial head ($\Delta = -3.9$ mm, $p = 0.001$) and DBT cross-sectional area ($\Delta = -50.2$ mm^2, $p = 0.003$).

Conclusion.—The quality of functional outcome after anatomical elbow rehabilitation of DBT correlates with the extent of tendinous hypertrophy during the healing process.

▶ Distal biceps tendon ruptures can be repaired by using a number of methods, including suture anchors, bone tunnels, or a cortical button. The authors have evaluated a cohort of their postoperative patients with 3-T MRI and correlated the findings with functional outcomes by measuring elbow range of motion and maximum elbow flexion strength. In this cohort, the distal biceps tendon repair was performed using suture anchors. These patients were compared with a control group of patients undergoing MRI for elbow pathology not involving the distal biceps tendon. There was found to be a correlation between the hypertrophy of the tendon repair and the functional outcome.

The results are compatible with the findings of tendon repairs at other anatomic sites, including the Achilles tendon and the patellar tendon. Although these findings help to illustrate the process of tendon healing in the setting of surgical repair, there are some limitations to the study. The surgical technique may alter the measurements of the tendon at particular sites. For example, a suture anchor technique pulls the distal tendon to the near cortex of the radial tuberosity. The appositional nature of this repair would intuitively result in a larger area of tendon bulk at the repair site than a repair that pulls the tendon into the cortex, such as with a cortical button. Furthermore, the findings do not help to direct clinical decision making with respect to surgical indications or techniques for distal biceps tendon repair.

My preferred technique for distal biceps tendon repair is the cortical button. The intraosseous placement of the tendon and the favorable biomechanics of the cortical button make the rehabilitation of the repair more rapid and less burdensome. Some authors endorse an immediate range-of-motion protocol for this surgical technique. Regardless of technique, the biology of tendon healing needs to be respected with regards to strengthening. I generally counsel my patients that unrestricted lifting needs to be avoided for 12 weeks postoperatively. Although this study does not currently alter my management of these injuries, it may lead to future investigations into the process of tendon healing that can shorten the rehabilitation time for distal biceps tendon repair.

M. J. Richard

15 Pediatric Trauma

Common medial elbow injuries in the adolescent athlete
Leahy I, Schorpion M, Ganley T (Children's Hosp of Philadelphia Sports Medicine and Performance Ctr, PA; Children's Hosp of Philadelphia, PA)
J Hand Ther 28:201-211, 2015

Recently there has been increased year-round sports participation among children and adolescents with limited to no rest periods. This has led to increases in pediatric repetitive stress injuries, once considered a rarity. Whether in the throwing athlete or in the athlete that experiences repetitive axial loading; increased medial tension and overload syndromes can lead to stress reactions and fractures. This occurs in the developing athlete due to the bone being weaker than the surrounding tendons and ligaments. The medial elbow is a high stress area and is susceptible to many conditions including apophysitis, avulsion fractures and ulnar collateral ligament disruption. Valgus stress can cause injury to the medial elbow which can lead to increased lateral compression, Panner's disease and osteochondral lesions of the capitellum and olecranon. The purpose of this manuscript is to review common elbow disorders in the adolescent population, outline management and highlight important features of rehabilitation.

▶ This review of literature highlights common pediatric medial elbow injuries but also gives guidance for the full evaluation of the child, looking beyond the single area of pain in the local structures to complete a "thorough evaluation of the neuromuscular control of the core while performing upper extremity movements" (p. 201). The complexity of the anatomy of the pediatric elbow is covered, along with the reasoning for injuries in the growing "single sport intensity" of this population.

Highest rates of this condition are seen in those participating in baseball, tennis, and gymnastics. In these children, fractures, lateral and posterior physeal avulsion injuries, prevalence of overuse injuries, Panner's disease, and osteochondral lesions are more often reported.

Radiograph examples are well presented in this review. The maturity of the skeleton is at risk, and sports with forces focused to the medial elbow are suspect. Therefore, the necessity of the whole body to produce and absorb the forces must be assessed and included in the intervention plan for these children. This plan includes scapular and core strength, joint mobility including laxity of the shoulder, activity and strength of scapular muscles, patellofemoral stability, synergistic core activation, and breathing mechanics.

Specific acute-, intermediate-, and late-phase rehabilitation guidelines are included. After movement coordination is achieved in the late phase, sport-specific rehabilitation can be addressed.

The course of medial elbow injuries in the adult focuses on rest and activity modification. For the pediatric client, more care should be placed toward the cause of the overuse injury because of the developing skeleton and muscular control. This review gives evidence-based guidance for the clinician treating the up-and-coming athlete to keep them in the game of life and to prevent life-altering injury.

V. H. O'Brien, OTD, OTR/L, CHT

Biomechanical Analysis of Screws Versus K-Wires for Lateral Humeral Condyle Fractures
Schlitz RS, Schwertz JM, Eberhardt AW, et al (Univ of Alabama at Birmingham)
J Pediatr Orthop 35:e93-e97, 2015

Background.—Good outcomes have been described for pediatric lateral condyle fractures treated by open reduction and fixation using either screws or Kirschner wires (K-wires). No studies have compared the biomechanical properties of the 2 fixation methods. We hypothesized that screw fixation would be more biomechanically stable than K-wire fixation.

Methods.—Synthetic humerus models were used for biomechanical testing, following a previously published protocol. A miter saw was used to make an oblique cut to simulate a Milch type II fracture. Fractures were anatomically reduced and fixed with either 2 divergent 0.062-inch K-wires placed bicortically or a 4.0-mm lag screw placed obliquely (perpendicular to the fracture line). Specimens were then embedded in polymethyl methacrylate bone cement for testing. Mechanical testing using displacement control was performed applying compression or distraction from 0 to 1.5 mm at a rate of 0.5 mm/s for 10 cycles. The maximum force was calculated based on the maximum force averaged over the 10 cycles. Stiffness was calculated based on the slope of the force-displacement curve of the 10th cycle. A 2-sample t test was used to determine significant differences between the stiffness and maximum force comparing the K-wire and screw groups. A P-value of <0.05 was considered statistically significant.

Results.—Stiffness and maximum force in tension testing were significantly greater with screw fixation compared with K-wire fixation. Testing in compression revealed statistically significant increased maximum force and a trend towards increased stiffness.

Conclusion.—Screw fixation in a synthetic bone model of pediatric lateral condyle fractures (Milch type II) provides increased biomechanical stability of the construct as compared with K-wires.

Clinical Relevance.—If similar effects were seen in vivo, increased biomechanical stability with screw fixation could decrease the occurrence of complications such as loss of reduction and nonunion.

▶ Pediatric lateral condyle fractures displaced > 2 mm should be treated with anatomic reduction and internal fixation, most commonly stabilized with Kirschner wires (k-wire).[1,2] Failure to maintain adequate reduction can lead to malunion, nonunion, avascular necrosis, ulnar nerve palsy, growth disturbance, or deformity. Deforming forces include compression or shear from joint reactive forces or tension from extensor musculature pull.

Screw fixation as an alternative to k-wires has been reported. A series by Li et al[3] compared k-wire and screw fixation for lateral condyle fractures. No difference was noted in fracture healing, but there was a higher rate of complications in the k-wire group.

The authors designed a biomechanical study to test the strength of fixation of both screws and k-wire fixation. Synthetic humerus models were fixed using either screw or k-wire construct and then sent through mechanical testing. Standardized lateral condyle Milch type II fractures were simulated. Fractures were fixed using 1 of the 2 methods. K-wires were placed with 60 degrees of divergence because this was reported by Bloom et al[4] to be the strongest construct biomechanically. A single screw was used (Fig 1).

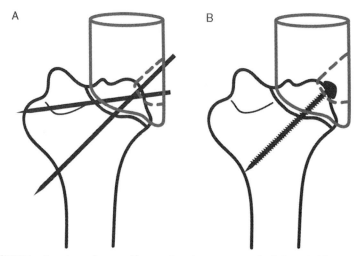

FIGURE 1.—Experimental set up. After creation of an osteotomy simulating a Milch type II lateral condyle fracture, a jig is used to place fixation with either 2 divergent 60-degree pins (A) or 1 60-degree cannulated screw (B). Polymethyl methacrylate (PMMA) was used to pot the distal fragment as shown by the gray lines. The dashed lines indicate where PMMA was removed to allow access to the distal fixation for testing. (Reprinted from Schlitz RS, Schwertz JM, Eberhardt AW, et al. Biomechanical analysis of screws versus k-wires for lateral humeral condyle fractures. *J Pediatr Orthop.* 2015;35:e93-e97, with permission Wolters Kluwer Health, Inc.)

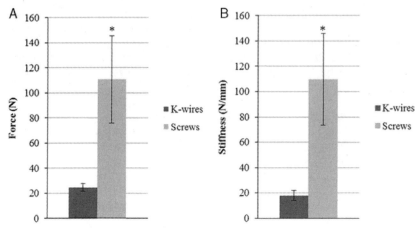

FIGURE 3.—Tension testing of simulated lateral condyle fractures fixed with Kirschner wires (K-wires) or cannulated screw. Results are averaged over 10 cycles of testing with 6 specimens per group. A, Maximum force. B. Stiffness. *$P < 0.05$ compared with K-wires. (Reprinted from Schlitz RS, Schwertz JM, Eberhardt AW, et al. Biomechanical analysis of screws versus k-wires for lateral humeral condyle fractures. *J Pediatr Orthop.* 2015;35:e93-e97, with permission Wolters Kluwer Health, Inc.)

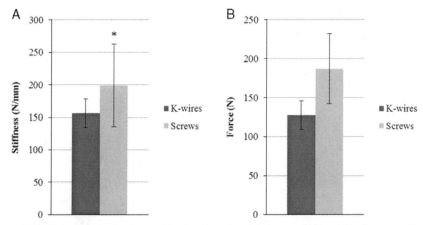

FIGURE 4.—Compression testing of simulated lateral condyle fractures fixed with Kirschner wires (K-wires) or cannulated screw. Results are averaged over 10 cycles of testing with 6 specimens per group. A, Maximum force. B, Stiffness. *$P < 0.05$ compared with K-wires. (Reprinted from Schlitz RS, Schwertz JM, Eberhardt AW, et al. Biomechanical analysis of screws versus k-wires for lateral humeral condyle fractures. *J Pediatr Orthop.* 2015;35:e93-e97, with permission Wolters Kluwer Health, Inc.)

The authors found a significant difference for both tension and maximal force for testing in tension ($P < .01$; Fig 3). Maximum force for screw was 110.8 N compared with 24.7 N for k-wire. Stiffness was also higher in screw fixation at 109.8 N compared with 18 N. In compression, only maximum force was significantly increased in screw fixation (187.0 N vs 127.8 N; Fig 4).

The authors conclude that screw fixation of lateral condyle fractures offers biomechanically superior fixation compared with to the standard k-wire using a synthetic bone model. Advantages of screw fixation include internal hardware, compression across the fracture site, and potential ability to move the patient sooner due to stronger internal fixation. Disadvantages included potential need for removal of hardware, especially in younger pediatric patients. There exists a theoretical risk of growth disturbance, but this has not been reported in the literature. Additionally, the pediatric fracture fragment may be primarily cartilaginous, which could make fixation difficult and lead to pull through in the distal fragment. The relative amount of bone and cartilage should be considered and may influence the surgeon to choose k-wire or screw fixation. Limitations of the study include a synthetic model, which may not correlate with in vivo conditions.

This article shows biomechanical superiority at the fracture site of screw fixation over k-wires in simulated pediatric lateral condyle fractures (Milch Type II), especially under tension. The authors report that the clinical significance is unclear but may be beneficial to help decrease risk of nonunion and allow earlier mobilization in the pediatric population. Future clinical trials are indicated.

M. A. O'Shaughnessy, MD

References

1. Flynn JC, Richards JF Jr, Saltzman RI. Prevention and treatment of non-union of slightly displaced fractures of the lateral humeral condyle in children. An end-result study. *J Bone Joint Surg Am*. 1975;57:1087-1092.
2. Foster DE, Sullivan JA, Gross RH. Lateral humeral condylar fractures in children. *J Pediatr Orthop*. 1985;5:16-22.
3. Li WC, Xu RJ. Comparison of Kirschner wires and AO cannulated screw internal fixation for displaced lateral humeral condyle fracture in children. *Int Orthop*. 2012;36:1261-1266.
4. Bloom T, Chen LY, Sabharwal S. Biomechanical analysis of lateral humeral condyle fracture pinning. *J Pediatr Orthop*. 2011;31:130-137.

Screw Fixation of Lateral Condyle Fractures: Results of Treatment

Shirley E, Anderson M, Neal K, et al (Nemours Children's Clinic, Jacksonville, FL)
J Pediatr Orthop 35:821-824, 2015

Background.—Fixation of lateral condyle distal humeral fractures has traditionally been achieved with K-wires. Screw fixation provides the advantage of compression across the fracture site, but the results of screw fixation and risk of iatrogenic physeal damage are not well defined. This study was designed to evaluate the efficacy of screw fixation for lateral condyle fractures.

Methods.—A retrospective study of patients with lateral condyle elbow fractures treated using screw fixation at a single institution was undertaken. Patients 12 years and younger with isolated fractures were included. Clinical notes were examined for residual symptoms, alignment, range of motion, and complications. Radiographs were reviewed for healing and growth arrest.

Results.—Ninety-six patients who were treated over a 7-year period met inclusion criteria. Mean patient age was 5.8 years (range, 2 to 12 y). Fifty-four patients required open reduction; 42 patients underwent a closed reduction. Mean follow-up was 28.1 weeks (range, 4.9 to 417 wk). The overall complication rate was 19% and was 5% when lateral overgrowth was excluded as a complication. Initial fracture union was achieved in 99% of patients. One patient required revision fixation with a bone graft. Hardware was symptomatic with prominence or loss of flexion in 4% of patients. There were no cases of growth arrest or alterations of the carrying angle. For patients with final follow-up >12 months, the mean extension loss was 2 degrees (range, 0 to 25 degrees) and the mean loss of flexion was 8 degrees (range, 0 to 25 degrees).

Conclusion.—Screw fixation of lateral condyle fractures results in satisfactory union with a low risk of complications at early follow-up.

Level of Evidence.—This study was a retrospective case series performed to investigate the results of treatment, level IV.

▶ Displaced pediatric lateral condyle fractures are traditionally stabilized with k-wires. The authors sought to evaluate the efficacy and safety profile of an alternative treatment, screw fixation (Fig 1), using a retrospective review of pediatric patients with lateral condyle fractures treated at 1 institution. Screw placement varied based on the size of the metaphyseal fragment (screw across the metaphysis vs across the capitellar growth plate), and although the trajectory pattern was classified, the potential growth arrest was analyzed as a single

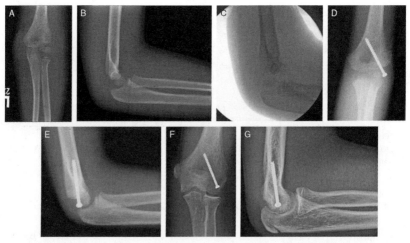

FIGURE 1.—A–G, Preoperative anteroposterior (AP) (A) and lateral (B) radiographs of a 6-year-old boy with type II lateral condyle fracture. Intraoperative lateral view (C) demonstrating fracture instability and displacement. Immediate postoperative AP (D) and lateral (E) radiographs following closed reduction and screw fixation. Absence of angular deformity on 8-year follow-up AP (F) and lateral (G) radiographs at age 14 years. (Reprinted from Shirley E, Anderson M, Neal K, et al. Screw fixation of lateral condyle fractures: results of treatment. *J Pediatr Orthop.* 2015;35:821-824, with permission from Wolters Kluwer Health, Inc.)

group of patients. The complication rate after screw fixation in this series was 18.8% with majority of complications attributable to lateral overgrowth (13%). Notably, there were no postoperative infections. Although hardware removal is recommended, the authors found that many patients did not arrange for this intervention, and they recommend early removal to avoid losing patients to follow-up. In their relatively short (average 28.1 weeks) follow-up period, there were no growth-plate related complications. A cost comparison is mentioned, comparing the return to the operating room for screw removal to the cost of possible pin-site infection, noting screw removal remains the more expensive treatment option. Screw fixation of lateral condyle fractures appears to be a safe treatment option that may decrease the potential postoperative loss of reduction and certainly lowers the risk of postoperative pin-site infection with no significant increased risk of growth-plate related complications.

F. G. Fishman, MD

Intra-articular Radial Head Fractures In the Skeletally Immature Patient: Complications and Management
Ackerson R, Nguyen A, Carry PM, et al (Univ of Colorado, Aurora; The Children's Hosp Colorado, Aurora)
J Pediatr Orthop 35:443-448, 2015

Background.—Intra-articular (IARH) and extra-articular (EARH) radial head fractures in skeletally immature patients are rare injuries that have not been well studied. The objective of this study was to investigate the rate of complications associated with IARH fractures relative to EARH fractures in pediatric patients treated at a tertiary referral children's hospital.

Methods.—With IRB approval, Current-Procedural Terminology codes were used to identify all patients who underwent management of radial head and/or neck fractures between 2005 and 2012. A retrospective chart review was used to collect variables related to: demographics, fracture type, treatment method(s), complications, need for physical/occupational therapy, and the need for subsequent surgery. Mid-P exact tests and logistic regression analyses were used to compare differences in the incidence of complications, need for physical therapy (PT), and need for revision surgery between the IARH and EARH fracture groups.

Results.—Among the 311 patients included in the cohort, 12 (3.86%) were affected by IARH fractures and 299 (96.14%) were affected by EARH fractures. The mean age at the time of injury was 11.46 (± 3.09) years and 8.32 (± 3.31) years in the IARH and EARH group, respectively. The estimated incidence of complications was significantly ($P < 0.0001$) higher in the IARH group (50 per 100) compared with the EARH group (1.34 per 100). A significantly ($P < 0.0001$) greater proportion of the subjects with IARH fractures also required revision surgery (25% IARH vs. 0% EARH) and PT (50% IARH vs. 19.59% EARH).

Conclusions.—Compared with EARH fractures, IARH fractures were associated with a significantly higher rate of complications, greater need for PT, and greater need for surgical intervention. The significant complication rate associated with pediatric IARH fractures necessitates an increased awareness of this fracture pattern and prompt, aggressive diagnostic and treatment modalities.

Level of Evidence.—Therapeutic studies: Level III.

▶ The authors of this study performed a retrospective review of pediatric patients with radial head and neck fractures to investigate the potential complications associated with the diagnosis and treatment of intraarticular radial head fractures (IARH) compared with extraarticular radial head (EARH) fractures. Their findings that there were more complications associated with IARH than EARH and that more patients with IARH required revision surgery and therapy to improve postinjury stiffness are somewhat intuitive (Fig 3). Because of the intraarticular nature of these injuries and the decreased remodeling potential of an injury involving the articular surface compared with a nonarticular injury in proximity to the physis, the discrepancy in outcomes and complications is understandable. The authors highlight that the differences in complications were compounded by the relatively low rate of appropriate recognition of the intraarticular nature of the injury at the time of initial evaluation. Based on

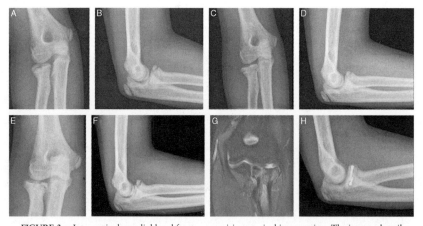

FIGURE 3.—Intra-articular radial head fracture requiring surgical intervention. The images describe a 13-year-old, elite level, female gymnast who injured her elbow during a tubing accident. A and B, Anteroposterior and lateral radiographs at presentation 1.5 months post initial injury reveal a Salter-Harris III fracture of radial epiphysis with mild displacement. Treatment consisted of casting. C and D, Anterorposterior and lateral radiographs 3.5 months postinjury show some potential evidence of osseous healing. Patient was cleared for gradual return to gymnastics. E and F, Eighteen months postinjury, patient was unable to participate in gymnastics due to worsening pain. Anteroposterior and lateral radiographs reveal nonunion of the radial head fracture and posterior subluxation of the radiocapitallar joint. G, T1-weighted, coronal plane MRI image demonstrate displacement of the radial head fracture and joint incongruity. H, Patient underwent open reduction and internal fixation for anatomic joint alignment as demonstrated on the lateral radiograph. MRI indicates magnetic resonance imaging. (Reprinted from Ackerson R, Nguyen A, Carry PM, et al. Intra-articular radial head fractures in the skeletally immature patient: complications and management. *J Pediatr Orthop.* 2015;35:443-448, with permission from Wolters Kluwer Health, Inc.)

the results reported in this study, it may behoove the pediatric practitioner to have a high suspicion for intraarticular radial head injuries and a low threshold for obtaining secondary imaging studies to further assess the injury and hopefully decrease the complication rates associated with IARH fractures.

F. G. Fishman, MD

Outcome of Displaced Fractures of the Distal Metaphyseal-Diaphyseal Junction of the Humerus in Children Treated With Elastic Stable Intramedullary Nails

Marengo L, Canavese F, Cravino M, et al (Regina Margherita Children's Hosp, Torino, Italy; Univ Hosp Estaing, Clermont-Ferrand, France; et al)
J Pediatr Orthop 35:611-616, 2015

Background.—The main objective of this study was to retrospectively evaluate the clinical and radiographic outcomes of displaced distal humeral metaphyseal-diaphyseal junction fractures in children treated by elastic stable intramedullary nailing (ESIN).

Methods.—During the study period, 14 consecutive children with fractures of the distal humeral metaphyseal-diaphyseal junction were surgically treated by ESIN. All patients underwent full-length preoperative and postoperative anteroposterior and lateral radiographs of the injured humerus. One year after the index surgery, patients were asked to answer the short version of the Disabilities of the Arm, Shoulder and Hand outcome questionnaire (Quick DASH).

Results.—During the study period, fractures of the distal metaphyseal-diaphyseal humeral junction represented 1.5% (16/1100) of all humeral fractures. Fourteen patients underwent surgery and met the inclusion criteria. The male to female ratio was 1:1. The average patient age at the time of injury was 9.7 years (range, 3.6 to 13.7 y). The left and right sides were equally affected. The mean follow-up was 28.1 months (range, 20 to 38 mo). Radiologically, no secondary displacement, nail migration, loss of fixation, consolidation delay, nonunion, or refracture was noted. None of the patients showed signs of growth arrest on either radiologic or clinical assessment. All patients returned to their previous daily and sport activities without discomfort or difficulty, and they were free of pain at their last follow-up visits. The injured elbow range of motion was comparable with that of the contralateral side at the last follow-up visit in all patients. The mean Quick DASH score was 0.81 (range, 0 to 6.8).

Conclusions.—We recommend surgery for displaced fractures of the distal humeral metaphyseal-diaphyseal junction. ESIN results in stable reduction, good rotational control, and faster mobilization.

Level of Evidence.—Level IV.

▶ Fractures of the metaphyseal-diaphyseal junction in children are relatively rare and in younger children may be amenable to closed treatment if an

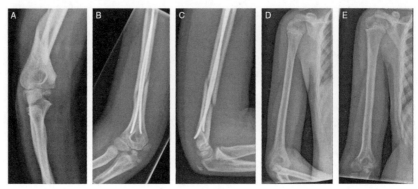

FIGURE 1.—Fracture of the distal metaphyseal-diaphyseal junction of the humerus (A); postoperative radiographs (B, C); final result after hardware removal (D, E). (Reprint from Marengo L, Canavese F, Cravino M, et al. Outcome of displaced fractures of the distal metaphyseal-diaphyseal junction of the humerus in children treated with elastic stable intramedullary nails. *J Pediatr Orthop.* 2015;35:611-616, with permission from Wolters Kluwer Health, Inc.)

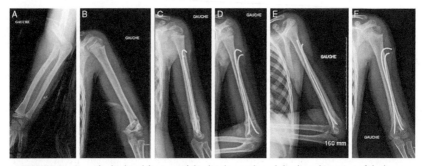

FIGURE 2.—Severely displaced fracture of the distal metaphyseal-diaphyseal junction of the humerus (A, B); intermediate postoperative radiographs showing good callus formation (B, C); final result before hardware removal (D, E). (Reprint from Marengo L, Canavese F, Cravino M, et al. Outcome of displaced fractures of the distal metaphyseal-diaphyseal junction of the humerus in children treated with elastic stable intramedullary nails. *J Pediatr Orthop.* 2015;35:611-616, with permission from Wolters Kluwer Health, Inc.)

appropriate reduction is possible. Surgical treatment for unstable fractures or fractures of this pattern in older children can be challenging. Cross pinning can be technically difficult secondary to the obliquity required to cross the fracture site. The authors in this study review the results of elastic stable intramedullary nailing (ESIN) for displaced distal humeral metaphyseal-diaphyseal fractures in children at 3 institutions. They describe a surgical technique in which 2 elastic nails are precontoured and inserted from proximal to distal, engaging both the lateral and medial columns distally (Figs 1 and 2). They found that rotational alignment was well controlled but that the ESIN was unable to fully control flexion and extension of the distal fragment, but that this did not portend functional limitations and was eventually remodeled as the child grew. Based on this small collection of patients, the technique of ESIN for distal humeral metaphyseal-diaphyseal fractures in skeletally mature patients appears to be a safe surgical technique for stabilizing these unstable fractures.

F. G. Fishman, MD

A Swollen Hand With Blisters: A Case of Compartment Syndrome in a Child

Rios-Alba T, Ahn J (Cleveland Clinic, OH; Univ of Chicago Med Ctr, IL)
Pediatr Emerg Care 31:425-426, 2015

The accurate identification of compartment syndrome in the emergency department is essential to timely treatment and prevention of long-term sequela. Recognizing compartment syndrome is not straightforward, especially in the pediatric population. In addition to communication barriers that exist with children, the classic signs of pain, pallor, paresthesia, paralysis, and pulselessness are not always present, making its diagnosis a challenge. We report a case of a child with compartment syndrome to the left hand due to compression from an ACE wrap. The existing literature on compartment syndrome in children is reviewed (Fig 1).

▶ The authors present a case of compartment syndrome developing in a child after parents wrapped the hand with an ACE bandage to prevent thumb sucking. Compartmental pressures measured in the operating room were 80 mm Hg, and fasciotomies were performed. This case report attempts to highlight the

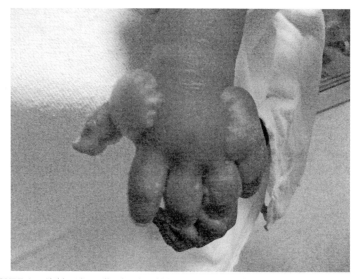

FIGURE 1.—Child with swollen hand and blisters. (Reprinted from Rios-Alba T, Ahn J. A swollen hand with blisters: a case of compartment syndrome in a child. *Pediatr Emerg Care*. 2015;31:425-426, with permission from Wolters Kluwer Health, Inc.)

difficulty in diagnosing compartment syndrome in a pediatric patient (Fig 1). The orthopedic community is aware of the risk of compartment syndrome in pediatric patients with high-energy injuries, especially supracondylar humerus fractures. Likewise, orthopedic surgeons are aware that children often do not display the typical signs and symptoms classically seen in compartment syndrome. This unique case involves a compression device and may provide some pause if ACE bandages or Coban wrapping are applied to children. The information presented has been written about previously in the pediatric and hand literature; however, this article provides a direct line to the pediatric emergency room physicians.

E. Lawler, MD

Imaging of the elbow in children with wrist fracture: an unnecessary source of radiation and use of resources?

Golding LP, Yasin Y, Singh J, et al (Wake Forest Univ Baptist Health, Winston-Salem, NC; et al)
Pediatr Radiol 45:1169-1173, 2015

Background.—Anecdotally accepted practice for evaluation of children with clinically suspected or radiographically proven wrist fracture in many urgent care and primary care settings is concurrent imaging of the forearm and elbow, despite the lack of evidence to support additional images. These additional radiographs may be an unnecessary source of radiation and use of health care resources.

Objective.—Our study assesses the necessity of additional radiographs of the forearm and elbow in children with wrist injury.

Materials and Methods.—We reviewed electronic medical records of children 17 and younger in whom wrist fracture was diagnosed in the emergency department. We identified the frequency with which additional radiographs of the proximal forearm and distal humerus demonstrated another site of acute injury.

Results.—We identified 214 children with wrist fracture. Of those, 129 received additional radiographs of the elbow. Physical examination findings proximal to the wrist were documented in only 16 (12%) of these 129 children. A second injury proximal to the wrist fracture was present in 4 (3%) of these 129 children, all of whom exhibited physical examination findings at the elbow. No fractures were documented in children with a negative physical examination of the elbow.

Conclusion.—Although elbow fractures occasionally complicate distal forearm fractures in children, our findings indicate that a careful physical evaluation of the elbow is sufficient to guide further radiographic investigation. Routine radiographs of both the wrist and elbow in children with distal forearm fracture appear to be unnecessary when an appropriate physical examination is performed.

▶ The mantra of orthopedic surgery is to image the joint above and below the injury. The medical community is now re-evaluating this philosophy because of concerns about radiation exposure and the increased health care costs of unnecessary imaging. This article retrospectively reviews 129 children with radiographically diagnosed distal forearm fractures to determine whether imaging of the elbow added any additional diagnostic information aside from physical examination findings. Radiographs of the proximal forearm/elbow were ordered in 63% of the children. Sixteen children (12%) had documented physical examination findings of elbow injury, and 4 children (3%) had radiographic evidence of injury. No fractures were seen on children with negative examination findings.

This study is limited in that the physical examination findings had to be gleaned from the medical record; thus, the data are not standardized. Six patients without documented elbow examination were assumed to have positive examination findings. Additionally, the nature of the medical record does not dictate that records are completed prior to the results of radiographs being available, which may bias the data.

Regardless, the information presented should empower us in our practices and in our education of residents that the patient's physical examination should guide our imaging protocols.

Along a similar vein, the Amsterdam Wrist Rules have been developed in the adult and pediatric population in an attempt to determine indications for obtaining wrist radiographs in both adult and pediatric patients with wrist trauma. These evidence-based studies, which include external validation models, will help avoid even further imaging in unlikely clinical scenarios.[1,2]

Although a more robust study with standardized data collection along with blinded evaluation would likely have a greater impact on the orthopedic community as a whole, I will use these data in my current practice.

As an orthopedic faculty member involved in resident education, this study helps emphasize the importance of patient evaluation including mechanism of injury and complete upper extremity examination in the emergency room setting.

E. Lawler, MD

References

1. Walenkamp MM, Bentohami A, Slaar A, et al. The Amsterdam wrist rules: the multicenter prospective derivation and external validation of a clinical decision rule for the use of radiography in acute wrist trauma. *BMC Musculoskelet Disord.* 2015;16:389.
2. Slaar A, Walenkamp MMJ, Bentohami A, et al. A clinical decision rule for the use of plain radiography in children after acute wrist injury: development and external validation of the Amsterdam Pediatric Wrist Rules. *Pediatric Radiology.* 2016;46: 50-60.

Fishtail deformity — a delayed complication of distal humeral fractures in children

Narayanan S, Shailam R, Grottkau BE, et al (Massachusetts General Hosp, Boston)
Pediatr Radiol 45:814-819, 2015

Background.—Concavity in the central portion of the distal humerus is referred to as fishtail deformity. This entity is a rare complication of distal humeral fractures in children.

Objective.—The purpose of this study is to describe imaging features of post-traumatic fishtail deformity and discuss the pathophysiology.

Materials and Methods.—We conducted a retrospective analysis of seven cases of fishtail deformity after distal humeral fractures.

Results.—Seven children ages 7–14 years (five boys, two girls) presented with elbow pain and history of distal humeral fracture. Four of the seven

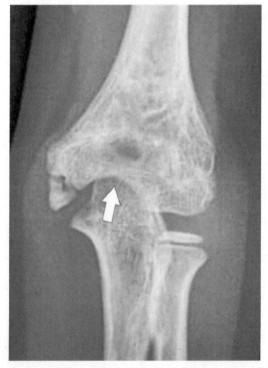

FIGURE 1.—Patient No. 1, a 7-year-old girl who had a grade three supracondylar fracture at age 3 that was treated with pinning. She presented with intermittent elbow pain. Anteroposterior radiograph of left elbow shows fishtail deformity with concave lateral trochlear bony defect (*arrow*). (Reprinted from Narayanan S, Shailam R, Grottkau BE, et al. Fishtail deformity — a delayed complication of distal humeral fractures in children. *Pediatr Radiol.* 2015;45:814-819, with permission from Springer-Verlag Berlin Heidelberg.)

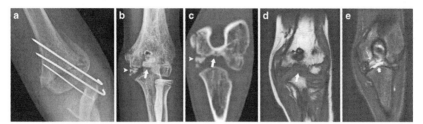

FIGURE 2.—Patient No. 3, a 12-year-old boy who had a grade 3 supracondylar fracture at age 6 that was treated with pinning. He presented with pain, clicking and mild flexion deformity. **a** Anteroposterior (AP) radiograph at age 6 shows healing supracondylar fracture after pinning. **b** AP radiograph at age 12 shows central distal humeral defect (*arrow*) with fragmented trochlear ossification medially (*arrowhead*), which is also seen on (**c**) corresponding coronal reformatted CT image. **d** Coronal T1-W MR image shows underdeveloped lateral trochlea (*arrow*). **e** Coronal T2-W fat-saturated MR image shows mild T2 hyperintensity of the trochlea laterally (*thin arrow*) and joint fluid (*thick arrow*). (Reprinted from Narayanan S, Shailam R, Grottkau BE, et al. Fishtail deformity — a delayed complication of distal humeral fractures in children. *Pediatr Radiol.* 2015;45:814-819, with permission from Springer-Verlag Berlin Heidelberg.)

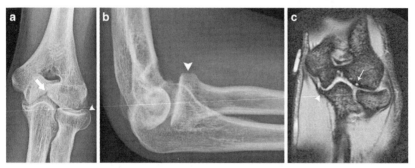

FIGURE 3.—Patient No. 5, an 8-year-old boy with a history of medial condylar fracture treated with casting at age 2. He presented with pain and swelling of the elbow. **a** Anteroposterior and (**b**) lateral radiographs show wedge-shaped central defect in the distal humerus (*arrow*) and enlargement and volar subluxation of the radial head (*arrowheads*). **c** Coronal 2-D gradient-echo MR image shows joint space narrowing, ulnar osteophyte (*arrowhead*) and subchondral cyst in the capitellum (*arrow*). (Reprinted from Narayanan S, Shailam R, Grottkau BE, et al. Fishtail deformity — a delayed complication of distal humeral fractures in children. *Pediatr Radiol.* 2015;45:814-819, with permission from Springer-Verlag Berlin Heidelberg.)

children had limited range of motion. Five children had prior grade 3 supracondylar fracture treated with closed reduction and percutaneous pinning. One child had a medial condylar fracture and another had a lateral condylar fracture; both had been treated with conservative casting. All children had radiographs, five had CT and three had MRI. All children had a concave central defect in the distal humerus. Other imaging features included joint space narrowing with osteophytes and subchondral cystic changes in four children, synovitis in one, hypertrophy or subluxation of the radial head in three and proximal migration of the ulna in two.

Conclusion.—Fishtail deformity of the distal humerus is a rare complication of distal humeral fractures in children. This entity is infrequently

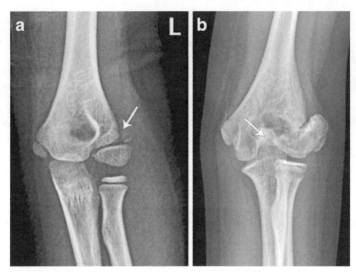

FIGURE 4.—Patient No. 6, an 11-year-old boy who had lateral condylar fracture at age 3 that was treated with casting; the boy was lost to follow-up. **a** Anteroposterior radiograph shows a lateral condylar fracture (*arrow*) with some displacement. **b** He returned 2 years after the initial fracture with elbow pain. Anteroposterior radiograph shows non-union of the lateral condylar fracture and fishtail deformity (*arrow*). (Reprinted from Narayanan S, Shailam R, Grottkau BE, et al. Fishtail deformity — a delayed complication of distal humeral fractures in children. *Pediatr Radiol.* 2015;45:814-819, with permission from Springer-Verlag Berlin Heidelberg.)

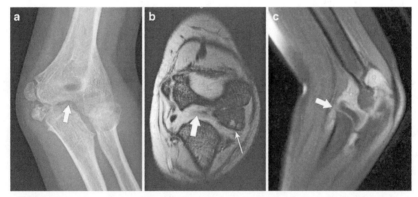

FIGURE 5.—Patient No. 7, an 11-year-old boy with pain and stiffness after supracondylar fracture at age 5. **a** Oblique radiograph shows fishtail deformity (*arrow*). **b** Coronal MR multiplanar gradient recalled acquisition in the steady state shows subchondral cysts in the capitellum (*thin arrow*) and concavity in the lateral trochlea (*thick arrow*). **c** Sagittal T2-W fat-saturated MR image shows hyperintense synovial inflammation (*asterisks*) and subluxation of the radial head (*arrow*). (Reprinted from Narayanan S, Shailam R, Grottkau BE, et al. Fishtail deformity — a delayed complication of distal humeral fractures in children. *Pediatr Radiol.* 2015;45:814-819, with permission from Springer-Verlag Berlin Heidelberg.)

TABLE 1.—Summary of Seven Cases With Fishtail Deformity Post Distal Humeral Fracture

No:	Age (y)	Sex	Clinical Exam	Initial Fracture			Imaging	Treatment and follow-up
				Age (years)	Type	Treatment		
1	7	F	Pain	3	Left supracondylar Grade 3	Closed reduction and percutaneous pinning	XR-fishtail deformity	Lateral epiphysiodesis to prevent overgrowth of lateral column. Persistent elbow clicking postoperatively
2	14	F	Pain, limited extension, increased carrying angle	6	Right supracondylar Grade 3	Closed reduction and percutaneous pinning	XR, CT, MRI-fishtail deformity, joint space narrowing with osteophytes and subchondral cystic changes in the capitellum, radial head and medial trochlea. Enlargement of radial head	Contracture release, debridement with resection of osteophytes and loose bodies. No recent follow-up
3	12	M	Pain, mild flexion deformity	6	Left supracondylar Grade 3	Closed reduction and percutaneous pinning	XR, CT, MRI -fishtail deformity with mildly increased T2 signal in trochlea, subchondral cyst in capitellum and medial trochlea, and proximal migration of ulna	Arthroscopy and debridement. Ablation of radial-capitellar physis. Occasional locking post-operatively
4	11	M	Mild pain	6	Left supracondylar Grade 3	Closed reduction and percutaneous pinning	XR, CT-fishtail deformity	No follow-up
5	8	M	Limited range of movement, varus deformity	2	Left medial condylar fracture	Casting	XR, CT-fishtail deformity, volar subluxation and hypertrophy of the radial head, subchondral cysts in capitellum. Proximal migration of the ulna, joint space narrowing and osteophytes	Persistent pain and synovitis requiring steroid injections and ulnar nerve decompression
6	11	M	Intermittent pain	3	Left lateral condylar fracture	Casting	XR, CT-Non-united lateral condylar fracture and wedge- shaped fishtail deformity	Conservative management, no recent follow-up
7	11	M	Pain, stiffness, limited range of motion	5	Left supracondylar Grade 3	Closed reduction and percutaneous pinning	XR, MRI-fishtail deformity, volar subluxation of the radial head, subchondral cystic changes in the capitellum. Synovitis and joint space narrowing	Conservative management, persistent flexion contracture with limited range of motion

XR radiograph, *CT* computed tomography, *MRI* magnetic resonance imaging
Reprinted from Narayanan S, Shailam R, Grortkau BE, et al. Fishtail deformity — a delayed complication of distal humeral fractures in children. *Pediatr Radiol.* 2015;45:814-819, with permission from Springer-Verlag Berlin Heidelberg.

reported in the radiology literature. Awareness of the classic imaging features can result in earlier diagnosis and appropriate treatment.

▶ This article aims to draw attention to the rare phenomenon of fishtail deformity by describing the corresponding imaging features and discussing the pathophysiology responsible. The authors performed a retrospective chart review of 7 children with fishtail deformity and history of distal humeral fracture (Table 1). Age at initial injury was 2 to 6 years, and they presented 4 to 8 years later with symptoms of pain or stiffness in the elbow. Five of 7 had type III supracondylar humerus fractures treated with closed reduction and percutaneous pinning, one had a lateral condyle fracture treated with casting, and one had a medial condyle fracture treated with casting. All patients had radiographs with the characteristic concave distal humeral defect secondary to underdeveloped lateral trochlear ossification center. Other imaging findings included joint space narrowing, cartilage loss, subchondral cysts, osteophytes, volar subluxation of the radial head, and/or proximal migration of the ulna. Four of the 7 patients ultimately had subsequent surgery to address symptoms resulting from this deformity. Surgical procedures were not standardized. The pathophysiology behind fishtail deformity is likely caused by avascular necrosis of the lateral trochlea owing to its vulnerable blood supply that has been described in several prior studies cited within this report. Once the deformity is noted on radiographs, CT or MRI can be performed to better evaluate nonossified portions of the distal humerus, the synovium, or loose bodies within the joint (Figs 1-5). Children can present with pain, clicking, limited range of motion, or cubitus valgus. Those that have volar subluxation of the radial head as well as proximal migration of the ulna or greater trochlear defect tend to be more symptomatic and have a larger amount of disability related to the elbow. The differential diagnosis includes a normal preossification center of the trochlea, idiopathic osteonecrosis (rare), osteochondritis dissecans (more well circumscribed defect on MRI without history of fracture), and epiphyseal dysplasia (usually bilateral and also involving other joints). Although this study does not inform about potential treatment options for this deformity, it does provide insight into the development of this complication after displaced and nondisplaced fractures and those treated operatively and nonoperatively. Further study is needed to determine optimal treatment and monitoring, but certainly educating families on the need for early return to the physician with the development of symptoms within the elbow after distal humerus fracture could potentially lead to earlier diagnosis and treatment.

E. J. Gauger, MD

Intra-articular Radial Head Fractures in the Skeletally Immature Patient: Complications and Management
Ackerson R, Nguyen A, Carry PM, et al (Univ of Colorado, Anschutz Med Campus, Aurora; Children's Hosp Colorado, Aurora; et al)
J Pediatr Orthop 35:443-448, 2015

Background.—Intra-articular (IARH) and extra-articular (EARH) radial head fractures in skeletally immature patients are rare injuries that have not been well studied. The objective of this study was to investigate the rate of complications associated with IARH fractures relative to EARH fractures in pediatric patients treated at a tertiary referral children's hospital.

Methods.—With IRB approval, Current-Procedural Terminology codes were used to identify all patients who underwent management of radial head and/or neck fractures between 2005 and 2012. A retrospective chart review was used to collect variables related to: demographics, fracture type, treatment method(s), complications, need for physical/ occupational therapy, and the need for subsequent surgery. Mid-P exact tests and logistic regression analyses were used to compare differences in the incidence of complications, need for physical therapy (PT), and need for revision surgery between the IARH and EARH fracture groups.

Results.—Among the 311 patients included in the cohort, 12 (3.86%) were affected by IARH fractures and 299 (96.14%) were affected by EARH fractures. The mean age at the time of injury was 11.46 (± 3.09) years and 8.32 (± 3.31) years in the IARH and EARH group, respectively. The estimated incidence of complications was significantly ($P < 0.0001$) higher in the IARH group (50 per 100) compared with the EARH group (1.34 per 100). A significantly ($P < 0.0001$) greater proportion of the subjects with IARH fractures also required revision surgery (25% IARH vs. 0% EARH) and PT (50% IARH vs. 19.59% EARH).

Conclusions.—Compared with EARH fractures, IARH fractures were associated with a significantly higher rate of complications, greater need for PT, and greater need for surgical intervention. The significant complication rate associated with pediatric IARH fractures necessitates an increased awareness of this fracture pattern and prompt, aggressive diagnostic and treatment modalities.

Level of Evidence.—Therapeutic studies: Level III.

▶ This article is a retrospective review of pediatric radial head and neck fractures over an 8-year period. The authors note a higher incidence of complications in intra-articular radial head fractures compared with extra-articular radial head fractures. It is important to note that only 12 of the 311 fractures were intra-articular fractures. Additionally, the complications noted (Table 2) included 2 patients that had chondral injuries, which may have occurred at the time of the injury and therefore are not true "complications" but rather unrecognized injuries. The authors do note that 25% of intra-articular fractures had the intra-articular component missed on the initial evaluation. Ultimately, I

TABLE 2.—Complications Among Proximal Radius Fractures

Sex	Age	Injury	MOI	Concomitant Injury	Initial Treatment	Complications	Treatment
F	7.9	Intra (SH IV)	Tripped	None	Closed reduction	Osteochondral defect + pain with motion	A
M	13.6	Intra (SH III)	Bike	None	Immobilization only	Fibrous nonunion	B + D
F	9.9	Intra (SH IV)	Bike	None	Immobilization only	Full thickness chondral loss + contracture	E
M	13.5	Intra (SH IV)	Tubing	None	Immobilization only	Contracture	F
F	7.1	Extra (SH II)	Fall from swing	None	ORIF	Pain with motion	A
F	12.9	Extra	Trampoline	Medial epicondyle fracture	Closed reduction in OR	Contracture	A
F	9.2	Extra (SH I)	Trampoline	None	Closed reduction	Heterotopic ossification + nonunion	G

A indicates physical therapy; B, debridement; D, chondroplasty; E, excision of radial head; F, open nonunion takedown with internal fixation of radial head; G, conservative management.
Reprinted from Ackerson R, Nguyen A, Carry PM, et al. Intra-articular radial head fractures in the skeletally immature patient: complications and management. *J Pediatr Orthop.* 2015;35:443-448, with permission from Wolters Kluwer Health, Inc.

agree with the authors that pediatric intra-articular radial head fractures are a subset of fractures that require special attention. Although the authors recommend advanced imaging for these fractures, my preference is to use an elbow arthrogram to assess the amount of displacement and aid in determining the appropriate treatment. More aggressive initial intervention may yield better outcomes, but future studies are needed to confirm this. The poor outcomes associated with pediatric intra-articular radial head fractures may be due to the initial injury itself because likely more force is required to create these fractures.

J. M. Abzug, MD

16 Congenital

Soft-Tissue Surgery for Camptodactyly Corrects Skeletal Changes
Netscher DT, Hamilton KL, Paz L (Baylor College of Medicine, Houston, TX)
Plast Reconstr Surg 136:1028-1035, 2015

Background.—This study demonstrates the potential for radiographic and clinical improvement with surgical correction of camptodactyly. Although historically these radiographic changes have been held to be permanent, the authors encourage surgical intervention for digits with severe flexion contracture or progressive radiographic changes before skeletal maturity is reached.

Methods.—The authors assessed 18 consecutively operated fingers in nine skeletally immature patients in whom advanced radiographic articular changes had occurred. Mean preoperative flexion contracture was 63 degrees (range, 35 to 105 degrees). The average age of the patients was 11 years (range, 4 to 15 years) at the time of surgery. Clinical response to surgery was studied, but radiographic articular changes were followed postoperatively as a primary outcome.

Results.—Each patient demonstrated the classic preoperative radiographic joint changes on radiographic films at the affected proximal interphalangeal or distal interphalangeal joint. All patients had substantial clinical improvement postoperatively. Two digits had extensive radiographic damage, requiring proximal interphalangeal joint arthrodesis. Fifteen of the remaining 16 digits (94 percent) had substantial improvement or full restoration of radiographic articular congruency at average follow-up of 9 months (range, 3 to 18 months). The only joint that did not remodel fully was the one that did not have complete clinical correction.

Conclusions.—Even in patients with severe radiographic changes from camptodactyly, surgery can effectively improve range of motion. Once radiographic articular changes become apparent, surgical correction should be undertaken not only to prevent further joint damage but also to reverse these radiographic changes before skeletal maturity is reached.

Clinical Question/Level of Evidence.—Therapeutic, IV.

▶ Camptodactyly is a nontraumatic flexion contracture of the finger. Lateral radiographs will often demonstrate a flattening of the head of the proximal

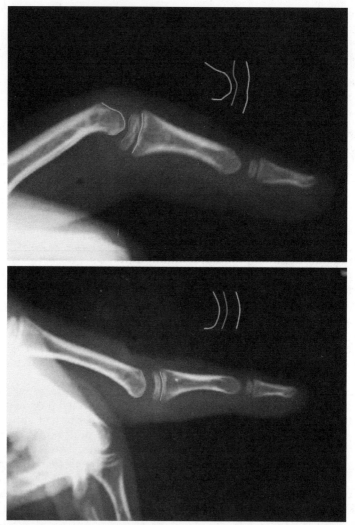

FIGURE 2.—Restoration of articular concentricity in camptodactyly following treatment. The concentricity that is lost before treatment (*above*) returns over time (*below*). (Reprinted from Netscher DT, Hamilton KL, Paz L. Soft-tissue surgery for camptodactyly corrects skeletal changes. *Plast Reconstr Surg* 2015;136:1028-1035, with permission from American Society of Plastic Surgeons.)

phalanx and base of the middle phalanx, resulting in a "beaked" appearance and a dorsal subluxation of the proximal phalanx and volar subluxation of the middle phalanx. Historically, these characteristic radiographic abnormalities were thought to be permanent. The goal of the current study was to follow radiographs of skeletally immature patients after surgical treatment of camptodactyly to assess for correction of these radiographic abnormalities.

Eighteen fingers in 9 patients were prospectively followed. All patients were skeletally immature, nonsyndromic, and exhibited radiographic joint changes. All patients underwent soft tissue surgical correction at an average of 11 years of age (range 4-15). Each finger was assessed radiographically and clinically preoperatively with anteroposterior (AP) and lateral radiographs, range of motion at the metacarpophalangeal (MP), proximal interphalangeal (PIP), and distal interphalangeal (DIP) joints.

Surgery was offered to patients with functional impairment and a contracture of 30 degrees or greater. Contraindications to surgery included contractures less than 30 degrees, nonprogressive flexion contractures, and skeletal maturity. The surgical technique is described and was limited to soft tissue release without boney intervention (p. 1030).

Patients had regular follow-up and were evaluated in the same manner as the preoperative evaluation. The concentricity of the affected joints was measured (Fig 2). Follow-up averaged 15 months, and reversal of skeletal changes was noted at an average of 9 months (range 3-18 months) after surgery. The mean flexion contracture improved from 62 degrees preoperatively to 4 degrees postoperatively. Two fingers required fusion at the PIP because the joint surfaces were considered unsalvageable. Active PIP motion averaged 85 degrees. Two digits required intrinsic transfer to achieve full extension. Fifteen of 16 nonfused joints demonstrated apparent full reversal of skeletal changes. One digit had persistent but improved joint incongruency, and this digit's flexion contracture did not fully resolve.

The study is limited by its small size and the difficulty of quantifying the radiographic changes. The authors conclude that the presence of radiographic changes associated with camptodactyly are indications for more timely surgical intervention because soft tissue correction will induce skeletal remodeling and correction of the articular changes.

K. Kollitz, MD

Pediatric Trigger Digits

Bauer AS, Bae DS (Boston Children's Hosp, MA)
J Hand Surg Am 40:2304-2309, 2015

Pediatric trigger thumb presents not at birth but early in childhood. Most evidence suggests that it is caused by a developmental size mismatch between the flexor pollicis longus tendon and its sheath. Patients generally present with the thumb interphalangeal joint locked in flexion. Surgical reviews report near universally excellent outcomes after open release of the A1 pulley. However, recent reports indicate that there may be a role for nonsurgical treatment for families that are willing to wait several years for possible spontaneous resolution of the deformity. Triggering in digits other than the thumb in children is generally associated with an underlying diagnosis including anatomic abnormalities of the tendons, and metabolic, inflammatory, and infectious etiologies. Although some have advocated nonsurgical treatment, surgery is often necessary to address the underlying anatomic etiology. More extensive surgery beyond simple A1 pulley release is often required, including release of the A3 pulley and resection of a slip of the flexor digitorum superficialis tendon.

▶ This review discusses treatment of pediatric trigger thumbs and digits. It is concise and well written, highlighting the recent advancements of the past 3 years regarding the treatment of these conditions. Based on several of the articles cited, my practice has changed over the past few years. Although surgical release of the A1 pulley is a straightforward and reliable procedure with excellent outcomes, the recent articles noting substantial improvements in range of motion of the thumb with observation alone have led me to recommend this to most parents. Therefore, surgical release is reserved for older children (> 4 years) and children whose parents have tried prolonged stretching (> 1 year) without substantial gains. Regarding trigger digits, I prefer to begin my release with an oblique incision that can be extended as needed to release the A3 pulley or more commonly excise a slip of the flexor digitorum superficialis tendon.

J. M. Abzug, MD

Safety and Efficacy of Derotational Osteotomy for Congenital Radioulnar Synostosis
Simcock X, Shah AS, Waters PM, et al (Children's Hosp, Boston, MA; Children's Hosp of Philadelphia, PA)
J Pediatr Orthop 35:838-843, 2015

Background.—Congenital radioulnar synostosis (CRUS) refers to an abnormal connection between the radius and ulna due to embryological failure of separation. Derotational osteotomy has been advocated for children with functional limitations, although historically this procedure has been associated with a 36% complication rate including compartment syndrome and loss of correction.

Methods.—A retrospective evaluation of consecutive patients who underwent derotational osteotomy for CRUS at a single institution was performed. Children with functional limitations secondary to excessive pronation were indicated for surgery with a goal of correction to 10 to 20 degrees of pronation. All patients were treated with a standardized surgical technique including careful subperiosteal elevation, rotational osteotomy at the level of the synostosis, control of the osteotomy fragments, appropriate pinning techniques, and prophylactic forearm fasciotomies. Electronic medical records, preoperative radiographs, and postoperative radiographs were reviewed.

Results.—Derotational osteotomy was performed in 31 forearms in 26 children (13 bilateral, 13 unilateral) with a mean age of 6.8 years (range, 3.0 to 18.8 y). The mean clinical follow-up was 46 months (range, 6 to

148 mo). The mean preoperative pronation deformity was 85 degrees (range, 60 to 100 degrees). The mean correction achieved was 77 degrees (range, 40 to 95 degrees), resulting in a mean final position of 8 degrees of pronation (range, 0 to 30 degrees). All patients successfully achieved union by 8 weeks postoperatively. There were no cases of compartment syndrome, vascular compromise, or loss of fixation. The overall complication rate was 12% (2 transient anterior interosseous nerve palsies, 1 transient radial nerve palsy, 1 symptomatic muscle herniation). Both transient anterior interosseous nerve palsies occurred in patients with rotational corrections exceeding 80 degrees.

Conclusions.—Derotational osteotomy can be safely and effectively performed in children with CRUS. Meticulous surgical technique, including control of the osteotomy, judicious pin fixation, and prophylactic fasiotomies, may diminish the risk of neurovascular compromise and loss of correction. Transient anterior interosseous nerve palsies occurred, and may be related to large rotational corrections.

Level of Evidence.—Level IV—case series.

▶ The authors address the safety and efficacy of a single-stage derotational osteotomy for the treatment of functionally limiting congenital radioulnar

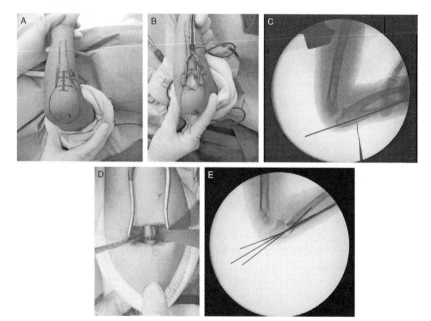

FIGURE 2.—A, Longitudinal incision at the site of synostosis identified by fluoroscopy. B, Intramedullary K-wire introduced at the olecranon apophysis. C, Intramedullary K-wire advanced distal to the synostosis on x-ray. D, Osteotomy around K-wire. E, Derotation with longitudinal and oblique fixation. Full flexion and extension was achieved clinically despite the mild osseous flexion deformity. (Reprinted from Simcock X, Shah AS, Waters PM, et al. Safety and efficacy of derotational osteotomy for congenital radioulnar synostosis. *J Pediatr Orthop.* 2015;35:838-843, with permission from Wolters Kluwer Health, Inc.)

synostosis (CRUS). If unilateral, CRUS is generally well tolerated with minimal functional limitations. However, if present bilaterally or unilaterally with the forearm in hyperpronation, CRUS can interfere with activities of daily living. Although a relatively rare anomaly, many techniques to reposition the forearm as derotational osteotomies through the synostosis have previously been described with high complication rates (including compartment syndrome, nerve palsies, loss of correction, and nonunion). This study demonstrates that a meticulous technique (Fig 2) can achieve appropriate derotation of the forearm while avoiding the historically reported complications. In particular, the authors recommend an intramedullary k wire to avoid translation of the bone fragments during the osteotomy, fixation with k wires after the osteotomy (and a cast), and prophylactic forearm fasciotomies. Based on the results reported of this sizeable patient population (in light of the rarity of the anomaly), this technique is a safe and effective method to address CRUS.

F. G. Fishman, MD

Results of Treatment of Delta Triphalangeal Thumbs by Excision of the Extra Phalanx

Wang AA, Hutchinson DT (Univ of Utah, Salt Lake City)
J Pediatr Orthop 35:474-477, 2015

Background.—We examined the long-term results of treatment of delta triphalangeal thumbs by excision of the delta ossicle alone with respect to range of motion (ROM), pain, and angulation at the interphalangeal (IP) joint.

Methods.—We retrospectively reviewed charts to identify patients who had Woods type I delta triphalangeal thumbs and underwent treatment by excision of the extra ossicle. Patients with >2 years' follow-up were then brought in for examination and radiographs.

Results.—We identified 21 thumbs in 14 patients. All patients with bilateral thumb involvement, except 1, had them treated at the same surgery. The average age at surgery was 22 months (range, 5 to 69 mo). Preoperatively, 2 patients had tip radial angulation, averaging 53 degrees. The other 19 thumbs were deviated tip ulnarly with an average preoperative angulation of 40 degrees (range, 20 to 85 degrees). All patients had pinning of the IP joint for an average of 4.5 weeks (range, 3 to 9 wk), and 14 thumbs had collateral ligament repair. We obtained follow-up data >2 years on 14 thumbs in 10 patients. The average follow-up was 6.7 years (range, 2 to 17 y). Average ROM at final follow-up was <−4-degree extension (range, −20 to 0 degrees) to 56-degree flexion (range, 30 to 82 degrees). Average clinical angulation was <1 degree (range, 0 to 10 degrees) and the average radiographic angulation was 7 degrees (range, 0 to 25 degrees). No degenerative changes were noted. There were no complaints of pain and 1 patient had persistent IP instability. No other surgeries had been performed on the affected thumbs and there were no other complications.

Conclusions.—Delta triphalangeal thumbs treated by excision of the extra ossicle can be expected to yield good long-lasting results with acceptable thumb IP ROM and no pain. Clinical appearance of the thumb with regard to angulation tends to be superior to radiographic findings. We prefer this method in treating Woods type I delta triphalangeal thumbs.
Level of Evidence.—IV.

▶ Traditionally, children with Wood type 1 (triangularly shaped delta phalanx) triphalangeal thumbs are treated with either excision of the delta phalanx at a younger age or with angular correction and resection of the extra joint performed on older children. The authors of this study retrospectively reviewed the radiographic and clinical outcomes of their series of patients who underwent excision of the delta phalanx with pinning of the interphalangeal (IP) joint and reconstruction of the collateral ligament. The long-term results of this relatively simple procedure are excellent with minimal residual clinical deviation of the digit, no pain, and an arc of motion of the new IP joint of approximately 60 degrees. The average age of the patients in this study at the time of surgery was 22 months, suggesting the best results may be found in younger children who undergo this procedure secondary to the high potential for remodeling.

F. G. Fishman, MD

Applying the Patient-Reported Outcomes Measurement Information System to Assess Upper Extremity Function among Children with Congenital Hand Differences
Waljee JF, Carlozzi N, Franzblau LE, et al (Univ of Michigan Med School, Ann Arbor)
Plast Reconstr Surg 136:200e-207e, 2015

Background.—Few studies have evaluated self-assessment tools among children with congenital hand differences. The authors compared three upper extremity disability instruments with the Patient-Reported Outcomes Measurement Information System (PROMIS) Pediatric Upper Extremity Item Bank.
Methods.—Thirty-three children (aged 6 to 17 years) with congenital hand differences completed the Pediatric Outcomes Data Collection Instrument; the Michigan Hand Outcomes Questionnaire; the Disabilities of the Arm, Shoulder, and Hand questionnaire; and the PROMIS Upper Extremity short form and computerized adaptive test. Hand function was also assessed, and construct validity and feasibility were examined.
Results.—PROMIS demonstrated good construct validity. Short form and computerized adaptive test were highly correlated with Disabilities of the Arm, Shoulder, and Hand questionnaire scores ($r = 0.80$, $p < 0.001$) and Pediatric Outcomes Data Collection Instrument domains ($r = 0.70$, $p < 0.001$). PROMIS was moderately correlated with the

Michigan Hand Outcomes Questionnaire ($r = 0.40$, $p < 0.05$). PROMIS scores also correlated with grip ($r = 0.60$, $p < 0.001$) and pinch strength ($r = 0.50$, $p < 0.001$). Compared with the Pediatric Outcomes Data Collection Instrument and the Disabilities of the Arm, Shoulder, and Hand and Michigan Hand Outcomes questionnaires, PROMIS required the least time to complete with fewer children requiring assistance.

Conclusion.—The Patient-Reported Outcomes Measurement Information System is highly correlated with both functional assessment and self-reported function among children with congenital hand differences.

▶ The Pediatric Upper Extremity Item Data Bank of the Patient Reported Outcomes Measurement Information System (PROMIS) was compared with 3 different outcomes scores in 33 patients with congenital upper extremity differences. The PROMIS captures many aspects of health-related quality of life. Previous studies examined the utility of the PROMIS Physical Function with the Disabilities of the Arm, Shoulder and Hand Questionnaire (DASH) in adult patients and noted strong correlation and reliability with decreased time burden.[1] In this study, the authors compared responses to the PROMIS Pediatric Upper Extremity Item Bank with the Michigan Hand Outcomes Questionnaire (MHQ), the DASH, and the Pediatric Outcomes Data Collection Instrument (PODCI). All participants completed both the computer adaptive test and the paper-and-pencil short form of PROMIS. The study found a high correction between PROMIS and both the DASH and the PODCI in all domains except mobility. The correlation with the MHQ was moderate. The computer adaptive testing and short form of the PROMIS were more feasible for children and required significantly less time to complete than other measures. Fewer children needed assistance to fill out the PROMIS.

This study is an important step in applying the PROMIS system to children with upper extremity differences. The study is limited in size in addition to its inclusion of only patients who had undergone surgery for their condition. The relative ease of obtaining data, especially in patients aged 7 and older, in addition to the decreased time burden, make this an important outcomes measure moving forward in congenital upper extremity surgery. Application to other conditions including nonoperative treatment is a natural extension for further research.

This is an important article for anyone who participates in pediatric upper extremity research and is interested in using the PROMIS system.

E. Lawler, MD

Reference

1. Tyser AR, Beckmann J, Franklin JD, et al. Evaluation of the PROMIS physical function computer adaptive test in the upper extremity. *J Hand Surg Am.* 2014; 39:2047-2051.

Bone lengthening of the radius with temporary external fixation of the wrist for mild radial club hand
Takagi T, Seki A, Mochida J, et al (Natl Ctr for Child Health and Development, Setagaya-ku, Tokyo, Japan; Tokai Univ School of Medicine, Isehara, Kanagawa, Japan)
J Plast Reconstr Aesthetic Surg 67:1688-1693, 2014

Background.—We report the utility of a surgical approach to treat mild (Bayne type I or II) radial club hand with a combination of radial bone lengthening and temporary external fixation between the ulna and the metacarpals.

Methods.—We evaluated five radial club hands that received a new procedure involving radius lengthening with external fixation to support the radial side of the wrist. The evaluation included an assessment of radial deficiency deformity recurrence from the anteroposterior radiographs and a measurement of the passive range of wrist motion with the use of a goniometer before surgery and at the time of the final follow-up. We recorded complications such as infection and nerve palsy.

Results.—The healing index of the radius was from 72.2 to 298.9 day/cm (mean, 176.8 day/cm). The mean radial/ulnar deviation was 84.0/−14.0° before surgery and 37.0/13.0° at the time of the final follow-up. No correction loss was detected during the follow-up. All patients were able to hold and bring an object to the mouth after surgery. No patient had a postoperative infection and there were no cases of nerve palsy.

Conclusions.—All cases demonstrated a better range of motion despite a poor healing index in the present series. Our novel technique can be performed for cases with mild radial deficiency and with mild radius deficiency including growth plate injuries.

▶ Radial longitudinal deficiency (RLD) exists in a wide range of severity. Milder forms (Bayne type I, short distal radius, or II, hypoplastic radius) may be surgically treated with distraction osteogenesis of the radius; however, if soft tissue lengthening on the radial side of the wrist is not undertaken, the radial deviation deformity of the wrist is likely to occur.

The authors describe a new technique for radial lengthening using soft tissue release at the radial side of the wrist and radial lengthening supported by an external fixator placed between the ulna and metacarpals to help prevent recurrence of wrist deformity. They report a case series of 5 patients with mild RLD (1 with Bayne type I and 4 with Bayne type II) treated with the described technique of soft tissue release and radial lengthening (p 1689). Two patients had thrombocytopenia absent radius syndrome. The average age at the time of surgery was 36 months, and the follow-up period ranged from 25 to 55 months.

Outcomes measured included an assessment of radial deficiency recurrence and passive range of motion of the wrist. Healing index was calculated as number of days required to heal 1 cm of additional length.

They report no postoperative complications. Results for each patient are reported in Table 1. No correction loss was detected during the follow-up period. Radial lengthening ranged from 5.1 to 16.8 mm.

TABLE 1.—Data on the Patients

	Bayne's Classification	Gender	Affected Side	Age at the Time of Operation (months)	Follow-up Period (months)	Pre		Post		Extended Length of the Radius (mm)	External Fixator Duration (days)	Healing Index (day/cm)
						Radial Deviation	Ulnar Deviation	Radial Deviation	Ulnar Deviation			
Case 1	I	M	R	21	44	40	20	70	0	5.1	72	142.0
Case 2	II	F	R	37	55	60	0	90	−10	5.3	134	252.8
Case 3	II	F	R	22	37	30	30	110	−10	16.8	198	118.2
Case 4	II	M	L	59	25	40	0	80	−40	15.2	110	72.2
Case 5	II	M	R	41	31	15	15	70	−10	5.6	168	298.9
Mean				36.0	38.4	37.0	13.0	84.0	−14.0	9.6	136.4	176.8

Reprinted from Takagi T, Seki A, Mochida J, et al. Bone lengthening of the radius with temporary external fixation of the wrist for mild radial club hand. *J Plast Reconstr Aesthetic Surg.* 2014;67:1688-1693, with permission from British Association of Plastic, Reconstructive and Aesthetic Surgeons.

The authors' reported technique is appropriate only for milder forms of RLD. In the short term, concomitant lengthening of the radius and radial soft tissue release may prevent recurrence of radial deviation of the wrist. The authors hypothesize that because the technique maintains the growth plate, the correction will be maintained as the child ages. Longer-term follow-up is needed to evaluate the durability and results of this method.

K. Kollitz, MD

Addressing muscle performance impairments in cerebral palsy: Implications for upper extremity resistance training
Moreau NG, Gannotti ME (Louisiana State Univ Health Sciences Ctr, New Orleans; Univ of Hartford, West Hartford, CT)
J Hand Ther 28:91-100, 2015

Study Design.—Case study and literature review.

Introduction.—Muscle performance consists of not only strength but also muscle power, rate of force development, and endurance. Therefore, resistance training programs should address not only the force-generating capacity of the muscle but also the ability to produce force quickly.

Purpose.—To discuss the National Strength and Conditioning Association's resistance training guidelines for youth as specifically related to optimal dosing for muscle strength versus muscle power. Dosing parameters of frequency, volume, intensity, duration, and velocity are discussed independently for strength and power.

Methods.—We describe how resistance training principles can be applied to the upper extremity in CP through a case study. The case describes an individual with spastic CP, who has a severe motor disability and is non-ambulatory, but has been able to perform resistance training focused on speed, power, and strength.

Discussion.—Recommendations to optimize the dosing of this individual's resistance training program are made.

▶ This review of evidence-based strengthening and conditioning to improve muscle performance in the population of pediatrics, and specifically in the diagnosis of cerebral palsy, is well defined, with dosing parameters for velocity, frequency, resistance, and repetition. In this diagnosis, loss of function is not always singly related to lack of strength; however, "muscle power and rate of force development are more impaired than strength and are related to activity limitations and functional performance." (p. 91) Although strengthening is often part of the standard rehabilitation plan of care, changes in function are not always seen as the desired result at the end of the course of strengthening rehabilitation. It is also noted, in this diagnosis, when a specific muscle is weak, if strengthening that is not of the proper dosage, that is, repetitive low-load activities, minimal changes will be noted and may be a reason for the lack of progress. Possible reasoning for a clinician's reticence to provide strengthening in this population to maximal ranges may be related to the understanding of how a muscle with spasticity will respond. This review shows that proper conditioning does not increase spasticity but may improve strength, function, and quality of life.

The review and case report also lay the foundation for viewing rehabilitation of the apparent lack of strength and improvement of function to be linked to the proper dosage of frequency, resistance, and repetition relying on the parameters laid out by the recommendations of National Strength and Conditioning Association for children and adolescents. The review also notes the variety of ways to provide resistance, such as stretch bands and free weights, available to every therapy clinic and that the formation of the rehabilitation plan is specific to each person. However, proper form of performance is essential. This finding echoes current evidence for the neuromuscular re-education over traditional strengthening. Quality of performance is more important than quantity in novel learning of muscle performance.[1]

The case report is of a man with several medical issues related to nutrition, mental health, bone density health, and back pain with scoliosis, with years of medical intervention since his infancy. The case report shows the value of proper muscle power strengthening for this person with the diagnosis of cerebral palsy to improve their quality of life and functional ability. The review is limited in the lack of a self-reported outcome tool. By the end of his 2 years of training, at age 20, noted in the supplemental videos provided, he states he progressed in strength, had reduction of pain, and improved in function and quality of life. He reports his progress from a significant lack of elbow extension to being able to fully extend his left arm and now is able to write. The changes noted were not completed at this stage of his life through progressive orthoses, or by surgery, but through this conditioning program. Occupational and physical therapists are qualified consulting professionals to promote the improvement of functional strength in this population. The tables provided give a foundation for moving rehabilitation beyond strengthening to positive functional changes related to the improvement of muscle power and rate of force development.

V. H. O'Brien, OTD, OTR/L, CHT

Reference

1. Boudreau SA, Farina D, Falla D. The role of motor learning and neuroplasticity in designing rehabilitation approaches for musculoskeletal pain disorders. *Manual Therapy.* 2010;15:410-414.

Congenital Radial Nerve Palsy
Song X, Abzug JM (Univ of Maryland School of Medicine, Timonium)
J Hand Surg Am 40:163-165, 2015

Background.—Isolated congenital radial nerve palsy almost always results in complete nerve recovery even if the condition appeared to be severe at the onset. The low incidence and spontaneous recovery typical of this disorder have contributed to a lack of knowledge about the condition's true incidence.

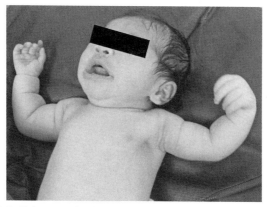

FIGURE 1.—Left-sided congenital radial nerve palsy in an infant as demonstrated by the left-sided wrist drop. (Reprinted from Song X, Abzug JM. Congenital radial nerve palsy. *J Hand Surg Am.* 2015;40:163-165, with permission from ASSH.)

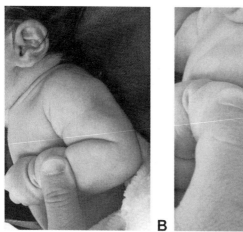
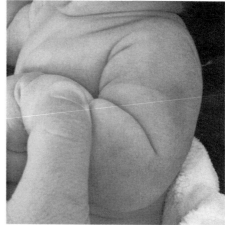

A   **B**

FIGURE 2.—Skin dimpling and ecchymosis present at the left lateral mid humerus level in an infant with a congenital radial nerve palsy. **A** Lateral view. **B** Frontal view. (Reprinted from Song X, Abzug JM. Congenital radial nerve palsy. *J Hand Surg Am.* 2015;40:163-165, with permission from ASSH.)

Evaluation.—The clinician should obtain a complete birth history, including the infant's weight, mode of delivery, use of any assistive devices, and immediate function noted in the extremity. Physical examination focuses on identifying which nerve roots and/or or peripheral nerves are nonfunctional, checking for fractures, and eliciting flexor functions of the upper extremity to differentiate the condition from brachial plexus birth palsy (BPBP). BPBP is characterized by a lack of grasp reflex or weak hand grip, abnormal shoulder and elbow motion, impaired shoulder abduction and elbow extension on Moro reflex testing, and abnormal asymmetric tonic neck reflex response. Congenital radial nerve palsies are commonly indicated by some form of discoloration or skin change at the mid-humeral level of the affected limb. A subcutaneous nodule is commonly found, which is revealed on biopsy to contain fat necrosis.

Treatment and Outcome.—Observation, physical therapy, including passive range of motion exercises, and the use of nighttime wrist splinting are the accepted course of treatment for congenital radial nerve palsy. Stretching exercises or stimulation of active movement may also be helpful. Spontaneous resolution and complete recovery is common even with no intervention. Average time to recovery is 9 weeks, with a range of 1 to 40 weeks.

Clinical Summary.—If congenital radial nerve palsy is suspected, the clinician should assess the infant for skin changes. If present, subcutaneous nodules can be subjected to histologic biopsy and will reveal fat necrosis, which is consistent with isolated compression as the underlying etiology of the disorder. The next step is to differentiate the condition from BPBP through a thorough physical examination. Most congenital radial nerve palsies resolve spontaneously with or without treatment.

▶ The authors present a concise summary of the diagnosis of congenital radial nerve palsy including physical examination findings to help differentiate this diagnosis from a brachial plexus birth palsy. The article is a reiteration and update of the findings of Monica et al.[1] This review of the literature notes 55 cases (compared with the previous 31). The important pearls are: (1) Radial nerve palsy will not involve shoulder function. (2) Subcutaneous nodule or erythema or induration may be noted at or around the midlateral humeral region (Figs 1 and 2). (3) Universally complete resolution is noted with or without therapy/splinting. Although not adding new information, it brings to light an uncommon diagnosis and helps both pediatricians and hand surgeons in counseling and treating patients.

E. Lawler, MD

Reference

1. Monica JT, Waters PMH, Bae DS. Radial nerve palsy in the newborn: a report of four cases and literature review. *J Pediatric Orthop.* 2008;28:460-462.

Syndactyly Web Space Reconstruction Using the Tapered M-to-V Flap: A Single-Surgeon, 30-Year Experience

Mericli AF, Black JS, Morgan RF (Univ of Virginia Health System, Charlottesville)
J Hand Surg Am 40:1755-1763, 2015

Purpose.—To describe the technique and results of the tapered M-to-V flap for syndactyly web space construction.

Methods.—We reviewed a single-surgeon, single-institution experience of all syndactyly reconstructions performed between 1982 and 2013. Demographic data and patient characteristics were recorded. Complications included flap loss, graft loss, web creep, infection, restricted range of motion, and digit deviation.

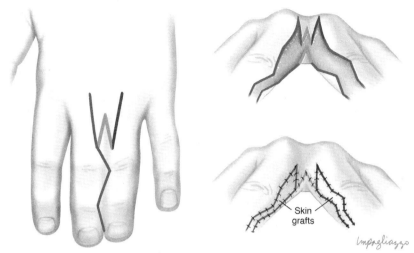

FIGURE 1.—Illustrated stepwise technique of the tapered M-to-V flap for syndactyly web space reconstruction. The release begins proximally along one side of the M flap (blue line). The partially incised M flap is advanced toward the palmar surface to determine the length needed. The central portion of the M flap and corresponding palmar V-shaped flap are incised to match the height of the V to the depth of the M (green line). Finally, the flap width is determined by incising the third portion of the M flap (purple line). (For interpretation of the references to color in this figure legend, the reader is referred to web version of this article). (Reprinted from Mericli AF, Black JS, Morgan RF. Syndactyly web space reconstruction using the tapered M-to-V flap: a single-surgeon, 30-year experience. *J Hand Surg Am.* 2015;40:1755-1763, with permission from American Society for Surgery of the Hand.)

Results.—A total of 138 web spaces were reconstructed in 93 patients. There were 89 primary congenital hand and 32 foot syndactylies. Four patients had an acquired simple incomplete syndactyly and 13 patients had secondary reconstructions. The complication rate was 14%. The most common complication was web creep resulting from partial skin graft loss (12 web spaces; 9%). There were no total flap losses. Univariate analysis revealed no factor to be predictive of an elevated complication rate. Average follow-up was 2.6 years (range, 6 mo to 26 y).

Conclusions.—The tapered M-to-V flap proved to be a reliable and versatile technique for web space reconstruction, offering several advantages over the standard rectangular flap method of repair, such as ease of intraoperative adjustment, a z-plasty at the palmodigital crease to minimize scar contracture, and better color match.

Type of Study/Level of Evidence.—Therapeutic IV.

▶ This is a 30-year retrospective review of a single surgeon's experience using a tapered M to V flap reconstruction for the treatment of syndactyly (Fig 1). Numerous flap designs exist for syndactyly reconstruction, and this technique is 1 more than can be added to the armamentarium. Some potential advantages of this flap are that it can be performed using a cut-as-you-go approach to optimize flap length and width. Furthermore, skin color may be better matched with this technique. It is important to note that the results including the outcomes and complications, may not be replicated, because this article only included the results from a single surgeon who had perfected this technique. Additionally, only 6 patients with complex syndactyly had this technique performed, and therefore future studies in this population would need to be conducted to have a better understanding of the outcomes and complications in this subset. The article discusses the use of skin graft from the groin region. My preference is to take skin graft from the volar wrist flexion crease because the color match on the digits is quite good and avoids the need to go to the leg.

J. M. Abzug, MD

Stability of the Basal Joints of the New Thumb After Pollicization for Thumb Hypoplasia
Trist ND, Tonkin MA, van der Spuy DJ, et al (Univ of Sydney, Australia)
J Hand Surg Am 40:1318-1326, 2015

Purpose.—To investigate the presence or absence of union of the new trapezium to the retained metacarpal base after pollicization and to relate this to stability of the new trapezium and the new carpometacarpal joint.

Methods.—Thirty-six patients (46 pollicizations) were assessed at clinical review. Mean time from surgery to review was 96 months (range, 9–260 mo). Clinical assessment measured range of motion (ROM) at the carpometacarpal joint, stability of the carpometacarpal joint, and extrinsic and intrinsic strength of both hands. Radiological review evaluated 3 parameters: bony union between the new trapezium and retained metacarpal base, stability of the new trapezium in relationship to the metacarpal base, and carpometacarpal joint stability.

Results.—There was radiographic nonunion between the new trapezium and the retained metacarpal base in 8 (1 treated) of 46 pollicizations. Relative risk of instability of the new trapezium was 39 times more likely if nonunion was present. Nine pollicizations were unstable at the carpometacarpal joint, 8 in those with union and 1 with nonunion. Relative risk of instability was 1.4 times more likely for those with union. For patients with nonunion, ROM and grip strength variables were reduced but only grip strength reached statistical significance. In patients with carpometacarpal joint instability, ROM and grip strength variables were reduced but none of the variables reached statistical significance.

Conclusions.—This study suggests that when the surgeon is attempting to obtain union of the new trapezium to the retained metacarpal base, failure to do so results in a poorer thumb with a significantly increased risk of trapezial instability and decreased grip strength. There is a mildly increased risk of carpometacarpal joint instability with union, but significantly poorer function as a consequence of this has not been demonstrated.

Type of Study/Level of Evidence.—Therapeutic IV.

▶ This is a retrospective review assessing the stability of the carpometacarpal joint (CMC) of a newly pollicized thumb. All of the pollicizations were performed by the senior author, using a single technique. Forty-six polliciza-tions were assessed clinically for instability; however, this assessment was per-formed by 2 trainees. The radiographic assessment was performed by the senior author and another trainee. The authors were able to conclude that pollicized digits that went on to nonunion had decreased grip strength and more instabil-ity. It is important to note that this may not be clinically relevant, because only 1 of these patients required a revision procedure. Currently, those of us who per-form pollicizations still struggle to obtain objective outcomes following the pro-cedure. Hopefully, future studies will provide objective assessment tools to permit comparison of various techniques and allow us to provide better answers to questions like the one posed in this article: what is the effect of instability of the CMC joint after a pollicization?

J. M. Abzug, MD

Use of an Axial Flap to Increase the Girth of Wassel IV Thumb Reconstructions
Dautel G, Perrin P (Univ Hosp, Nancy, France)
J Hand Surg Am 40:1327-1332, 2015

Purpose.—To investigate the use of a flap supplied by the radial collat-eral artery of the radial duplicate in Wassel type IV thumb duplications. We hypothesized that such a flap was viable and would make it possible to increase the girth of the reconstructed thumb.

Methods.—We operated on 17 thumbs in 16 children with type IV thumb duplication using a procedure that included the dissection of a long, narrow strip of skin and soft tissue harvested on the radial side of the radial duplicate. The girth of the reconstructed thumb was measured clinically and compared with that of the contralateral thumb. The width of the soft tissues and bony structures was also measured by x-ray and compared with the opposite side. Furthermore, children, caregivers, and the investigator assessed the overall cosmetic result using a visual analog scale score.

Results.—All flaps fully survived. The average girth of the reconstructed thumb relative to the healthy contralateral thumb ranged from 92% to 103%, depending on the level of measurement. The mean visual analog scale score was 8.3 (children), 8.2 (caregivers), and 8.8 (investigator).

Conclusions.—An axial patterned flap proved to be viable and effective in improving the volume and contour of the reconstructed thumb.

Clinical Relevance.—In radial polydactyly, each of the thumbs has a typically smaller girth than the contralateral thumb. Our clinical and radiological measurements showed the efficacy of this reconstruction in increasing the volume and girth of the reconstructed thumb, even though the skeleton of the ulnar duplicate remained thinner.

Type of Study/Level of Evidence.—Therapeutic IV.

▶ Wassel type IV is the most common form of thumb duplication. Excision of the usually smaller radial duplicate, followed by reconstruction of the key elements such as the radial collateral ligament and reinsertion of the thenar muscles, is widely accepted as the procedure of choice for such thumbs.

The reconstructed thumb is nevertheless usually smaller, albeit in varying degrees, than the contralateral normal thumb. This article describes the use of a flap based on the radial duplicate to increase the girth of the final thumb. This is done with the goal of making the size of the reconstructed thumb as close to the normal contralateral thumb as possible.

This goal is laudable but usually impossible to achieve completely. As the authors acknowledge, the ulnar duplicate skeletal structures and nail are invariably asymmetrical in varying degrees compared with the other side. Although adding a flap can address overall girth, the nail and skeletal structures remain smaller. This is borne out in their study, where the width of the reconstructed thumb is narrower at the nail level and wider at the metacarpal head, where the 2 duplicates articulate. In addition, skin and soft tissue are added on the radial side only. If the flap is excessively bulky, it risks introducing radioulnar asymmetry to the reconstruction. Nevertheless, where soft tissue on the radial side is deficient compared with the ulnar side, some form of skin and soft tissue flap from the radial duplicate can help improve the symmetry. There is a wide variety in clinical appearance of a Wassel IV thumb. The initial form would have as much impact on final appearance as the surgical reconstruction itself. Therefore, the requirement for additional skin and soft tissue is also variable. In many cases, a racquet type incision would already allow sufficient skin and soft tissue bulk for closure, while minimizing the final scars.

Aiming for a bigger reconstructed thumb may not be necessary from the viewpoint of both patient satisfaction and function. There is differing evidence on the importance of the relative size of the reconstructed thumb. Although the reported visual scores appear to be acceptable, there is no comparison group available in this study. In my view, given an acceptable thumb size (which would roughly be a nail size at least as large as the index finger nail), symmetry between ulnar and radial aspects of the thumb is more noticeable and of greater concern to patients and parents compared with size similarity between sides.

A. Chong, MD

Short-term and Long-term Clinical Results of the Surgical Correction of Thumb-in-Palm Deformity in Patients With Cerebral Palsy
Alewijnse JV, Smeulders MJC, Kreulen M (Academic Med Ctr, Amsterdam, The Netherlands; et al)
J Pediatr Orthop 35:825-830, 2015

Background.—Thumb-in-palm deformity disturbs a functional grip of the hand in patients with cerebral palsy. Reported recurrence rates after surgical correction are contradicting and earlier studies are limited to short-term follow-up. Therefore, the aim of this retrospective clinical outcome study is to evaluate the success rate of surgical correction of thumb-in-palm deformity around 1 year and at a minimum of 5 years follow-up. In addition, long-term patient satisfaction of the treatment is evaluated.

Methods.—Patients with cerebral palsy who underwent a surgical correction for their thumb-in-palm deformity between April 2003 and April 2008 at the Academic Medical Center in Amsterdam were included. All patients were classified into 4 categories according to the assessment system of the Committee on Spastic Hand Evaluation. The result of surgery was considered "short-term successful" and "long-term successful" when, respectively, short-term and long-term classification was better compared with preoperative. The association between the patient satisfaction outcomes and the long-term clinical outcomes were statistically analyzed.

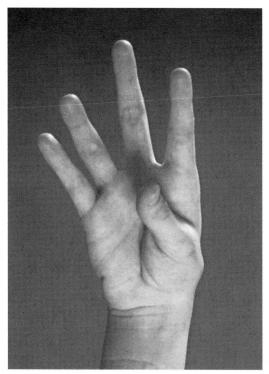

FIGURE 1.—Typical preoperative example of a type 1 thumb-in-palm deformity with metacarpal adduction without MCP or IP involvement. This patient did not have a MCP hyperextension instability. When asked to close the hand, the tip of the thumb will end between the fingers. IP indicates interphalangeal; MCP, metacarpophalangeal. (Reprinted from Alewijnse JV, Smeulders MJC, Kreulen M. Short-term and long-term clinical results of the surgical correction of thumb-in-palm deformity in patients with cerebral palsy. *J Pediatr Orthop.* 2015;35:825-830, with permission from Wolters Kluwer Health, Inc.)

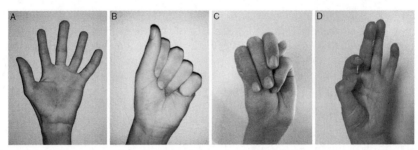

FIGURE 2.—Long-term thumb positions: (A) group 4, the thumb has full potential to abduct (note the subcutaneous course of the rerouted extensor pollicis longus) and (B) a normal lateral pinch; (C) group 1, a full recurrence with the thumb flexed and adducted in the hand without the possibility of a lateral pinch grip; (D) postoperative flexed position of the interphalangeal joint in a group 1 result. (Reprinted from Alewijnse JV, Smeulders MJC, Kreulen M. Short-term and long-term clinical results of the surgical correction of thumb-in-palm deformity in patients with cerebral palsy. *J Pediatr Orthop.* 2015;35:825-830, with permission from Wolters Kluwer Health, Inc.)

Results.—Data were collected from 39 patients and their charts. The success rate was 87% at short-term follow-up, which in the long term decreased to 80%. Interestingly, thumb position deteriorated in 29% of the patients between short-term and long-term follow-up. In the long term, 74% of the patients were satisfied with the position of their thumb and 87% would undergo the surgery again. Both these outcomes were statistically significant associated with the long-term success rate ($P < 0.05$).

Conclusions.—The surgical correction of thumb-in-palm deformity has a high clinical success rate and patient satisfaction in the long term. However, it should be taken into account that the clinical result around 1 year postoperative cannot be considered final.

Level of Evidence.—Level IV.

▶ The authors of this study sought to evaluate the short-term (1-year) and long-term (minimum 5-year follow-up) success rate of surgical correction of thumb-in-palm deformity in patients with hemiplegic spastic cerebral palsy and type I (metacarpal adduction contracture with or without MCP instability) thumb in palm deformities (Figs 1 and 2). Patients with cerebral palsy are a challenging population in which to perform outcomes-based research secondary to the variability of presentation. The authors were quite specific in their inclusion criteria, although the surgical procedures performed did vary between patients. A successful result in this study was based on physical examination findings or photographs demonstrating maintenance of the thumb out of the palm and the satisfaction rate of the patient. The results of this study do not address improved dexterity of the thumb or improvements in hand function. The authors caution that although they found a high success rate at 1 year after the surgery, deterioration in the position of the thumb was noted in up to 29% of the patients at the time of long-term follow-up.

F. G. Fishman, MD

17 Shoulder: Rotator Cuff

A Randomized, Double-Blinded, Placebo-Controlled Clinical Trial Evaluating the Effectiveness of Daily Vibration After Arthroscopic Rotator Cuff Repair
Lam PH, Hansen K, Keighley G, et al (Univ of New South Wales, Sydney, Australia)
Am J Sports Med 43:2774-2782, 2015

Background.—Rotator cuff repair is a common method to treat rotator cuff tears; however, retear rates remain high. High-frequency, low-magnitude vibration has been demonstrated to promote new bone formation in both animal models and in humans.

Hypothesis.—This type of mechanical stimulation applied postoperatively will enhance tendon-to-bone healing and reduce postoperative retear rates.

Study Design.—Randomized controlled trial; Level of evidence, 1.

Methods.—A randomized, double-blinded, placebo-controlled clinical trial was conducted to investigate the effects of 5 minutes of 80-Hz vibration applied daily after arthroscopic rotator cuff repair for 6 months on postoperative rotator cuff healing. The primary outcome was ultrasound-assessed repair integrity at 6 months after repair. Recruited patients were randomized into 2 groups: one group received a vibration device that oscillated at 80 Hz, and the other group received a placebo device.

Results.—The postoperative retear rates of both groups were similar (9.1% [5/55] in the vibration group, and 9.3% [5/54] in the placebo group) at 6 months as determined by ultrasound imaging. Vibration did provide acute pain relief at 6 weeks after surgery (visual analog scale [VAS] score, 2.24 ± 0.29 cm) compared with placebo (VAS score, 3.67 ± 0.48 cm) ($P < .003$). Six months after surgery, both groups had significant reductions in pain during overhead activities, at rest, and during sleep and overall shoulder pain compared with before surgery ($P < .001$). Both the vibration and placebo groups had significant increases in shoulder strength with abduction in the scapular plane, adduction, liftoff, internal rotation, and external rotation 6 months after surgery. Statistical analysis showed that vibration was not a contributing factor at improving these parameters in these periods.

Conclusion.—High-frequency, low-magnitude vibration did provide acute pain relief on application 6 weeks after arthroscopic rotator cuff repair surgery. However, vibration did not improve tendon-to-bone healing, shoulder range of motion, shoulder strength, or shoulder pain with activities, at rest, and at night when compared with placebo.

▶ Vibration therapy has been demonstrated to improve bone formation in human and animal models, and interest in this modality for rotator cuff tears has emerged. Retear rates are high after rotator cuff repair, and the authors sought to determine whether vibration therapy could improve healing after cuff repair. Specifically, the study looked at whether mechanical stimulation would enhance tendon-to-bone healing and reduce postoperative retear rates.

Postoperative healing begins with fibrovascular interface tissue formation between tendon and bone[1] followed by bony ingrowth into the interface tissue and later collagen fiber formation at the tendon-bone interface.[2] Several animal and human studies have shown high-frequency, low-magnitude vibration therapy increases vascularity, promotes new bone formation, and improves bone density. It has been shown to increase muscle strength, flexibility, and stability and reduce pain. Post—anterior cruciate ligament reconstruction, tendon healing was improved with vibration therapy in increased stability and higher peak torque.[3]

The authors designed a prospective, randomized, double-blinded, placebo-controlled trial in 120 patients. Sixty received a sham device, and 60 received the therapeutic device. Patients had full-thickness rotator cuff tears or partial thickness (>50%) supraspinatus tear converted to full thickness at time of operation. Patients underwent arthroscopic repair with a knotless suture anchors with an inverted mattress construct by the senior author.

Postoperatively, patients underwent the same rehabilitation protocol and used either the active or placebo vibration device for daily use.

Postoperative follow-up visits occurred at 1, 6, 12, and 24 weeks. At each visit, various questionnaires and passive range of motion and shoulder strength were assessed. At 6 months, each participant underwent ultrasound evaluation by a blinded musculoskeletal-trained ultrasonagrapher to assess integrity of the rotator cuff, tendon thickness, footprint dimensions, bursal thickness, and posterior capsule thickness.

One hundred and twenty patients (57 women, 63 men) with an average age of 28 (range 24-91) were included with 109 at final follow-up at 6 months. Retear rate was 9.2% (10 patients), with 5 in each group. The mean VAS score at 6 weeks was significantly lower in the vibration group (2.24 vs 3.67, $P < .003$). At 6 months, both groups had significantly lower visual analog scale pain scores compared with the 6-week visit; however, there was no significant difference between placebo and test groups. At 6 months, both groups had a significant reduction in pain and difficulties with overhead activities compared with preoperatively ($P < .001$), but there was no difference between groups. Similar improvements were noted in both groups relating to stiffness, pain at night, pain at rest, and frequency of extreme pain at 6-month follow-up but there was no difference between the groups. Range of motion and shoulder strength were improved in both groups, and no difference was noted. Postoperative ultrasound at 6 months showed both groups had similar findings.

The authors conducted a well-designed randomized blinded placebo controlled study to test the effects of vibration therapy on healing and pain relief after arthroscopic rotator cuff repair. The only statistically significant finding was that acute pain relief was improved with vibration at the 6-week point but was similarly improved in the placebo group at all other time points. Motion, pain, and strength were all similarly improved in both groups at final follow-up. Retear rates were similar between the 2 groups and averaged 9.2% in this study.

Therefore, high-frequency, low-magnitude vibration did not improve bone-tendon healing and did not improve strength, range of motion, or pain at final follow-up of 6 months. It did result in improved pain relief at 6 weeks, which was not sustained long term.

M. O'Shaughnessy, MD

References

1. Rodeo SA, Arnoczky SP, Torzilli PA, Hidaka C, Warren RF. Tendon-healing in a bone tunnel. A biomechanical and histological study in the dog. *J Bone Joint Surg Am.* 1993;75:1795-1803.
2. Oguma H, Murakami G, Takahashi-Iwanaga H, Aoki M, Ishii S. Early anchoring collagen fibers at the bone-tendon interface are conducted by woven bone formation: light microscope and scanning electron microscope observation using a canine model. *J Orthop Res.* 2001;19:873-880.
3. Brunetti O, Filippi GM, Lorenzini M, et al. Improvement of posture stability by vibratory stimulation following anterior cruciate ligament reconstruction. *Knee Surg Sports Traumatol Arthrosc.* 2006;14:1180-1187.

Preoperative Deltoid Size and Fatty Infiltration of the Deltoid and Rotator Cuff Correlate to Outcomes After Reverse Total Shoulder Arthroplasty

Wiater BP, Koueiter DM, Maerz T, et al (Beaumont Health System, Royal Oak, MI)
Clin Orthop Relat Res 473:663-673, 2015

Background.—Reverse total shoulder arthroplasty (RTSA) allows the deltoid to substitute for the nonfunctioning rotator cuff. To date, it is unknown whether preoperative deltoid and rotator cuff parameters correlate with clinical outcomes.

Questions/Purposes.—We asked whether associations exist between 2-year postoperative results (ROM, strength, and outcomes scores) and preoperative (1) deltoid size; (2) fatty infiltration of the deltoid; and/or (3) fatty infiltration of the rotator cuff.

Methods.—A prospective RTSA registry was reviewed for patients with cuff tear arthropathy or massive rotator cuff tears, minimum 2-year followup, and preoperative shoulder MRI. Final analysis included 30 patients (average age, 71 ± 10 years; eight males, 22 females). Only a small proportion of patients who received an RTSA at our center met inclusion and minimum followup requirements (30 of 222; 14%); however, these patients were found to be similar at baseline to the overall group of patients who underwent surgery in terms of age, gender, and preoperative outcomes scores. The cross-sectional area of the anterior, middle, and posterior deltoid was measured on axial proton density-weighted MRI. Fatty infiltration of the deltoid, supraspinatus, infraspinatus, teres minor, and subscapularis were quantitatively assessed on sagittal T1-weighted MR images. Patients were followed for Constant-Murley score, American Shoulder and Elbow Surgeons (ASES) scores, subjective shoulder value, pain, ROM, and strength. Correlations of muscle parameters with all outcomes measures were calculated.

Results.—Preoperative deltoid size correlated positively with postoperative Constant-Murley score (67.27 ± 13.07) ($\rho = 0.432$, $p = 0.017$), ASES (82.64 ± 14.25) ($\rho = 0.377$; $p = 0.40$), subjective shoulder value (82.67 ± 17.89) ($\rho = 0.427$; $p = 0.019$), and strength (3.72 pounds ± 2.99 pounds) ($\rho = 0.454$; $p = 0.015$). Quantitative deltoid fatty infiltration (7.91% ± 4.32%) correlated with decreased postoperative ASES scores ($\rho = -0.401$; $p = 0.047$). Quantitative fatty infiltration of the infraspinatus (30.47% ± 15.01%) correlated with decreased postoperative external rotation (34.13° ± 16.80°) ($\rho = -0.494$; $p = 0.037$).

Conclusions.—Larger preoperative deltoid size correlates with improved validated outcomes scores, whereas fatty infiltration of the deltoid and infraspinatus may have deleterious effects on validated outcomes scores and ROM after RTSA. The current study is a preliminary exploration of this topic; future studies should include prospective enrollment and standardized MRI with a multivariate statistical approach. Quantitative information attained from preoperative imaging not only holds diagnostic value, but, should future studies confirm our findings, also might provide prognostic value. This information may prove beneficial in preoperative patient counseling and might aid preoperative and postoperative decision-making by identifying subpopulations of patients who may benefit by therapy aimed at improving muscle properties.

Level of Evidence.—Level III, prognostic study.

▶ This study is an extension of previous studies looking at the quality of the teres minor and clinical outcomes. The concepts are applied to deltoid volume and fatty atrophy. It is unclear whether deltoid size is a surrogate for patient size. Ultimately, the study reinforces that the quality of the deltoid is important for outcomes of reverse arthroplasty.

N. Chen

Which patients do not recover from shoulder impingement syndrome, either with operative treatment or with nonoperative treatment? Subgroup analysis involving 140 patients at 2 and 5 years in a randomized study
Ketola S, Lehtinen J, Rousi T, et al (Coxa Hosp for Joint Replacement, Tampere, Finland; Hatanpää Hosp, Tampere, Finland; Kanta-Häme Central Hosp, Hämeenlinna, Finland; et al)
Acta Orthop 86:641-646, 2015

Background and Purpose.—Shoulder impingement syndrome is common, but treatment is controversial. Arthroscopic acromioplasty is popular even though its efficacy is unknown. In this study, we analyzed stage-II shoulder impingement patients in subgroups to identify those who would benefit from the operation.

Patients and Methods.—In a previous randomized study, 140 patients were either treated with a supervised exercise program or with arthroscopic acromioplasty followed by a similar exercise program. The patients were followed up at 2 and 5 years after randomization. Self-reported pain was used as the primary outcome measure.

Results.—Both treatment groups had less pain at 2 and 5 years, and this was similar in both groups. Duration of symptoms, marital status (single), long periods of sick leave, and lack of professional education appeared to increase the risk of persistent pain despite the treatment. Patients with impingement with radiological acromioclavicular (AC) joint degeneration also had more pain. The patients in the exercise group who later wanted operative treatment and had it did not get better after the operation.

Interpretation.—The natural course probably plays a substantial role in the outcome. Based on our findings, it is difficult to recommend arthroscopic acromioplasty for any specific subgroup. Regarding operative treatment, however, a concomitant AC joint resection might be recommended if there are signs of AC joint degeneration. Even more challenging for the development of a treatment algorithm is the finding that patients who do not recover after nonoperative treatment should not be operated either.

▶ Well-done prospective studies on operative versus nonoperative treatments in orthopedics are lacking. Many published studies examine the outcome of different operative interventions, without inclusion of nonsurgical (or "conservative") treatments. Even more rare is a longer term follow-up of such a study.

This report is the rare exception in that it uses randomized treatment data on operative and nonoperative treatment for impingement syndrome with 2- and 5-year follow-up.

This group of patients had preoperative imaging to evaluate the rotator cuff before randomization. The current study did not describe the operative findings.

Previously reported was that operative treatment for impingement did not produce different outcomes from nonoperative treatment. This study looked at the subgroups of patients in both groups that did not get better.

Approximately one-third of each group did not get better. The two-thirds of the group who felt better at follow-up did so regardless of the treatment administered to them.

Overall, there was a negative correlation between work satisfaction and pain.

Although it was a small subset in the group undergoing surgery, patients with acromioclavicular (AC) arthritis on imaging had more pain than those without. The data did not include any physical examination findings at the AC joint.

The subgroup of nonoperative patients who did not get better and then went on to surgery did not get better; as a group, they had more self-reported pain, disability, pain at night, days with pain, and Strengths and Difficulties Questionnaire score (all without statistical significance) than the other patients.

R. Papandrea, MD

Chronic Degeneration Leads to Poor Healing of Repaired Massive Rotator Cuff Tears in Rats

Killian ML, Cavinatto LM, Ward SR, et al (Washington Univ, St Louis, MO; Univ of California, San Diego, La Jolla; et al)
Am J Sports Med 43:2401-2410, 2015

Background.—Chronic rotator cuff tears present a clinical challenge, often with poor outcomes after surgical repair. Degenerative changes to the muscle, tendon, and bone are thought to hinder healing after surgical repair; additionally, the ability to overcome degenerative changes after surgical repair remains unclear.

Purpose/Hypothesis.—The purpose of this study was to evaluate healing outcomes of muscle, tendon, and bone after tendon repair in a model of chronic rotator cuff disease and to compare these outcomes to those of acute rotator cuff injuries and repair. The hypothesis was that degenerative rotator cuff changes associated with chronic multitendon tears and muscle unloading would lead to poor structural and mechanical outcomes after repair compared with acute injuries and repair.

Study Design.—Controlled laboratory study.

Methods.—Chronic rotator cuff injuries, induced via detachment of the supraspinatus (SS) and infraspinatus (IS) tendons and injection of botulinum toxin A into the SS and IS muscle bellies, were created in the shoulders of rats. After 8 weeks of injury, tendons were surgically reattached to the humeral head, and an acute, dual-tendon injury and repair was performed on the contralateral side. After 8 weeks of healing, muscles were examined histologically, and tendon-to-bone samples were examined microscopically, histologically, and biomechanically and via micro—computed tomography.

Results.—All repairs were intact at the time of dissection, with no evidence of gapping or ruptures. Tendon-to-bone healing after repair in our chronic injury model led to reduced bone quality and morphological disorganization at the repair site compared with acute injuries and repair.

SS and IS muscles were atrophic at 8 weeks after repair of chronic injuries, indicating incomplete recovery after repair, whereas SS and IS muscles exhibited less atrophy and degeneration in the acute injury group at 8 weeks after repair. After chronic injuries and repair, humeral heads had decreased total mineral density and an altered trabecular structure, and the repair had decreased strength, stiffness, and toughness, compared with the acute injury and repair group.

Conclusion.—Chronic degenerative changes in rotator cuff muscles, tendons, and bone led to inferior healing characteristics after repair compared with acute injuries and repair. The changes were not reversible after repair in the time course studied, consistent with clinical impressions.

Clinical Relevance.—High retear rates after rotator cuff repair are associated with tear size and chronicity. Understanding the mechanisms behind this association may allow for targeted tissue therapy for tissue degeneration that occurs in the setting of chronic tears.

▶ High retear rates after rotator cuff repair are associated with tear size and chronicity. Chronic tears have poorer operative outcomes as the degenerative changes in the muscle, tendon, and bone are thought to hinder healing. Understanding the mechanism behind this association may allow for targeted tissue therapy for tissue degeneration that occurs in the setting of chronic rotator cuff tears.

A controlled laboratory study using a rat model was designed to evaluate healing outcomes of muscle, tendon, and bone after tendon repair in a model of chronic rotator cuff disease compared with an acute tear model. The hypothesis was that the chronic tear model would exhibit poor structural and mechanical outcomes after repair compared to the acute injury model.

The rodent model for chronic degenerative tears was created by releasing supraspinatus (SS) and infraspinatus (IS) and then injecting botulinum toxin A into the muscle bellies to accelerate atrophy and fibrosis to mimic chronic degenerative changes. The contralateral shoulder underwent sham operation with exposure of both tendons and closure at the index procedure. Cuff repair was performed 8 weeks after injury with contralateral acute release and repair performed at the same anesthetic. This allowed side-to-side comparison of tendon to bone healing after repair of a chronic versus acute tear injury model.

Results of the study showed that all repairs were intact at the time of dissection without evidence of rupture. However, tendon to bone healing in the chronic model resulted in reduced bone quality and morphologic disorganization at the repair site. The SS and IS muscles showed persistent atrophy at 8 weeks compared with the acute model indicating incomplete recovery. Bony analysis of the humeral head showed decreased bone mineral density in addition to altered trabecular structure in the chronic model (Fig 1). Finally, the tendon repair exhibited decreased strength, stiffness, and toughness in the chronic repair group (Fig 2).

Overall, the study found that chronic degenerative tear rat model exhibited inferior healing characteristics of muscle, tendon, and bone compared with the acute tear model, and these changes were not reversible after repair.

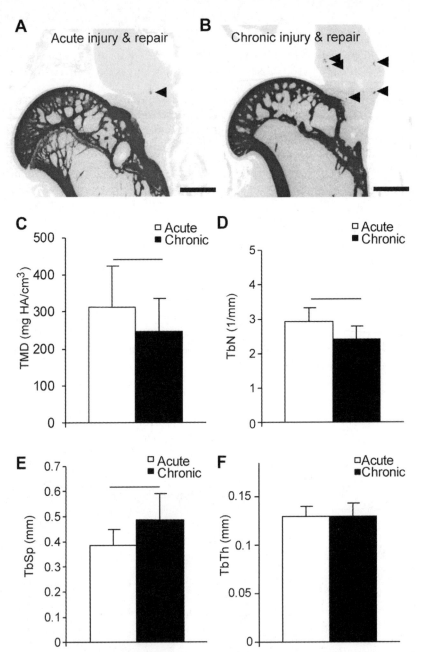

FIGURE 1.—Representative micro−computed tomographic reconstructions of 0.5 mm−thick coronal sections of proximal humeri after (A) acute injuries and repair and (B) chronic injuries and repair. Arrowheads indicate localized heterotopic ossifications in the tendon/scar. Trabecular bone morphometric outcomes for (C) tissue mineral density (TMD), (D) trabecular number (TbN), and (E) trabecular spacing (TbSp) were significantly different between acute and chronic groups. (F) No differences in trabecular thickness (TbTh) between groups were observed. Lines indicate significant differences between acute and chronic groups ($P < .05$). Scale bar in A and B = 2 mm. Data are presented as mean + upper 95% CI. (Reprinted from Killian ML, Cavinatto LM, Ward SR, et al. Chronic degeneration leads to poor healing of repaired massive rotator cuff tears in rats. *Am J Sports Med.* 2015;43:2401-2410, with permission from The Author(s).)

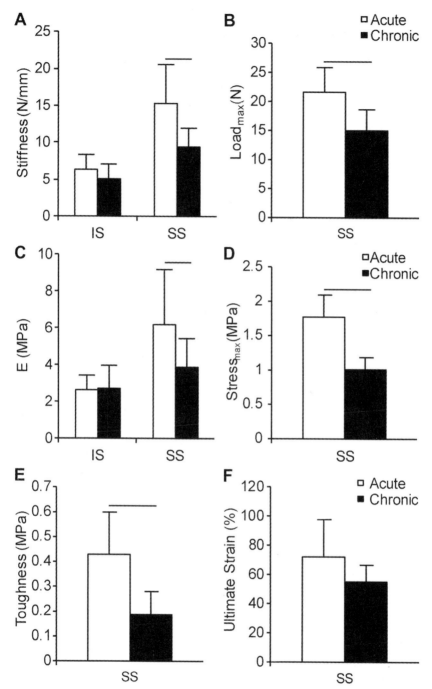

FIGURE 2.—Mechanical outcomes for uniaxial tensile tests of infraspinatus (IS) and supraspinatus (SS) tendon-to-bone attachments of the acute injury and repair group and chronic injury and repair group. (A) Stiffness (N/mm) for IS and SS attachments, (B) maximum load to failure (Load$_{max}$, N) for SS attachments, (C) Young modulus (MPa) for IS and SS attachments, (D) maximum stress to failure of SS attachments (Stress$_{max}$, MPa), (E) toughness (MPa) of SS attachments, and (F) ultimate strain (%) of SS attachments. Lines indicate significant differences between acute and chronic groups ($P < .05$). Data are presented as mean + upper 95% CI. (Reprinted from Killian ML, Cavinatto LM, Ward SR, et al. Chronic degeneration leads to poor healing of repaired massive rotator cuff tears in rats. *Am J Sports Med*. 2015;43:2401-2410, with permission from The Author(s).)

The authors conclude that the current animal study supports the clinical impression that chronic tears are more difficult to repair because of long-standing retraction and structural changes to the muscle; additionally, healing is not guaranteed after repair. The authors' data can serve as a foundation for further study directed at targeted treatment modalities for the degeneration seen in the setting of chronic tears.

M. O'Shaughnessy, MD

A Systematic Review of the Psychometric Properties of Patient-Reported Outcome Instruments for Use in Patients with Rotator Cuff Disease
Huang H, Grant JA, Miller BS, et al (Univ of Michigan, Ann Arbor; Dalhousie Univ, Saint John, New Brunswick, Canada; et al)
Am J Sports Med 43:2572-2582, 2015

Background.—Many patient-reported outcome instruments (or questionnaires) have been developed for use in patients with rotator cuff disease. Before an instrument is implemented, its psychometric properties should be carefully assessed, and the methodological quality of papers that investigate a psychometric component of an instrument must be carefully evaluated. Together, the psychometric evidence and the methodological quality can then be used to arrive at an estimate of an instrument's quality.

Purpose.—To identify patient-reported outcome instruments used in patients with rotator cuff disease and to critically appraise and summarize their psychometric properties to guide researchers and clinicians in using high-quality patient-reported outcome instruments in this population.

Study Design.—Systematic review.

Methods.—Systematic literature searches were performed to find English-language articles concerning the development or evaluation of a psychometric property of a patient-reported outcome instrument for use in patients with rotator cuff disease. Methodological quality and psychometric evidence were critically appraised and summarized through 2 standardized sets of criteria.

Results.—A total of 1881 articles evaluating 39 instruments were found per the search strategy, of which 73 articles evaluating 16 instruments were included in this study. The Constant-Murley score, the DASH (Disability of the Arm, Shoulder, and Hand), and the Shoulder Pain and Disability Index were the 3 most frequently evaluated instruments. In contrast, the psychometric properties of the Korean Shoulder Scoring System, Shoulder Activity Level, Subjective Shoulder Value, and Western Ontario Osteoarthritis Shoulder index were evaluated by only 1 study each. The Western Ontario Rotator Cuff Index was found to have the best overall quality of psychometric properties per the established criteria, with positive evidence found in internal consistency, reliability, content validity, hypothesis testing, and responsiveness. The DASH, Shoulder Pain and Disability Index, and Simple Shoulder Test had good evidence in support of internal consistency, reliability, structural validity, hypothesis testing, and responsiveness. Inadequate methodological quality was found across many studies, particularly in internal consistency, reliability, measurement error, hypothesis testing, and responsiveness.

Conclusion.—More high-quality methodological studies should be performed to assess the properties in all identified instruments.

▶ This systematic review highlights the important topic of patient-reported outcomes in rotator cuff surgery with specific attention to the psychometric properties of different outcome measures. As the authors highlight, when choosing a patient-reported outcome measure, it is important to choose one that measures in a valid, reliable, and responsive manner. Little work has been done in this area in the past, and given the frequency of rotator cuff pathology and the burden this disease process places on society, this is a timely and important study. The authors found a total of 16 patient-reported outcome measures that have been used to assess patients after rotator cuff surgery. Their analysis in this study demonstrates that the WORC (Western Ontario Rotator Cuff) tool had the highest rating among all of the instruments. This was followed by the Disability of the Arm, Shoulder, and Hand; the Shoulder Pain and Disability Index; and the Simple Shoulder Test. The authors also found methodological differences that limited the conclusions that could be drawn. They highlight the need for future work on this area.

J. Macalena, MD

The Optimum Tension for Bridging Sutures in Transosseous-Equivalent Rotator Cuff Repair: A Cadaveric Biomechanical Study

Park JS, McGarry MH, Campbell ST, et al (Korea Univ Anam Hosp, Seoul; Veterans Affairs Long Beach Healthcare System, Long Beach, CA; et al)
Am J Sports Med 43:2118-2125, 2015

Background.—Transosseous-equivalent (TOE) rotator cuff repair can increase contact area and contact pressure between the repaired cuff tendon and bony footprint and can show higher ultimate loads to failure and smaller gap formation compared with other repair techniques. However, it has been suggested that medial rotator cuff failure after TOE repair may result from increased bridging suture tension.

Purpose.—To determine optimum bridging suture tension in TOE repair by evaluating footprint contact and construct failure characteristics at different tensions.

Study Design.—Controlled laboratory study.

Methods.—A total of 18 fresh-frozen cadaveric shoulders, randomly divided into 3 groups, were constructed with a TOE configuration using the same medial suture anchor and placing a Tekscan sensing pad between the repaired rotator cuff tendon and footprint. Nine of the 18 shoulders were used to measure footprint contact characteristics. With use of the

Tekscan measurement system, the contact pressure and area between the rotator cuff tendon and greater tuberosity were quantified for bridging suture tensions of 60, 90, and 120 N with glenohumeral abduction angles of 0° and 30° and humeral rotation angles of 30° (internal), 0°, and 30° (external). TOE constructs of all 18 shoulders then underwent construct failure testing (cyclic loading and load to failure) to determine the yield load, ultimate load, stiffness, hysteresis, strain, and failure mode at 60 and 120 N of tension.

Results.—As bridging suture tension increased, contact force, contact pressure, and peak pressure increased significantly at all positions ($P < .05$ for all). Regarding contact area, no significant differences were found between 90 and 120 N at all positions, although there were significant differences between 60 and 90 N. The construct failure test demonstrated no significant differences in any parameters according to various tensions ($P > .05$ for all).

Conclusion.—Increasing bridging suture tension to over 90 N did not improve contact area but did increase contact force and pressure. Bridging suture tension did not significantly affect ultimate failure loads.

Clinical Relevance.—Considering the risks of overtensioning bridging sutures, it may be clinically more beneficial to keep bridging suture tension below 90 N.

▶ The transosseous-equivalent rotator cuff repair is a commonly used technique that was developed to preserve contact of the tendon footprint and allow early postoperative rehabilitation.[1] Using a cadaver model, the authors of this study attempted to understand how the bridging suture tension affects the tendon contact force, pressure, and area as well as the construct failure.

The results of this study were not unexpected. The authors hypothesized that a threshold exists over which the bridging suture tension would not affect the contact pressure and area of the tendon. Although the contact pressure did increase with increasing bridging suture tension, there was a threshold of 90 N after which the contact area of the tendon remained stable. The authors also posited that the failure characteristics of the construct would not be dependent on the bridging suture tension, which was the finding of this study. A prior study found that the bridging sutures reduce blood flow to the tendon.[2] Out of concern for the impact this reduction in blood flow may have on tendon healing, the authors recommend against tensioning the bridging sutures over 90 N.

Although this study presents a nice evaluation of the transosseous-equivalent rotator cuff repair construct, there are challenges in applying its findings to the clinical setting. First, it is difficult to know if the bridging suture tension is optimized during surgery. The authors found that when performing a rotator cuff repair with the Versa-lok, the maximal suture tension by the senior surgeon was 120 N. Therefore, 90 N (the threshold determined in the study) is 75% of maximum tension. However, the maximal suture tension may vary from surgeon to surgeon, and most surgeons will not be using a tensiometer to determine this. Another challenge arises because the study uses a cadaver model, and tendon healing could not be evaluated (a limitation recognized by the authors). Finally, the most critical factor in the success of a rotator cuff repair is the quality of the tendon tissue. The cadaveric shoulders were relatively young and did not have gross evidence of rotator cuff pathology. Therefore, the construct failure testing in this study may not accurately reflect the types of failures seen in clinical practice.

E. Kinnucan, MD

References

1. Park MC, ElAttrache NS, Ahmad CS, Tibone JE. "Transosseous-equivalent" rotator cuff repair technique. *Arthroscopy.* 2006;22:1360.e1-5.
2. Christoforetti JJ, Krupp RJ, Singleton SB, Kissenberth MJ, Cook C, Hawkins RJ. Arthroscopic suture bridge transosseus equivalent fixation of rotator cuff tendon preserves intratendinous blood flow at the time of initial fixation. *J Shoulder Elbow Surg.* 2012;21:523-530.

Prolotherapy for Refractory Rotator Cuff Disease: Retrospective Case-Control Study of 1-Year Follow-Up

Lee D-H, Kwack K-S, Rah UW, et al (Ajou Univ School of Medicine, Suwon, Republic of Korea)
Arch Phys Med Rehabil 96:2027-2032, 2015

Objective.—To determine the efficacy of prolotherapy for refractory rotator cuff disease.

Design.—Retrospective case-control study.

Setting.—University-affiliated tertiary care hospital.

Participants.—Patients with nontraumatic refractory rotator cuff disease (N = 151) who were unresponsive to 3 months of aggressive conservative treatment. Of the patients, 63 received prolotherapies with 16.5% dextrose 10-ml solution (treatment group), and 63 continued conservative treatment (control group).

Interventions.—Not applicable.

Main Outcome Measures.—Visual analog scale (VAS) score of the average shoulder pain level for the past 1 week, Shoulder Pain and Disability Index (SPADI) score, isometric strength of the shoulder abductor, active range of motion (AROM) of the shoulder, maximal tear size on ultrasonography, and number of analgesic ingestions per day.

Results.—Over 1-year follow-up, 57 patients in the treatment group and 53 in the control group were analyzed. There was no significant difference between the 2 groups in age, sex, shoulder dominance, duration of symptoms, and ultrasonographic findings at pretreatment. The average number of injections in the treatment group is 4.8 ± 1.3. Compared with the control group, VAS score, SPADI score, isometric strength of shoulder abductor, and shoulder AROM of flexion, abduction, and external rotation showed significant improvement in the treatment group. There were no adverse events.

Conclusions.—To our knowledge, this is the first study to assess the efficacy of prolotherapy in rotator cuff disease. Prolotherapy showed improvement in pain, disability, isometric strength, and shoulder AROM in patients with refractory chronic rotator cuff disease. The results suggest positive outcomes, but one should still take caution in directly interpreting it as an effective treatment option, considering the limitations of this non-randomized retrospective study. To show the efficacy of prolotherapy, further studies on prospective randomized controlled trials will be required.

▶ In this retrospective nonblinded study, the authors attempted to show the efficacy of using prolotherapy in refractory rotator cuff disease. None of these patients responded to aggressive conservative treatments including the use of nonsteroidal anti-inflammatory medications, opioids, and tricyclic medications as well as an aggressive institutional exercise programs followed by a home exercise program. Patients underwent corticosteroid injections and the potential for suprascapular nerve blocks if their pain level was greater than or equal to 5. A total of 151 patients were selected to participate in the study; 63 self-adopted the prolotherapy and 88 adopted other treatments, which ultimately boiled down to 63 patients willing to undergo continued conservative care. In the treatment group, patients underwent sonographically guided injections of 16.5% dextrose. These injections were administered at 0, 2, and 5 weeks and then every 4 weeks thereafter. Limitations were placed on the number of injections.

Although the use of prolotherapy has been around for many years, there are very few systematic reviews of its efficacy. This study, although retrospective, does show that there is a positive trend in treatment of recalcitrant rotator cuff disease using this modality. Unfortunately, this study is limited by the fact that it is retrospective, and the patients were self-allocated and not randomized. There also was no systematic review of patient compliance with conservative intervention.

This study does raise the question of potential alternative treatment for recalcitrant rotator cuff symptoms. This may be a viable alternative if the patient does not respond to standard aggressive conservative care.

J. Brault, DO

Arthroscopic Partial Repair of Irreparable Rotator Cuff Tears: Preoperative Factors Associated with Outcome Deterioration over 2 Years
Shon MS, Koh KH, Lim TK, et al (Natl Med Ctr, Seoul, South Korea; Inje Univ, Goyang, South Korea; Eulji Univ School of Medicine, Seoul, South Korea; et al)
Am J Sports Med 43:1965-1975, 2015

Background.—Arthroscopic partial repair is a treatment option in irreparable large-to-massive rotator cuff tears without arthritic changes. However, there are indications that arthroscopic partial repair does not yield satisfactory outcomes.

Purpose.—To report the clinical and radiographic results of arthroscopic partial repairs in patients with irreparable large-to-massive cuff tears. In addition, an analysis was performed regarding preoperative factors that may influence patient outcomes and patient-rated satisfaction over time.

Study Design.—Case series; Level of evidence, 4.

Methods.—From 2005 to 2011, a total of 31 patients who underwent arthroscopic partial repair for irreparable large-to-massive cuff tears were retrospectively evaluated. Partial repair was defined as posterior cuff tissue repair with or without subscapularis tendon repair to restore the transverse force couple of the cuff. Pain visual analog scale (PVAS), questionnaire results (American Shoulder and Elbow Surgeons [ASES] and Simple Shoulder Test [SST]), and radiographic changes (acromiohumeral distance and degenerative change) were assessed preoperatively, at first follow-up (roughly 1 year postoperatively), and at final follow-up (>2 years postoperatively). Patients rated their satisfaction level at each postoperative follow-up as well. Preoperative factors that might influence outcomes, such as patient demographics, tear size, and fatty infiltration, were investigated.

Results.—The preoperative, first follow-up, and final follow-up results for mean PVAS (5.13, 2.13, and 3.16, respectively) and questionnaires (ASES: 41.97, 76.37, and 73.78; SST: 3.61, 6.33, and 6.07, respectively) improved significantly (all $P < .05$). Radiographic evaluation showed no difference compared with preoperative status. Nevertheless, patient-rated satisfaction at final evaluation was inferior: 16 good responses ("very satisfied" and "satisfied") and 15 poor responses ("rather the same" and "dissatisfied"). Despite initial improvements in both groups ($P < .05$), patients with poor satisfaction demonstrated statistically significant deterioration in mean PVAS (from 2.07 to 4.67), questionnaire scores (ASES: from 74.56 to 59.80; SST: from 5.11 to 3.81), and acromiohumeral distance (from 7.19 to 5.06 mm) between the first and final follow-up (all $P < .05$). Patients with good satisfaction showed no significant difference or they improved ($P > .05$) from the first to the final follow-up. Among preoperative factors, fatty infiltration of the teres minor was identified as the only statistically significant factor affecting patient-rated satisfaction ($P = .007$).

Conclusion.—This study showed that arthroscopic partial repair may produce initial improvement in selected outcomes at 2-year follow-up. However, about half of the patients in the study were not satisfied with their outcomes, which had deteriorated over time. Preoperative fatty infiltration of the teres minor was the only factor that correlated with worse final outcomes and poor satisfaction after arthroscopic partial repair.

▶ Irreparable rotator cuff tears represent a particular challenge to upper extremity surgeons. For older patients with irreparable tears accompanied by arthritic changes, reverse arthroplasty has become a popular option. However, in the patient without arthritis, surgical options are limited and include debridement with or without subacromial decompression, tenotomy or tenodesis of the long

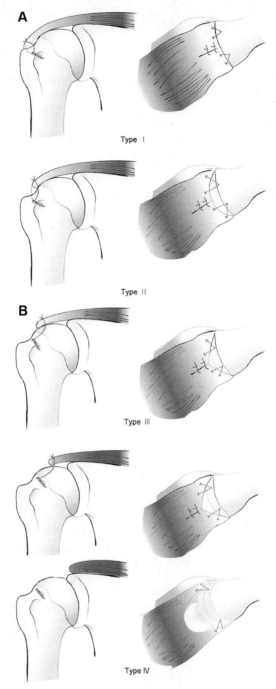

FIGURE 1.—Schematic drawing showing (A) type I and II repairs as complete repairs and (B) type III and IV repairs as incomplete repairs with unrepaired defect and uncovered footprint. (Reprinted from Shon MS, Koh KH, Lim TK, et al. Arthroscopic partial repair of irreparable rotator cuff tears: preoperative factors associated with outcome deterioration over 2 years. Am J Sports Med 2015;43:1965-1975, with permission from The Author(s).)

head of the biceps, latissimus or pectoralis transfer, and allograft reconstruction. A partial repair called *force couple repair* was proposed by Burkhart et al.[1]

This study aimed to evaluate outcomes of patients treated with arthroscopic partial repair. Patients were included if they had large to massive cuff tears that underwent partial repair. Partial repair is not the same as incomplete repair, and the authors of the study took care to only evaluate patients with what were deemed type IV repairs (Fig 1): incomplete repair with a substantial unrepaired defect that entailed moderate to extensive exposure of the humeral head greater than 10 mm after only partial repair. Partial repair was defined as posterior cuff tissue repair (infraspinatus and teres minor) with or without subscapularis tendon repair to restore the transverse force couple of the remaining cuff, which demonstrated irreparable infraspinatus tendon with severe retraction, atrophy, and fatty infiltration.

Thirty-one patients met inclusion criteria and were available for final follow-up (>2 years postoperative). Results showed improved pain visual analog scale (PVAS), and questionnaire results improved significantly (*P* < .05). Radiographs showed no difference between preoperative and postoperative films. Patient-related satisfaction was disappointing at final follow-up with 16 good responses (either very satisfied or satisfied) and 15 poor results (rather the same and dissatisfied). Both groups showed initial improvements, yet over time the poor-result patients had a significant decline in PVAS, questionnaire, and acromiohumeral distance (*P* < .05). When evaluating preoperative factors and final outcome, the only statistically significant factor affecting patient-rated satisfaction was fatty infiltration of teres minor (*P* < .007).

Overall, the authors conclude that arthroscopic partial repair of large to massive cuff tears led to initial improvements in pain scores and function; however, in longer-term follow-up, half of the patients were not satisfied with their outcome. Preoperative teres minor fatty infiltration was a significant risk factor for poor outcome.

M. O'Shaughnessy, MD

Reference

1. Burkhart SS, Nottage WM, Ogilvie-Harris DJ, Kohn HS, Pachelli A. Partial repair of irreparable rotator cuff tears. *Arthroscopy.* 1994;10:363-370.

Effectiveness of Botulinum Toxin for Shoulder Pain Treatment: A Systematic Review and Meta-Analysis
Wu T, Fu Y, Song HX, et al (Zhejiang Univ, Hangzhou, People's Republic of China; Alxa League Central Hosp, Inner Mongolia Autonomous Region, People's Republic of China; et al)
Arch Phys Med Rehabil 96:2214-2220, 2015

Objective.—To evaluate the current evidence of the effectiveness of botulinum toxin (BTX) treatment for shoulder pain.

Data Sources.—Ovid MEDLINE In-Process and Other Non-Indexed Citations, Ovid MEDLINE, Ovid EMBASE, Web of Science, and Scopus were searched from inception through week 18 of 2015.

Study Selection.—Randomized controlled trials comparing the clinical efficacy (pain intensity and shoulder range of motion [ROM]) of BTX injection to conventional therapy (steroid or placebo injection) were included.

Data Extraction.—Two reviewers independently screened abstracts and full texts. The results of the pain intensity and shoulder ROM were extracted and presented in the form of mean and SD. We constructed random-effects models and calculated the mean difference (MD) for continuous outcomes. A total of 219 articles were identified, of which 9 articles were eligible for the final analysis.

Data Synthesis.—The analysis indicated a statistically significant decreased pain score in the BTX therapy group compared with the control group, with the MD $= 1.35$ (95% confidence interval [CI], .80−1.91; $P < .001$; $I^2 = 81\%$). Patients who received BTX therapy were more likely to have a significant increase in shoulder abduction ROM than patients in the control group, with the MD $= 8.02$ (95% CI, 1.17−14.88, $P = .02$, $I^2 = 89\%$).

Conclusions.—Compared with conventional (steroid or placebo injection) therapy, BTX injections have beneficial effects for adult patients with shoulder pain, evidenced by improved pain scores and ROM.

▶ Over the last 20 years, one has heard rumors of botulism toxin (BTX) injections being used with great effect for various pain problems in various parts of the anatomy. Shoulder pain is one of those vexing problems that may lend itself to BTX treatment as well. Thankfully, Wu et al performed a meta-analysis to sort through the evidence regarding BTX injections and shoulder pain.

Of course, the devil is in the details, and these authors cast a broad net in their search, with the only relevant inclusion criteria being that these were randomized, controlled trials on humans. Outcomes were pain (visual analog scale), numeric rating scales, and shoulder range of motion (ROM).

As one can imagine, there are many types of shoulder pain as well as many types of BTX injections. Injections were either intramuscular, intra-articular (presumably into the gleno-humeral joint), or subacromial. The intra-articular injections were done under fluoroscopic guidance. Only the subacromial injections were done under ultrasound guidance. These latter injections were to treat subacromial bursitis or shoulder impingement syndrome. In the end, only 9 studies were included, and 6 of these were to treat shoulder pain from spasticity or stroke. One studied pain from arthritis, presumably from the gleno-humeral joint. One looked at patients with adhesive capsulitis. And only one looked at shoulder impingement.

I suspect that the readers of this YEAR BOOK would be most interested in the studies on arthritis, capsulitis, and impingement. In short, (1) BTX was more effective than placebo for gleno-humeral arthritis at 1-month follow up, (2) BTX injections were equal to steroid injections for increasing ROM and for the relief of pain from adhesive capsulitis, and (3) in treating shoulder impingement, BTX offered more prolonged relief than treatment with steroid injections.[1-3]

K. Bengtson, MD

References

1. Singh JA, Mahowald ML, Noorbaloochi S. Intra-articular botulinum toxin A for refractory shoulder pain: a randomized, double-blinded, placebo-controlled trial. *Transl Res.* 2009;153:205-216.
2. Joo YJ, Yoon SJ, Kim CW, et al. A comparison of the short-term effects of a botulinum toxin type A and triamcinolone acetate injection on adhesive capsulitis of the shoulder. *Ann Rehabil Med.* 2013;37:208-214.
3. Lee JH, Lee SH, Song SH. Clinical effectiveness of botulinum toxin type B in the treatment of subacromial bursitis or shoulder impingement syndrome. *Clin J Pain.* 2011;27:523-528.

Early mobilisation following mini-open rotator cuff repair: a randomised control trial
Sheps DM, Bouliane M, Styles-Tripp F, et al (Univ of Alberta, Edmonton, Canada)
Bone Joint J 97-B:1257-1263, 2015

This study compared the clinical outcomes following mini-open rotator cuff repair (MORCR) between early mobilisation and usual care, involving initial immobilisation. In total, 189 patients with radiologically-confirmed full-thickness rotator cuff tears underwent MORCR and were randomised to either early mobilisation (n = 97) or standard rehabilitation (n = 92) groups. Patients were assessed at six weeks and three, six, 12 and 24 months postoperatively. Six-week range of movement comparisons demonstrated significantly increased abduction ($p = 0.002$) and scapular plane elevation ($p = 0.006$) in the early mobilisation group, an effect which was not detectable at three months ($p > 0.51$) or afterwards. At 24 months post-operatively, patients who performed pain-free, early active mobilisation for activities of daily living showed no difference in clinical outcomes from patients immobilised for six weeks following MORCR. We suggest that the choice of rehabilitation regime following MORCR may be left to the discretion of the patient and the treating surgeon.

▶ Postoperative protocol after full-thickness rotator cuff repair is typically immobilization for 6 weeks followed by progressive rehabilitation over 6 to 12 months. Significant variability exists among surgeons regarding rehabilitation protocol.

Delaying active movement may predispose patients to stiffness and may delay recovery and return to work. Conversely, inadequate immobilization may result in incomplete healing and increased risk for retear. One study found a statistically significant increased retear rate in a subgroup of patients (medium and large tears) undergoing early passive motion.[1] Alternatively, animal models for anterior cruciate ligament reconstruction and flexor tendon repair have shown that early mobilization improved healing rates.[2,3] Three systematic reviews have compared early passive motion and immobilization after arthroscopic rotator cuff repair and showed improvement in early range of motion (ROM) in the early-motion group; however, the improvement did not persist at 1 year.[1,4,5]

Although more rotator cuff injuries are being repaired arthroscopically, surveys indicate that mini-open rotator cuff repair (MORCR) is still performed in approximately 40% of surgical cases. No randomized controlled trial has evaluated early active motion versus immobilization following mini-open rotator cuff repair.

The authors conducted a randomized, controlled, double-blind multicenter superiority trial. Patients were randomized to standard rehabilitation (SR) consisting of 6 weeks of immobilization or early active movement termed early mobilization (EM). The primary outcome was shoulder ROM but pain, abduction strength, and health-related quality-of-life scores (HRQOL) were also evaluated. SR consisted of sling for 6 weeks with no active movement of the shoulder; EM consisted of sling as needed and active movement for activities of daily living as soon as pain allowed.

The study was powered to detect a 10-degree change in ROM. One hundred and sixty-five patients with documented (ultrasound or MRI) full-thickness tear completed the 24-month follow-up and were included in the final analysis. The majority of patients (136 of 189) had medium or large size tears, with no significant difference in clinical or radiographic parameters between groups. Multiple fellowship-trained shoulder surgeons were involved with providing care, and patients were drawn from a large urban area.

Both groups commenced passive and self-assisted exercises on postoperative day 1. The SR group was told to wear the sling at all times except when performing the passive or self-assisted exercises. The EM group continued the same passive and self-assisted exercise but was allowed to perform any activity as long as it did not cause pain. They were instructed to avoid resisted activities and allowed to wear the sling for comfort only. At 6 weeks, both groups converged into the same rehabilitation protocol.

Results of the study showed that the EM group had improved abduction ($P = .002$) and scapular plane elevation ($P = .006$) at 6 weeks, but at 3 months the group showed no significant difference ($P > .51$). Shoulder pain at either activity or rest was not significantly different between groups at any time, with both groups noting improvement at 6 weeks that continued up to 24 months. HRQOL scores were improved in both groups at 24 months. Reinjury was documented in 7 patients (4 EM, 3 SR) within 1 year of surgery. Other complications were noted in 37 patients (17 EM and 20 SR, $P = .47$).

This well-designed, randomized clinical trial shows that EM after MORCR was associated with quicker recovery of abduction and scapular elevation early compared with SR; however, the gains equilibrated by the 3-month visit. The authors conclude that EM and SR have equivalent outcomes at intermediate-term follow-up, and therefore rehabilitation protocol may be reasonably left to the discretion of the surgeon. Future trials are indicated to determine whether there are any differences in healing rates that may influence long-term outcomes.

M. O'Shaughnessy, MD

References

1. Chang KV, Hung CY, Han DS, Chen WS, Wang TG, Chien KL. Early versus delayed passive range of motion exercise for arthroscopic rotator cuff repair: a meta-analysis of randomized controlled trials. *Am J Sports Med.* 2015;43: 1265-1273.
2. Gelberman RH, Woo SL, Lothringer K, Akeson WH, Amiel D. Effects of early intermittent passive mobilization on healing canine flexor tendons. *J Hand Surg Am.* 1982;7:170-175.
3. Shelbourne KD, Klotz C. What I have learned about the ACL: utilizing a progressive rehabilitation scheme to achieve total knee symmetry after anterior cruciate ligament reconstruction. *J Orthop Sci.* 2006;11:318-325.
4. Riboh JC, Garrigues GE. Early passive motion versus immobilization after arthroscopic rotator cuff repair. *Arthroscopy.* 2014;30:997-1005.
5. Chan K, MacDermid JC, Hoppe DJ, et al. Delayed versus early motion after arthroscopic rotator cuff repair: a meta-analysis. *J Shoulder Elbow Surg.* 2014; 23:1631-1639.

Clinical Outcomes of Modified Mason-Allen Single-Row Repair for Bursal-Sided Partial-Thickness Rotator Cuff Tears: Comparison With the Double-Row Suture-Bridge Technique

Shin S-J, Kook S-H, Rao N, et al (Ewha Womans Univ Mokdong Hosp, Seoul, Korea)
Am J Sports Med 43:1976-1982, 2015

Background.—Various repair techniques have been reported for the operative treatment of bursal-sided partial-thickness rotator cuff tears. Recently, arthroscopic single-row repair using a modified Mason-Allen technique has been introduced.

Hypothesis.—The arthroscopic, modified Mason-Allen single-row technique with preservation of the articular-sided tendon provides satisfactory clinical outcomes and similar results to the double-row suture-bridge technique after conversion of a partial-thickness tear to a full-thickness tear.

Study Design.—Cohort study; Level of evidence, 3.

Methods.—A retrospective study was conducted on 84 consecutive patients with symptomatic, bursal-sided partial-thickness rotator cuff tears involving more than 50% thickness of the tendon. A total of 47 patients were treated by the modified Mason-Allen single-row repair technique, preserving the articular-sided tendon, and 37 patients were treated by the double-row suture-bridge repair technique after conversion to a full-thickness tear. The clinical and functional outcomes were evaluated using the American Shoulder and Elbow Surgeons (ASES) and Constant scores and a visual analog scale (VAS) for pain and satisfaction of patients. Magnetic resonance imaging (MRI) was used to analyze the integrity of tendons at 6-month follow-up. Patients were followed up for a mean of 32.5 months.

Results.—In the 47 patients treated with the modified Mason-Allen suture technique, the VAS score decreased from a preoperative mean of 5.3 ± 0.3 to 0.9 ± 0.5 at the time of final follow-up. There was a statistically significant increase in the mean ASES score (from 45.4 ± 2.9 to 88.6 ± 4.5) and mean Constant score (from 66.9 ± 2.6 to 88.1 ± 2.4) (*P* < .001). Four of 47 patients (8.5%) demonstrated retears at 6-month postoperative MRI. There was no statistical difference in terms of functional outcomes and the retear rate compared with those of patients with the suture-bridge repair technique (3 patients, 8.1%). However, the mean number of suture anchors used in the patients with modified Mason-Allen suture repair (1.2 ± 0.4) was significantly fewer than that in the patients with suture-bridge repair (3.2 ± 0.4) (*P* < .01).

Conclusion.—The modified Mason-Allen single-row repair technique that preserved the articular-sided tendon provided satisfactory clinical outcomes in patients with symptomatic, bursal-sided partial-thickness rotator cuff tears. Despite a fewer number of suture anchors, the shoulder functional outcomes and retear rate in patients after modified Mason-Allen repair were comparable with those of patients who underwent double-row suture-bridge repair. Therefore, the modified Mason-Allen single-row repair technique using a triple-loaded suture anchor can be considered as an effective treatment in patients with bursal-sided partial-thickness rotator cuff tears.

▶ The authors report a retrospective study on patients undergoing high-grade partial bursal-sided rotator cuff tear repair using either a modified Mason Allen stitch with a single triple-loaded anchor through a limited window or conversion to a full-thickness tear and repair using a double row configuration with either 3 or 4 anchors. No differences in functional scores, pain, and retear (based on MRI) were observed. As might be expected, 2 fewer anchors were required in the modified Mason Allen group.

As discussed by the authors, several approaches to the surgical management of partial bursal sided tears have been proposed. Conversion to a full-thickness tear likely represents the technically less demanding option, as it allows for more straightforward suture passing and visualization. Based on this study, repair of the bursal-sided tear, while preserving most of the articular-sided fibers using a modified Mason Allen technique, does appear to provide the more cost-effective alternative. However, this technique may be more technically demanding. No information of surgical time is provided to further elucidate this finding. Although retear rates were similar, no detail is provided on how outcomes were affected in this subset of patients and as to how the selected technique played a role in the type and configuration of the retear.

P. Streubel, MD

Early Versus Delayed Passive Range of Motion after Rotator Cuff Repair: A Systematic Review and Meta-analysis

Kluczynski MA, Nayyar S, Marzo JM, et al (The State Univ of New York, Buffalo)
Am J Sports Med 43:2057-2063, 2015

Background.—Postoperative rehabilitation has been shown to affect healing of the rotator cuff after surgical repair. However, it is unknown whether an early or delayed rehabilitation protocol is most beneficial for healing.

Purpose.—To determine whether early versus delayed passive range of motion (PROM) affects rotator cuff (RC) retear rates after surgery.

Study Design.—Systematic review and meta-analysis.

Methods.—A systematic review of the literature published between January 2003 and February 2014 was conducted. Retear rates were compared for early (within 1 week after surgery) versus delayed (3-6 weeks after surgery) PROM using χ^2 or Fisher exact tests as well as relative risks (RR) and 95% CIs. In the first analysis, data from evidence level 1 studies that directly compared early versus delayed PROM were pooled; and in the second analysis, data from level 1 to 4 studies that did not directly compare early versus delayed PROM were pooled. The second analysis was stratified by tear size and repair method.

Results.—Twenty-eight studies (1729 repairs) were included. The first analysis of level 1 studies did not reveal a significant difference in retear rates for early (13.7%) versus delayed (10.5%) PROM ($P = .36$; RR = 1.30 [95% CI, 0.74-2.30]). The second analysis revealed that for ≤3 cm tears, the risk of retear was lower for early versus delayed PROM for transosseous (TO) plus single-row anchor (SA) repairs (18.7% vs 28.2%, $P = .02$; RR = 0.66 [95% CI, 0.47-0.95]). For >5 cm tears, the risk of retear was greater for early versus delayed PROM for double-row anchor (DA) repairs (56.4% vs 20%, $P = .002$; RR = 2.82 [95% CI, 1.31-6.07]) and for all repair methods combined (52.2% vs 22.6%, $P = .01$; RR = 2.31 [95% CI, 1.16-4.61]). There were no statistically significant associations for tears measuring <1 cm, 1 to 3 cm, 3 to 5 cm, and >3 cm.

Conclusion.—Evidence is lacking with regard to the optimal timing of PROM after RC repair; however, this study suggests that tear size may be influential.

▶ This article aids shoulder surgeons in counseling patients whether to start with early or delayed rehabilitation depending on rotator cuff tear size. One conclusion is that caution should be taken with larger tears. The strength of this article is that several level 1 studies were included with significant results. Level 1 to 4 studies that did not directly compare early versus delayed rehabilitation were also included but analyzed separately. The main weakness of the study is that all data analyses are pooled into a large group of patients. There are so many different variables that influence outcomes and make group recommendations not suitable for an individual basis recommendation. So we can tell the patient about expected results on a pool of patients, but we cannot guarantee that same result for an individual. I do tell patients about the data published on the literature, but my decision whether to start early or delay rehabilitation continues to be determined on an individual basis taking into account patient-specific factors (tear size, tendon quality, and fixation method).

J. P. Simone, MD

Smoking Predisposes to Rotator Cuff Pathology and Shoulder Dysfunction: A Systematic Review
Bishop JY, Santiago-Torres JE, Rimmke N, et al (The Ohio State Univ, Columbus)
Arthroscopy 31:1598-1605, 2015

Purpose.—To investigate the association of smoking with rotator cuff (RTC) disease and shoulder dysfunction, defined as poor scores on shoulder rating scales.

Methods.—A systematic review was performed using a search strategy based on "shoulder AND [smoke OR smoking OR nicotine OR tobacco]." English-language clinical or basic science studies testing the association of smoking and shoulder dysfunction on shoulder rating scales or disease of the soft tissue of the shoulder were included. Level V evidence studies and articles reporting only on surgery outcomes, subjective symptoms, adhesive capsulitis, or presence of fracture or oncologic mass were excluded.

Results.—Thirteen studies were included, comprising a total of 16,172 patients, of whom 6,081 were smokers. All 4 clinical studies addressing the association between smoking and patient-reported shoulder symptoms and dysfunction in terms of poor scores on shoulder rating scales (i.e., Simple Shoulder Test; University of California, Los Angeles shoulder scale; and self-reported surveys) confirmed this correlation with 6,678 patients, of whom 1,723 were smokers. Two of four studies documenting provider-reported RTC disease comprised 8,461 patients, of whom 4,082 were smokers, and found a time- and dose-dependent relation of smoking with RTC tears and a correlation of smoking with impingement syndrome. Smoking was also reported in 4 other articles to be associated with the prevalence of larger RTC tears or tears with pronounced degenerative changes in 1,033 patients, of whom 276 were smokers, and may accelerate RTC degeneration, which could result in tears at a younger age. In addition, 1 basic science study showed that nicotine increased stiffness of the supraspinatus tendon in a rat model.

Conclusions.—Smoking is associated with RTC tears, shoulder dysfunction, and shoulder symptoms. Smoking may also accelerate RTC degeneration and increase the prevalence of larger RTC tears. These correlations suggest that smoking may increase the risk of symptomatic RTC disease, which could consequently increase the need for surgical interventions.

TABLE 1.—Clinical Studies on Smoking and Patient-Reported Symptoms and Shoulder Dysfunction

Authors	Journal	No. of Patients (Mean Age, yr)	Pertinent Findings
McRae et al.[11] (2011)	*J Shoulder Elbow Surg*	54 (58.2)	Smoking was associated with poor shoulder function and pain scores. Smoking was correlated with SST scores ($P = .003$) and had a greater correlation when combined with female sex and work-related injury ($P < .001$). However, there was no correlation with ASES scores ($P = .184$).
Rechardt et al.[12] (2010)	*BMC Musculoskelet Disorders*	6,237 (51.9)	Patients with unilateral shoulder pain (OR, 1.9; 95% CI, 1.3 to 2.9) and bilateral shoulder pain (OR, 1.8; 95% CI, 1.0 to 3.1) were more likely to be currently smoking men who had smoked for >20 pack-years and women who had smoked for 10 to 20 pack-years, respectively. Smoking was not associated with chronic RTC tendinitis.
Kane et al.[13] (2010)	*Sports Health*	163	Shoulder pain and loss of function were found to be proportional to smoking. Smokers had worse mean scores on the Subjective Shoulder Rating System assessment ($P = .005$), Shoulder Rating Questionnaire ($P = .0008$), and Oxford Shoulder Questionnaire ($P = .0042$). Smokers also reported lower active range of motion in both the left and right shoulders ($P = .024$). No significant difference was found between smokers of <1 pack per day and smokers of ≥1 pack per day.
Mallon et al.[14] (2004)	*J Shoulder Elbow Surg*	224 (52.3)	Preoperative scores showed that smokers had higher pain scores ($P < .0001$) and lower UCLA scores ($P = .00025$) than nonsmokers.

Editor's Note: Please refer to original journal article for full references.
ASES, American Shoulder and Elbow Surgeons; CI, confidence interval; OR, odds ratio; RTC, rotator cuff; SST, Simple Shoulder Test; UCLA, University of California, Los Angeles shoulder scale.
Reprinted from Bishop JY, Santiago-Torres JE, Rimmke N, et al. Smoking predisposes to rotator cuff pathology and shoulder dysfunction: a systematic review. *Arthroscopy.* 2015;31:1598-1605, with permission from Arthroscopy Association of North America.

TABLE 2.—Clinical Studies on Smoking and Provider-Reported Rotator Cuff Disease

Authors	Journal	No. of Patients (Mean Age, yr)	Pertinent Findings
Baumgarten et al.[15] (2010)	*Clin Orthop Relat Res*	584 (57.7)	This study showed a time- and dose-dependent relation between smoking and RTC tears. The correlation increased when smoking occurred within 10 yr of presentation (OR, 4.24; CI, 1.75 to 10.25; $P = .0006$) and was significant in patients with a history of smoking 1 to 2 packs per day (OR, 1.66; $P = .009$) and even greater for 2 packs per day (OR, 3.35; $P = .0007$). Ultrasonography was used to diagnose RTC tears.
Fehringer et al.[16] (2008)	*J Shoulder Elbow Surg*	104 (71.4)	No statistically significant association of smoking with increasing RTC tear prevalence was found ($P = .52$) in 200 shoulders from 104 patients aged ≥65 yr. Ultrasonography was used to diagnose RTC tears.
Tangtrakulwanich and Kapbird[17] (2012)	*World J Orthop*	302 (50)	Current smokers were at greater risk of impingement syndrome compared with nonsmokers (OR, 6.8; 95% CI, 1.2 to 39). Impingement syndrome was diagnosed with a lidocaine subacromial injection test
Titchener et al.[18] (2014)	*J Shoulder Elbow Surg*	7,471 (55)	Current smoking status was not associated with a diagnosis of RTC disease (OR, 1.03; CI, 0.91 to 1.15), whereas a history of smoking was associated with RTC disease (OR, 1.24; CI, 1.10 to 1.39). This effect disappeared after adjustment for number of general practice consultation rate per year (OR, 1.09; CI, 0.96 to 1.23).

Editor's Note: Please refer to original journal article for full references.
CI, confidence interval; OR, odds ratio; RTC, rotator cuff.
Reprinted from Bishop JY, Santiago-Torres JE, Rimmke N, et al. Smoking predisposes to rotator cuff pathology and shoulder dysfunction: a systematic review. *Arthroscopy.* 2015;31:1598-1605, with permission from Arthroscopy Association of North America.

TABLE 3.—Studies on Smoking and Degree of Rotator Cuff Pathology

Authors	Journal	Type of Study or No. of Patients (Mean Age, yr)	Pertinent Findings
Basic science study			
Ichinose et al.[19] (2010)	Acta Orthop	Animal model (rat)	Nicotine caused an increase in the calculated elastic modulus of the supraspinatus tendon ($P < .05$).
Clinical studies			
Carbone et al.[20] (2012)	J Shoulder Elbow Surg	408 (59)	The analysis resulted in a finding suggestive of significance of an increase in the severity of RTC tears as the average number of cigarettes smoked increased ($P = .099$). When combining type II, III, and IV tears (SCOI classification), the authors showed that increasing tear severity was associated with increasing daily numbers of cigarettes ($P = .04$). In addition, the total number of cigarettes smoked over a lifetime differed significantly between patients with a small tear and those with at least a type II tear ($P = .032$).
Kane et al.[21] (2006)	Orthopedics	Cadaveric study, 36 (75)	Macroscopic RTC tears were more likely in cadavers with a history of smoking, and the presence of advanced microscopic RTC pathology was more than twice as likely in cadavers with a history of smoking. The data were not statistically significant.
Kukkonen et al.[22] (2014)	Scand J Med Sci Sports	564 (59.8)	Smokers were significantly younger, with equally large tears, compared with nonsmokers ($P < .001$). There was no significant difference in preoperative Constant score ($P = .075$) or mean size of intraoperatively measured tendon tear ($P = .5$) in smokers v nonsmokers.
Lundgreen et al.[23] (2014)	Arthroscopy	25 (55.6)	Samples of the supraspinatus muscle were obtained arthroscopically in patients undergoing surgery for full-thickness RTC tears. Those with a smoking history of at least half a pack per day had a longer duration of symptoms (19 months v 11 months, $P < .05$), were younger (52 yr [SD, 6.4 yr] v 58 yr [SE, 5.8 yr]; $P < .01$), and had more advanced degeneration with a higher Bonar score (13.5 v 9, $P < .001$) than nonsmokers. The study also showed increased density of apoptotic cells ($P < .024$), reduced tenocyte density ($P < .019$), and upregulation of proliferative activity ($P < .0001$) in tendons of patients with a smoking history.

Editor's Note: Please refer to original journal article for full references.

RTC, rotator cuff; SCOI, Southern California Orthopedic Institute.

Reprinted from Bishop JY, Santiago-Torres JE, Rimmke N, et al. Smoking predisposes to rotator cuff pathology and shoulder dysfunction: a systematic review. *Arthroscopy.* 2015;31:1598-1605, with permission from Arthroscopy Association of North America.

Level of Evidence.—Level IV, systematic review of Level II through IV studies.

▶ This report is a systematic review of 13 level II through IV studies analyzing the association between smoking with shoulder dysfunction and rotator cuff (RTC) disease. The authors divide the extant literature into 3 categories focusing on the relationship between smoking and (1) patient-reported symptoms and shoulder dysfunction (Table 1), (2) provider-reported RTC disease (Table 2) and (3) degree of RTC pathology (Table 3). The comprehensive review found that smoking is associated with higher prevalence of shoulder dysfunction and symptoms, increased risk of RTC degeneration, increased risk of RTC tears at a younger age, and larger tears. There were mixed results regarding whether smokers have a higher prevalence of RTC tears. It is known that the RTC has a region of relative hypovascularity, and nicotine causes hypoxia. The authors include a basic science study showing that nicotine increased the elastic modulus of the supraspinatus tendon, altering its mechanical properties. Although not proven in this systematic review, it is extremely plausible that smoking can lead to increased prevalence of rotator cuff tears. A well-designed prospective case series could shed light on this subject.

This comprehensive review provides a summary of the best known evidence available indicating that smoking has a detrimental effect on shoulder function and predisposes to rotator cuff conditions. It has been my practice to counsel all my patients on the multitude of profound negative effects that smoking has on their general health as well as specific musculoskeletal effects. In an elective setting, I strongly recommend cessation of smoking (including cigarettes, cigars, electronic cigarettes, and nicotine patches) as part of a comprehensive nonoperative management plan prior to discussing surgical options, as there is also evidence that smoking status is associated with poor clinical and healing outcomes in RTC repair.

E. Gauger, MD

Outcome of Large to Massive Rotator Cuff Tears Repaired With and Without Extracellular Matrix Augmentation: A Prospective Comparative Study
Gilot GJ, Alvarez-Pinzon AM, Barcksdale L, et al (Cleveland Clinic Florida, Weston)
Arthroscopy 31:1459-1465, 2015

Purpose.—To compare the results of arthroscopic repair of large to massive rotator cuff tears (RCTs) with or without augmentation using an extracellular matrix (ECM) graft and to present ECM graft augmentation as a valuable surgical alternative used for biomechanical reinforcement in any RCT repair.

Methods.—We performed a prospective, blinded, single-center, comparative study of patients who underwent arthroscopic repair of a large to massive RCT with or without augmentation with ECM graft. The primary outcome was assessed by the presence or absence of a retear of the previously repaired rotator cuff, as noted on ultrasound examination. The secondary outcomes were patient satisfaction evaluated preoperatively and postoperatively using the 12-item Short Form Health Survey, the American Shoulder and Elbow Surgeons shoulder outcome score, a visual analog scale score, the Western Ontario Rotator Cuff index, and a shoulder activity level survey.

Results.—We enrolled 35 patients in the study: 20 in the ECM-augmented rotator cuff repair group and 15 in the control group. The follow-up period ranged from 22 to 26 months, with a mean of 24.9 months. There was a significant difference between the groups in terms of the incidence of retears: 26% (4 retears) in the control group and 10% (2 retears) in the ECM graft group ($P = .0483$). The mean pain level decreased from 6.9 to 4.1 in the control group and from 6.8 to 0.9 in the ECM graft group ($P = .024$). The American Shoulder and Elbow Surgeons score improved from 62.1 to 72.6 points in the control group and from 63.8 to 88.9 points ($P = .02$) in the treatment group. The mean Short Form 12 scores improved in the 2 groups, with a statistically significant difference favoring graft augmentation ($P = .031$), and correspondingly, the Western Ontario Rotator Cuff index scores improved in both arms, favoring the treatment group ($P = .0412$).

Conclusions.—The use of ECM for augmentation of arthroscopic repairs of large to massive RCTs reduces the incidence of retears, improves patient outcome scores, and is a viable option during complicated cases in which a significant failure rate is anticipated.

Level of Evidence.—Level III, prospective, blinded, nonrandomized, comparative study.

▶ This study shows encouraging results in favor of extracellular matrix augmentation for the treatment of large to massive rotator cuff tears. Significantly higher repair integrity, American Shoulder and Elbow Surgeons score, Short Form 12, and Western Ontario Rotator Cuff index scores were reported at a minimum 22-month follow-up for patients undergoing augmentation compared with those undergoing repair only. Of note, no full-thickness tears were observed in patients undergoing augmentation, which stands in contrast to several previous studies showing high rates of structural failure after repair of large and massive rotator cuff tears.

Although baseline characteristics were overall similar, it is not clear on what basis tears were deemed to require augmentation versus partial repair. Furthermore, it is unclear how fatty atrophy was distributed in the 2 groups. Given the lack of randomization, an inherent selection bias may have existed at the time of treatment selection.

Despite the lack of randomization, this study provides important comparative data that will aid in finding the role of augmentation during repair of complex rotator cuff tears.

P. Streubel, MD

Low Serum Vitamin D Is Not Correlated With the Severity of a Rotator Cuff Tear or Retear After Arthroscopic Repair

Ryu KJ, Kim BH, Lee Y, et al (Yonsei Univ College of Medicine, Seoul, Republic of Korea; CHA Univ, Seongnam-si, Kyeonggi-do, Republic of Korea)
Am J Sports Med 43:1743-1750, 2015

Background.—Despite the essential role of vitamin D in muscle function, the prevalence of vitamin D deficiency has been reported to be very high. Recently, low vitamin D level was found to correlate with fatty degeneration of the rotator cuff tendon in humans and to negatively affect early healing at the rotator cuff repair site in an animal study. However, the effects of vitamin D level on severity of rotator cuff tear and healing after surgical repair have not been documented.

Purpose.—To evaluate (1) the prevalence of vitamin D deficiency among patients who underwent arthroscopic repair for a full-thickness rotator cuff tear, (2) the relationship of vitamin D level with severity of the rotator cuff tear, and (3) surgical outcomes after repair.

Study Design.—Cohort study; Level of evidence, 2.

Methods.—A consecutive series of 91 patients (age, 50-65 years) who underwent arthroscopic rotator cuff repair for full-thickness, small-sized to massive tears were evaluated. Preoperative serum vitamin D levels (25-hydroxyvitamin) were analyzed to detect correlations with the features of a preoperative rotator cuff tear as well as postoperative structural and functional outcomes. All patients were followed clinically for a minimum of 1 year.

Results.—Preoperative vitamin D levels were deficient (<20 ng/mL) in 80 subjects (88%), insufficient (20-30 ng/mL) in 8 subjects (9%), and normal (>30 ng/mL) in 3 subjects (3%). No correlation was found between preoperative tear size ($P=.23$), extent of retraction ($P=.60$), degree of fatty infiltration of each cuff muscle ($P>.50$ each), or the global fatty infiltration index ($P=.32$). Similarly, no correlations were detected between vitamin D level and postoperative Sugaya type ($P=.66$) or any of the functional outcome scores ($P>.50$ each).

Conclusion.—Low serum vitamin D level was not related to tear size, extent of retraction, or the degree of fatty infiltration in cuff muscles. It also had no significant relationships with postoperative structural integrity and functional outcomes after arthroscopic repair. The results suggest that low serum vitamin D level is not a significant risk factor for the severity of rotator cuff tear or poor healing after repair.

▶ The purpose of this study was to (1) look at the prevalence of vitamin D deficiency in a group of patients undergoing arthroscopic rotator cuff repair, (2) determine if there was a relationship between rotator cuff tear size and vitamin D status, and (3) determine the relationship, if any, between vitamin D status and functional outcome of these rotator cuff repairs. Although this research exemplifies the exuberance of vitamin D deficiency (88%) and insufficiency (9%), it does not adequately address the other stated purposes.

The small sample size was problematic, but more importantly the inclusion criteria for this study are weak. For instance, the researchers did not identify when the preoperative vitamin D was obtained. Was it within 2 days or 2 weeks or 2 years of the surgery? Day-of-surgery vitamin D would have been consistent or a postoperative vitamin D would have added value. The comorbidities of these participants were not addressed in either the inclusion or exclusion criteria.

Overall, the study design was poor. This research has added to the preexisting body of knowledge reporting the prevalence of vitamin D deficiency and insufficiency.

I will not change my practice based on the information in this research.

L. Fitton, CNP

Traumatic Supraspinatus Tears in Patients Younger Than 25 Years
Dilisio MF, Noel CR, Noble JS, et al (Creighton Univ Orthopaedics, Omaha, NE; Crystal Clinic Orthopaedic Ctr, Akron, OH)
Orthopedics 38:e631-e634, 2015

Traumatic rotator cuff tears in patients younger than 25 years are rare events, with few reports in the literature. When compared with the more mature shoulder, the young, healthy supraspinatus tendon is a robust tendon that is able to absorb a significant amount of energy before tendon failure. Therefore, the diagnosis of a rotator cuff tear can be often overlooked in this population due to the patient's age. This is a report of traumatic supraspinatus repairs in patients younger than 25 years. Nine patients younger than 25 years were identified with a posttraumatic supraspinatus tear as visualized during routine diagnostic shoulder arthroscopy. These 9 patients represented 0.33% of all rotator cuff repairs during a 9-year period. Average patient age was 19.1 years (±3.7 years; range, 13 to 25 years). Magnetic resonance imaging failed to diagnose a rotator cuff tear in 50% of the patients. Mean delay from injury to surgery was 6.6 months. All tears were arthroscopically repaired. Concomitant anterior instability pathology was demonstrated among 66.7% of the patients. No complications were reported. At latest follow-up, all patients reported minimal to no shoulder pain and were tolerating strenuous work, activities, and sports without significant complaints. Even with advanced imaging, the diagnosis of a rotator cuff tear can often be missed in this patient population. Although clinical outcomes can be good, care must be taken to broaden the diagnostic differential in young patients with posttraumatic shoulder pain.

▶ Medical students are taught to think of horses when hoof beats are heard but never to forget the occasional zebra that shows up. Full-thickness rotator cuff tears in patients younger than 25 years are zebras. Despite the public's perception that young people get rotator cuff tears, treating physicians know it's uncommon.

This study of full-thickness posttraumatic supraspinatus tears in patients younger than 25 represents less than 1% of the tears treated surgically by the treating physicians. Eight of 9 of the patients had an MRI examination, of which, only 50% showed a full-thickness tear of the supraspinatus.

All patients sustained a single traumatic event. Four patients had a full-thickness tear, and the other 5 patients had a high-grade tear with more than 50% thickness. Six of 9 patients had concomitant anterior instability condition.

Seven of 9 patients had physical examination signs consistent with instability, whereas only 5 of 9 patients had weakness on examination when testing the rotator cuff. All nine patients had pain with extremes of motion and resisted forward flexion.

R. Papandrea, MD

Botulinum Toxin is Detrimental to Repair of a Chronic Rotator Cuff Tear in a Rabbit Model

Gilotra M, Nguyen T, Christian M, et al (Univ of Maryland, Baltimore)
J Orthop Res 33:1152-1157, 2015

Re-tear continues to be a problem after rotator cuff repair. Intramuscular botulinum toxin (Botox) injection can help optimize tension at the repair site to promote healing but could have an adverse effect on the degenerated muscle in a chronic tear. We hypothesized that Botox injection would improve repair characteristics without adverse effect on the muscle in a chronic rotator cuff tear model. The supraspinatus tendon of both shoulders in 14 rabbits underwent delayed repair 12 weeks after transection. One shoulder was treated with intramuscular Botox injection and the other with a saline control injection. Six weeks after repair, outcomes were based on biomechanics, histology, and magnetic resonance imaging. Botox-treated repairs were significantly weaker (2.64 N) than control repairs (5.51 N, $p = 0.03$). Eighty percent of Botox-treated repairs and 40% of control repairs healed with some partial defect. Fatty infiltration of the supraspinatus was present in all shoulders (Goutallier Grade 3 or 4) but was increased in the setting of Botox. This study provides additional support for the rabbit supraspinatus model of chronic cuff tear, showing consistent fatty infiltration. Contrary to our hypothesis, Botox had a negative effect on repair strength and might increase fatty infiltration.

▶ Rotator cuff repair outcomes have been studied extensively, and unfortunately failure rates are relatively high. Tear chronicity and larger tear size are associated with higher repair failure rates. Research continues in a search for modifiable patient factors and improved repair techniques to improve tendon healing and reduce retear rates. Many authors seek to determine the ideal postoperative rehabilitation protocol. Postoperative protocols seek to gain return of motion and function while also providing adequate protection of the repair to promote tendon healing. This study sought to determine if improved healing would be achieved if repair site tension was decreased with intramuscular

Botox injection. This study found Botox-treated repairs were weaker than controls.

In a study by Galatz et al[1] it was shown with a rat model that intramuscular Botox and immobilization had a detrimental effect on tendon healing. Galatz et al evaluated an acute tear, whereas this study by Gilotra et al evaluated a chronic tear in a rabbit model. Together these studies show that removal of load on either an acute or chronic tear negatively affects healing of the repaired tendon. These findings suggest that exposing a repair to some load is beneficial. This information may lead surgeons to use a more liberal rehabilitation protocol including initiating range of motion at an earlier date.

A. K. Harrison, MD

Reference

1. Galatz LM, Charlton N, Das R, et al. Complete removal of load is detrimental to rotator cuff healing. *J Shoulder Elbow Surg.* 2009;18:669-675.

Does Rotator Cuff Repair Improve Psychologic Status and Quality of Life in Patients With Rotator Cuff Tear?

Cho C-H, Song K-S, Hwang I, et al (Keimyung Univ, Daegu, Korea; et al)
Clin Orthop Relat Res 473:3494-3500, 2015

Background.—Recently, psychological status, patient-centered outcomes, and health-related quality of life (HRQoL) in patients with scheduled or who underwent orthopaedic surgeries have been emphasized. The relationship between preoperative psychological status and postoperative clinical outcome in patients with rotator cuff repair has not yet been investigated.

Questions/Purposes.—The primary objective of this study was to investigate changes in psychological status (depression, anxiety, insomnia) and HRQoL after rotator cuff repair. The secondary objective was to assess whether preoperative depression, anxiety, and insomnia predict clinical outcome after rotator cuff repair.

Methods.—Forty-seven patients who underwent rotator cuff repair prospectively completed the visual analog scale (VAS) pain score, the UCLA Scale, the American Shoulder and Elbow Surgeons' Scale (ASES), the Hospital Anxiety and Depression Scale (HADS), the Pittsburgh Sleep Quality Index (PSQI), and the World Health Organization Quality-of-life Scale Abbreviated Version (WHOQOL-BREF) before surgery and at 3, 6, and 12 months after surgery. Repeated-measures analysis of variance was used to evaluate the serial changes in psychological parameters and outcome measurements. The chi-square test was also used to compare preoperative and postoperative prevalence of depression, anxiety, and insomnia. Finally, multiple regression analysis was applied to determine the relationship between preoperative psychological status and postoperative clinical outcome.

Results.—With surgery, depression, anxiety, and insomnia decreased, whereas quality of life increased. The mean HADS-D and HADS-A scores and the mean PSQI score decreased from 3.7 ± 3.3, 4.3 ± 4.3, and 6.6 ± 3.6, respectively, before surgery to 2.1 ± 2.3, 1.4 ± 2.4, and 4.2 ± 3.3, respectively, at 12 months after surgery (HADS-D mean difference 1.6 [95% confidence interval {CI}, 0.6–2.6], $p = 0.003$; HADS-A mean difference 2.9 [1.5–4.4], $p < 0.001$; PSQI mean difference 2.4 [1.3–3.4], $p < 0.001$). The mean WHOQOL-BREF score increased from 60.4 ± 11.0 before surgery to 67.4 ± 11.8 at 12 months after surgery (mean difference −7.0 [95% CI, −10.7 to −3.4], $p < 0.001$). At 12 months after surgery, there were decreases in the prevalence of depression (six of 47 [22.8%] versus three of 47 [6.4%], $p = 0.002$), anxiety (11 of 47 [23.4%] versus two of 47 [4.3%], $p = 0.016$), and insomnia (33 of 47 [70.2%] versus 20 of 47 [42.6%], $p = 0.022$). Preoperative HADS-depression, HADS-anxiety, and PSQI scores did not correlate with the VAS pain score, UCLA, or ASES scores at 12 months after surgery.

Conclusions.—Psychological status and HRQoL improved with decreasing pain and increasing functional ability from 3 months after surgery. Preoperative depression, anxiety, and insomnia did not predict poor outcome after rotator cuff repair. Our findings suggest that successful rotator cuff repair may improve psychological status and HRQoL.

Level of Evidence.—Level II, prospective study.

▶ Patient-reported outcomes and changes in quality of life after surgical procedures are increasingly important measures and topics of study. Although there is literature documenting that patients' psychological health affects rotator cuff repair outcomes, there is limited study documenting changes in psychological status or any relationship between preoperative psychological state and postoperative outcome. These authors found that rotator cuff repair improved psychological status and health-related quality of life.

This article is timely and relevant to current practice as surgeons look to identify patients for whom surgery will lead to a relatively predictable positive result. It has long been known that patient factors play a role in surgical outcomes, and there is increasing evidence that patient psychological health affects outcomes for various procedures. Understanding these factors is an important aspect of surgical decision making with the patient. In addition, health care will need to increasingly show value; therefore, it is important to establish the effect of surgery on quality of life. This study found that after rotator cuff repair, patients had improved depression, anxiety, and insomnia. It is equally important that preoperative psychological status did not affect outcome measures. Preoperative anxiety and depression should not be considered a contraindication for rotator cuff repair or assumed to be associated with poorer postoperative outcomes. In fact, rotator cuff repair may improve some patients' psychological health.

A. K. Harrison, MD

What Is the Prevalence of Senior-athlete Rotator Cuff Injuries and Are They Associated With Pain and Dysfunction?

McMahon PJ, Prasad A, Francis KA (Univ of Pittsburgh, PA; Univ of Pittsburgh Med Ctr, PA)
Clin Orthop Relat Res 472:2427-2432, 2014

Background.—Older individuals with rotator cuff injuries may have difficulties not only with activities of daily living, but also with sports activities.

Questions/Purposes.—(1) How frequent and severe are rotator cuff abnormalities, as identified by ultrasound, in senior athletes? (2) To what degree does the severity of ultrasound-identified rotator cuff pathology correlate with pain and shoulder dysfunction?

Methods.—We assessed pain and shoulder function in 141 elite athletes older than 60 years of age (median age, 70 years; range 60—84) at the Senior Olympics who volunteered to participate. An ultrasound evaluation of the rotator cuff of the dominant shoulder was performed by an experienced musculoskeletal radiologist in all of these elite athletes. We then determined the relationship between ultrasound findings and shoulder pain and shoulder function as assessed with the Disabilities of the Arm, Shoulder and Hand (DASH) and American Shoulder and Elbow Surgeons (ASES) scores.

Results.—There were 20 shoulders with a normal cuff (14.2% [20 of 141], of which 5% [one of 20] were painful), 23 with tendinosis (16.3% [23 of 141], of which 30% [six of 20] were painful), 68 with a partial-thickness rotator cuff tear (48.2% [68 of 141], of which 32% [20 of 63] were painful), and 30 with a full-thickness rotator cuff tear (21.3% [30 of 141], of which 25% [seven of 28] were painful). Only 5% of athletes (one of 20) with a normal cuff on ultrasound evaluation reported shoulder pain, whereas 30% of athletes (33 of 111) with any degree of rotator cuff damage on ultrasound evaluation reported shoulder pain, This resulted in an odds ratio of 8.0 (95% confidence interval, 1.0—62.5). The proportion of patients who had pain was not different in those with different severities of rotator cuff pathology. Neither the ASES nor the DASH was different in those with different severities.

Conclusions.—The frequency of full-thickness rotator cuff tears in senior athletes was 21.3% (30 of 141). Pain was a predictor of rotator cuff injury but not of its severity. The odds of having shoulder pain was eight times greater in those athletes with any rotator cuff damage as compared with those without any rotator cuff damage. Those with pain had poorer shoulder function but the ASES and DASH were poor predictors of the severity of rotator cuff pathology. Rotator cuff tears in older individuals are often not painful and may not need to be repaired for successful participation in athletics.

Level of Evidence.—Level II, prognostic study. See Guidelines for Authors for a complete description of levels of evidence.

▶ The title is a bit ambitious, but this article is a nice addition to the literature. By looking at a group of athletes at the Senior Olympics, the authors give us a better understanding of rotator cuff disease in the ever-increasing population of senior athletes in our practice.

We already know that occurrences of rotator cuff conditions increase steadily with age. However, it is nice to be reassured that most rotator cuff disease (65% to 75%) remains asymptomatic even in high-demand seniors. Moreover, just like their younger counterparts, the severity of rotator cuff disease in seniors does not correspond with the severity of symptoms.

K. Bengston, MD

Fluoroquinolones Impair Tendon Healing in a Rat Rotator Cuff Repair Model: A Preliminary Study

Fox AJS, Schär MO, Wanivenhaus F, et al (Hosp for Special Surgery, NY)
Am J Sports Med 2014;42:2851-2859

Background.—Recent studies suggest that fluoroquinolone antibiotics predispose tendons to tendinopathy and/or rupture. However, no investigations on the reparative capacity of tendons exposed to fluoroquinolones have been conducted.

Hypothesis.—Fluoroquinolone-treated animals will have inferior biochemical, histological, and biomechanical properties at the healing tendon-bone enthesis compared with controls.

Study Design.—Controlled laboratory study.

Methods.—Ninety-two rats underwent rotator cuff repair and were randomly assigned to 1 of 4 groups: (1) preoperative (Preop), whereby animals received fleroxacin for 1 week preoperatively; (2) pre- and postoperative (Pre/Postop), whereby animals received fleroxacin for 1 week preoperatively and for 2 weeks postoperatively; (3) postoperative (Postop), whereby animals received fleroxacin for 2 weeks postoperatively; and (4) control, whereby animals received vehicle for 1 week preoperatively and for 2 weeks postoperatively. Rats were euthanized at 2 weeks postoperatively for biochemical, histological, and biomechanical analysis. All data were expressed as mean ± standard error of the mean (SEM). Statistical comparisons were performed using either 1-way or 2-way ANOVA, with $P < .05$ considered significant.

Results.—Reverse transcriptase quantitative polymerase chain reaction (RTqPCR) analysis revealed a 30-fold increase in expression of matrix metalloproteinase (MMP)-3, a 7-fold increase in MMP-13, and a 4-fold increase in tissue inhibitor of metalloproteinases (TIMP)-1 in the Pre/Postop group compared with the other groups. The appearance of the healing enthesis in all treated animals was qualitatively different than that in controls. The tendons were friable and atrophic. All 3 treated groups showed significantly less fibrocartilage and poorly organized collagen at the healing enthesis compared with control animals. There was a significant difference in the mode of failure, with treated animals demonstrating an intrasubstance failure of the supraspinatus tendon during testing. In contrast, only 1 of 10 control samples failed within the tendon substance. The healing enthesis of the Pre/Postop group displayed significantly reduced ultimate load to failure compared with the Preop, Postop, and control groups. There was no significant difference in load to failure in the Preop group compared with the Postop group. Pre/Postop animals demonstrated significantly reduced cross-sectional area compared with the Postop and control groups. There was also a significant reduction in area between the Preop and control groups.

Conclusion.—In this preliminary study, fluoroquinolone treatment negatively influenced tendon healing.

Clinical Relevance.—These findings indicate that there was an active but inadequate repair response that has potential clinical implications for patients who are exposed to fluoroquinolones before tendon repair surgery.

▶ In this study, the authors show that alterations in inflammatory-driven extracellular matrix remodeling may contribute to fluoroquinolone-induced tendon damage and that fluoroquinolones have no effect on extracellular matrix production but rather promote the production of a lower quality matrix. Their histologic results indicate that fibrocartilage formation and collagen organization at the repair site were deleteriously altered by the administration of fluoroquinolones, whether the drug was administered preoperatively, postoperatively, or both. All animals treated with this antibiotic had a significant reduction in fibrocartilage and Sharpey's fibers at the healing site, thereby indicating inferior osseous integration of tendon to bone. They found that fluoroquinolone-treated tendons had significantly reduced load to failure in a cross-sectional area compared with control specimens, and they noted a predilection for midsubstance rupture of the tendon as opposed to the control animals in which the ruptures occurred at the repair site. The authors did not detect any differences in stiffness, Young's modulus, maximum stress, or energy to failure among the groups; thus, they suggested that longer periods after surgery may be required to examine alterations in biomechanical properties rather than the single time point of 2 weeks postoperatively used to examine the effects of the antibiotic. At the time of harvest, the preoperative-only group showed no evidence of systematic fluoroquinolone antibiotic in the serum; however, there were statistically significant changes in both reduction in tendon cross-sectional area and the area of fibrocartilage at the point of healing. The usual mode of failure was intrasubstance failure of the tendon after repair. The authors suggest that fluoroquinolone administration preoperatively has a negative influence on the overall success of the repair. They noted that the use of the antibiotic postoperatively had an even more deleterious effect compared with that of the preoperative state. The authors then speculated their results applying their model to humans, recommending delaying surgery by at least 6 weeks if a patient had taken pre-operative fluoroquinolone antibiotics. However, they admit that this recommendation is relatively arbitrary. The limitations of this study are as follows: The antibiotic chosen, fleroxacin, was intentionally chosen because of its known deleterious properties on tendons, yet the drug is not a commonly used fluoroquinolone antibiotic in humans; therefore, this antibiotic is not representative of the class in general. The authors also noted that the rats treated with the antibiotic all had postoperative weight loss consistent with general malaise along with reduced feeding and lethargy. This finding may also be one of the reasons why the tendons failed, relating to the systematic effects of poor nutrition. Their model was that of an acute injury, whereas most rotator cuff repair and tendon repairs done in humans are done for chronic tendinopathy and chronic tears. The tissue in these states is not representative of the acute, traumatic injury; therefore, this finding may not be generally applicable to the repair of chronic tendon tears. Finally, the animal study was done only once at a single snapshot in time (the 2-week period). Longer periods, and perhaps longer periods of antibiotic administration, may be necessary to understand the deleterious effects of fluoroquinolones on tendon repair. There are existing models that look at the repair of chronic tendon tears, and this study should likely be repeated using a chronic injury and repair model.

A. B. Shafritz, MD

Platelet-Rich Plasma for Arthroscopic Repair of Medium to Large Rotator Cuff Tears: A Randomized Controlled Trial

Jo CH, Shin JS, Shin WH, et al (Seoul Natl Univ College of Medicine, Korea)
Am J Sports Med 43:2102-2110, 2015

Background.—Two main questions about the use of platelet-rich plasma (PRP) for regeneration purposes are its effect on the speed of healing and the quality of healing. Despite recent numerous studies, evidence is still lacking in this area, especially in a representative patient population with medium to large rotator cuff tears.

Purpose.—To assess the efficacy of PRP augmentation on the speed and quality of healing in patients undergoing arthroscopic repair for medium to large rotator cuff tears.

Study Design.—Randomized controlled trial; Level of evidence, 1.

Methods.—A total of 74 patients scheduled for arthroscopic repair of medium to large rotator cuff tears were randomly assigned to undergo either PRP-augmented repair (PRP group) or conventional repair (conventional group). In the PRP group, 3 PRP gels (3 × 3 mL) were applied to each patient between the torn end and the greater tuberosity. The primary outcome was the Constant score at 3 months after surgery. Secondary outcome measures included the visual analog scale (VAS) for pain, range of motion (ROM), muscle strength, overall satisfaction and function, functional scores, retear rate, and change in the cross-sectional area (CSA) of the supraspinatus muscle.

Results.—There was no difference between the 2 groups in the Constant score at 3 months ($P > .05$). The 2 groups had similar results on the VAS for pain, ROM, muscle strength, overall satisfaction and function, and other functional scores (all $P > .05$) except for the VAS for worst pain ($P = .043$). The retear rate of the PRP group (3.0%) was significantly lower than that of the conventional group (20.0%) ($P = .032$). The change in 1-year postoperative and immediately postoperative CSAs was significantly different between the 2 groups: -36.76 ± 45.31 mm^2 in the PRP group versus -67.47 ± 47.26 mm^2 in the conventional group ($P = .014$).

Conclusion.—Compared with repairs without PRP augmentation, the current PRP preparation and application methods for medium to large rotator cuff repairs significantly improved the quality, as evidenced by a decreased retear rate and increased CSA of the supraspinatus, but not the speed of healing. However, further studies may be needed to investigate the effects of PRP on the speed of healing without risking the quality.

▶ The use of platelet-rich plasma (PRP) in rotator cuff repair is thought to potentially accelerate the speed of healing at early time points and to improve the quality of healing over time. The authors sought to evaluate 2 main potentials of PRP gel application on healing after rotator cuff repair: (1) whether it could accelerate the speed of healing measured by the Constant score at 3 months and (2) whether it could improve the quality of healing with assessment of the retear rate at 12 months after repair. Inclusion criteria were medium to large tears, which were randomly allocated to undergo traditional arthroscopic cuff repair (conventional group) versus arthroscopic cuff repair with PRP gel inserted at the bone-tendon interface placed after placement of the medial row anchors, followed by tying the medial knots and placement of the lateral row anchors.

The authors state that the most important findings of the study are that the application of PRP for rotator cuff repair in patients with medium to large rotator cuff tears improved the quality of healing but did not accelerate the speed of healing. Patients in the PRP group did not show higher Constant scores at 3 months. The only positive clinical finding was that the PRP group showed lower visual analog (VAS) measures of the worst pain than the conventional group ($P = .043$). Furthermore, American Shoulder And Elbow Surgeons, UCLA, and Shoulder Pain and Disability Index scores and VAS pain scores at rest and at night and mean pain scores significantly improved only in the conventional group at 3 months after surgery. However, the PRP group showed significant improvement in both structural outcomes compared with the conventional group: a 6-fold lower retear rate and a lower decrease in the measured surface area of the supraspinatus muscle. These results are in line with results of previous studies in different populations. Neither group showed any improvement or differences in clinical outcomes at 3 to 12 months after surgery compared with the control groups, but findings suggested improved structural outcomes at 1 year after repair. The authors suggest that the application of

PRP for rotator cuff repair is worthwhile, even though it may not provide improved clinical outcomes in the early period.

E. Cheung, MD

Early Versus Delayed Passive Range of Motion After Rotator Cuff Repair: A Systematic Review and Meta-analysis
Kluczynski MA, Nayyar S, Marzo JM, et al (State Univ of New York, Buffalo)
Am J Sports Med 43:2057-2063, 2015

Background.—Postoperative rehabilitation has been shown to affect healing of the rotator cuff after surgical repair. However, it is unknown whether an early or delayed rehabilitation protocol is most beneficial for healing.

Purpose.—To determine whether early versus delayed passive range of motion (PROM) affects rotator cuff (RC) retear rates after surgery.

Study Design.—Systematic review and meta-analysis.

Methods.—A systematic review of the literature published between January 2003 and February 2014 was conducted. Retear rates were compared for early (within 1 week after surgery) versus delayed (3-6 weeks after surgery) PROM using χ^2 or Fisher exact tests as well as relative risks (RR) and 95% CIs. In the first analysis, data from evidence level 1 studies that directly compared early versus delayed PROM were pooled; and in the second analysis, data from level 1 to 4 studies that did not directly compare early versus delayed PROM were pooled. The second analysis was stratified by tear size and repair method.

Results.—Twenty-eight studies (1729 repairs) were included. The first analysis of level 1 studies did not reveal a significant difference in retear rates for early (13.7%) versus delayed (10.5%) PROM ($P=.36$; RR = 1.30 [95% CI, 0.74-2.30]). The second analysis revealed that for 3 cm tears, the risk of retear was lower for early versus delayed PROM for transosseous (TO) plus single-row anchor (SA) repairs (18.7% vs 28.2%, $P=.02$; RR = 0.66 [95% CI, 0.47-0.95]). For >5 cm tears, the risk of retear was greater for early versus delayed PROM for double-row anchor (DA) repairs (56.4% vs 20%, $P=.002$; RR = 2.82 [95% CI, 1.31-6.07]) and for all repair methods combined (52.2% vs 22.6%, $P=.01$; RR = 2.31 [95% CI, 1.16-4.61]). There were no statistically significant associations for tears measuring <1 cm, 1 to 3 cm, 3 to 5 cm, and >3 cm.

Conclusion.—Evidence is lacking with regard to the optimal timing of PROM after RC repair; however, this study suggests that tear size may be influential.

▶ This was a systematic review looking at retear rates after rotator cuff repair (RCR). Background information includes the fact that retear rates after RCR have been reported to be as high as at least 20% in tears > 3 cm in size and at least 70% in tears > 5 cm in size. Factors that have been identified as influential to cuff healing include age, medical comorbidities, surgical technique, nicotine use, activity level, bone quality, rotator cuff tissue quality, tear size, and rehabilitation protocols. Animal studies have shown that early passive range of motion can promote type III collagen synthesis at the tendon-bone interface and allows for early collagen crosslinking. Rehabilitation protocols have frequently been based on expert opinion rather than scientific rationale. It is thought that perhaps early motion is critical to prevent postoperative adhesions but to protect integrity of the repair. In the past, clinical trials looking at early motion found no difference in healing and no difference in shoulder stiffness between early and delayed motion, but these studies have lower numbers of participants. The retear rate after analysis of Level I studies in this article found that there was no significant difference in retear rates in early versus late passive range of motion groups. However, for tear sizes > 5 cm, the retear rate was significantly higher, accounting for all repair techniques. This implies that for larger tears, it may be prudent to not start an early passive range of motion protocol.

E. Cheung, MD

18 Shoulder: Trauma

Long stem reverse shoulder arthroplasty and cerclage for treatment of complex long segment proximal humeral fractures with diaphyseal extension in patients more than 65 years old
Garofalo R, Flanagin B, Castagna A, et al (Shoulder Service F Miulli Hosp Acquaviva Delle Fonti-BA Italy; Shoulder Ctr Baylor Univ Med Ctr at Dallas; Shoulder and Elbow Unit IRCCS Humanitas Inst Milan Italy; et al)
Injury 46:2379-2383, 2015

Introduction.—Treatment of long segment proximal humeral fractures with extension below the surgical neck into the diaphysis remains a significant challenge for orthopaedic surgeons. The purpose of this paper was to evaluate the clinical and radiological outcomes following primary long-stem RSA with cerclage fixation for complex long segment proximal humeral fractures with diaphyseal extension in patients more than 65 years old.

Material and Methods.—Between February 2010 and March 2013, 22 patients who suffered a complex proximal humerus fracture with extended diaphyseal involvement underwent surgery with long-stem RSA and cerclages fixation. There were 17 female and 5 male patients, and the mean age was 77.2 years at time of surgery (range 65–84 years). All patients had a 3 or 4-part proximal humerus fracture or a two part fracture with a split of humeral head, with extension to the proximal diaphysis. Clinical and radiographic follow-up was performed on all 22 patients at 6 weeks, at 3, 6, and 12 months postoperatively, and then at 2 years. Clinical evaluation consisted of the shoulder rating Constant scale. X ray evaluation was done to evaluate fracture healing and eventually humeral and glenoid component loosening or other complications.

Results.—No infections were reported, neither other serious complications. Two patients developed a seroma and one patient developed chronic pain at that was treated with referral to pain management. No patients were lost at follow-up. At final follow-up, average active elevation was 132.5° (range 100°–140°), external rotation 30° (range 55°–10°). Average abduction was 120° (range 90°–135°). The mean adjusted Constant score was 72/100 (range 64–82). All fractures were healed within 3 months after surgery. No loosening of the humeral or glenoid components and no episodes of dislocation/instability were observed in this series. We did not observe scapular notching in any patient on the x-ray at most recent follow-up.

Conclusion.—Long-stem RSA with cerclages wire fixation represents a viable treatment option for complex long-segment displaced proximal humerus fractures with diaphyseal extension in patients older than 65 years. Our results suggest clinical outcomes at two years of follow up are satisfactory with an acceptable complication rate.

▶ The authors present a relatively large cohort of patients who underwent reverse total shoulder arthroplasty (RTSA) for the management of complex proximal humerus fracture with diaphyseal extension. These injuries represent the most severe end of the spectrum of proximal humerus fractures with a high potential for complications. The results are encouraging, supporting RTSA as a reliable alternative for the treatment of these fractures. No instability was observed, and overall satisfactory range of motion, pain control, and overall function were achieved. However, the readership should be reminded that cases were performed by highly experienced shoulder surgeons, raising the question of whether results are reproducible in less experienced hands.

A very detailed description of the surgical technique is provided. However, the results section is less concise. Specifically, little detail is provided on the final assessment of the humeral component. One of the many difficulties encountered in this clinical scenario is obtaining an optimal cement mantle. Because placement of the stem is frequently distal to the isthmus of the humeral shaft, cement plugs are usually unable to resist distal cement migration, frequently leading to less than ideal cement mantles. According to the Materials and Methods section, Sperling's criteria[1] were used to determine humeral component loosening. Although no loosening is reported, 2 of the provided pictures raise concerns for the potential of humeral stems at risk.

P. Streubel, MD

Reference

1. Sperling JW, Cofield RH, O'Driscoll SW, Torchia ME, Rowland CM. Radiographic assessment of ingrowth total shoulder arthroplasty. *J Shoulder Elbow Surg.* 2000;9:507-513.

Multicenter Randomized Clinical Trial of Nonoperative Versus Operative Treatment of Acute Acromio-Clavicular Joint Dislocation
The Canadian Orthopaedic Trauma Society ()
J Orthop Trauma 29:479-487, 2015

Objective.—To perform a randomized clinical trial of operative versus nonoperative treatment of acute acromio-clavicular (AC) joint dislocations using modern surgical fixation and both patient-based and surgeon-based outcome measures to determine which treatment method was superior.

Design.—Prospective, randomized.

Setting.—Multicenter.

Patients/Participants.—Eight-three patients with acute (<28 days from the time of injury) complete (grade III, IV, and V) dislocations of the AC joint.

Intervention.—Patients were randomized to operative repair with hook plate fixation versus nonoperative treatment (operative repair, 40; nonoperative treatment, 43).

Main Outcome Measurements.—Disabilities of the Arm, Shoulder and Hand (DASH) score at 1 year after injury. Assessment also included a complete clinical assessment, evaluation of the constant score, and a radiographic evaluation at 6 weeks, and at 3, 6, 12, and 24 months.

Results.—There were no demographic differences between the 2 groups, and the mechanisms of injury were similar between the 2 groups. The DASH scores (a disability score, lower score is better) were significantly better in the nonoperative group at 6 weeks (operative, 45; nonoperative, 31; $P = 0.014$) and 3 months (operative, 29; nonoperative, 16; $P = 0.005$). There were no significant differences between the groups at 6 months (operative, 14; nonoperative, 12; $P = 0.442$), 1 year (operative, 9; nonoperative, 9; $P = 0.997$), or 2 years (operative, 5; nonoperative, 6; $P = 0.439$) after injury. Constant scores were similar (better scores in the nonoperative group at 6 weeks, 3 months, and 6 months; $P = 0.0001$; and no difference thereafter). Although radiographic results were better in the operative group, the reoperation rate was significantly lower in the nonoperative group ($P < 0.05$).

Conclusions.—Although hook plate fixation resulted in superior radiographic alignment, it was not clinically superior to nonoperative treatment of acute complete dislocations of the AC joint. The nonoperative group had better early scores, although both groups improved from a significant level of initial disability to a good or excellent result (mean DASH score, 5–6; mean constant score, 91–95) at 2 years. At present, there is no clear evidence that operative treatment with the currently available hook plate improves short-term outcome for complete AC joint dislocations.

▶ The authors present an interesting study comparing operative versus nonoperative treatment for acute acromioclavicular joint dislocation. This study is significant because there is still no consensus on which is the best treatment modality for this type of lesion. The main strength of the study is its comparative design. The same surgery and the same nonoperative protocol were done for all patients. It is not easy to have so many cases when inclusion criteria are strict. The main weakness involves grouping types III, IV, and V for operative treatment. Previous studies have shown similar results for type III lesions. There is no comparative study like this one for type V lesions only. As a reader, I would have liked to know how this subgroup of patients did. But as a whole, it is good to know that in the short-term nonoperative treatment will do better, and final results will be the same for both types of treatment (Figs. 3-5), as long

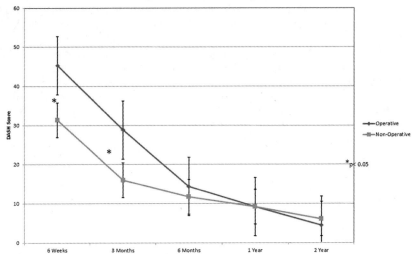

FIGURE 3.—DASH scores of the operative and nonoperative groups (mean scores; error bars represent standard error of the mean; SEM). DASH scores were significantly lower (better) in the nonoperative group at 6 and 12 weeks postoperatively. *Editor's note*: A color image accompanies the online version of this article. (Reprinted from The Canadian Orthopaedic Trauma Society. Multicenter randomized clinical trial of nonoperative versus operative treatment of acute acromio-clavicular joint dislocation. *J Orthop Trauma*. 2015;29:479-487, with permission from Wolters Kluwer Health, Inc.)

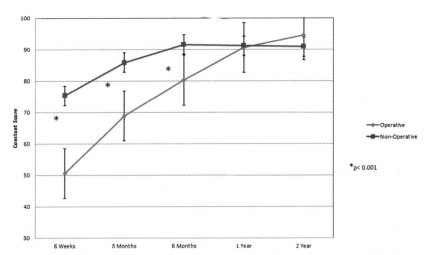

FIGURE 4.—Constant scores of the operative and nonoperative groups (mean scores and SEM bars). Constant scores were significantly better (higher) in the nonoperative group at 6 and 12 weeks postoperatively. *Editor's note*: A color image accompanies the online version of this article. (Reprinted from The Canadian Orthopaedic Trauma Society. Multicenter randomized clinical trial of nonoperative versus operative treatment of acute acromio-clavicular joint dislocation. *J Orthop Trauma*. 2015;29:479-487, with permission from Wolters Kluwer Health, Inc.)

Return to Work

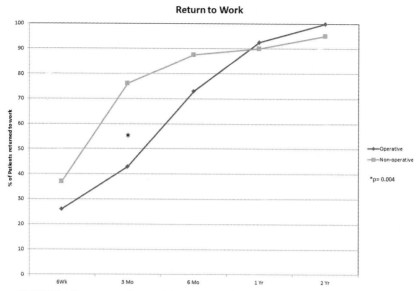

FIGURE 5.—Return-to-work rates of the operative and nonoperative groups. Patients in the nonoperative group returned to work more quickly than those in the operative group, although by a year after injury, almost all patients had returned to their preinjury work status. *Editor's note*: A color image accompanies the online version of this article. (Reprinted from The Canadian Orthopaedic Trauma Society. Multicenter randomized clinical trial of nonoperative versus operative treatment of acute acromio-clavicular joint dislocation. *J Orthop Trauma*. 2015;29:479-487, with permission from Wolters Kluwer Health, Inc.)

as the patient understands that cosmetic results will be different. Long-term follow-up is needed to draw further conclusions. In general, I treat type III lesions nonoperatively and types IV, V, and VI with surgery. With new evidence such as that presented in this study, counseling for nonoperative treatment in the last group is an option.

J. P. Simone, MD

A Comparison of the Charlson and Elixhauser Comorbidity Measures to Predict Inpatient Mortality After Proximal Humerus Fracture

Menendez ME, Ring D (Harvard Med School, Boston, MA)
J Orthop Trauma 29:488-493, 2015

Objectives.—Proximal humerus fractures are very common in infirm elderly patients and are associated with appreciable inpatient mortality. We sought to compare the discriminative ability of the Charlson and Elixhauser comorbidity measures for predicting inpatient mortality after proximal humerus fractures.

Methods.—Data from the Nationwide Inpatient Sample (2002—2011) were obtained. We constructed 2 main multivariable logistic regression models, with inpatient mortality as the dependent variable and 1 of the

2 comorbidity scores, as well as age and sex, as independent variables. A base model that contained only age and sex was also evaluated. The predictive performance of the Charlson and Elixhauser comorbidity measures was assessed and compared using the area under the receiver operating characteristic curve (AUC) derived from these regression models.

Results.—Elixhauser comorbidity adjustment provided better discrimination of inpatient mortality [AUC = 0.840, 95% confidence interval (CI), 0.828–0.853] than the Charlson model (AUC = 0.786, 95% CI, 0.771–0.801) and the base model without comorbidity adjustment (AUC = 0.722, 95% CI, 0.705–0.740). In terms of relative improvement in predictive ability, the Elixhauser score performed 46% better than the Charlson score.

Conclusions.—Given that inadequate comorbidity risk adjustment can unfairly penalize hospitals and surgeons that care for a disproportionate share of infirm and sick patients, wider adoption of the Elixhauser measure for mortality prediction after proximal humerus fracture—and perhaps other musculoskeletal injuries—merits to be considered.

▶ Because reimbursement of hospitals and physicians is increasingly tied to patient outcomes, predictors of outcome are necessary to create a basis for the measurement of performance. The use of comorbidity measures for specific conditions has become more commonplace in nonorthopedic specialties. Using data from the Nationwide Inpatient Sample, the authors of this study compared 2 comorbidity measures for patients with a diagnosis of proximal humerus fracture. In this study, the Elixhauser comorbidity measure provided better discrimination of inpatient mortality than the Charlson index. Based on this finding, the authors suggest that the Elixhauser comorbidity measure may provide a more accurate picture when considering patient outcomes for proximal humerus fracture and other forms of shoulder trauma.

W. T. Payne, MD

The Interrater and Intrarater Agreement of a Modified Neer Classification System and Associated Treatment Choice for Lateral Clavicle Fractures
Cho C-H, Oh JH, Jung G-H, et al (Keimyung Univ School of Medicine, Daegu, South Korea; Seoul Natl Univ College of Medicine, Seongnam, South Korea; Kosin Univ School of Medicine, Busan, South Korea; et al)
Am J Sports Med 43:2431-2436, 2015

Background.—As there is substantial variation in the classification and diagnosis of lateral clavicle fractures, proper management can be challenging. Although the Neer classification system modified by Craig has been widely used, no study has assessed its validity through inter- and intrarater agreement.

Purpose.—To determine the inter- and intrarater agreement of the modified Neer classification system and associated treatment choice for lateral clavicle fractures and to assess whether 3-dimensional computed tomography (3D CT) improves the level of agreement.

Study Design.—Cohort study (diagnosis); Level of evidence, 3.

Methods.—Nine experienced shoulder specialists and 9 orthopaedic fellows evaluated 52 patients with lateral clavicle fractures, completing fracture typing according to the modified Neer classification system and selecting a treatment choice for each case. Web-based assessment was performed using plain radiographs only, followed by the addition of 3D CT images 2 weeks later. This procedure was repeated 4 weeks later. Fleiss κ values were calculated to estimate the inter- and intrarater agreement.

Results.—Based on plain radiographs only, the inter- and intrarater agreement of the modified Neer classification system was regarded as fair (κ = 0.344) and moderate (κ = 0.496), respectively; the inter- and intrarater agreement of treatment choice was both regarded as moderate (κ = 0.465 and 0.555, respectively). Based on the plain radiographs and 3D CT images, the inter- and intrarater agreement of the classification system was regarded as fair (κ = 0.317) and moderate (κ = 0.508), respectively; the inter- and intrarater agreement of treatment choice was regarded as moderate (κ = 0.463) and substantial (κ = 0.623), respectively. There were no significant differences in the level of agreement between the plain radiographs only and plain radiographs plus 3D CT images for any κ values (all *P* > .05).

Conclusion.—The level of interrater agreement of the modified Neer classification system for lateral clavicle fractures was fair. Additional 3D CT did not improve the overall level of interrater or intrarater agreement of the modified Neer classification system or associated treatment choice. To eliminate a common source of disagreement among surgeons, a new classification system to focus on unclassifiable fracture types is needed.

▶ Surgeons continue to exert effort into categorizing injuries for both reporting and treatment decisions. The spectrum of injuries that results from trauma rarely is such that it can be truly compartmentalized into a classification system of only a few types. With limited categories, there will always be injuries that defy classification.

Studies that look to measure agreement in a classification often force the subjects to place an injury into some category, even when the subject knows that the injury is such that it does not truly fit into any of the predetermined categories. This study included images of their "case 1," which perfectly demonstrate the difficulty of a system that does not include a pattern demonstrated on images.

The conclusion that a new classification is needed is not a surprise, given the fair agreement on classification and the finding that 3-dimensional compute tomography images did not improve classification.

R. Papandrea, MD

Surgical Versus Conservative Treatments for Displaced Midshaft Clavicular Fractures: A Systematic Review of Overlapping Meta-Analyses

Zhao J-G, Wang J, Long L (Tianjin Hosp, China)
Medicine (Baltimore) 94:e1057, 2015

Multiple meta-analyses have been performed to compare surgical and conservative interventions for treating displaced midshaft clavicular fractures. But conclusions are discordant.

The purposes of current study were (1) to conduct a systematic review of meta-analyses comparing surgical and conservative interventions for the treatment of displaced midshaft clavicular fractures, (2) to help decision makers interpret and choose among discordant meta-analyses, and (3) to provide treatment recommendations through the best available evidence.

We searched the Cochrane library, PubMed, and EMBASE databases to identify meta-analyses comparing surgical and conservative treatments for the displaced midshaft clavicular fractures. Two investigators independently scanned titles and abstracts to exclude irrelevant articles and identify meta-analyses that met the eligibility criteria. The methodological quality of the meta-analysis was independently assessed by the two investigators using the Oxford Centre for Evidence-based Medicine Levels of Evidence and the Assessment of Multiple Systematic Reviews (AMSTAR) tool. The Jadad decision algorithm was applied to determine which of the included studies provided the best available evidence.

Six meta-analyses met the eligibility criteria in this systematic review. AMSTAR scores ranged from 5 to 10. The Jadad decision-making tool suggests that the highest quality review should be selected based on the publication characteristics of the primary trials, the methodology of the primary trials, the language restrictions, and whether analysis of data on individual patients was included in the study. As a result, we selected a high-quality Cochrane review.

This systematic review of overlapping meta-analyses comparing surgical and conservative treatments suggests that surgical treatment provides a lower rate of overall treatment failure and a better functional outcome, but is associated with more implant-related complications. Hence, treatment should be individualized, with careful consideration of the advantages and disadvantages of each treatment method and of patient preferences.

▶ The authors correctly highlight the discordance in previously published meta-analyses comparing the surgical and nonsurgical treatment of displaced, midshaft clavicle fractures. They reviewed 6 meta-analyses published between 2012 and 2014 and applied the Jaddad Decision Algorithm[1] to determine which study provided the best available evidence to guide treatment decisions. Ultimately, the Cochrane review by Lenza[2] was determined to have the highest quality of included studies. However, the conclusion of that review does not solve this clinical question. The data remain inconclusive, and each patient should be treated individually. This review, in my opinion, underscores the limitations of meta-analyses in providing quality treatment guidelines. Even a well-executed meta-analysis can have significant bias and limited applicability, if the included studies are flawed. I commend the authors for attempting to achieve clarity on this clinical question, but despite 6 meta-analyses on the same question in a 2-year time span, they reached a rather lackluster conclusion.

A. T. Moeller, MD

References

1. Jadad AR, Cook DJ, Browman GP. A guide to interpreting discordant systematic review. *CMAJ.* 1997;156:1411-1416.
2. Lenza M, Buchbinder R, Johnston RV, Belloti JC, Faloppa F. Surgical verus conservative interventions for treating fractures of the middle third of the clavicle. *Cochrane Database Systematic Rev.* 2013;6:CD009363.

Bilateral weighted radiographs are required for accurate classification of acromioclavicular separation: An observational study of 59 cases
Ibrahim EF, Forrest NP, Forester A (Charing Cross Hosp, London, United Kingdom)
Injury 46:1900-1905, 2015

Introduction.—Misinterpretation of the Rockwood classification system for acromioclavicular joint (ACJ) separations has resulted in a trend towards using unilateral radiographs for grading. Further, the use of weighted views to 'unmask' a grade III injury has fallen out of favour. Recent evidence suggests that many radiographic grade III injuries represent only a partial injury to the stabilising ligaments. This study aimed to determine (1) whether accurate classification is possible on unilateral radiographs and (2) the efficacy of weighted bilateral radiographs in unmasking higher-grade injuries.

Methods.—Complete bilateral non-weighted and weighted sets of radiographs for patients presenting with an acromioclavicular separation over a 10-year period were analysed retrospectively, and they were graded I—VI according to Rockwood's criteria. Comparison was made between grading based on (1) a single antero-posterior (AP) view of the injured side, (2) bilateral non-weighted views and (3) bilateral weighted views. Radiographic measurements for cases that changed grade after weighted views were statistically compared to see if this could have been predicted beforehand.

Results.—Fifty-nine sets of radiographs on 59 patients (48 male, mean age of 33 years) were included. Compared with unilateral radiographs, non-weighted bilateral comparison films resulted in a grade change for 44 patients (74.5%). Twenty-eight of 56 patients initially graded as I, II or III were upgraded to grade V and two of three initial grade V patients were downgraded to grade III. The addition of a weighted view further upgraded 10 patients to grade V. No grade II injury was changed to grade III and no injury of any severity was downgraded by a weighted view. Grade III injuries upgraded on weighted views had a significantly greater baseline median percentage coracoclavicular distance increase than those that were not upgraded (80.7% vs. 55.4%, $p = 0.015$). However, no cut-off point for this value could be identified to predict an upgrade.

Conclusions.—The accurate classification of ACJ separation requires weighted bilateral comparative views. Attempts to predict grade on a single AP radiograph result in a gross underestimation of severity. The value of bilateral weighted views is to 'unmask' a grade V injury, and it is recommended as a first-line investigation.

▶ The authors present a retrospective radiographic study to determine whether acromioclavicular joint (ACJ) separation can be accurately classified based on unilateral radiographs and the efficacy of weighted bilateral radiographs in unmasking higher-grade injuries. Compared with unilateral radiographs, nonweighted bilateral radiographs showed that 28 of 56 (50%) injuries initially classified as Rockwood I, II, or III were upgraded to grade V, and 2 of 3 (66%) injuries classified as grade V were downgraded to grade III, refuting the ability for unilateral films to accurately determine the grade of injury. When comparing nonweighted versus weighted bilateral films, an additional 10 grade III injuries were upgraded to grade V with no injuries being downgraded. If the assumption is made that most surgeons would treat grade I, II, and III injuries nonoperatively and grade V operatively, 27 of 59 (46%) patients would have been advised for nonoperative treatment based on unilateral radiographs and operative treatment based on bilateral weighted radiographs. The authors conclude that accurate ACJ separation classification requires weighted bilateral radiographs with unilateral images underestimating the severity of the injury.

Given the variability in the relationship between the articular surface of the clavicle and acromion (overriding, underriding, incongruent) and the normal variation in the coracoclavicular distance, it is my practice to routinely get bilateral anteroposterior radiographs, preferably on the same film, and to focus primarily on the coracoclavicular distance. The radiographic protocol in my clinic is to obtain a weighted bilateral view that can occasionally be difficult in the acute setting secondary to discomfort and muscle spasm. Furthermore, I always obtain an axillary lateral view to identify a potential grade IV injury, which was mentioned in the study but not analyzed for the results. I am in agreement with the authors that further studies correlating MRI with radiographs and ultimately with clinical outcomes would be extremely helpful in determining the optimal management of ACJ separation.

E. Gauger, MD

Reverse shoulder arthroplasty as a salvage procedure after failed internal fixation of fractures of the proximal humerus: outcomes and complications
Hussey MM, Hussey SE, Mighell MA (Florida Orthopaedic Inst)
Bone Joint J 97-B:967-972, 2015

Failed internal fixation of a fracture of the proximal humerus produces many challenges with limited surgical options. The aim of this study was to evaluate the clinical outcomes after the use of a reverse shoulder arthroplasty under these circumstances. Between 2007 and 2012, 19 patients (15 women and four men, mean age 66 years; 52 to 82) with failed internal fixation after a proximal humeral fracture, underwent implant removal and reverse shoulder arthroplasty (RSA). The mean follow-up was 36 months (25 to 60). The mean American Shoulder and Elbow Score improved from 27.8 to 50.1 ($p = 0.019$). The mean Simple Shoulder Test score improved from 0.7 to 3.2 ($p = 0.020$), and the mean visual analogue scale for pain improved from 6.8 to 4.3 ($p = 0.012$). Mean forward flexion improved from 58.7° to 101.1° ($p < 0.001$), mean abduction from 58.7° to 89.1° ($p = 0.012$), mean external rotation from 10.7° to 23.1° ($p = 0.043$) and mean internal rotation from buttocks to L4 ($p = 0.034$). A major complication was recorded in five patients (26%) (one intra-operative fracture, loosening of the humeral component in two and two peri-prosthetic fractures). A total of 15 patients (79%) rated their outcome as excellent or good, one (5%) as satisfactory, and three (16%) as unsatisfactory.

An improvement in outcomes and pain can be expected when performing a RSA as a salvage procedure after failed internal fixation of a fracture of the proximal humerus. Patients should be cautioned about the possibility for major complications following this technically demanding procedure.

▶ Management of failed operative treatment of proximal humerus fractures represents one of the most difficult clinical scenarios in shoulder surgery. The study by Hussey et al further supports this notion. The authors present a consecutive series of patients treated by a single surgeon with reverse total shoulder arthroplasty (RTSA) for treatment of failed operative fixation of proximal humerus fractures. Although 84% of patients rated their overall outcomes as either excellent, good, or satisfactory, only modest improvements in shoulder function were achieved based on average American Shoulder and Elbow Score (ASES) and Simple Shoulder Test (SST) scores. The 2.3-point improvement in SST scores barely reached the minimal clinically significant difference as reported by Tashjian et al.[1] Furthermore, the average visual analogue scale score for pain only improved from 6.8 to 4.3. This difference, although significant, suggests that, on average, patients cannot reliably be counseled on RTSA, predictably offering a pain-free shoulder in this setting. The modest improvement in function and pain comes with a major complication occurring in one-quarter of patients and 16% requiring an additional surgical intervention.

The utility of operative treatment of displaced proximal humerus fractures has recently come under increased scrutiny with increasing levels of evidence.[2] This study further underlines the need for carefully selecting patients for operative proximal humerus fracture fixation, as failure of such treatment currently has no easy solution.

P. Streubel, MD

References

1. Tashjian RZ, Deloach J, Green A, Porucznik CA, Powell AP. Minimal clinically important differences in ASES and simple shoulder test scores after nonoperative treatment of rotator cuff disease. *J Bone Joint Surg Am.* 2010;92:296-303.
2. Rangan A, Handoll H, Brealey S, et al. PROFHER Trial Collaborators. Surgical vs nonsurgical treatment of adults with displaced fractures of the proximal humerus: the PROFHER randomized clinical trial. *JAMA.* 2015;313:1037-1047.

Midterm outcome and complications after minimally invasive treatment of displaced proximal humeral fractures in patients younger than 70 years using the Humerusblock
Tauber M, Hirzinger C, Hoffelner T, et al (Paracelsus Med Univ, Salzburg, Austria; et al)
Injury 46:1914-1920, 2015

Introduction.—The Humerusblock (HB) represents a minimally invasive implant allowing for the stabilisation of proximal humeral fractures after closed or percutaneous reduction. The aim of the study was to perform a general clinical and radiological midterm follow-up focusing on the quality and complications in a large series of patients of younger age (<70 years).

Patients and Methods.—A total of 126 patients with an average age of 53.6 years treated surgically using the HB device were evaluated clinically using the Constant score (CS) and radiologically by biplanar radiographs after a mean follow-up time of 59 months. Thirty-three patients had a two-part fracture, 58 a three-part fracture and 35 a four-part fracture. Ultrasound imaging for bilateral rotator cuff evaluation was performed, and complications regarding implant failure, revision rate and post-traumatic avascular necrosis (AVN) were analysed.

Results.—The average CS was 77.3 points for the affected shoulder and 86.5 points for the unaffected shoulder ($P = 0.001$). The subjective shoulder value was 84.2%. Two-part fractures achieved 77.5 points, three-part fractures 81.7 points and four-part fractures 69.8 points. Surgical neck non-union was observed in 1.3% and AVN was observed in 11% associated with a CS of 46.4 points. Implant failure occurred in 9.6%. Varus malposition was present in 36%, and it was clinically relevant when exceeding 25°.

Conclusion.—Percutaneous fracture treatment using the HB achieves good functional outcomes with an acceptable complication rate. The rate of AVN was surprisingly high, especially in four-part fractures (26%), which presumably is due to the longer follow-up period. Varus malalignment was clinically relevant when exceeding 25°.

Study Design.—Retrospective case series (evidence-based medicine (EBM) level IV).

▶ In this report, the authors sought to study the outcomes of patients younger than 70 years who underwent minimally invasive open reduction and fixation of displaced proximal humerus fractures using a specially designed device called the Humerusblock. A total of 126 patients with an average age of 53.6 years

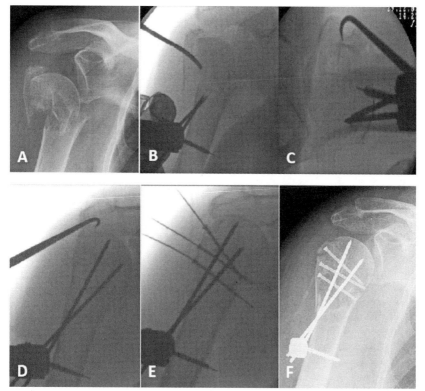

FIGURE 2.—(A) Valgus-impacted three-part fracture with displacement of the greater tuberosity and humerus shaft at the surgical neck level. (B) Intraoperative fluoroscopy imaging with the HB positioned at the humerus shaft. The K-wires are drilled until the surgical neck. The valgus-impacted articular segment is percutaneously reduced using an elevator. (C) An axillary view is performed to check the correct rotation of the humeral head and relationship between the head and shaft. Rotation can be controlled using a hook retractor. (D) After fixation of the articular segment by the two K-wires, the greater tuberosity is reduced by a hook retractor pulling it inferiorly and anteriorly. (E) Percutaneous fixation of the greater tuberosity is performed using cannulated screws. (F) Post-operative a.p. view shows anatomic fracture reduction with a centered glenohumeral joint. (Reprinted from Tauber M, Hirzinger C, Hoffelner T, et al. Midterm outcome and complications after minimally invasive treatment of displaced proximal humeral fractures in patients younger than 70 years using the Humerusblock. *Injury.* 2015;46:1914-1920, with permission from Elsevier.)

were treated with this device. Mean follow-up time was 59 months. The average constant score was 73.3 points for the postoperative shoulder and 86.5 points for the unaffected shoulder. Subjective shoulder value was 84.2%. Implant failure was noted in 9.6%. Even though these fractures were initially repaired anatomically with these devices, varus malposition occurred in 36% of patients. Varus malposition became clinically relevant affecting the patient's outcome if it exceeded 25°.

The Humerusblock device was developed by Synthes in Europe and was introduced in 1999 (Fig 2). This device is not approved for use in the United States. The device uses 2 locked 2.2-mm crossing k-wires inside a machined block that is affixed to cortical bone with a 4-mm screw. The device could be used in isolation or in association with cannulated percutaneous screws.

The authors report their results grouped by fracture type: 2-part, 3-part, and 4-part fractures. They summated their complications and postoperative range of motion as well. The authors noted that malunion occurred in 45 patients with an average of 13.4°. Fourteen patients (9.6%), had implant failure with loss of reduction and needed revision surgery (not simply hardware removal). Sixteen patients had avascular necrosis noted at final follow-up. In addition, the k-wires had to be repositioned or removed from the Humerusblock in 14 patients (9.3%) occurring at an average of 29.9 days (range, 16.4 days).

This study shows the advantages and limitations of the Humerusblock device. It is not available for use in the United States. The senior author is a known pioneer in treating proximal humerus fractures percutaneously. This report is of the senior author's series of patients, and the results may not be generalizable to other orthopedic surgeons. The authors concluded that excellent and good results were obtained from most patients with acceptable complication rates. The authors felt that they had a surprisingly high rate of avascular necrosis in 4-part valgus-impacted proximal humerus fractures. It is not clear whether the senior author is still using this device.

A. B. Shafritz, MD

Deltoid Tuberosity Index: A Simple Radiographic Tool to Assess Local Bone Quality in Proximal Humerus Fractures
Spross C, Kaestle N, Benninger E, et al (Kantonsspital St. Gallen, Switzerland)
Clin Orthop Relat Res 473:3038-3045, 2015

Background.—Osteoporosis may complicate surgical fixation and healing of proximal humerus fractures and should be assessed preoperatively. Peripheral quantitative CT (pQCT) and the Tingart measurement are helpful methods, but both have limitations in clinical use because of limited availability (pQCT) or fracture lines crossing the area of interest (Tingart measurement). The aim of our study was to introduce and validate a simple cortical index to assess the quality of bone in proximal humerus fractures using AP radiographs.

Questions/Purposes.—We asked: (1) How do the deltoid tuberosity index and Tingart measurement correlate with each other, with patient age, and local bone mineral density (BMD) of the humeral head, measured by pQCT? (2) Which threshold values for the deltoid tuberosity index and Tingart measurement optimally discriminate poor local bone quality of the proximal humerus? (3) Are the deltoid tuberosity index and Tingart measurement clinically applicable and reproducible in patients with proximal humerus fractures?

Methods.—The deltoid tuberosity index was measured immediately above the upper end of the deltoid tuberosity. At this position, where the outer cortical borders become parallel, the deltoid tuberosity index equals the ratio between the outer cortical and inner endosteal diameter. In the first part of our study, we retrospectively measured the deltoid tuberosity index on 31 patients (16 women, 15 men; mean age, 65 years; range, 22–83 years) who were scheduled for elective surgery other than fracture repair. Inclusion criteria were available native pQCT scans, AP shoulder radiographs taken in internal rotation, and no previous shoulder surgery. The deltoid tuberosity index and the Tingart measurement were measured on the preoperative internal rotation AP radiograph. The second part of our study was performed by reviewing 40 radiographs of patients with proximal humerus fractures (31 women, nine men; median age, 65 years; range, 22–88 years). Interrater (two surgeons) and intrarater (two readings) reliabilities, applicability, and diagnostic accuracy were assessed.

Results.—The correlations between radiograph measurements and local BMD (pQCT) were strong for the deltoid tuberosity index (r = 0.80; 95% CI, 0.63–0.90; $p < 0.001$) and moderate for the Tingart measurement (r = 0.67; 95% CI, 0.42–0.83; $p < 0.001$). There was moderate correlation between patient age and the deltoid tuberosity index (r = 0.65; $p < 0.001$), patient age and the Tingart measurement (r = 0.69; $p < 0.001$), and patient age and pQCT (r = 0.73; $p < 0.001$). The correlation between the deltoid tuberosity index and the Tingart measurement was strong (r = 0.84; $p < 0.001$). We determined the cutoff value for the deltoid tuberosity index to be 1.44, with the area under the curve = 0.87 (95% CI, 0.74–0.99). This provided a sensitivity of 0.88 and specificity of 0.80. For the Tingart measurement, we determined the cutoff value to be 5.3 mm, with the area under the curve = 0.83 (95% CI, 0.67–0.98), which resulted in a sensitivity of 0.81 and specificity of 0.85. The intraobserver reliability was high and not different between the Tingart measurement (intraclass correlation coefficients [ICC] = 0.75 and 0.88) and deltoid tuberosity index (ICC = 0.88 and 0.82). However, interobserver reliability was higher for the deltoid tuberosity index (ICC = 0.96; 95% CI, 0.93–0.98) than for the Tingart measurement (ICC = 0.85; 95% CI, 0.69–0.93). The clinical applicability on AP radiographs of fractures was better for the deltoid tuberosity index ($p = 0.025$) because it was measureable on more of the radiographs (77/80; 96%) than the Tingart measurement (69/80; 86%).

Conclusions.—The deltoid tuberosity index correlated strongly with local BMD measured on pQCT and our study evidence shows that it is a reliable, simple, and applicable tool to assess local bone quality in the proximal humerus. We found that deltoid tuberosity index values consistently lower than 1.4 indicated low local BMD of the proximal humerus. Furthermore, the use of the deltoid tuberosity index has important advantages over the Tingart measurement regarding clinical applicability in patients with proximal humerus fractures, when fracture lines obscure the Tingart measurement landmarks. However, further studies are needed to assess the effect of the deltoid tuberosity index measurement and osteoporosis on treatment and outcome in patients with proximal humerus fractures.

Level of Evidence.—Level IV, diagnostic study.

▶ In this study, the authors sought to determine a simple way to measure bone mineral density and bone quality in patients who sustained a proximal humerus

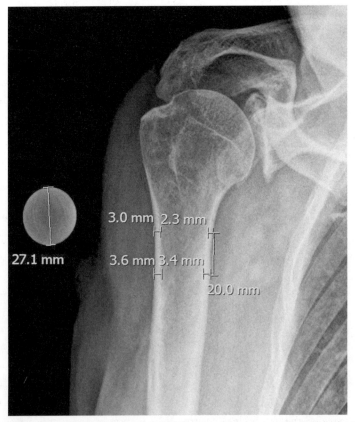

FIGURE 1.—The two levels of combined cortical thickness are level 1, at the proximal diaphysis where the medial and the lateral endosteal cortical borders become parallel; and level 2, which is 2 cm distal to level 1. The sum of the means of the two levels is calculated and must be corrected for magnification error. (Reprinted from Spross C, Kaestle N, Benninger E, et al. Deltoid tuberosity index: a simple radiographic tool to assess local bone quality in proximal humerus fractures. *Clin Orthop Relat Res.* 2015;473:3038-3045, with permission from The Association of Bone and Joint Surgeons.)

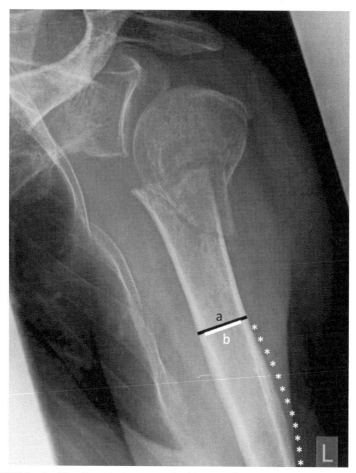

FIGURE 2.—An AP radiograph shows a proximal humerus fracture in a 75-year-old patient. The proximal diaphysis is fractured, which complicates the definition of the levels for the Tingart measurement. The deltoid tuberosity index is measured directly proximal to the deltoid tuberosity (asterisks), where the outer cortical borders become parallel. At this level, the ratio between the outer cortical and the inner endosteal diameter is calculated (a/b). (Reprinted from Spross C, Kaestle N, Benninger E, et al. Deltoid tuberosity index: a simple radiographic tool to assess local bone quality in proximal humerus fractures. *Clin Orthop Relat Res.* 2015;473:3038-3045, with permission from The Association of Bone and Joint Surgeons.)

fracture. Low bone mineral density and poor bone quality may compromise efforts of open reduction internal fixation or bone healing in terms of maintenance of fracture fragment reduction and hardware viability in those treated operatively. To determine a simple method for measuring bone quality in the proximal humerus, the authors studied cortical bone thickness at the deltoid tuberosity insertion point on the humerus, as this is a relatively constant point that can be readily evaluated. Current limitations in assessing bone quality in the proximal humerus at the time of fracture include fractures going through the bone fragments that are traditionally used to determine bone mineral density. The authors

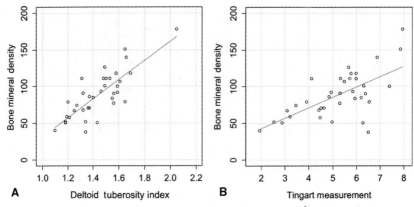

FIGURE 3.—The correlations between (A) bone mineral density (mg/cm³) and the deltoid tuberosity index and (B) bone mineral density and the Tingart measurement are shown. (Reprinted from Spross C, Kaestle N, Benninger E, et al. Deltoid tuberosity index: a simple radiographic tool to assess local bone quality in proximal humerus fractures. *Clin Orthop Relat Res.* 2015;473:3038-3045, with permission from The Association of Bone and Joint Surgeons.)

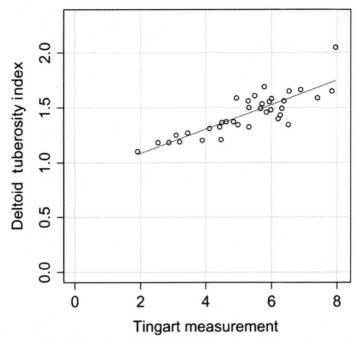

FIGURE 4.—The correlation between the deltoid tuberosity index and Tingart measurement is shown. (Reprinted from Spross C, Kaestle N, Benninger E, et al. Deltoid tuberosity index: a simple radiographic tool to assess local bone quality in proximal humerus fractures. *Clin Orthop Relat Res.* 2015;473:3038-3045, with permission from The Association of Bone and Joint Surgeons.)

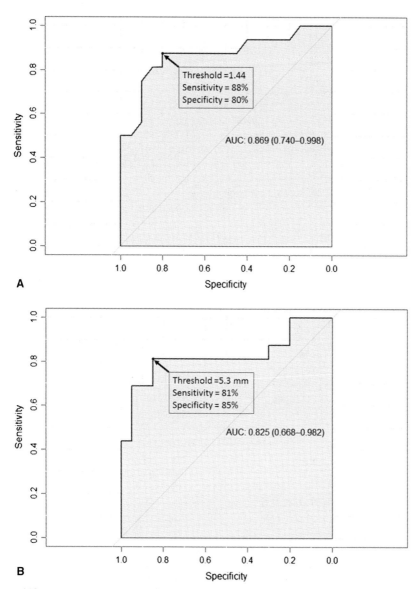

FIGURE 5.—Receiver operating characteristic curves for (A) the deltoid tuberosity index and (B) the Tingart measurement are shown. AUC = area under the curve. (Reprinted from Spross C, Kaestle N, Benninger E, et al. Deltoid tuberosity index: a simple radiographic tool to assess local bone quality in proximal humerus fractures. *Clin Orthop Relat Res.* 2015;473:3038-3045, with permission from The Association of Bone and Joint Surgeons.)

note 3 techniques to measure bone mineral density in the proximal humerus: dual-energy x-ray absorptiometry (DEXA) scan, quantitative CT scan, and the Tingart measurement. The Tingart measurement, described in Figure 1, measures cortical thickness in 2 places in the proximal humerus, but requires magnification correction. The Tingart measurement was previously correlated with DEXA measurements; however, Tingart measurements on a fractured proximal humerus are difficult to obtain, as fracture fragments may preclude accurate measurements, and arm rotational position can be variable. As a result, the investigators developed the deltoid tuberosity index to substitute for the Tingart measurement. The deltoid tuberosity is rarely fractured, and, with the arm in internal rotation, the common position in which the arm is immobilized in a sling, the deltoid tuberosity index can be regularly and reproducibly obtained. Calculation of the deltoid tuberosity index is shown in Figure 2. To test the accuracy, dependability, and reliability of this measurement, 2 sets of patients were evaluated: patients without fractures in whom the Tingart measurement and deltoid tuberosity index could be reliably measured and the interobserver reliability determined, and those with proximal humerus fractures. The receiver operator curves for these measurements are shown in Figures 3 and 4. The specificity and sensitivity for these measures are shown in Figure 5. The authors ultimately showed a correlation for the deltoid tuberosity index at 0.96 and the Tingart measurement at 0.85. In addition, they found that the deltoid tuberosity index could be performed reliably on more patients with fractures than could the Tingart measurement.

There are numerous limitations to this study. There is no defined threshold value for osteoporosis of the proximal humerus, either by DEXA or peripheral quantitative CT measurements. There is no convincing literature published suggesting that osteoporosis surrounding proximal humeral fractures is truly associated with poor outcomes. The authors were not able to provide absolute Tingart measurement values for patients with fractures because magnification correction was not available.

This report does show that deltoid tuberosity index and the Tingart measurement correlate well to local bone mineral density of the proximal humerus as measured by quantitative CT scans. Compared with the Tingart measurement, the deltoid tuberosity index is advantageous, as it serves as a reliable tool to get an impression of local bone quality on an anteroposterior radiograph. The authors believe that the deltoid tuberosity index, therefore, could serve as a useful tool in future studies of proximal humerus fractures to determine whether local bone mineral density has an effect on the outcome of treatment of proximal humerus fractures.

A. B. Shafritz, MD

Transosseous braided-tape and double-row fixations are better than tension band for avulsion-type greater tuberosity fractures
Brais G, Ménard J, Mutch J, et al (Université de Montréal, Canada; Hôpital du Sacré-Cœur de Montréal Res Ctr, Canada; et al)
Injury 46:1007-1012, 2015

Introduction.—The optimal treatment for avulsion-type greater tuberosity fractures is yet to be determined. Three fixation methods are tested: tension band with #2 wire suture (TB), double-row suture bridge with anchors (DR), and simple transosseous fixation with braided tape (BT).

Materials and Methods.—Twenty-four porcine proximal humeri were randomised into three groups: TB, DR and BT. A standardised greater tuberosity (GT) osteotomy was performed at 90° to the humeral diaphysis axis. A mechanical testing machine was used to simulate supraspinatus contraction. The force required to produce 3 mm and 5 mm displacement, as well as complete failure was measured with an axial load cell. Also, three cycles of shoulder flexion/extension with 25 N of supraspinatus contraction were performed. Maximum GT fragment translation and rotation amplitude during one cycle were measured.

Results.—During supraspinatus contraction, DR and BT groups ($p < 0.05$) were superior to TB group for both displacements. The BT technique had the strongest maximal load to failure (BT = 466 N; DR = 386 N; TB = 320 N). For the flexion/extension, DR and BT groups had less displacement and rotation than TB group (anterio-posterior displacement: BT = 2.0 mm, DR = 1.9 mm, TB = 5.8 mm; anterio-posterior angular displacement: BT = 1.4°, DR = 1.0°, TB = 4.8°). No significant difference was observed between DR and BT groups, except for the medio-lateral rotation favouring the DR group.

Conclusion.—In conclusion, BT and DR are good fixation methods to treat displaced avulsion-type greater tuberosity fractures. They have similar mechanical properties, and are stronger and more stable that the TB construct. Potential advantages of the BT over the DR may be a lower cost and easier surgery.

Level of Evidence.—Basic science study (LEVEL II).

▶ The objective of this study is to compare the biomechanical properties of 3 fixation techniques for avulsion-type greater tuberosity fractures: the tension band, the transosseous braided tape, and the double row suture bridge (Figs

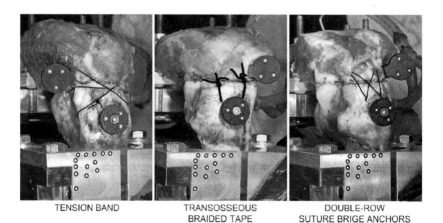

| TENSION BAND | TRANSOSSEOUS BRAIDED TAPE | DOUBLE-ROW SUTURE BRIGE ANCHORS |

FIGURE 1.—Pictures of the three different constructs: tension band with #2 suture (left); two simple transosseous braided tape sutures (centre); double row suture bridge with anchors (right). (Reprinted from Brais G, Ménard J, Mutch J, et al. Transosseous braided-tape and double-row fixations are better than tension band for avulsion-type greater tuberosity fractures. *Injury.* 2015;46:1007-1012, with permission from Elsevier.)

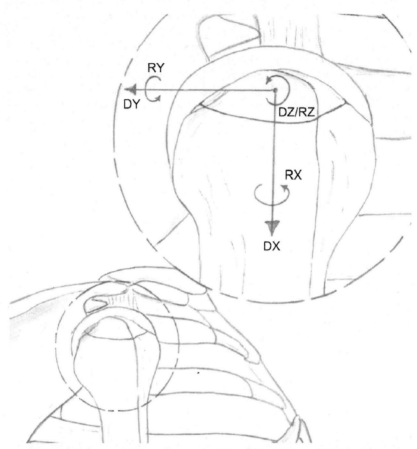

FIGURE 4.—Displacement and rotation nomenclature. Displacement and rotation in the supero-inferior axis are represented by DX and RX, respectively. Displacement and rotation in the antero-posterior axis are represented by DY and RY, respectively. Displacement and rotation in the medio-lateral axis are represented by DZ and RZ, respectively. (Reprinted from Brais G, Ménard J, Mutch J, et al. Trans-osseous braided-tape and double-row fixations are better than tension band for avulsion-type greater tuberosity fractures. *Injury*. 2015;46:1007-1012, with permission from Elsevier.)

1 and 4). The study has a straightforward design, and the authors use a previously validated model and method of measuring fracture displacement and rotation.

As with any biomechanical study, the findings must be considered in the context of clinical relevance. The authors report that the tension band technique leads to a greater average maximal displacement of the greater tuberosity fragment compared with the other techniques. The magnitude of this difference is at least 2 mm in most cases. Previous literature reported that a 2-mm gap in a fracture leads to less axial stiffness and a prolonged time for ossification.[1] Therefore, this difference in displacement may be clinically relevant in terms of gap formation and fracture healing.

Greater tuberosity fractures tend to occur in younger patients with good bone quality; this rationale is used to justify the choice of a young porcine shoulder model. However, the results of this study may not translate well when treating an elderly patient. Another factor to consider is that the biomechanical testing was performed at 0° of abduction and ±15° of flexion/extension. Depending on the rehabilitation protocol and the compliance of the patient, it is possible that a recently repaired greater tuberosity fracture could experience a greater degree of abduction and flexion/extension than the motion evaluated in this study.

It can be a challenge to apply the findings of a biomechanical study to the care of patients. However, this report presents convincing evidence that the transosseous braided tape and double row suture bridge techniques are superior to tension band fixation for greater tuberosity fractures. It is unclear whether the transosseous braided tape and double row suture bridge techniques are equal to each other in the clinical setting, and further research is needed.

E. Kinnucan, MD

Reference

1. Mark H, Nilsson A, Nannmark U, Rydevik B. Effects of fracture fixation stability on ossification in healing fractures. *Clin Orthop Relat Res*. 2004;419:245-250.

Outcomes After Hemiarthroplasty for Proximal Humerus Fracture Are Significantly Affected by Hand Dominance
LeBlanc JEM, MacDermid JC, Faber KJ, et al (Univ of Western Ontario, London, Canada)
J Orthop Trauma 29:379-383, 2015

Objectives.—Hand dominance has been reported to be an important factor affecting outcomes after upper extremity trauma but remains unstudied after hemiarthroplasty for fracture. This study determined whether dominance affected outcomes after hemiarthroplasty for proximal humerus fractures.

Design.—Retrospective cohort study.

Setting.—Tertiary care referral center.

Patients.—Sixty-one patients, after hemiarthroplasty for proximal humerus fracture, returned for comprehensive assessment and were divided into 2 groups: dominant (DOM) shoulder affected (n = 25) and non-dominant (non-DOM) shoulder affected (n = 36).

Intervention.—Fracture-specific proximal humeral hemiarthroplasty for displaced proximal humerus fractures.

Main Outcome Measures.—Patients were assessed with self-reported outcomes (visual analog scale pain, American Shoulder and Elbow Surgeons shoulder score, disability of the arm, shoulder, and hand questionnaire, simple shoulder test, and short form 12) and objective (range-of-motion and hand-held dynamometer strength) testing.

Results.—At 49 months of mean follow-up, there were no significant differences between groups for gender, age, follow-up time, or visual analog scale pain ($P > 0.256$). The DOM-affected group had significantly worse scores for American Shoulder and Elbow Surgeons shoulder score ($P = 0.043$), disability of the arm, shoulder, and hand questionnaire ($P = 0.039$), and simple shoulder test ($P = 0.021$). The DOM-affected group also had consistently higher correlations between self-reported and objective outcomes than the non-DOM group.

Conclusions.—Patients who underwent hemiarthroplasty for fracture on their DOM shoulders had significantly poorer outcomes than patients with non-DOM—sided injuries. Although positive outcomes can be expected after hemiarthroplasty, patients should be instructed that they may have less satisfactory function and strength if their injury was on the DOM side.

Level of Evidence.—Prognostic Level II. See Instructions for Authors for a complete description of levels of evidence.

▶ Hand dominance is known to be an independent factor that influences the outcomes of traumatic injury to the upper extremity. The purpose of the study was to determine whether hand dominance affected outcomes after hemiarthroplasty for proximal humerus fractures. Sixty-one patients were retrospectively reviewed after hemiarthroplasty for proximal humerus fractures and were divided into 2 groups; 25 patients fractured the dominant side, and 36 patients fractured the nondominant side. Primary outcomes assessed were self-reported visual analog scale for pain, American Shoulder and Elbow Surgeons shoulder score (ASES), Disabilities of the Arm, Shoulder and Hand (DASH), Simple Shoulder Test (SST), and Short Form 12. Objective measures included range of motion and hand-held dynamometer strength testing.

TABLE 2.—DOM Versus Non-DOM Group Outcomes (Independent *t* tests)

Outcome	Group	P	Mean (SD)	d
Pain VAS	Non-DOM	0.143	0.9 (2)	
	DOM		1.8 (3)	
ASES	Non-DOM	0.043	80 (16)	0.54
	DOM		66 (24)	
DASH	Non-DOM	0.039	23 (17)	0.55
	DOM		35 (24)	
SST	Non-DOM	0.021	9 (3)	0.63
	DOM		7 (3)	
SF-12 physical	Non-DOM	0.102	42 (11)	
	DOM		37 (11)	
SF-12 mental	Non-DOM	0.069	55 (10)	
	DOM		49 (16)	

Bold indicates statistically significant values ($P < 0.05$).
Reprinted from LeBlanc JEM, MacDermid JC, Faber KJ, et al. Outcomes after hemiarthroplasty for proximal humerus fracture are significantly affected by hand dominance. *J Orthop Trauma.* 2015;29:379-383, with permission from Wolters Kluwer Health, Inc.

The surgical technique and rehabilitation protocol used were described. Follow-up averaged 49 months. The 2 groups (dominant and nondominant arm) were similar in terms of sex, age, follow-up time, and fracture type. Both groups had similar levels of pain at last follow-up; however, patients with the dominant hand affected had significantly worse scores on the ASES, DASH, and SST (Table 2); these differences met or exceeded the established minimum clinically important differences. There were no significant differences in objective measures of strength and range of motion except for a deficit in forward elevation strength in the dominant-arm group. The authors then correlated strength and range of motion with self-reported outcomes. Objective functional measures were more predictive of self-reported function and disability when the dominant side was affected.

When the nondominant arm was affected, ASES, DASH, and SST scores were at normal or near-normal age-adjusted values. The authors hypothesize that overall function as measured on these self-reported scores is primarily determined by the dominant arm. Although all patients who undergo hemiarthroplasty can expect good pain relief and will have similar strength and range of motion regardless of which side is affected, those whose dominant arm was fractured should be counseled that they will experience more disability or impairment than if their nondominant arm had been affected.

K. Kollitz, MD

19 Shoulder: Miscellaneous

The Effect of Cartilage Injury After Arthroscopic Stabilization for Shoulder Instability
Krych AJ, Sousa PL, King AH, et al (Mayo Clinic, Rochester, MN)
Orthopedics 38:e965-e969, 2015

This study was undertaken to (1) determine the incidence of articular cartilage injuries in patients with instability of the glenohumeral joint, (2) determine whether recurrent dislocations increased the risk of articular damage, and (3) correlate these injuries with postoperative clinical outcomes. A cohort was identified of consecutive patients who underwent diagnostic magnetic resonance imaging and shoulder arthroscopy for glenohumeral instability with documented dislocation or subluxation between 1997 and 2006 at a single institution. Patients with moderate or severe osteoarthritis were excluded. Arthroscopic findings were recorded, including lesion location and Outerbridge grade. The American Shoulder and Elbow Surgeons Standardized Shoulder Assessment Form (ASES) was used to assess outcome in 61 patients who were available for follow-up. Outcomes were compared between shoulders with and without articular lesions. A total of 87 shoulders (83 patients) met the inclusion criteria, with 69 (83%) men and 14 (17%) women. Mean age was 26.1 years (range, 18-64 years), and mean follow-up was 36 months (range, 33-39 months). Cartilage injuries were found in 56 shoulders (64%). Previously documented shoulder dislocation requiring closed reduction ($P = .046$) and the number of discrete dislocations ($P = .032$) were significant for glenoid injury. A greater number of dislocations was associated with higher-grade lesions of the glenohumeral joint ($P < .001$). Overall, mean ASES score was 89.6 (range, 37-100). In patients with an articular cartilage lesion, mean ASES score was 90.4 (range, 58-100) compared with 88.1 (range, 37-100) in those without this injury ($P = .75$). Although clinical outcomes were not significantly affected, further investigation is warranted to establish a relationship between these injuries and longer-term outcomes.

▶ This article is a retrospective review of 87 shoulders in 83 patients who underwent MRI evaluation and arthroscopic shoulder stabilization to determine

TABLE 1.—Incidence and Location of Glenohumeral Articular Cartilage Lesions Confirmed by Arthroscopy

Lesion Location	Lesions, No.	Incidence, %
Either joint surface	56	64
All glenoids	55	63
All humeri	23	26
Surfaces		
No articular lesions	31	36
Both surfaces involved	22	25
One surface Involved	34	39
Glenoid alone	33	38
Humeral alone	1	1
Total	87	100

Reprinted from Krych AJ, Sousa PL, King AH, et al. The effect of cartilage injury after arthroscopic stabilization for shoulder instability. *Orthopedics*. 2015;38:e965-e969, with permission from SLACK Incorporated.

TABLE 2.—Location and Grade of Glenohumeral Articular Cartilage Lesions Confirmed by Arthroscopy[a]

Lesion	Glenoid Articular Lesion		Humeral Articular Lesion		Lesions on Both Surfaces	
	Joints, No.	Incidence, %	Joints, No.	Incidence, %	Joints, No.	Incidence, %
No lesions present	32	37	64	74	-	-
Lesion, any grade	55	63	23	26	22	25
Grade 1	7	8	4	4	2	2
Grade 2	21	24	12	14	8	9
Grade 3	17	20	5	6	5	6
Grade 4	10	11	2	2	7	8
Total	87	100	87	100	87	100

[a]All incidence rates reflect the total number of joints (N = 87). In the case of multiple articular lesions, the lesion grade represents the lesion with the highest grade.
Reprinted from Krych AJ, Sousa PL, King AH, et al. The effect of cartilage injury after arthroscopic stabilization for shoulder instability. *Orthopedics*. 2015;38:e965-e969, with permission from SLACK Incorporated.

TABLE 3.—Incidence and Location of Articular Cartilage Lesions Confirmed by Arthroscopy in Patients With and Without a Documented History of Shoulder Dislocation[a]

Lesion Location	Documented Dislocation		Documented Subluxation	
	Joints, No.	Incidence, %	Joints, No.	Incidence, %
No articular lesions	20	31	11	50
Any lesion, any location	45	69	11	50
Glenoid lesion only	27	41	6	27
Humeral lesion only	0	0	1	5
Both surfaces involved	18	28	4	18
Total	65	75	22	25

[a]All incidence rates reflect the total number of joints (N = 87).
Reprinted from Krych AJ, Sousa PL, King AH, et al. The effect of cartilage injury after arthroscopic stabilization for shoulder instability. *Orthopedics*. 2015;38:e965-e969, with permission from SLACK Incorporated.

TABLE 4.—Midterm American Shoulder and Elbow Surgeons Score and Number of Dislocations Stratified by Grade of Glenohumeral Articular Lesions Confirmed by Arthroscopy[a]

Lesion	Joints, No.	Dislocations, Mean	ASES Score Assessment	
			Mean Score	SD
No articular lesion	22	1.6	88.1	16.3
Lesion, any grade	39	5.3	90.4	9.7
Grade 1	4	0.75	81.2	7.7
Grade 2	14	3.3	88.5	11.5
Grade 3	12	7.8	93.2	8.5
Grade 4	8	7.9	95.0	3.6
All shoulders	61	3.9	89.6	12.4

Abbreviation: ASES, American Shoulder and Elbow Surgeons.
[a]In the case of multiple articular lesions, the lesion grade represents the lesion with the highest grade on either joint surface.
Reprinted from Krych AJ, Sousa PL, King AH, et al. The effect of cartilage injury after arthroscopic stabilization for shoulder instability. *Orthopedics.* 2015;38:e965-e969, with permission from SLACK Incorporated.

the following: (1) the incidence of articular cartilage injuries in patients with glenohumeral instability, (2) whether recurrent dislocations increased the risk of cartilage damage, and (3) whether postoperative outcomes are affected by cartilage injury (Tables 1-4). Cartilage lesions were found in 56 shoulders (64%). The location of the cartilage injury was categorized based on its presence on the humeral head or glenoid, but the exact location and size of the lesion were not presented. Of note, Hill-Sachs lesions were present in 76% of the shoulders but were not considered articular cartilage injuries, potentially because nonengaging Hill-Sachs lesions do not articulate with the glenoid. A history of dislocation versus subluxation was associated with a higher rate of cartilage injury. Also, patients with more dislocations had increased likelihood of cartilage damage and higher grade cartilage lesions, which makes intuitive sense. Interestingly, there was no statistical difference in clinical outcomes when comparing groups with and without articular cartilage injury. As pointed out by the authors, further studies with longer term outcomes may shed light on the effect of articular cartilage injury on clinical outcomes. It would have been interesting to investigate what percentage of articular cartilage injuries seen with arthroscopy were detected by preoperative MRI. In my practice, I have a low threshold for operative management of traumatic glenohumeral instability, particularly in younger patients in whom the potential for further instability events, and as demonstrated by this article increased likelihood of cartilage injury, is markedly higher.

E. Gauger, MD

Arthroscopic Capsulolabral Reconstruction for Posterior Shoulder Instability in Patients 18 Years Old or Younger

Wooten CJ, Krych AJ, Schleck CD, et al (Mayo Clinic, Rochester, MN; et al)
J Pediatr Orthop 35:462-466, 2015

Purpose.—The purpose of this study was to determine clinical outcomes for pain, function, instability, and return to activity level and sport in patients 18 years old or younger, treated with arthroscopic capsulolabral reconstruction for posterior instability of the shoulder.

Methods.—We retrospectively reviewed 22 athletes (25 shoulders) with unidirectional recurrent posterior shoulder instability treated with arthroscopic posterior capsulolabral reconstruction from 2002 to 2009. The study group included 19 males and 3 females with a mean age of 17 years. Patients were evaluated at a mean of 63 months postoperatively with American Shoulder and Elbow Surgeons (ASES) composite scores and subset scores for pain, stability, and function, as well as Marx activity scores. Statistical analysis was performed for continuous and categorical variables with significance set at $\alpha = 0.05$.

Results.—The overall mean postoperative ASES and Marx scores were 74.3 (SD ± 20) and 14.8 (SD ± 3.2), respectively. Twenty-three shoulders were stable at the time of final follow-up (92%). Two shoulders had traumatic recurrent episodes of posterior instability. Return to sport at the same level was achieved in 67% of athletes. Overall postoperative ASES scores were significantly higher in male patients ($P = 0.04$), those with traumatic injuries ($P = 0.03$), and in contact athletes ($P < 0.01$). Postoperative Marx scores were significantly higher in male patients ($P < 0.01$). Preoperative and postoperative range of motion were assessed and without significant difference.

Conclusion.—Arthroscopic capsulolabral reconstruction is an effective treatment for symptomatic unidirectional posterior glenohumeral instability in 18 years old or younger. In distinction to treatment of anterior instability, outcomes in this series were improved in males, contact athletes, and patients with a traumatic etiology of posterior glenohumeral instability.

Level of Evidence.—Level IV.

▶ The study is a retrospective case series of 22 athletes (25 shoulders) 18 years old or younger who were treated for isolated posterior shoulder instability with arthroscopic posterior labral repair and posterior capsular shift if there was capsular laxity (76% patients). The primary purpose was to determine the clinical outcomes at a mean of 63 months postoperatively. The authors do an excellent job at describing the preoperative clinical and radiographic evaluation, operative treatment and postoperative rehabilitation. Ninety-two percent of patients were stable at final follow-up determined by a subjective stability scale with 67% of patients returning to the same level of sport participation. Several risk factors were associated with statistically significant improved outcomes, including male patients, patients with traumatic injuries, and contact athletes. Despite the statistical significance, I would be careful in concluding that males and contact athletes consistently do better because there were only 3 female patients included in the study, and participation in contact sports puts patients at risk for recurrent injury. Furthermore, atraumatic posterior instability is likely related to some level of hyperlaxity or mild multidirectional instability and inherently more difficult to treat. A detailed table with individual patient characteristics and outcomes as well as inclusion of Beighton criteria would have been helpful.

Posterior shoulder instability is extremely common in my patient population, which consists predominantly of young (17- to 24-year-old) active-duty military and contact athletes. The typical presentation is difficulty doing push-ups or bench press and, contrary to anterior instability, can present as pain more than subjective instability. The jerk test and posterior load and shift are integral in diagnosis and are discussed in the article. I will always order an MRI arthrogram to evaluate for concomitant pathology, such as bony defects, and have the patient undergo intensive physical therapy aimed at periscapular muscular stabilization and rotator cuff strengthening before discussing surgical management.

E. Gauger, MD

Operative Management Options for Traumatic Anterior Shoulder Instability in Patients Younger Than 30 Years

Davis DE, Abboud JA (Thomas Jefferson Univ, Philadelphia, PA)
Orthopedics 38:570-576, 2015

Anterior instability of the glenohumeral joint is a relatively common problem in the young population. Identification and treatment is essential to reduce the risk of recurrent instability, whether that is re-dislocation or subluxation events. Nonoperative treatment for first-time dislocations was the classic option; however, a relatively high rate of recurrent dislocations has led to earlier operative management in some cases. Surgical treatment through either an open or arthroscopic approach has continued to be an area of research and debate. The decision depends partly on the exact etiology of the instability and the extent of soft tissue or bony deficiency. As arthroscopic techniques and experience improve, surgical procedures for arthroscopic anterior shoulder instability continue to evolve. This review serves as an in-depth overview of the treatment options for traumatic anterior shoulder instability in the patient younger than 30 years, generally focusing on non-rotator cuff—associated etiologies for recurrent instability.

▶ In this continuing medical education review article, the authors' educational objectives are to discuss the evaluation of the young patient with an instability event, to describe the injury patterns and pathology leading to anterior shoulder instability, to explain the operative options for shoulder instability based on pathology, and to review postoperative rehabilitation for patients undergoing operative treatment of instability. The incidence of anterior shoulder instability was reported at 23 per 100,000 patients with a rate of recurrent instability after traumatic dislocation of 19% in the general population, but in adolescents the reported rate was as high as 92%.

TABLE 1.—Summary of Studies Comparing Open Versus Arthroscopic Procedures for Bankart Lesion Repair

Study	Study Type	Recurrence	Complications
Pulavarti et al[33]	Cochrane Database review of RCTs of open vs arthroscopic Bankart repair (N = 3)	Open: 5.9% Arthroscopic: 7.6%	1 arthroscopic long thoracic nerve injury, 1 arthroscopic broken hardware, 1 open broken hardware
Archetti Netto et al[34]	RCT of arthroscopic vs open Bankart repair	Open: 0% Arthroscopic: 11.8%	1 superficial wound infection in open surgery
Freedman et al[35]	Meta-analysis: arthroscopic vs open Bankart repair (N = 6)	Open: 3.4% Arthroscopic: 12.6%	No significant difference in infection, hardware failure, loss of motion requiring surgery, or nerve injury
Mohtadi et al[36]	Meta-analysis: arthroscopic vs open Bankart repair (N = 11)	Open: 7.6% Arthroscopic: 17.5%	Not reported

Editor's Note: Please refer to original journal article for full references.
Abbreviation: RCT, randomized, controlled trial.
Reprinted from Davis DE, Abboud JA. Operative management options for traumatic anterior shoulder instability in patients younger than 30 years. *Orthopedics*. 2015;38:570-576, with permission from SLACK Incorporated.

TABLE 2.—Summary of Results of the Latarjet Procedure

Study	Procedure	Outcomes	Complications
Schmid et al[37]	Latarjet procedure (N = 49)	No redislocations; 14% recurrent subluxation; Constant score: 80.1-84.6 (P =.061); Simple Shoulder Test: 53.4-73.5 (P <.001)	12% complication rate: 4 delayed wound healing, 1 frozen shoulder, 1 malunion of coracoid to glenoid rim
Hovelius et al[38]	Bristow-Latarjet procedure (N = 319)	5% recurrent dislocation; 13% recurrent subluxation; recurrence rate decreased from 18% to 4% when capsular shift added to closure	5 shoulders underwent screw removal, 1 removal of a loose anchor, 1 arthroplasty (intraoperative complications not reported)
Cerciello et al[39]	Latarjet in soccer players (N = 28)	1/28 redislocation; average return to soccer = 8 mo; Duplay score at final follow-up = 91.2	1 axillary nerve palsy in patient with dislocation

Editor's Note: Please refer to original journal article for full references.
Reprinted from Davis DE, Abboud JA. Operative management options for traumatic anterior shoulder instability in patients younger than 30 years. *Orthopedics.* 2015;38:570-576, with permission from SLACK Incorporated.

In this comprehensive review article, the authors do an excellent job of discussing the classification of anterior instability and the evaluation of the patient, including specific instability tests and calculation of the instability severity index score to help clarify the best treatment option to reduce the risk of recurrence: arthroscopic versus open stabilization procedures. The authors discuss imaging studies including plain film evaluation and MRI. They point out the need for obtaining a CT scan in the event that bone loss is thought to occur either on the glenoid side or the humeral side.

The authors describe the classic arthroscopic Bankart procedure and the treatment of instability with glenoid bone loss using the Bristow and Latarjet procedures. They review management options of humeral bone loss: tamping out Hill-Sachs lesions and the remplissage procedure. The authors then provide an overview of postoperative rehabilitation. They present the results of operative versus nonoperative treatment, the results of Bankart repair (soft tissue and bony), and results after Bristow and Latarjet procedures (Tables 1 and 2). Finally, instability rates after surgery and other complications are cited. A comprehensive bibliography is available.

A. B. Shafritz, MD

Does External Rotation Bracing for Anterior Shoulder Dislocation Actually Result in Reduction of the Labrum? A Systematic Review

Jordan RW, Saithna A, Old J, et al (Univ Hosps Coventry & Warwickshire, United Kingdom; Pan Am Clinic, Winnipeg, Manitoba, Canada; et al)
Am J Sports Med 43:2328-2333, 2015

Background.—External rotation (ER) bracing has been shown to improve labral reduction in cadaveric studies, but this has not translated to universal improvement in re-dislocation rates in clinical series.

Purpose.—To systematically review and critically appraise the literature that investigates how well the labrum is actually reduced by ER in patients who have had an anterior shoulder dislocation.

Study Design.—Systematic review.

Methods.—We conducted a systematic review of the literature using the online databases Medline, EMBASE, and the Cochrane Controlled Trial Register. Studies were included if they reported on the difference in labral reduction after ER and internal rotation bracing in patients who had a traumatic anterior shoulder dislocation.

Results.—Of the 6 studies included, 5 assessed labral reduction on magnetic resonance imaging and 1 arthroscopically. Each study reported an overall improvement in labral reduction with ER, but anatomic reduction was not commonly achieved. This was despite the use of extreme positions that are unlikely to be well tolerated.

Conclusion.—External rotation results in anatomic reduction of the labrum in only 35% of cases. We postulate that failure to reduce the labrum may be a contraindication to ER bracing and propose further study to determine whether acute MRI could be used to help identify patients in whom ER achieves labral reduction in a comfortable position. This approach also has the advantage of avoiding the significant inconvenience of ER bracing in those in whom the labrum does not reduce and are therefore theoretically less likely to benefit. However, it is a novel strategy with significant resource implications and therefore warrants further study.

▶ Although more than 90% of patients have a Bankart lesion after primary traumatic anterior shoulder dislocation, recurrent instability is not universally seen in these patients. Some studies found that recurrent instability rates are lower with Bankart repair when compared with immobilization alone. Despite this finding, surgical management for first-time dislocators is not universally accepted, and many investigators favor a trial of nonoperative treatment. In an effort to improve nonoperative outcomes, Itoi et al[1] proposed via their cadaveric study that bracing in external rotation (ER) improved anatomic reduction of the labrum. Clinical studies of ER bracing have not shown the same success, however, and many authors suggest reasons for this, including the extreme degree of ER bracing required or poor patient compliance.

This article adds important information to the available literature in that this review concluded that ER bracing does not often anatomically reduce the labrum (anatomic reduction was only achieved in 35% of cases). These authors also make the excellent point that the degree of ER bracing in many MRI studies exceeds what is often used in clinical studies. Therefore, increasing patient bracing is not likely to improve patient compliance and, as this review showed, may not actually reduce the labrum anatomically.

This article makes an excellent conclusion that failure to reduce the labrum is a contraindication for bracing. The authors suggest that perhaps acute MRI in ER would identify those patients in whom anatomic reduction of the labrum is achieved, and this subset of patients could be appropriate candidates for this nonoperative treatment. Further study into this area is needed to assist our patients with decision making and treatment for first-time shoulder dislocations.

A. K. Harrison, MD

Reference

1. Itoi E, Hatakeyama Y, Pradhan RL, Kido T, Sato K. Position of immobilization after dislocation of the shoulder: a cadaveric study. *J Bone Joint Surg Am*. 1999; 81:385-390.

A Qualitative Investigation of Return to Sport After Arthroscopic Bankart Repair: Beyond Stability
Tjong VK, Devitt BM, Murnaghan ML, et al (Univ of Toronto, Ontario, Canada; et al)
Am J Sports Med 43:2005-2011, 2015

Background.—Arthroscopic shoulder stabilization is known to have excellent functional results, but many patients do not return to their preinjury level of sport, with return to play rates reported between 48% and 100% despite good outcome scores.

Purpose.—To understand specific subjective psychosocial factors influencing a patient's decision to return to sport after arthroscopic shoulder stabilization.

Study Design.—Case series; Level of evidence, 4.

Methods.—Semistructured qualitative interviews were conducted with patients aged 18 to 40 years who had undergone primary arthroscopic shoulder stabilization and had a minimum 2-year follow-up. All patients participated in sport before surgery without any further revision operations or shoulder injuries. Qualitative data analysis was performed in accordance with the Strauss and Corbin theory to derive codes, categories, and themes. Preinjury and current sport participation was defined by type, level of competition, and the Brophy/Marx shoulder activity score. Patient-reported pain and shoulder function were also obtained.

Results.—A total of 25 patients were interviewed, revealing that fear of reinjury, shifts in priority, mood, social support, and self-motivation were found to greatly influence the decision to return to sport both in patients who had and had not returned to their preinjury level of play. Patients also described fear of sporting incompetence, self-awareness issues, recommendations from physical therapists, and degree of confidence as less common considerations affecting their return to sport.

Conclusion.—In spite of excellent functional outcomes, extrinsic and intrinsic factors such as competing interests, kinesiophobia, age, and internal stressors and motivators can have a major effect on a patient's decision to return to sport after arthroscopic shoulder stabilization. The qualitative methods used in this study provide a unique patient-derived perspective into postoperative recovery and highlight the necessity to recognize and address subjective and psychosocial factors rather than objective functional outcome scores alone as contributing to a patient's decision to return to play.

▶ This excellent case series of patients undergoing arthroscopic shoulder stabilization delves into an important and underreported consequence of injury: psychosocial factors. The authors identified 25 patients who underwent arthroscopic shoulder stabilization who scored well on standard functional outcome measures. They found that the most important factor regarding their lack of return to sport was not a lack of shoulder function but a variety of intrinsic and extrinsic factors. The authors highlight 5 patient-derived themes: competing interest, psychological motivators, fear of reinjury, social support, and advancing age as reasons to not return to sport. This article shows us that the orthopedic surgeon should be wary of the significant contribution of patient's psychological and sociologic recovery after shoulder reconstructive surgery.

J. Macalena, MD

Complications Associated With Arthroscopic Labral Repair Implants: A Case Series

Felder JJ, Elliott MP, Mair SD (Univ of Kentucky, Lexington)
Orthopedics 38:439-443, 2015

Arthroscopic labral repair in the shoulder has become commonplace in recent years. A variety of implants have evolved in parallel with arthroscopic techniques. Any orthopedic implant that is placed in close proximity to the joint has the potential to cause subsequent damage to the articular surface if it is left prominent or dislodges secondary to improper surgical technique. This article focuses on a series of implant-related complications of labral surgery and their subsequent management. Additionally, correct patient selection and surgical technique are discussed.

▶ This article provides case reviews of 4 patients who sustained complications after arthroscopic labral repair. The first case demonstrated significant chondral wear of the humeral head after intraarticular placement of a 3.5-mm screw. This screw head damaged the humeral head and caused tendinosis to the biceps. The screw was removed and the symptoms abated. Cases 2 and 3 demonstrated implants that had broken free during a strenuous event postoperatively and became dislodged. Both of these cases were treated with implant excision using an arthroscopic technique. The final case showed an implant within the midportion of the glenoid. This metal implant had caused chondral wear to the surrounding glenoid and humeral head. The most important lesson from this case series is to always place your implants carefully. Also a high index of suspicion should be had when postoperative patients complain of locking or catching symptoms. Postoperative imaging can be an important adjunct to assess anchor placement.

J. Macalena, MD

Arthroscopic Stabilization of Posterior Shoulder Instability Is Successful in American Football Players

Arner JW, McClincy MP, Bradley JP (Univ of Pittsburgh Med Ctr, PA)
Arthroscopy 31:1466-1471, 2015

Purpose.—To evaluate subjective and objective clinical outcomes of arthroscopic posterior capsulolabral repair for the treatment of symptomatic unidirectional posterior shoulder instability in American football players.

Methods.—Fifty-six consecutive American football players with unidirectional posterior shoulder instability underwent an arthroscopic posterior capsulolabral repair with or without suture anchors. Patients were evaluated, with return to play as the primary outcome measure supplemented with the American Shoulder and Elbow Surgeons (ASES) scoring system.

Stability, range of motion, strength, pain, and function were also assessed with subjective scales.

Results.—At a mean follow-up of 44.7 months postoperatively, 93% returned to sport and 79% returned to sport at the same level. Significant improvements (*P* < .01) were seen between preoperative and postoperative evaluations in ASES score and subjective scores of stability, range of motion, strength, pain, and function. Excellent or good results (ASES score > 60; stability < 6) were achieved in 96.5% of athletes, and 96% were satisfied with their operations.

Conclusions.—Arthroscopic capsulolabral repair for unidirectional posterior shoulder instability is effective in American football players because it improves stability, pain, and joint function, which optimizes the likelihood of successful return to play.

Level of Evidence.—Case series; Level of evidence, IV.

▶ The authors submit a well-done case series with 56 patients regarding the arthroscopic treatment of posterior shoulder instability. Return to play was the primary endpoint, and the authors showed a 93% return to play and a 79% return to play at the same level. Statistically significant improvements in American Shoulder and Elbow Surgeons scores and subjective improvements in stability, range of motion, strength, pain, and function. This cohort did identify 2 failures, both with continued symptoms of instability. Specifically, posterior instability patients in this cohort had lower rate of failure than a similar study of all comers as published by Bradley in 2013.[1] Limitations of this study include the fact that it only covers American Football players. Further, no direct control group for technique or nonoperative management was used.

J. Macalena, MD

Reference

1. Bradley JP, McClincy MP, Arner JW, Tejwani SG. Arthroscopic capsulolabral reconstruction for posterior instability of the shoulder: a prospective study of 200 shoulders. *Am J Sports Med.* 2013;41:2005-2014.

Anterior Shoulder Instability Is Associated with an Underlying Deficiency of the Bony Glenoid Concavity
Moroder P, Ernstbrunner L, Pomwenger W, et al (Paracelsus Med Univ, Salzburg, Germany; et al)
Arthroscopy 31:1223-1231, 2015

Purpose.—To determine whether anterior shoulder instability is associated with an inherent deficiency of the bony glenoid concavity, which results in a reduced bony shoulder stability ratio (BSSR).

Methods.—In this case-control study, we searched the institutional database for patients treated for unilateral recurrent anterior shoulder instability. We included 30 consecutive patients with atraumatic instability, 30 consecutive patients with traumatic instability, and 36 matched healthy controls, for a total of 96 shoulders. Computed tomography images of the unaffected shoulders of the instability patients were compared with images of the ipsilateral shoulders of age- and sex-matched healthy controls for differences in glenoid morphology. By use of a mathematical formula based on Pythagorean trigonometric identities, the mean BSSRs of the different groups were calculated and compared. Validation of the formula was accomplished by finite element analysis.

Results.—The mean BSSR of atraumatic instability patients was 17.9% ± 8.5% and therefore significantly lower than the mean BSSR of 31.1% ± 7.5% of the control group (13.2%; 95% confidence interval [CI], 9.1% to 17.4%; $P < .001$). The mean BSSR of the traumatic instability group was higher, at 23.9% ± 8.5% ($P = .007$), but still showed a

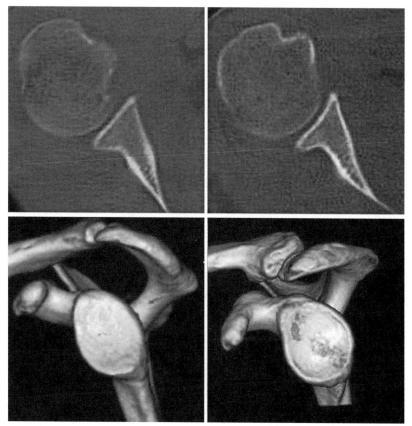

FIGURE 1.—Exemplary axial and 3-dimensional computed tomography images of different glenoid concavity shapes encountered in clinical practice. (Reprinted from Moroder P, Ernstbrunner L, Pomwenger W, et al. Anterior shoulder instability is associated with an underlying deficiency of the bony glenoid concavity. *Arthroscopy.* 2015;31:1223-1231, with permission from Arthroscopy Association of North America.)

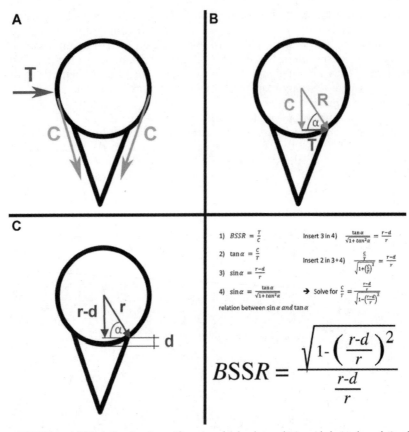

FIGURE 2.—(A) The ball-and-socket configuration of a glenohumeral joint with depicted translational force (T) and compressive force (C). (B) The compressive force vector (C) and the translational force vector (T) form a right triangle, with the resulting force vector as the hypotenuse (R). (C) An identical right triangle is described by geometrical entities of the ball-and-socket configuration including the radius (r) and the concavity depth (d), or combinations thereof. (D) Mathematical considerations based on Pythagorean trigonometric identities put the right triangle of the force vectors in relation to the right triangle of the geometrical entities to determine the bony shoulder stability ratio (BSSR), which is the ratio for the maximal translational force (T) against which a shoulder can be stabilized by a given concavity-compression force (C). (Reprinted from Moroder P, Ernstbrunner L, Pomwenger W, et al. Anterior shoulder instability is associated with an underlying deficiency of the bony glenoid concavity. *Arthroscopy.* 2015;31:1223-1231, with permission from Arthroscopy Association of North America.)

deficit of 7.2% (95% CI, 2.8% to 11.7%; $P=.002$) compared with controls. The atraumatic instability group showed a mean reduction of 0.9 mm (95% CI, 0.6 to 1.1 mm; $P<.001$) in concavity depth and a decrease of 2.9° (95% CI, 0.4° to 5.3°; $P=.021$) in concavity retroversion, whereas the traumatic instability patients had a reduction of 0.4 mm (95% CI, 0.1 to 0.8 mm; $P=.006$) in concavity depth. Neither of the instability groups differed significantly from their respective controls in terms of glenoid concavity diameter, head radius, or glenoid vault morphology.

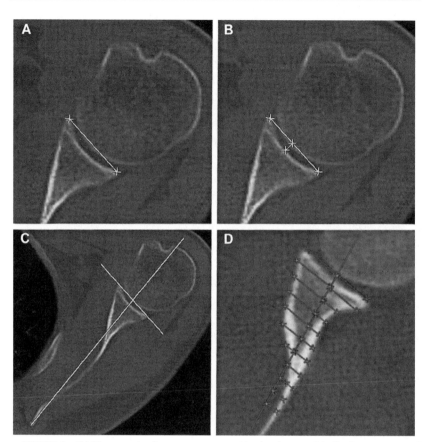

FIGURE 4.—(A) The concavity diameter was measured by drawing a straight line from one apex of the concavity to the opposite apex. (B) The depth was defined as the distance from the deepest point of the concavity to the diameter line. (C) The version was determined by drawing a tangential line on the concavity and a line running from the medial border of the scapula through the middle of the concavity. The anteromedial angle formed by the 2 lines was used to measure the concavity version. (D) Example of measurements performed to determine the tapering of the glenoid vault from lateral to medial. The vault extent was measured in 5-mm steps from lateral to medial parallel to the tangential line of the glenoid concavity and in relation to its midpoint. All the different measurements were performed in the standardized axial imaging plane illustrated in Fig 2. (Reprinted from Moroder P, Ernstbrunner L, Pomwenger W, et al. Anterior shoulder instability is associated with an underlying deficiency of the bony glenoid concavity. *Arthroscopy.* 2015;31:1223-1231, with permission from Arthroscopy Association of North America.)

Conclusions.—Anterior shoulder instability is associated with an inherent flattening of the bony glenoid concavity, which significantly decreases the BSSR. The deficiency appears to be more pronounced in patients with atraumatic instability than in patients with traumatic instability.

Level of Evidence.—Level III, case-control study.

▶ It is well known that patients with a bony injury to the anterior glenoid (bony bankart) are predisposed to recurrent shoulder instability. It leads from this knowledge that patients with inherent bony deficiency of the glenoid are also predisposed to anterior instability. This well-conceived case control study looked at 96 shoulders with either traumatic instability or atraumatic instability. Unaffected contralateral shoulders were used as the control group. The authors used the data obtained from this study to define the Bony Shoulder Stability Ratio (BSSR)—an inherent measure of the bony depth and width of the glenoid. To add validity to their study, the authors then performed a finite element analysis. Patients in this study with atraumatic instability had the lowest BSRR (reaching statistical significance). Traumatic instability patients also had a BSRR that was statistically significantly less than that in the control group. These data suggest a predisposition to instability when the BSRR is decreased. Flattening of the glenoid was the largest contribution to the decreased BSRR (Figs 1, 2, and 4). This study, as the authors concede, does not account for the contribution of the cartilage or the labrum. Further work will be necessary in the setting of humeral sided lesions (Hill-Sachs deformity).

J. Macalena, MD

Posterior Instability of the Shoulder: A Systematic Review and Meta-analysis of Clinical Outcomes
DeLong JM, Jiang K, Bradley JP (Med Univ of South Carolina, Charleston; Univ of Pittsburgh Med Ctr, PA; Burke and Bradley Orthopedics, Pittsburgh, PA)
Am J Sports Med 43:1805-1817, 2015

Background.—To date, there are no reports in the literature of a systematic review and meta-analysis for posterior instability of the shoulder.

Purpose.—The primary objective was to systematically capture, critically evaluate, and perform a meta-analysis of all available literature on arthroscopic clinical outcomes to provide insight and clinical recommendations for unilateral posterior shoulder instability. The secondary objective was to use the same means to assess clinical outcome literature for open treatment, of which a subset of highly reported outcome measures were used to determine superiority of arthroscopic versus open procedures for unilateral posterior shoulder.

Study Design.—Systematic review, meta-analysis.

Methods.—A systematic search to obtain every available, published, level of evidence study reporting patient data for unidirectional posterior shoulder instability was performed by use of the Cochrane Database of Systematic Reviews, PubMed/Medline database, manual searches of high impact factor journals and conference proceedings, and secondary references appraised for studies meeting inclusion criteria.

Results.—The systematic search captured a total of 1035 publications. After initial exclusion criteria were applied, 607 abstracts were assessed for eligibility. Full-text articles were obtained for 324 articles, and a total of 53 unique publications (27 arthroscopic studies, 26 open studies) reporting clinical outcomes for unidirectional posterior shoulder instability met inclusion criteria and were included in the systematic review and meta-analysis.

Conclusion.—Well-defined and uniform shoulder outcome measures to assess posterior shoulder instability are lacking throughout the literature. However, arthroscopic procedures are shown to be an effective and reliable treatment for unidirectional posterior glenohumeral instability with respect to outcome scores, patient satisfaction, and return to play. Despite similar results of outcome measures to the overall athletic population, throwing athletes are less likely to return to their preinjury levels of sport compared with contact athletes or the overall athletic population. Evidence also indicates that arthroscopic stabilization procedures using suture anchors result in fewer recurrences and revisions than anchorless repairs in young adults engaging in highly demanding physical activity. Furthermore, the literature suggests that patients treated arthroscopically have superior outcomes compared with patients who undergo open procedures with respect to stability, recurrence of instability, patient satisfaction, return to sport, and return to previous level of play.

▶ Posterior instability of the shoulder is seen less frequently than anterior instability and may be associated with undefined vague shoulder pain and symptoms. However, the incidence of posterior instability has become increasingly recognized particularly in the competitive athletic population. Additionally challenging is that no single pathologic lesion occurs with posterior instability, and a variety of lesions often accompany this diagnosis. These patients are challenging to accurately diagnose, classify, and effectively treat. There has been a shift over the years away from open treatment toward arthroscopic management. The predominant arthroscopic intervention consists of posterior capsulolabral stabilization with anchor or anchorless suture fixation, often combined with capsular plication.[1]

The authors conducted a comprehensive systematic review of the available literature on unidirectional posterior shoulder instability, performing a meta-analysis of the current literature with regard to objective and subjective clinical outcomes following arthroscopic intervention. Secondarily, comparison was made between outcomes following arthroscopic versus open techniques.

Table 1 lists the primary and secondary outcomes in the analysis for arthroscopic treatment, comparing results of the total cohort (n = 815) and the subgroup of athletes, contact athletes, and overhead/throwing athletes. Of note, overall, patients had high subjective stability (91%) and satisfaction (94%). Recurrent instability was 8% and reoperation rate was 8%. Overall complication rate was 2.5%. Functional outcome measures were high with overall mean postoperative score of 90% of maximum score. Interestingly, the overhead/throwing athlete had the least favorable outcomes, with the highest rates of recurrent instability, lowest return to sport at any level, and a low rate of return to previous level of sport (58%).

Table 2 contrasts the outcomes of arthroscopic and open procedures. Taken as a whole, the data show a trend toward superior outcomes in the arthroscopic technique compared with open. Of note, the recurrence rate is lower (8% vs

TABLE 1.—Primary and Secondary Arthroscopic Outcomes—Posterior Shoulder Instability[a]

Outcome Measure	Total Population		Overall Athletes		Contact Athletes		Throwing/Overhead Athletes	
	% (SD)	n/N (Studies)[b]	% (SD)	n/N (Studies)[b]	% (SD)	n/N (Studies)[b]	% (SD)	n/N (Studies)[b]
Primary outcomes								
Recurrent instability	8.1 (±3.8)	66/815 (26)	8.6 (±4.8)	44/513 (15)	5.1 (±2.3)	9/178 (6)	12.1 (±1.5)	4/33 (3)
Revision/reoperation	7.6 (±3.5)	38/502 (19)	6.8 (±4.0)	26/381 (13)	6.2 (±2.9)	11/178 (6)	c	1/6 (2)
Persistent pain	12.3 (±2.2)	45/365 (18)	17.5 (±2.5)	18/103 (9)	c	1/1 (1)	c	4/4 (2)
Subjective stability	91.1 (±48.3)	637/699 (18)	91.9 (±58.2)	443/482 (11)	91.4 (±47.1)	160/175 (5)	89.3 (±16.3)	25/28 (2)
Return to sport (any level)	N/A	N/A	91.8 (±45.4)	561/611 (19)	89.3 (±42.4)	159/178 (6)	83.9 (±12.5)	26/31 (3)
Return to sport (previous level)	N/A	N/A	67.4 (±35.9)	368/546 (15)	71.9 (±32.6)	128/178 (6)	58.1 (±7.9)	18/31 (3)
Secondary outcomes								
Objective stability	95.1 (±10.5)	97/102 (7)	97.1 (±12.8)	68/70 (5)	92.9 (±4.2)	26/28 (4)	100c (±2.6)	13/13 (4)
Postoperative stiffness	c	2/8 (3)	c	2/8 (3)	c	1/1 (1)	c	1/1 (1)
Range of motion	90.4 (±52.7)	492/544 (15)	83.6 (±63.7)	285/341 (8)	97.1 (±49.1)	133/137 (5)	c	6/7 (3)
Muscle strength	64.4 (±36.6)	328/509 (9)	54.0 (±40.9)	174/322 (5)	53.6 (±31.9)	67/125 (3)	c	2/2 (2)
Patient satisfaction	93.8 (±51.8)	442/471 (13)	93.2 (±60.4)	341/366 (10)	92.4 (±52.5)	157/170 (4)	c	1/1 (1)

[a]N/A, not applicable.
[b]n/N, number of affected shoulders/total number reported (number of studies).
[c]Low-powered patient population.
Reprinted from DeLong JM, Jiang K, Bradley JP. Posterior instability of the shoulder: a systematic review and meta-analysis of clinical outcomes. *Am J Sports Med.* 201543:1805-1817, with permission from The Author(s).

TABLE 2.—Functional Outcome Measures—Posterior Shoulder Instability[a]

Outcome Measure	No. of Studies	No. of Shoulders	Mean Preoperative Score	Mean Postoperative Score	Maximum Score/Raw Points	Postoperative % of Ideal Maximum Score
ASES	9	524	53.63 (7 studies)	89.65	100	90
WD	2	21	37.4 (1 study)	80.45	100	80
Modified Conway	1	12	NR	NR	NR	NR
SST	3	70	9.3 (1 study)	11.57	12	96
VAS	2	49	3.5 (1 study)	0.9	10	91
Modified West Point Rowe	1	1	40	95	100	95
UCLA	2	30	16 (1 study)	31.8	35	91
Oxford	2	4	15 (1 study)	43	48	90
Bigliani	2	15	3 (1 study)	6.54	8	82
Rowe	2	46	35.6 (1 study)	94.8	100	95
SANE	3	54	NR	90.83	100	91
WOSI	3	81	NR	312.63	2100	85
PSS	1	5	NR	87	100	87
Neer-Foster	2	133	NR	97% Satisfactory	Satisfactory	97
Subjective Patient Shoulder Evaluation	1	33	NR	20.0	24	83
Wolf-Eakin	2	32	NR	22.3 (1 study)	24	93
L'Insalata	1	27	NR	90	100	90
SF-36	1	27	NR	50.4	50 (normal, healthy)	99
Constant-Murley	1	3	NR	NR	100	NR
Athletic Shoulder Outcome Rating	1	20	NR	83	100	83
Undefined scoring system	2	17	NR	NR	NR	NR

[a]ASES, American Shoulder and Elbow Score; NR, not reported; PSS, Penn Shoulder Score; SANE, Single Assessment Numeric Evaluation; SF-36, Short Form Health Survey; SST, Simple Shoulder Test; UCLA, University of California, Los Angeles Shoulder Rating Scale; VAS, Visual Analog Scale; WD, Walch-Duplay; WOSI, Western Ontario Shoulder Instability.
Reprinted from DeLong JM, Jiang K, Bradley JP. Posterior instability of the shoulder: a systematic review and meta-analysis of clinical outcomes. *Am J Sports Med.* 201543:1805-1817, with permission from The Author(s).

9%), patient satisfaction higher (94% vs 86%), and return to sport at previous level increased (67% vs 37%) (Table 2).

Several trends were discussed. Prior surgery did seem to lead to a higher chance of failure in several studies. Use of modern arthroscopic suture anchor appeared to provide more reliable outcomes than sutureless repair. Several studies in the review noticed postoperative failures were related to failure of initial diagnosis of multidirectional instability, underscoring the importance of accurate diagnosis at the time of surgery. The unique pathologic changes noted in the hyperlax patient had higher rates of failure, pointing toward the conclusion that these patients may represent a distinct population who require additional well-planned intervention. Early mobilization did seem to lead to inferior outcomes in a few studies and should be entertained with caution. Finally, the overhead/throwing athlete as a subgroup had substantially lower success rates and may require a specialized evaluation and outcome measure unique to the population. Future trials are indicated, in particular, prospective level-2 studies, which are lacking in the current literature.

The authors conducted a well-designed systematic review and were awarded the 2014 Systematic Review Award commending their efforts.

M. O'Shaughnessy, MD

Reference

1. Bradley JP, Forsythe B, Mascarenhas R. Arthroscopic management of posterior shoulder instability: diagnosis, indications, and technique. *Clin Sports Med.* 2008;27:649-670.

Arm Abduction Provides a Better Reduction of the Bankart Lesion During Immobilization in External Rotation After an Initial Shoulder Dislocation
Itoi E, Kitamura T, Hitachi S, et al (Tohoku Univ School of Medicine, Sendai, Japan; Kumamoto Orthopaedic Hosp, Japan; et al)
Am J Sports Med 43:1731-1736, 2015

Background.—Shoulder dislocation often recurs, especially in the younger population. Immobilization in external rotation, in which a Bankart lesion is displaced in the anterior, medial, and inferior directions, was introduced as a new method of nonoperative treatment, but its clinical efficiency is controversial. In terms of reducing the lesion, it is reasonable to incorporate not only external rotation, which makes the anterior soft tissues tight to push the lesion posteriorly and laterally, but also abduction, which makes the inferior soft tissues tight to push the lesion superiorly.

Hypothesis.—Abducting the arm during immobilization in external rotation will improve the reduction of a Bankart lesion.

Study Design.—Controlled laboratory study.

Methods.—There were 37 patients with initial shoulder dislocation enrolled in this study. After reduction, MRI was taken in 4 positions of the shoulder: adduction and internal rotation (Add-IR), adduction and external rotation (Add-ER), 30° of abduction and 30° of external rotation (Abd-30ER), and 30° of abduction and 60° of external rotation (Abd-60ER). On radial slices, the separation, displacement of the labrum, and opening angle of the capsule were measured.

Results.—Add-ER improved the reduction of the anterior labrum but not the inferior labrum when compared with Add-IR. Both Abd-30ER and Abd-60ER improved the reduction of the inferior labrum as compared with Add-IR. Furthermore, Abd-60ER improved the reduction more than Add-ER.

Conclusion.—Among the 4 positions tested, Abd-60ER is the best position in terms of reducing the Bankart lesion.

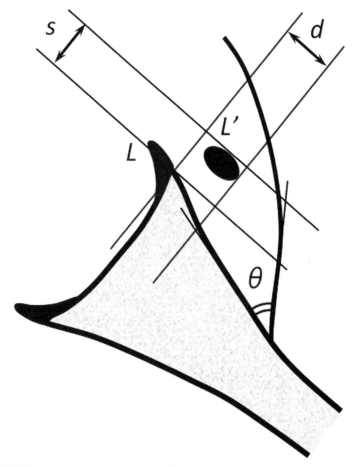

FIGURE 2.—Measured parameters on magnetic resonance imaging. d, displacement; L, original labrum; L′, displaced labrum; s, separation; θ, opening angle. (Reprinted from Itoi E, Kitamura T, Hitachi S, et al. Arm abduction provides a better reduction of the bankart lesion during immobilization in external rotation after an initial shoulder dislocation. *Am J Sports Med.* 2015;43:1731-1736, with permission from The Author(s).)

Clinical Relevance.—Abducting the shoulder during immobilization in external rotation is demonstrated to improve the reduction of the Bankart lesion. Therefore, this position is expected to reduce the recurrence rate after initial dislocation of the shoulder. Future clinical trials are necessary.

▶ Bankart lesions following anterior shoulder dislocation can result in high recurrence rate, especially in young patients. Nonoperative management using immobilization is preferred to avoid the risks of operation if possible. Traditional teaching based on previous studies including cadaver and intraoperative observations found that the optimal arm position for Bankart lesion reduction is an adducted, internally rotated position. However, these data were based on arthroscopic visualization.

The authors' study disproves this commonly held belief, showing that, abduction and external rotation of 60° give the best results.

The study is a prospective series in which radiographic observer was blinded. Thirty-seven acute anterior dislocations with no evidence of fracture were enrolled, with 31 shoulders available for measurements (26 men, 5 women) average age of 19 (range, 13-32). Patients were seen for acute anterior dislocation and reduced by the clinician. They subsequently underwent MRI with the arm in 4 test positions. A cast mold was created to set the arm in the 4 study positions, using the same mold/support for each patient in attempt to standardize the intervention. The test positions included (1) adduction, 30° internal rotation; (2) adduction, 30° external rotation; (3) abduction 30°, external rotation 30°; and (4) 30° abduction, 60° external rotation. Radiographic measurements were taken from the MRI images to determine separation, displacement, and opening angle as diagramed in Fig 2 with the arm in each of the 4 test positions.

Authors discuss that clinical trials are warranted. Prior studies found that abduction is poorly tolerated and leads to high rates of noncompliance. Thus, although the study's data support the hypothesis that abduction, external rotation 60° is the best position to reduce the lesion, clinical studies are warranted to determine the best clinically acceptable position.

This study has the capability to change the nonoperative management and immobilization protocol for anterior shoulder dislocations resulting in Bankart lesions.

M. O'Shaughnessy, MD

Comparison of 3-Dimensional Computed Tomography–Based Measurement of Glenoid Bone Loss With Arthroscopic Defect Size Estimation in Patients with Anterior Shoulder Instability
Bakshi NK, Patel I, Jacobson JA, et al (Univ of Michigan, Ann Arbor; et al)
Arthroscopy 31:1880-1885, 2015

Purpose.—The purpose of this study was to compare four 3-dimensional (3D) computed tomography (CT) methods of measuring glenoid bone loss with the arthroscopic estimation of glenoid bone loss.

Methods.—Twenty patients with recurrent anterior shoulder instability underwent bilateral shoulder CT scans and were found to have glenoid bone loss. Arthroscopic estimation of glenoid bone loss was performed in all patients. Three-dimensional CT reconstruction was performed on the CT scans of each patient. The glenoid bone loss of each patient was measured using the surface area, Pico, ratio, and anteroposterior distance—from—bare area methods. The mean percent loss calculated with each method was compared with arthroscopy to determine the reliability of arthroscopy in the measurement of glenoid bone loss.

Results.—The mean percent bone loss calculated with arthroscopic estimation, surface area, Pico, ratio, and anteroposterior distance—from—bare area methods was 18.13% ± 11.81%, 12.15% ± 8.50% ($P = .005$), 12.77% ± 8.17% ($P = .002$), 9.50% ± 8.74% ($P < .001$), and 12.44% ± 10.68% ($P = .001$), respectively. Repeated-measures analysis of variance showed that the 3D CT methods and arthroscopy were

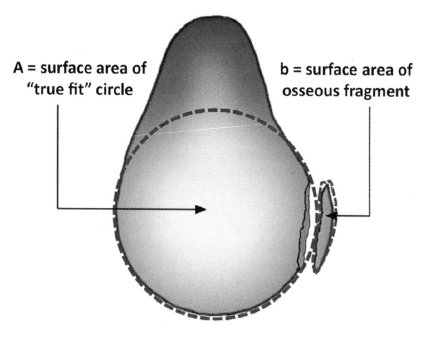

$$\text{Percent Bone Loss} = \frac{b}{A} \times 100\%$$

FIGURE 2.—Surface area method of measuring glenoid bone loss in a right glenoid. (Reprinted from Bakshi NK, Patel I, Jacobson JA, et al. Comparison of 3-dimensional computed tomography—based measurement of glenoid bone loss with arthroscopic defect size estimation in patients with anterior shoulder instability. *Arthroscopy.* 2015;31:1880-1885, with permission from Arthroscopy Association of North America.)

significantly different ($F_{4,76} = 13.168$, $P = .02$). The estimate using arthroscopy is 55% greater than the average of the 3D CT methods.

Conclusions.—Our findings suggest that arthroscopy significantly overestimates glenoid bone loss compared with CT and call into question its validity as a method of measurement. A more internally consistent and accurate method for the measurement of glenoid bone loss is necessary to appropriately diagnose and treat shoulder instability.

Level of Evidence.—Level IV, case series.

▶ This well-designed case series of 20 patients compared 4 different techniques to estimate glenoid bone loss on CT scans and then correlate the radiographic findings with arthroscopic findings. Contralateral shoulders were used as control groups. The 4 CT methods assessed included surface area, Pico, ratio, and distance from bare area as seen in Figures 2 through 4. The surface area method, Pico method, and distance from bare area method all produced bone loss at about 12%, whereas the ratio method estimated significantly less at 9% as seen in Table 2. All of these values were significantly

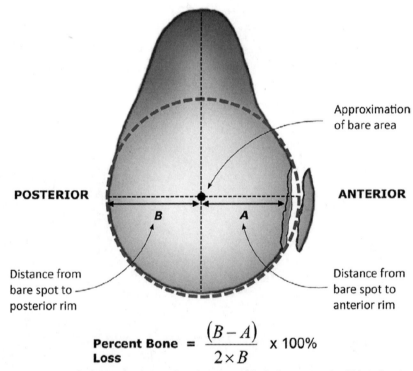

$$\text{Percent Bone Loss} = \frac{(B - A)}{2 \times B} \times 100\%$$

FIGURE 3.—Anteroposterior distance from bare area method of measuring glenoid bone loss in a right glenoid. (Reprinted from Bakshi NK, Patel I, Jacobson JA, et al. Comparison of 3-dimensional computed tomography–based measurement of glenoid bone loss with arthroscopic defect size estimation in patients with anterior shoulder instability. *Arthroscopy.* 2015;31:1880-1885, with permission from Arthroscopy Association of North America.)

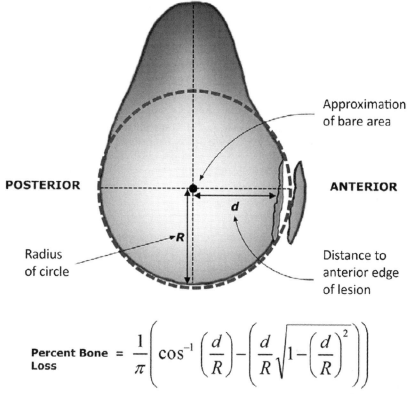

$$\text{Percent Bone Loss} = \frac{1}{\pi}\left(\cos^{-1}\left(\frac{d}{R}\right)-\left(\frac{d}{R}\sqrt{1-\left(\frac{d}{R}\right)^2}\right)\right)$$

FIGURE 4.—Ratio method of measuring glenoid bone loss in a right glenoid. (Reprinted from Bakshi NK, Patel I, Jacobson JA, et al. Comparison of 3-dimensional computed tomography—based measurement of glenoid bone loss with arthroscopic defect size estimation in patients with anterior shoulder instability. *Arthroscopy.* 2015;31:1880-1885, with permission from Arthroscopy Association of North America.)

TABLE 2.—Bone Loss Estimates by 3D CT and Arthroscopic Estimation

Method	Mean % Bone Loss	Paired 2-Tailed t Test Compared With Arthroscopic Estimation	95% CI
Surface area method	12.15 ± 8.50	$P = .005$	8.42-15.88
Pico method	12.77 ± 8.17	$P = .002$	9.19-16.35
AP distance—from—bare area method	12.44 ± 10.68	$P = .001$	7.76-17.12
Ratio method	9.50 ± 8.74	$P < .001$	5.67-13.33
Arthroscopic estimation	18.13 ± 11.81		12.95-23.31

NOTE. Repeated-measures analysis of variance showed $F_{4,76} = 13.168$ and $P < .05$.
AP, anteroposterior; CI, confidence interval; CT, computed tomography; 3D, 3-dimensional.
Reprinted from Bakshi NK, Patel I, Jacobson JA, et al. Comparison of 3-dimensional computed tomography—based measurement of glenoid bone loss with arthroscopic defect size estimation in patients with anterior shoulder instability. *Arthroscopy.* 2015;31:1880-1885, with permission from Arthroscopy Association of North America.

less than the arthroscopic technique, which produced a large value of approximately 18%. The authors conclude that the arthroscopic technique overestimated the amount of bone loss by 55% and recommend caution in using this technique. Further work is necessary on this topic to define the most valid technique to define glenoid bone loss.

J. Macalena, MD

The Effect of a Combined Glenoid and Hill-Sachs Defect on Glenohumeral Stability: A Biomechanical Cadaveric Study Using 3-Dimensional Modeling of 142 Patients
Arciero RA, Parrino A, Bernhardson AS, et al (Univ of Connecticut Health Ctr, Farmington; Naval Med Ctr, San Diego, CA; et al)
Am J Sports Med 43:1422-1429, 2014

Background.—Bone loss in anterior glenohumeral instability occurs on both the glenoid and the humerus; however, existing biomechanical studies have evaluated glenoid and humeral head defects in isolation. Thus, little is known about the combined effect of these bony lesions in a clinically relevant model on glenohumeral stability.

Hypothesis/Purpose.—The purpose of this study was to determine the biomechanical efficacy of a Bankart repair in the setting of bipolar (glenoid and humeral head) bone defects determined via computer-generated 3-dimensional (3D) modeling of 142 patients with recurrent anterior shoulder instability. The null hypothesis was that adding a bipolar bone defect will have no effect on glenohumeral stability after soft tissue Bankart repair.

Study Design.—Controlled laboratory study.

Methods.—A total of 142 consecutive patients with recurrent anterior instability were analyzed with 3D computed tomography scans. Two Hill-Sachs lesions were selected on the basis of volumetric size representing the 25th percentile (0.87 cm^3; small) and 50th percentile (1.47 cm^3; medium) and printed in plastic resin with a 3D printer. A total of 21 cadaveric shoulders were evaluated on a custom shoulder-testing device permitting 6 degrees of freedom, and the force required to translate the humeral head anteriorly 10 mm at a rate of 2.0 mm/s with a compressive load of 50 N was determined at 60° of glenohumeral abduction and 60° of external rotation. All Bankart lesions were made sharply from the 2- to 6-o'clock positions for a right shoulder. Subsequent Bankart repair with transosseous tunnels using high-strength suture was performed. Hill-Sachs lesions were made in the cadaver utilizing a plastic mold from the exact replica off the 3D printer. Testing was conducted in the following sequence for each specimen: (1) intact, (2) posterior capsulotomy, (3) Bankart lesion, (4) Bankart repair, (5) Bankart lesion with 2-mm glenoid defect, (6) Bankart repair, (7) Bankart lesion with 2-mm glenoid defect and Hill-Sachs lesion, (8) Bankart repair, (9) Bankart lesion with 4-mm glenoid defect and Hill-Sachs lesion, (10) Bankart repair, (11) Bankart lesion with 6-mm glenoid defect and Hill-Sachs lesion, and (12) Bankart repair. All sequences were used first for a medium Hill-Sachs lesion (10 specimens) and then repeated for a small Hill-Sachs lesion (11 specimens). Three trials were performed in each condition, and the mean value was used for data analysis.

Results.—A statistically significant and progressive reduction in load to translation was observed after a Bankart lesion was created and with the addition of progressive glenoid defects for each humeral head defect. For medium (50th percentile) Hill-Sachs lesions, there was a 22%, 43%, and 58% reduction in stability with a 2-, 4-, and 6-mm glenoid defect, respectively. For small (25th percentile) Hill-Sachs lesions, there was an 18%, 27%, and 42% reduction in stability with a 2-, 4-, and 6-mm glenoid defect, respectively. With a ≥2-mm glenoid defect, the medium Hill-Sachs group demonstrated significant reduction in translation force after Bankart repair ($P < .01$), and for the small Hill-Sachs group, a ≥4-mm glenoid defect was required to produce a statistical decrease ($P < .01$) in reduction force after repair.

Conclusion.—Combined glenoid and humeral head defects have an additive and negative effect on glenohumeral stability. As little as a 2-mm glenoid defect with a medium-sized Hill-Sachs lesion demonstrated a compromise in soft tissue Bankart repair, while small-sized Hill-Sachs lesions showed compromise of soft tissue repair with ≥4-mm glenoid bone loss.

Clinical Relevance.—Bipolar bony lesions of the glenoid and humeral head occur frequently together in clinical practice. Surgeons should be aware that the combined defects and glenoid bone loss of 2 to 4 mm or approximately 8% to 15% of the glenoid could compromise Bankart repair and thus may require surgical strategies in addition to traditional Bankart repair alone to optimize stability.

▶ This is a very well done biomechanical study. The authors went through extensive modeling to standardize and confirm the Hill-Sachs lesion size and shape based on actual data from 142 patients. The authors used previous studies' techniques, which have already been accepted and tested on a large sample.

Results showed what one would expect. The combination of Hill-Sachs lesions with glenoid bone loss leads to significant decrease in force required for dislocation.

This model and information will be useful for investigators to measure the benefit of treatments of combined bone loss including Remplissage and Latarjet bone grafts.

R. Papandrea, MD

Sporting Activity After Arthroscopic Bankart Repair for Chronic Glenohumeral Instability

Plath JE, Feucht MJ, Saier T, et al (Technische Universität München; Berufsgenossenschaftliche Unfallklinik Murnau; et al)

Arthroscopy 31:1996-2003, 2015

Purpose.—The purpose of this study was to collect detailed data on postoperative sporting activity after arthroscopic Bankart repair for chronic shoulder instability.

Methods.—Of 113 patients who underwent arthroscopic Bankart repair between February 2008 and August 2010, 81 met the inclusion criteria and were surveyed by a specially designed postal sport-specific questionnaire. Of these 81 patients, 66 (82%) were available for evaluation.

Results.—All previously active patients performed some activity at follow-up. Of 9 patients (56%) who had been inactive, 5 took up new activities postoperatively. Forty-four patients (66%) stated that surgery had (strongly) improved their sporting proficiency. Seventeen patients (26%) reported no impact, and 5 patients (8%) reported a further deterioration compared with preoperatively. The improvement in sporting proficiency was negatively correlated with the preoperative risk level ($\rho = 0.42$, $P < .001$), preoperative performance level ($\rho = 0.31$, $P = .012$), and preoperative Tegner scale ($\rho = 0.36$, $P = .003$), as well as hours of sporting activity per week ($\rho = 0.25$, $P = .042$), whereas age showed a positive correlation ($\rho = 0.28$, $P = .023$). There was no change in duration, frequency, number of disciplines, Tegner activity scale, risk category, or performance level.

Conclusions.—Arthroscopic Bankart repair provides a high rate of return to activity among patients treated for chronic shoulder instability. A number of previously inactive patients returned to activity postoperatively. However, one-third of patients reported no benefit from surgery in terms of sporting activity. The improvement in sporting proficiency was highly dependent on the demands on the shoulder in sports, as well as the age of the patient. Overall, there was no significant increase in duration, frequency, number of disciplines, Tegner activity scale, or performance level between preoperative and follow-up evaluation and no increased return to high-risk activities.

Level of Evidence.—Level IV, therapeutic case series.

▶ The authors of this retrospective study defined chronic instability of the shoulder as being present for more than 1 year. A routine arthroscopic Bankart repair was done.

Although the study did not focus on recurrence, a 10% recurrence rate was reported, with age at time of surgery being the only statistically significant risk factor for recurrence.

The study was conducted to examine the return to sport after the reconstruction.

Two-thirds of the group reported improvement in sporting proficiency, with more than 50% of previously inactive patients becoming active after surgery.

Although one-third of the group noted no improvement in sporting activity, or even further deterioration (8%), only 19% of this group that did not report improved sport activity stated the limitations were shoulder related.

R. Papandrea, MD

External Rotation Immobilization for Primary Shoulder Dislocation: A Randomized Controlled Trial
Whelan DB, Joint Orthopaedic Initiative for National Trials of the Shoulder (JOINTS) (Univ of Toronto, Ontario, Canada; et al)
Clin Orthop Relat Res 472:2380-2386, 2014

Background.—The traditional treatment for primary anterior shoulder dislocations has been immobilization in a sling with the arm in a position of adduction and internal rotation. However, recent basic science and clinical data have suggested recurrent instability may be reduced with immobilization in external rotation after primary shoulder dislocation.

Questions/Purposes.—We performed a randomized controlled trial to compare the (1) frequency of recurrent instability and (2) disease-specific quality-of-life scores after treatment of first-time shoulder dislocation using either immobilization in external rotation or immobilization in internal rotation in a group of young patients.

Methods.—Sixty patients younger than 35 years of age with primary, traumatic, anterior shoulder dislocations were randomized (concealed, computer-generated) to immobilization with either an internal rotation sling (n = 29) or an external rotation brace (n = 31) at a mean of 4 days after closed reduction (range, 1–7 days). Patients with large bony lesions or polytrauma were excluded. The two groups were similar at baseline. Both groups were immobilized for 4 weeks with identical therapy protocols thereafter. Blinded assessments were completed by independent observers for a minimum of 12 months (mean, 25 months; range, 12–43 months). Recurrent instability was defined as a second documented anterior dislocation or multiple episodes of shoulder subluxation severe enough for the patient to request surgical stabilization. Validated disease-specific quality-of-life data (Western Ontario Shoulder Instability index [WOSI], American Shoulder and Elbow Surgeons evaluation [ASES]) were also collected. Ten patients (17%, five from each group) were lost to followup. Reported compliance with immobilization in both groups was excellent (80%).

Results.—With the numbers available, there was no difference in the rate of recurrent instability between groups: 10 of 27 patients (37%) with the external rotation brace versus 10 of 25 patients (40%) with the sling redislocated or developed symptomatic recurrent instability ($p = 0.41$). WOSI scores were not different between groups ($p = 0.74$) and, although the difference in ASES scores approached statistical significance ($p = 0.05$), the magnitude of this difference was small and of uncertain clinical importance.

Conclusions.—Despite previous published findings, our results show immobilization in external rotation did not confer a significant benefit versus sling immobilization in the prevention of recurrent instability after primary anterior shoulder dislocation. Further studies with larger numbers may elucidate whether functional outcomes, compliance, or comfort with immobilization can be improved with this device.

Level of Evidence.—Level I, therapeutic study. See Instructions for Authors for a complete description of levels of evidence.

▶ It is a common scenario in the medical literature: a single group publishes a study or group of studies with an extraordinary finding—perhaps a finding that seems too good to be true, such as a 100% success rate. Thereafter, there is a substantial time gap in which other research groups struggle to put together a similar study to confirm or controvert these remarkable findings. In this case, a group out of Japan published a preliminary study in 2003 showing a 0% recurrence rate of anterior shoulder dislocations after immobilizing their patients with the shoulder in relative external rotation. The same group subsequently performed a larger, randomized study indicating an almost 40% risk reduction by immobilizing the shoulder in external rotation compared with internal rotation.

It wasn't until 2011 that a separate group was able to perform a similar study. However, this study failed to show a substantial difference between the 2 methods of immobilization after shoulder dislocation. In this article, Whelan et al weigh in on this perceived controversy in an attempt to provide a "tie-breaker" study. Unfortunately, their numbers were too small to show a meaningful difference between the 2 treatment groups. So, the controversy remains. Keep your eyes open for bigger and better studies in the future.

K. Bengston, MD

Latissimus Dorsi and Teres Major Transfer With Reverse Shoulder Arthroplasty Restores Active Motion and Reduces Pain for Posterosuperior Cuff Dysfunction
Shi LL, Cahill KE, Ek ET, et al (Univ of Chicago Hosps, IL; Univ of Melbourne, Australia; et al)
Clin Orthop Relat Res 473:3212-3217, 2015

Background.—In patients with rotator cuff dysfunction, reverse shoulder arthroplasty can restore active forward flexion, but it does not provide a solution for the lack of active external rotation because of infraspinatus and the teres minor dysfunction. A modified L'Episcopo procedure can be performed in the same setting wherein the latissimus dorsi and teres major tendons are transferred to the lateral aspect of proximal humerus in an attempt to restore active external rotation.

Questions/Purposes.—(1) Do latissimus dorsi and teres major tendon transfers with reverse shoulder arthroplasty improve external rotation function in patients with posterosuperior rotator cuff dysfunction? (2) Do patients experience less pain and have improved outcome scores after surgery? (3) What are the complications associated with reverse shoulder arthroplasty with latissimus dorsi and teres major transfer?

Methods.—Between 2007 and 2010, we treated all patients undergoing shoulder arthroplasty who had a profound external rotation lag sign and advanced fatty degeneration of the posterosuperior rotator cuff (infraspinatus plus teres minor) with this approach. A total of 21 patients (mean age 66 years; range, 58–82 years) were treated this way and followed for a minimum of 2 years (range, 26–81 months); none was lost to followup, and all have been seen in the last 5 years. We compared pre- and postoperative ranges of motion, pain, and functional status; scores were drawn from chart review. We also categorized major and minor complications.

Results.—Active forward flexion improved from 56° ± 36° to 120° ± 38° (mean difference: 64° [95% confidence interval {CI}, 45°–83°], $p < 0.001$). Active external rotation with the arm adducted improved from 6° ± 16° to 38° ± 14° (mean difference: 30° [95% CI, 21°–39°], $p < 0.001$); active external rotation with the arm abducted improved from 19° ± 25° to 74° ± 22° (mean difference: 44° [95% CI, 22°–65°], $p < 0.001$). Pain visual analog score improved from 8.4 ± 2.3 to 1.7 ± 2.1 (mean difference: −6.9 [95% CI, −8.7 to −5.2], $p < 0.001$), and Single Assessment Numeric Evaluation score improved from 28% ± 21% to 80% ± 24% (mean difference: 46% [95% CI, 28%–64%], $p < 0.001$). There were six major complications, five of which were treated operatively. Overall, three patients' latissimus and teres major transfer failed based on persistent lack of external rotation.

Conclusions.—In patients with posterior and superior cuff deficiency, reverse shoulder arthroplasty combined with latissimus dorsi and teres major transfer through a single deltopectoral incision can reliably increase active forward flexion and external rotation. Patients experience pain relief and functional improvement but have a high rate of complications; therefore, we recommend the procedure be limited to patients indicated for reverse who have profound external rotation loss and a high grade of infraspinatus/teres minor fatty atrophy.

Level of Evidence.—Level IV, therapeutic study.

▶ The authors present a retrospective review of 21 consecutive patients treated with reverse total shoulder arthroplasty and modified L'Episcopo procedure (Fig 1A-B), transferring the teres major and latissimus dorsi to the lateral aspect of the humerus to regain external rotation (ER). Patients were selected for tendon transfer if there was a 30° ER lag with the arm in either adduction or abduction. The previous literature consisted of small case series with short follow-up and lacked clearly defined surgical indications and technique. The current study involves 2 surgeons who performed all procedures through a single deltopectoral

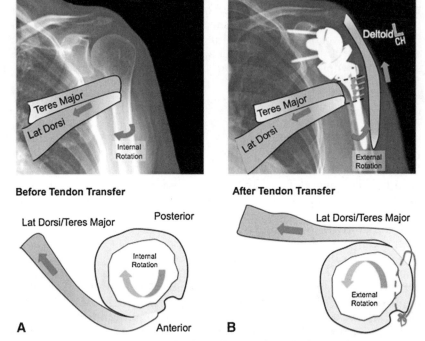

Before Tendon Transfer   **After Tendon Transfer**

FIGURE 1.—A–B Schematics are used to depict a latissimus dorsi ("lat dorsi") and teres major transfer in the setting of reverse shoulder arthroplasty. (A) Before the tendon transfer, the latissimus and teres major tendons attach on the anterior humerus and serve as internal rotators. (B) After the reverse shoulder replacement and tendon transfers, the latissimus and teres major tendons are rerouted from the posterior humerus and attached to the lateral humerus. They then serve as external rotators. (Reprinted from Shi LL, Cahill KE, Ek ET, et al. Latissimus dorsi and teres major transfer with reverse shoulder arthroplasty restores active motion and reduces pain for posterosuperior cuff dysfunction. *Clin Orthop Relat Res.* 2015;473:3212-3217, with permission from The Association of Bone and Joint Surgeons.)

approach with similar operative technique and postoperative protocol with 100% follow-up 2 years after surgery. There were significant improvements in active forward flexion and ER with the arm adducted and abducted (mean improvement 30° and 44°, respectively). Patients also had significant improvements in the Visual Analog Pain scale and Single Assessment Numeric Evaluation score. Forty-three percent of patients experienced a complication (3 minor and 6 major) and 3 patients' tendon transfers failed as defined by persistent ER lag of more than 30°. I am in agreement with the authors that the simultaneous tendon transfer with reverse total shoulder arthroplasty is indicated for patients with profound ER lag. What remains unclear is the amount of ER lag/posterosuperior cuff dysfunction that can be tolerated to avoid the morbidity associated with the tendon transfer, as it is not known what percentage of clinical improvement is caused by the reverse total shoulder and what percentage is secondary to the tendon transfer. Given the complexity of the procedure, it should be reserved for the experienced shoulder surgeon. The report does highlight the importance of preoperative evaluation for posterosuperior cuff dysfunction. Physical examination is paramount in determining the function of the posterosuperior cuff and in my clinical practice is augmented with MRI to evaluate for rotator cuff atrophy and, very rarely, EMG/NCS (Electromyography and Nerve Conduction Studies) in younger patients with profound atrophy to evaluate for nerve entrapment.

E. Gauger, MD

The Impact of Rotator Cuff Deficiency on Structure, Mechanical Properties, and Gene Expression Profiles of the Long Head of the Biceps Tendon (LHBT): Implications for Management of the LHBT During Primary Shoulder Arthroplasty

Kurdziel MD, Moravek JE, Wiater BP, et al (Beaumont Health System, Royal Oak, MI; et al)

J Orthop Res 33:1158-1164, 2015

The long head of the biceps tendon (LHBT) occupies a unique proximal intra-articular and distal extra-articular position within the human shoulder. In the presence of a rotator cuff (RC) tear, the LHBT is recruited into an accelerated role undergoing potential mechanical and biochemical degeneration. Intra-articular sections of the LHBT were harvested during primary shoulder arthroplasty from patients with an intact or deficient RC. LHBTs were stained (H&E, Alcian Blue) and subjected to histologic analysis using the semiquantitative Bonar scale and measurement of collagen orientation. LHBTs (n = 12 per group) were also subjected to gene-expression analyses via an RT^2-PCR Profiler Array quantifying 84 genes associated with cell-cell and cell-matrix interactions. LHBTs (n = 18 per group) were biomechanically tested with both stress-relaxation and load-to-failure protocols and subsequently modeled with the Quasilinear Viscoelastic (QLV) and Structural-Based Elastic (SBE) models. While no histologic differences were observed, significant differences in mechanical testing, and viscoelastic modeling parameters were found. PCR arrays identified five genes that were differentially expressed between RC-intact and RC-deficient LHBT groups. LHBTs display signs of pathology regardless of RC status in the arthroplasty population, which may be secondary to both glenohumeral joint arthritis and the additional mechanical role of the LHBT in this population.

▶ This study evaluated biceps specimens recovered at the time of arthroplasty using techniques evaluating mechanics, histology, and gene expression. There were changes in mechanical tissue properties and gene expression. Further studies are needed to understand and interpret these findings.

N. C. Chen, MD

Arthroscopic Tissue Culture for the Evaluation of Periprosthetic Shoulder Infection

Dilisio MF, Miller LR, Warner JJP, et al (Massachusetts General Hosp, Boston)
J Bone Joint Surg Am 96:1952-1958, 2014

Background.—Periprosthetic shoulder infections can be difficult to diagnose. The purpose of this study was to investigate the utility of arthroscopic tissue culture for the diagnosis of infection following shoulder arthroplasty. Our hypothesis was that culture of arthroscopic biopsy tissue is a more reliable method than fluoroscopically guided shoulder aspiration for diagnosing such infection.

Methods.—A retrospective review identified patients who had undergone culture of arthroscopic biopsy tissue during the evaluation of a possible chronic periprosthetic shoulder infection. The culture results of the arthroscopic biopsies were compared with those of fluoroscopically guided glenohumeral aspiration and open tissue biopsy samples obtained at the time of revision surgery.

Results.—Nineteen patients had undergone arthroscopic biopsy to evaluate a painful shoulder arthroplasty for infection. All subsequently underwent revision surgery, and 41% of those with culture results at that time had a positive result, which included *Propionibacterium acnes* in each case. All arthroscopic biopsy culture results were consistent with the culture results obtained during the revision surgery, yielding 100% sensitivity, specificity, positive predictive value, and negative predictive value. In contrast, fluoroscopically guided glenohumeral aspiration yielded a sensitivity of 16.7%, specificity of 100%, positive predictive value of 100%, and negative predictive value of 58.3%.

Conclusions.—Arthroscopic tissue biopsy is a reliable method for diagnosing periprosthetic shoulder infection and identifying the causative organism.

Level of Evidence.—Diagnostic Level I. See Instructions for Authors for a complete description of levels of evidence.

▶ This retrospective study examines the utility of culture of arthroscopic tissue biopsy in the evaluation of chronically painful shoulder arthroplasties. Nineteen patients underwent arthroscopic tissue biopsy at an average of 2 years from their original shoulder arthroplasty. In all patients, the cause of chronic pain was not known at the time of the surgery. No patient had elevated erythrocyte sedimentation rate, C-reactive protein, and white blood cell count (although some patients had slight elevations of 1 or 2 of those laboratory values). Arthroscopic tissue biopsy proved more sensitive at detecting infection than fluoroscopically guided aspiration, with 9 of 19 arthroscopic cultures positive and only 1 of 14 flouroscopically guided aspirates growing bacteria. In addition, arthroscopic tissue biopsy cultures correlated well with intraoperative cultures in the 7 cases in which both types of cultures were available.

Although not all patients had all 3 types of tests (flouroscopically guided aspirate, arthroscopic biopsy, intraoperative cultures), this small study strongly suggests that arthroscopically obtained tissue culture is more sensitive than fluoroscopically guided aspirate at detecting bacterial infection in shoulder arthroplasty. In these cases, the procedure involved minimal morbidity with no reported complications and minimal postoperative rehabilitation. Arthroscopic examination also provides the ability to evaluate other causes of chronic shoulder pain such as glenoid loosening, presence of synovitis or metallosis, and the integrity of the rotator cuff. Certainly, an arthroscopic tissue biopsy is not indicated in evaluation of all painful shoulder arthroplasties. The authors recognize that a limitation of the study is the selection bias in this patient group. Patients with more aggressive infections caused by other organisms (eg *Staphylococcus aureus*) may be more easily diagnosed with a combination of laboratory evaluation and fluoroscopically guided aspiration. But for a subset of those patients who may have a more indolent infection that manifests as a chronically painful shoulder with normal laboratory evaluation, arthroscopic tissue biopsy may prove a useful diagnostic tool.

C. Ward, MD

Conversion of Stemmed Hemi- or Total to Reverse Total Shoulder Arthroplasty: Advantages of a Modular Stem Design

Wieser K, Borbas P, Ek ET, et al (Univ of Zurich, Switzerland)
Clin Orthop Relat Res 473:651-660, 2014

Background.—If revision of a failed anatomic hemiarthroplasty or total shoulder arthroplasty is uncertain to preserve or restore satisfactory rotator cuff function, conversion to a reverse total shoulder arthroplasty has become the preferred treatment, at least for elderly patients. However, revision of a well-fixed humeral stem has the potential risk of loss of humeral bone stock, nerve injury, periprosthetic fracture, and malunion or nonunion of a humeral osteotomy with later humeral component loosening.

Questions/Purposes.—The purposes of this study were to determine whether preservation of a modular stem is associated with (1) less blood loss and operative time (2) fewer perioperative and postoperative complications, including reoperations and revisions and/or (3) improved Constant and Murley scores and subjective shoulder values for conversion to a reverse total shoulder arthroplasty compared with stem revision.

Methods.—Between 2005 and 2011, 48 hemiarthroplasties and eight total shoulder arthroplasties (total = 56 shoulders 54 patients) were converted to an Anatomical™ reverse total shoulder arthroplasty system without (n = 13) or with (n = 43) stem exchange. Complications and revisions for all patients were tallied through review of medical and surgical records. The outcomes scores included the Constant and Murley score and the subjective shoulder value. Complete clinical followup was available on 80% of shoulders (43 patients 45 of 56 procedures, 32 with and 13 without stem exchange) at a minimum of 12 months (mean, 37 months range, 12—83 months).

Results.—Blood loss averaged 485 mL (range, 300–700 mL SD, 151 mL) and surgical time averaged 118 minutes (range, 90–160 minutes SD, 21 minutes) without stem exchange and 831 mL (range, 350–2000 mL SD, 400 mL) and 176 minutes (range, 120–300 minutes SD, 42 minutes) with stem exchange ($p = 0.001$). Intraoperative complications (8% versus 30% odds ratio [OR], 5.2) and reinterventions (8% versus 14% OR, 1.9) were substantially fewer in patients without stem exchange. The complication rate leading to dropout from the study was substantial in the stem revision group (six patients 43 shoulders [14%]), but there were no complication-related dropouts in the stem-retaining group. If, however, such complications could be avoided, with the numbers available we detected no difference in the functional outcome between the two groups.

Conclusions.—Patients undergoing revision of stemmed hemiarthroplasty or total to reverse total shoulder arthroplasty without stem exchange had less intraoperative blood loss and operative time, fewer intraoperative complications, and fewer revisions than did patients whose index revision procedures included a full stem exchange. Therefore modularity of a shoulder arthroplasty system has substantial advantages if conversion to reverse total shoulder arthroplasty becomes necessary and should be considered as prerequisite for stemmed shoulder arthroplasty systems.

Level of Evidence.—Level III, therapeutic study.

▶ In this study, the authors seek to determine the value of a platform stem in total shoulder arthroplasty. The idea behind such a stem is convertibility between uses for humeral fractures, anatomic shoulder arthroplasty, and reverse total shoulder arthroplasty. The theoretical benefit of such a stem is to make revision shoulder surgery easier by allowing retention of a well-fixed humeral component. Prior studies found that significant complications occur when a well-fixed humeral stem is removed including humeral fractures and prolonged operating times regardless of whether the stem is bony ingrowth or potted in bone cement. Although implant manufacturers have produced convertible humeral stems, few reports evaluate the utility of a convertible humeral stem in humans. In this study, revision shoulder arthroplasties performed from 2005 to 2011 in Switzerland were evaluated. Fifty-six shoulders in 54 patients underwent revision. Thirteen index arthroplasties were performed using a convertible stem (23%); the other 43 required stem extraction and exchange. Twenty percent of patients were lost to follow-up. The minimum follow-up was 1 year. The outcome measures reported included a Constant-Murley score and subjective shoulder value. Intraoperative complications as well as operating times were noted. In their results, the authors showed that removing a well-fixed humeral stem added approximately 1 hour to the surgical time and increased blood loss significantly. Intraoperative complications were 5 times more likely if stem exchange had to be performed. Although the number of patients with convertible stems studied is small (13 convertible stems were evaluated), the authors did show that there were significantly increased intraoperative complications, blood loss, and operating time associated with having to remove a well-fixed humeral stem; therefore, use of platform stem in shoulder arthroplasty may be preferable if future revision surgery is a possibility.

A. B. Shafritz, MD

Preoperative Deltoid Size and Fatty Infiltration of the Deltoid and Rotator Cuff Correlate to Outcomes After Reverse Total Shoulder Arthroplasty
Wiater BP, Koueiter DM, Maerz T, et al (Beaumont Health System, Royal Oak, MI)
Clin Orthop Relat Res 473:663-673, 2014

Background.—Reverse total shoulder arthroplasty (RTSA) allows the deltoid to substitute for the nonfunctioning rotator cuff. To date, it is unknown whether preoperative deltoid and rotator cuff parameters correlate with clinical outcomes.

Questions/Purposes.—We asked whether associations exist between 2-year postoperative results (ROM, strength, and outcomes scores) and preoperative (1) deltoid size; (2) fatty infiltration of the deltoid; and/or (3) fatty infiltration of the rotator cuff.

Methods.—A prospective RTSA registry was reviewed for patients with cuff tear arthropathy or massive rotator cuff tears, minimum 2-year followup, and preoperative shoulder MRI. Final analysis included 30 patients (average age, 71 ± 10 years; eight males, 22 females). Only a small proportion of patients who received an RTSA at our center met inclusion and minimum followup requirements (30 of 222; 14%); however, these patients were found to be similar at baseline to the overall group of patients who underwent surgery in terms of age, gender, and preoperative outcomes scores. The cross-sectional area of the anterior, middle, and posterior deltoid was measured on axial proton density-weighted MRI. Fatty infiltration of the deltoid, supraspinatus, infraspinatus, teres minor, and subscapularis were quantitatively assessed on sagittal T1-weighted MR images. Patients were followed for Constant-Murley score, American Shoulder and Elbow Surgeons (ASES) scores, subjective shoulder value, pain, ROM, and strength. Correlations of muscle parameters with all outcomes measures were calculated.

Results.—Preoperative deltoid size correlated positively with postoperative Constant-Murley score (67.27 ± 13.07) ($\rho = 0.432$, $p = 0.017$), ASES (82.64 ± 14.25) ($\rho = 0.377$; $p = 0.40$), subjective shoulder value (82.67 ± 17.89) ($\rho = 0.427$; $p = 0.019$), and strength (3.72 pounds ± 2.99 pounds) ($\rho = 0.454$; $p = 0.015$). Quantitative deltoid fatty infiltration (7.91% ± 4.32%) correlated with decreased postoperative ASES scores ($\rho = -0.401$; $p = 0.047$). Quantitative fatty infiltration of the infraspinatus (30.47% ± 15.01%) correlated with decreased postoperative external rotation (34.13° ± 16.80°) ($\rho = -0.494$; $p = 0.037$).

Conclusions.—Larger preoperative deltoid size correlates with improved validated outcomes scores, whereas fatty infiltration of the deltoid and infraspinatus may have deleterious effects on validated outcomes scores and ROM after RTSA. The current study is a preliminary exploration of this topic; future studies should include prospective enrollment and standardized MRI with a multivariate statistical approach. Quantitative information attained from preoperative imaging not only holds diagnostic value, but, should future studies confirm our findings, also might provide prognostic value. This information may prove beneficial in preoperative patient counseling and might aid preoperative and postoperative decision-making by identifying subpopulations of patients who may benefit by therapy aimed at improving muscle properties.

Level of Evidence.—Level III, prognostic study.

▶ This article is an exploration of whether Constant-Murley or American Shoulder and Elbow Surgeons scores have a correlation to fatty atrophy of the deltoid or rotator cuff on MRI and are an extension of previous studies that show a correlation between fatty atrophy and functional outcomes. The authors also looked at preoperative deltoid size and found a correlation between the deltoid size and outcomes.

The results are as expected; they are consistent with prior literature.[1,2] Although these studies reinforce our understanding of the biomechanics of reverse arthroplasty, the larger issue is how are these findings modifiable? In patients with fatty atrophy of the teres minor, reverse arthroplasty with latissimus transfer is an option. What is the role of preoperative therapy? In patients with preoperative deltoid atrophy, is there a benefit to different arthroplasty designs?

N. C. Chen, MD

References

1. Greiner SH, Back DA, Herrmann S, Perka C, Asbach P. Degenerative changes of the deltoid muscle have impact on clinical outcome after reversed total shoulder arthroplasty. *Arch Orthop Trauma Surg.* 2010;130:177-183.
2. Simovitch RW, Helmy N, Zumstein MA, Gerber C. Impact of fatty infiltration of the teres minor muscle on the outcome of reverse total shoulder arthroplasty. *J Bone Joint Surg Am.* 2007;89:934-939.

A novel osteotomy in shoulder joint replacement based on analysis of the cartilage/metaphyseal interface
Harrold F, Malhas A, Wigderowitz C (Univ of Dundee, Scotland, United Kingdom)
Clin Biomech (Bristol, Avon) 29:1032-1038, 2014

Background.—The accuracy of reconstruction is thought to impact on functional outcome following glenohumeral joint arthroplasty. The objective of this study was to define an area of minimal anatomic variation at the cartilage/metaphyseal interface of the proximal humerus to optimize the osteotomy of the humeral head, enabling accurate reconstruction with a prosthetic component.

Methods.—Hand held digitization and 3D surface laser scanning techniques were used to digitize 24 cadaveric arms and determine the normal geometry. Each humeral head was then examined to identify the most consistent anatomical landmarks for the ideal osteotomy plane to optimize humeral component positioning.

Findings.—The novel, posterior referencing, osteotomy resulted in a mean increase in retroversion of only 0.4° when compared to the original geometry. A traditional anterior referencing osteotomy, by comparison, produced a mean increase in retroversion of 11°. In addition, the novel osteotomy only increased axial diameter by 0.71 mm and head height by 0.02 mm compared to an anterior referencing osteotomy (3.0 mm and 2.7 mm respectively).

Interpretation.—The traditional osteotomy, referencing the anterior border of the cartilage/metaphyseal interface potentially resulted in an increase in prosthetic head size and retroversion. The novel osteotomy, referencing from the posterior cartilage/metaphyseal interface enabled a more accurate recovery of head geometry. Importantly, the increase in retroversion created by the traditional osteotomy was not replicated with the novel technique. Referencing from the posterior cartilage/metaphyseal interface produced a more reliable osteotomy, more closely matching the original humeral geometry.

Level of Evidence.—Basic Science, Anatomic study, Computer model.

▶ This review provides an excellent introduction and discussion regarding the reasons why anatomic shoulder replacement is desirable. The limitations of this study are that it is a 3-dimensional modeling study and is a theoretical summation study that was not practically executed. No actual surgical procedure was performed on these cadaveric specimens, and, therefore, reproducibility in human hands was not evaluated. In addition, this study shows the ideal line of osteotomy drawn using the landmarks; however, it does not take into account the kerf of the saw blade used, which would have an effect in vivo. In addition, the characteristics of the metaphyseal bone are not taken into account. Would significant osteoporosis or osteosclerosis in the metaphyseal bone affect the results? Would the landmarks evaluated be readily apparent to the surgeon in the diseased state? Many times after osteotomy is performed, a protective plate is applied to the metaphysis to prevent damage during retraction. Surgeons are aware that during glenoid preparation, the metaphysis of the proximal humerus can become crushed or plastically deformed from retractors and pressure. This would, therefore, change the geometry of the resected metaphysis and could lead to increased retroversion, increased anteversion, need for a thicker humeral head or a smaller diameter humeral head to reconstruct the anatomy. It has not been shown that anatomic reconstruction of the proximal humerus to the native state is accomplished with shoulder arthroplasty as the arthritic humeral head and neck no longer represent the native, normal anatomical condition. Long-term studies of the results of shoulder arthroplasty also have not proven that anatomic reconstruction of the proximal humerus is necessary to have a successful long-term outcome. Although it may be aesthetically pleasing to the surgeon to view an anatomic recreation of proximal humeral anatomy, the overall results of shoulder arthroplasty and patient outcomes are not found to be affected by this. Although numerous reports concerning cohorts of patients with failed shoulder arthroplasties have shown that anatomic malalignments may be implicated as the cause of failure, the fact remains that these anatomic malalignments have not been proven to be the cause of failure. Overall, this report provides a useful tool for surgeons who routinely replace proximal humeral anatomy. The findings suggest that the posterior reference point at which the articular cartilage meets the bare area should be used intraoperatively for those seeking to anatomically reconstruct the proximal humerus as an additional checkpoint and an additional landmark prior to performing the humeral osteotomy.

A. B. Shafritz, MD

Glenohumeral Pressure With Surface Replacement Arthroplasty Versus Hemiarthroplasty

Petraglia CA, Ramirez MA, Tsai MA, et al (MedStar Union Memorial Hosp, Baltimore, MD)
Orthopedics 37:e892-e896, 2014

It is not known whether significant differences in the glenohumeral center of pressure and contact pressure exist between surface replacement arthroplasty and hemiarthroplasty compared with the native joint. Twelve fresh-frozen cadaveric shoulders were dissected free of soft tissue, and the joint capsule was removed. The scapula was potted with the glenoid parallel to the ground. A pressure-sensitive sensor was placed in the glenohumeral joint, and each specimen was tested in sequence: intact, surface replacement, and hemiarthroplasty. Loading was done with a 440-N compression load at 0.5 Hz with the shoulder in 4 different positions. The center of pressure and contact pressure were measured at each position. The glenohumeral contact pressure with surface replacement was not different from intact pressure in 2 arm positions. Pressure with hemiarthroplasty was significantly different compared with the intact shoulder at all 4 arm positions and compared with the surface replacement group at 2 arm positions ($P \leq .05$). Change in the anterior-posterior center of pressure from intact was significantly smaller with surface replacement compared with hemiarthroplasty with the humerus at 0° flexion/0° abduction and at 0° flexion/90° abduction (1.11 ± 0.89 mm vs 2.38 ± 1.62 mm, $P = .02$, and 0.68 ± 0.50 mm vs 2.37 ± 2.0 mm, $P = .01$, respectively). Change in the superior-inferior center of pressure was significantly smaller with surface replacement vs hemiarthroplasty at 0° flexion/0° abduction and at 90° flexion/90° abduction (0.98 ± 1.16 mm vs 2.33 ± 1.38 mm, $P = .02$, and 1.50 ± 1.28 mm vs 2.90 ± 1.92 mm, $P = .04$, respectively). Compared with hemiarthroplasty, surface replacement arthroplasty more closely replicated the contact pressure and center of pressure in the intact glenohumeral joint.

▶ There are several limitations to this study. This is a cadaveric model using 12 specimens. The 12 specimens selected were normal shoulders. None of the specimens had severe glenohumeral arthritic changes; therefore, the results of this study are not likely to be generally applicable to significantly diseased shoulders. Although the authors note in their indications in the introduction and the discussion that surface replacement arthroplasty is best indicated for patients with isolated humeral head lesions without glenoid disease, the reality is that any humeral lesions are likely associated with some form of glenoid arthrosis. While in the normal state it might be easy for a surgeon to identify and recreate humeral anatomy as close to normal as possible, in the diseased state this task is much more challenging. Another limitation of this study is that the specimens were stripped of all the soft tissues surrounding the bone, and these soft tissue structures obviously provide constraint in the in vivo setting. In addition, the muscles and tendons of the rotator cuff as well as deltoid and other muscles surrounding the shoulder girdle provide additional vectors for force generation such that a cadaveric study may not be able to represent the in vivo characteristics of the shoulder joint. In the discussion, the authors cite intermediate outcomes of the Copeland surface replacement arthroplasty at 5- and 10-year intervals. Other studies have been published concerning surface replacement arthroplasty, which show no difference between that technique and humeral hemiarthroplasty, and other studies show inferior outcomes compared with stemmed arthroplasty. Finally, several surface replacement and many stemmed humeral systems are available; a future study should compare all implants against each other in the same testing apparatus to aid in reproducibility and assess comparability.

A. B. Shafritz, MD

Outcomes After Hemiarthroplasty for Proximal Humerus Fracture Are Significantly Affected by Hand Dominance
LeBlanc JEM, MacDermid JC, Faber KJ, et al (Univ of Western Ontario, London, Canada)
J Orthop Trauma 29:379-383, 2015

Objectives.—Hand dominance has been reported to be an important factor affecting outcomes after upper extremity trauma but remains unstudied after hemiarthroplasty for fracture. This study determined whether dominance affected outcomes after hemiarthroplasty for proximal humerus fractures.
Design.—Retrospective cohort study.
Setting.—Tertiary care referral center.
Patients.—Sixty-one patients, after hemiarthroplasty for proximal humerus fracture, returned for comprehensive assessment and were divided

into 2 groups: dominant (DOM) shoulder affected (n = 25) and non-dominant (non-DOM) shoulder affected (n = 36).

Intervention.—Fracture-specific proximal humeral hemiarthroplasty for displaced proximal humerus fractures.

Main Outcome Measures.—Patients were assessed with self-reported outcomes (visual analog scale pain, American Shoulder and Elbow Surgeons shoulder score, disability of the arm, shoulder, and hand questionnaire, simple shoulder test, and short form 12) and objective (range-of-motion and hand-held dynamometer strength) testing.

Results.—At 49 months of mean follow-up, there were no significant differences between groups for gender, age, follow-up time, or visual analog scale pain ($P > 0.256$). The DOM-affected group had significantly worse scores for American Shoulder and Elbow Surgeons shoulder score ($P = 0.043$), disability of the arm, shoulder, and hand questionnaire ($P = 0.039$), and simple shoulder test ($P = 0.021$). The DOM-affected group also had consistently higher correlations between self-reported and objective outcomes than the non-DOM group.

Conclusions.—Patients who underwent hemiarthroplasty for fracture on their DOM shoulders had significantly poorer outcomes than patients with non-DOM—sided injuries. Although positive outcomes can be expected after hemiarthroplasty, patients should be instructed that they may have less satisfactory function and strength if their injury was on the DOM side.

Level of Evidence.—Prognostic Level II. See Instructions for Authors for a complete description of levels of evidence.

▶ This study suggests that hemiarthroplasty for proximal humerus fracture can reliably relieve pain, but outcomes vary depending on multiple factors. Patients who underwent hemiarthroplasty for a proximal humerus fracture on their dominant (DOM) arm had significantly worse outcomes than patients with non-DOM-sided injuries. Additionally, the non-DOM group had average DASH and SF-12 scores near equivalent to age-matched population norms, whereas the DOM group had an approximately 50% worse DASH score and a 10% worse SF-12 score. This suggests that hemiarthroplasty for non-DOM-sided injuries is a satisfactory treatment option, and further study is required to determine whether other procedures (such as perhaps reverse shoulder arthroplasty in select patients) are better suited to DOM-sided injuries. As background information, the effect of hand dominance on the outcomes of trauma has been studied previously in distal radius fractures. Beaul et al demonstrated that patients who sustain distal radius fractures on their DOM arm have significantly higher levels of dysfunction in terms of general activities, including personal hygiene. However, in the nontrauma population, authors have demonstrated that outcomes after nonoperative treatment of generalized shoulder pain or after total shoulder arthroplasty are not affected by arm dominance. The differences noted in this study may influence management, especially because there is poor consensus on the optimum method of management of displaced proximal humerus fractures. The treating surgeon should be aware that patients undergoing hemiarthroplasty for a DOM-sided injury have substantially worse self-reported outcomes.

E. Cheung, MD

The Incidence of *Propionibacterium acnes* in Shoulder Arthroscopy

Chuang MJ, Jancosko JJ, Mendoza V, et al (Sports Clinic Orthopaedic Med Associates, Laguna Hills, CA; Saddleback Memorial Med Ctr, Laguna Hills, CA)
Arthroscopy 31:1702-1707, 2015

Purpose.—To document the skin colonization and deep tissue inoculation rates associated with arthroscopic shoulder surgery and how these rates differ with procedural and demographic factors.

Methods.—We prospectively recruited outpatient shoulder arthroscopy patients who agreed to participate and met the inclusion criteria from February 2013 to May 2014. All patients received routine antibiotic prophylaxis intravenously. Initial cultures were obtained before the skin preparation by swabbing the skin at the 3 standard portal sites: posterior, anterosuperior, and anterolateral. The skin preparation used 4% chlorhexidine scrub and 2% chlorhexidine gluconate/70% isopropyl alcohol paint applied to the entire shoulder. After completion of the arthroscopic procedure, a second culture was obtained through a cannula at the surgical site. All cultures were plated for 21 days using *Brucella* medium.

Results.—We enrolled 51 patients over a 15-month period. Cultures showed a 72.5% *Propionibacterium acnes* superficial colonization rate: 46.1% of female and 81.6% of male patients ($P = .027$). We identified a deep culture—positive inoculation rate of 19.6%, all with positive *P acnes* skin colonization. No correlation could be made concerning diagnosis, procedure, suture anchor use, age, or sex.

Conclusions.—The rate of skin colonization with *P acnes* is high at arthroscopic portals, especially in men. Despite standard skin preparation and prophylactic antibiotics, the rate of deep tissue inoculation with *P acnes* in shoulder arthroscopy is much higher than the rate of infection reported in the literature.

Clinical Relevance.—Shoulder arthroscopy introduces a significant amount of *P acnes* into the deep tissues.

▶ There is a growing body of literature showing a high incidence of *Propionibacterium acnes* in shoulder surgery. This article emphasizes that *P acnes* is commonly isolated even in shoulder arthroscopy. These findings should be regarded seriously and studied further.

N. C. Chen, MD

Expert Surgeons Can Be Distinguished From Trainees, and Surgical Proficiency Can Be Defined, Using Validated Metrics and Shoulder Models
Lubowitz JH, Provencher MT, Brand JC, et al ()
Arthroscopy 31:1635-1636, 2015

Experts at performing arthroscopic shoulder Bankart procedures can be distinguished from surgical trainees using validated metrics and a cadaveric or simulator model. The combination of performance metrics plus models generates a tool that can be used to precisely and accurately define a performance threshold and assess whether or not a surgeon is proficient at performing a procedure. A tool that can be used to judge surgical expertise has implications for training and credentialing. Experienced surgeons make fewer mistakes and are faster than novices.

▶ This editorial briefly comments on 3 separate articles published in *Arthroscopy* and written by the same authors. The authors designed and tested a set of metrics, a surgical simulator and a cadaver surgical model to test operator's safety and proficiency at performing an arthroscopic Bankart repair. The measurement variables, performance on a model, and performance on a cadaver were published in 3 consecutive separate reports.

The editorial lauds the authors for developing a means to critically and reliably evaluate surgeon's and student's expertise without putting a live patient at risk. They suggest that a person not meeting requirements could undergo remedial training and further education. The article wraps up stating that surgical simulation and training are topics of critical importance.

This editorial quickly summarizes the salient points of 3 articles. It obviously lacks the substance that the original articles possess but is worth reading nonetheless. Surgeon training and proficiency is a difficult and moving target in modern medicine. It is a great asset to have a start to standardized means to both teach and evaluate future surgeons.

N. A. Hoekzema, MD

Utility of the Instability Severity Index Score in Predicting Failure After Arthroscopic Anterior Stabilization of the Shoulder
Phadnis J, Arnold C, Elmorsy A, et al (Royal Surrey County Hosp, Guildford, United Kingdom)
Am J Sports Med 43:1983-1988, 2015

Background.—The redislocation rate after arthroscopic stabilization for anterior glenohumeral instability is up to 30%. The Instability Severity Index Score (ISIS) was developed to preoperatively rationalize the risk of failure, but it has not yet been validated by an independent group.

Purpose.—To assess the utility of the ISIS in predicting failure of arthroscopic anterior shoulder stabilization and to identify other preoperative factors for failure.

Study Design.—Case-control study; Level of evidence, 3.

Methods.—A case-control study was performed on 141 consecutive patients, comparing those who suffered failure of arthroscopic stabilization with those who had successful arthroscopic stabilization. The mean follow-up time was 47 months (range, 24-132 months). The ISIS was applied retrospectively, and an analysis was performed to establish independent risk factors for failure. A receiver operator coefficient curve was constructed to set a threshold ISIS for considering alternative surgery.

Results.—Of 141 patients, 19 (13.5%) suffered recurrent instability. The mean ISIS of the failed stabilization group was higher than that of the successful stabilization group (5.1 vs 1.7; $P < .001$). Independent risk factors for failure were Hill-Sachs lesion ($P < .001$), glenoid bone loss ($P < .001$), age <21 years at the time of surgery ($P < .001$), age at first dislocation ($P = .01$), competitive-level participation in sports ($P < .001$), and participation in contact or overhead sports ($P = .03$). The presence of glenoid bone loss carried the highest risk of failure (70%). There was a 70% risk of failure if the ISIS was ≥ 4, as opposed to a 4% risk of failure if the ISIS was <4.

Conclusion.—This is the first completely independent study to confirm that the ISIS is a useful preoperative tool. It is recommended that surgeons consider alternative forms of stabilization if the ISIS is ≥ 4.

▶ The Injury Severity Index Score (ISIS) is a method of stratifying which patients should undergo arthroscopic versus open anterior stabilization procedures. This study reported using the ISIS by an independent group in a case control study. The authors provide an independent assessment of the ISIS and provide evidence to support its utility in decision making.

N. C. Chen, MD

Assessment of the Postoperative Appearance of the Rotator Cuff Tendon Using Serial Sonography After Arthroscopic Repair of a Rotator Cuff Tear

Yoo HJ, Choi J-Y, Hong SH, et al (Seoul Natl Univ Hosp, Korea; et al)
J Ultrasound Med 34:1183-1190, 2015

Objectives.—The purpose of this study was to evaluate serial changes in sonographic findings of a rotator cuff tendon after rotator cuff repair.

Methods.—Sixty-five arthroscopically repaired rotator cuff tears (43 full-thickness tears and 22 partial-thickness tears) were retrospectively included in this study. Serial sonographic examinations were performed at 5 weeks, 3 months, and 6 months after surgery. The sonographic findings of the repaired tendon were assessed for a recurrent tear, tendon thickness, morphologic tendon characteristics, vascularity, and bursitis at each time point.

Results.—Four recurrent tears occurred within 3 months of surgery. The postoperative tendon thickness decreased from 5 weeks to 6 months after surgery ($P = .001$). There were significant changes in the morphologic tendon characteristics, including the echo texture, fibrillar pattern, and surface irregularity of the repaired tendon, from 5 weeks to 6 months after surgery ($P < .001$). Additionally, subacromial-subdeltoid bursitis and the vascularity of the repaired tendon decreased postoperatively over time.

Conclusions.—Serial sonography after arthroscopic rotator cuff repair was useful for monitoring the postoperative changes in a repaired tendon. The morphologic appearance of the repaired tendon and peritendinous soft tissue changes improved over time and nearly normalized within 6 months of surgery.

▶ This retrospective review assessed the utility of performing serial postoperative sonography after an arthroscopic repair. There is little in the literature regarding the postoperative changes seen as these repaired tendons heal. The use of ultrasound scan seems to be a reliable, inexpensive, clinic-based study that can accurately assess the morphologic changes seen within the healing tendon and the surrounding supporting tissue. Of note, the recurrent tears of the repaired tendon were infrequent, less than 4 of 65 (6%), but interestingly occurred within the first 3 months.

There were several limitations in the study, as pointed out by the authors. There was a subjective assessment of morphologic tendon characteristic change over the timeframe studied. Also, it was difficult to assess the patient's repaired tendon in the 5-week period secondary to pain and the limited motion. Also, the follow-up period for this type of repair was short at 6 months. Also not addressed was the level of the patient's pain and function at the evaluation.

Overall, this study shows the reliable and noninvasive way to assess the rotator cuff status after arthroscopic repair. Sonographic evaluation may prove to be a useful tool in postoperative assessment of the repaired tendons to direct postoperative rehabilitation and act as surveillance for recurrent tears.

J. Brault, MD

Outcome After Arthroscopic Decompression of Inferior Labral Cysts Combined With Labral Repair

Jeong J-J, Panchal K, Park S-E, et al (The Catholic Univ of Korea, Daejeon, South Korea)
Arthroscopy 31:1060-1068, 2015

Purpose.—To analyze the clinical and radiologic outcomes of arthroscopic cyst decompression and labral repair in patients with inferior paralabral cysts with chronic shoulder pain.

Methods.—Between March 2006 and September 2012, 16 patients who were identified as having inferior paralabral cysts presented with chronic shoulder pain. All patients underwent a thorough physical examination and preoperative magnetic resonance arthrographic evaluation. The mean age was 30 years (range, 17 to 50 years). The mean follow-up period was 38 months (range, 16 to 60 months). Clinical outcome scores (American Shoulder and Elbow Surgeons; University of California, Los Angeles; and Simple Shoulder Test) and passive shoulder range of motion were evaluated at last follow-up. Follow-up magnetic resonance imaging was performed at a mean of 8 months to determine the labral healing status and assess for cyst recurrence.

Results.—The incidence of isolated inferior paralabral cysts was 0.6% (16 of 2,656 cases). Of the patients, 8 had multiple cysts and 8 had a single cyst. The mean length and width of the cysts were 1.0 cm and 0.4 cm, respectively. Eight cases had a history of trauma, and 13 patients were involved in sports activities. Seventy-five percent of cases showed a positive relocation test. The mean American Shoulder and Elbow Surgeons; University of California, Los Angeles; and Simple Shoulder Test scores

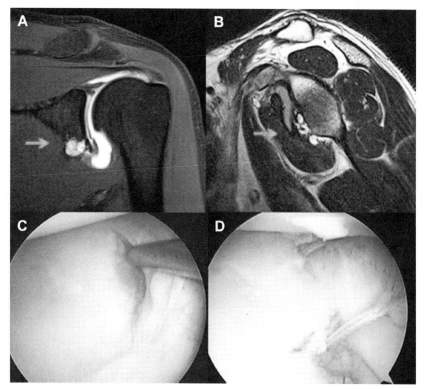

FIGURE 1.—A 21-year-old man had chronic right shoulder pain for the past 2 years. Two months earlier, he was injured while slipping and falling down and his pain was aggravated. (A, B) On magnetic resonance imaging, T2-weighted oblique coronal and oblique sagittal images show a 3 × 4–cm multiseptate cyst (arrows) at the anteroinferior aspect of the glenoid. (C) Arthroscopic findings in right shoulder with patient in lateral decubitus position. The arthroscope is in the posterior portal, showing an anteroinferior labral tear. (D) Cyst decompression and repair of the anteroinferior labral tear were performed. (Reprinted from Jeong J-J, Panchal K, Park S-E, et al. Outcome after arthroscopic decompression of inferior labral cysts combined with labral repair. *Arthroscopy.* 2015;31:1060-1068, with permission from the Arthroscopy Association of North America.)

TABLE 1.—Details of Patients With Inferior Paralabral Cysts

Patient No.	Age, yr	Trauma History	Sports	Dominant Arm	Operated Arm	No. of Cysts, Cyst Location, and Cyst Size	No. of Anchors	Labral Tear Location
1	32	No	Yes	R	L	Multiseptate, PI aspect, and 2.7 × 1.7 cm	3	PI (7-9 o'clock)
2	37	Yes	Yes	R	L	Multiseptate, AI aspect, and 0.7 × 0.9 cm	2	AI (3:30-5 o'clock)
3	17	Yes	Yes	R	R	Single, PI aspect, and 0.3 × 0.3 cm	2	PI (7-11 o'clock)
4	24	No	Yes	R	R	Multiseptate, AI aspect, and 1 × 0.5 cm	2	AI (4-7 o'clock)
5	21	Yes	Yes	R	L	Multiseptate, AI aspect, 2.0 × 0.5 cm	4	AI (3-7 o'clock)
6	44	No	No	R	R	Single, PI aspect, and 0.9 × 0.3 cm	2	PI (6-8 o'clock)
7	29	No	Yes	L	L	Single, AI aspect, and 0.3 × 0.3 cm	3	AI (5-7 o'clock)
8	21	No	Yes	L	L	Single, PI aspect, and 0.9 × 0.2 cm	2	PI (6-8 o'clock)
9	23	No	Yes	R	L	Multiseptate, PI aspect, and 0.9 × 0.3 cm	4	AI-PI (4-9 o'clock)
10	37	Yes	Yes	R	L	Single, PI aspect, and 0.3 × 0.4 cm	2	PI (5-8 o'clock)
11	37	Yes	Yes	R	R	Single, PI aspect, and 0.6 × 0.2 cm	4	AI-PI (3:30-9 o'clock)
12	25	Yes	Yes	R	L	Multiseptate, PI aspect, and 3.5 × 1.4 cm	5	PI (7-9 o'clock)
13	50	No	Yes	L	L	Multiseptate, PI and AI aspect, and 0.8 × 0.8 cm and 0.9 × 0.3 cm	2	AI-PI (5-8 o'clock)
14	36	Yes	Yes	R	R	Multiseptate, AI aspect, and 0.4 × 0.2 cm	2	AI (4-5 o'clock)
15	26	Yes	No	R	L	Single, PI aspect, and 0.3 × 0.2 cm	2	PI (7-8 o'clock)
16	23	No	No	R	L	Single, PI aspect, and 0.6 × 0.3 cm	2	PI (6-8 o'clock)

AI, anteroinferior; L, left; PI, posteroinferior; R, right.
Reprinted from Jeong J-J, Panchal K, Park S-E, et al. Outcome after arthroscopic decompression of inferior labral cysts combined with labral repair. Arthroscopy. 2015;31:1060-1068, with permission from the Arthroscopy Association of North America.

improved from 64, 22, and 8.7, respectively, preoperatively to 83, 31, and 10, respectively ($P < .001$), at final follow-up. Shoulder range of motion did not show any significant improvement. The location of the labral tear was as follows: anteroinferior tear in 5 cases, posteroinferior tear in 8 cases, and combined anteroinferior and posteroinferior tear in 3 cases. All cysts were found to be in association with a labral tear. A mean of 2.7 anchors were used for inferior labral repair. These cysts were found only in male patients. None of the patients showed any evidence of cyst recurrence on follow-up magnetic resonance imaging.

Conclusions.—Inferior labral tears treated with cyst decompression and labral repair showed satisfactory clinical results without any recurrence. Inferior paralabral cysts should be considered in the differential diagnosis in patients presenting with chronic shoulder pain, particularly active male patients.

Level of Evidence.—Level IV, therapeutic case series.

▶ This study shows results on arthroscopic decompression of inferior labral cysts combined with labral repair. This is a significant study showing a rare pathology. The study's main strength is that only patients with inferior labral conditions were included. All other possible causes of shoulder pain were excluded, and a significant time of nonoperative treatment was tried before undergoing surgery. This brings us to a low number of cases but with precise pathology. All patients improved significantly after surgery. Methods are very clear and reproducible. There are much data in this study suggesting epidemiology for inferior labral cysts. Besides surgical results, enough information is given to consider this pathology as a differential diagnosis for young active male patients. I treat patients with paralabral cysts in the same manner as the authors of this study (Fig 1, Tables 1 and 2). I try nonoperative methods as

TABLE 2.—Preoperative and Postoperative Clinical Results in Treatment of Inferior Paralabral Cysts

	Preoperative	Postoperative	P Value*
Clinical scores			
ASES	64 ± 16 (29 to 85)	83 ± 10 (65 to 98.5)	< .001
UCLA	22 ± 3.6 (14 to 25)	31 ± 2.5 (25 to 33)	< .001
SST	8.7 ± 2.3 (5 to 12)	10 ± 1.5 (6 to 12)	< .001
VAS pain	4.8 ± 1.3 (3.5 to 8)	1.6 ± 0.5 (1 to 4)	< .001
Shoulder ROM			
Forward flexion, °	168 ± 14 (130 to 180)	163 ± 15 (130 to 180)	.123
Abduction, °	169 ± 14 (130 to 180)	163 ± 15 (130 to 180)	.069
External rotation at side, °	43 ± 23 (0 to 90)	35 ± 26 (−5 to 90)	.204
Internal rotation at back	T10 vertebral level (L5 to T5)	T11 vertebral level (L2 to T7)	.151

NOTE. Data are presented as mean ± standard deviation (range) or mean (range).
ASES, American Shoulder and Elbow Society; ROM, range of motion; SST, Simple Shoulder Test; UCLA, University of California, Los Angeles; VAS, visual analog scale.
*$P < .05$ was deemed clinically significant.
Reprinted from Jeong J-J, Panchal K, Park S-E, et al. Outcome after arthroscopic decompression of inferior labral cysts combined with labral repair. *Arthroscopy.* 2015;31:1060-1068, with permission from the Arthroscopy Association of North America.

primary treatment. If this fails, I perform arthroscopic examination, cyst decompression, and labral repair.

J. P. Simone, MD

Demographic Analysis of Open and Arthroscopic Distal Clavicle Excision in a Private Insurance Database

Alluri RK, Kupperman AI, Montgomery SR, et al (David Geffen School of Medicine at UCLA, Los Angeles, CA)
Arthroscopy 30:1068-1074, 2014

Purpose.—The purpose of this study was to evaluate and quantify the demographic characteristics of patients undergoing open and arthroscopic distal clavicle excision (DCE) in the United States while also describing changes in practice patterns over time.

Methods.—Patients who underwent DCE from 2004 to 2009 were identified by Current Procedural Terminology (CPT) codes in a national database of orthopaedic insurance records. The year of procedure, age, sex, geographic region, and concomitant rotator cuff repair or subacromial decompression (SAD) were recorded for each patient. Results were reported as the incidence of procedures identified per 10,000 patients searched in the database.

Results.—Between 2004 and 2009, 73,231 DCEs were performed; 74% were arthroscopic and 26% were open. The incidence of arthroscopic DCE increased from 37.8 in 2004 to 58.5 in 2009 ($P < .001$), whereas the incidence of open DCE decreased from 21.1 in 2004 to 14.1 in 2009 ($P < .001$). Sixty-one percent of DCEs were performed in men ($P < .001$). Women were more likely to undergo an arthroscopic procedure ($P < .001$). Arthroscopic DCE was most common in patients aged 50 to 59 years ($P < .001$). Open DCE was most common in patients aged 60 to 69 years ($P < .001$). Open rotator cuff repair and SAD were concomitantly performed in 38% and 23% of open DCEs, respectively. Arthroscopic rotator cuff repair and SAD were concomitantly performed in 33% and 95% arthroscopic DCEs, respectively.

Conclusions.—This analysis of DCE using a private insurance database shows that arthroscopic DCEs progressively increased, whereas open DCEs concomitantly decreased between 2004 and 2009. The majority of DCEs were performed in men between the ages of 50 and 59 years. Both arthroscopic and open DCEs are frequently performed in conjunction with rotator cuff repair or SAD.

Level of Evidence.—Level IV, cross-sectional study.

▶ In this report, the authors provide a comprehensive introduction and background with historical information concerning the history, indications, and outcomes for patients undergoing both open and arthroscopic distal clavicle excision. Their results as shown in Fig 2 show a steady increase in the incidence of arthroscopic distal clavicle excision with concomitant decrease in open distal

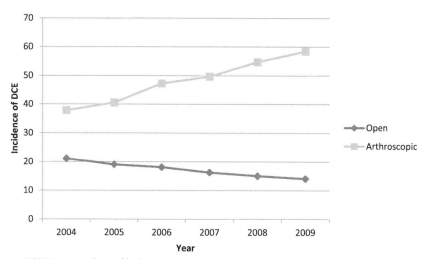

FIGURE 2.—Incidence of both open and arthroscopic distal clavicle excision (DCE) per year between 2004 and 2009. Incidence is defined as number of cases per 10,000 patients. (Reprinted from Alluri RK, Kupperman AI, Montgomery SR, et al. Demographic analysis of open and arthroscopic distal clavicle excision in a private insurance database. *Arthroscopy.* 2014;30:1068-1074, with permission from Arthroscopy Association of North America.)

clavicle excision. Interestingly, the overall incidence of distal clavicle excision has slowly and steadily increased during this 5-year period. The authors present a broad discussion concerning rationale for why this trend may be observed, suggesting that arthroscopic techniques have become more popular because of improved recovery, improved appearance, and improved strength with the operation. These reasons are not evaluated in this report. The authors present some limitations of their studies. Their largest limitation is that the Pearl Diver database is not a true cross section of the US population. The South is the greatest represented population in their database, whereas the Northeast was underrepresented. As a result, a true cross-sectional demographic of the United States population is not covered. In addition, they only queried a private insurance database; Medicare and Medicaid are not included. With patients older than 65 eligible for Medicare, the data curves may be quite skewed regarding patients 65 and older. The final limitation that the authors note is that the cross-sectional analysis is dependent on searching Current Procedural Terminology codes, and inaccurate coding could cause an error in data sampling. The authors conclude that both open and arthroscopic distal clavicle excisions are frequently performed in conjunction with rotator cuff repair or subacromial decompression. This article provides a snapshot as to trends in open versus arthroscopic distal clavicle excision surgery in the United States. It has many additional limitations that were not discussed. This article does not study indications or outcomes from the operation. It merely measures the number of times it has been performed. Because there are no control numbers, we do not know how the increase compares with the numbers of other types of surgeries performed during these years. Further, there is no information regarding the surgeons, whether they are subspecialty trained, subspecialty practicing, or general practitioners. There is no way of knowing the exact surgical technique used for any given procedure other than open or arthroscopic. Although we do know the age and sex of the patients that had these operations and whether they had additional procedures done concomitantly, we do not know the underlying pathologic diagnosis as to why the operation was being performed. The study only looks at patients who are privately insured. We do not know anything about and cannot generalize this study to patients who are in other insurance programs (eg, federal programs, uninsured patients, other private plans). The authors note that most patients who were studied were in Southern regions, and, therefore, geographic practice patterns are not accurately represented.

A. B. Shafritz, MD

The natural history of the rheumatoid shoulder: a prospective long-term follow-up study
van der Zwaal P, Pijls BG, Thomassen BJW, et al (Leiden Univ Med Ctr, The Netherlands; et al)
Bone Joint J 96-B;1520-1524, 2014

The purpose of this study was to evaluate the natural history of rheumatoid disease of the shoulder over an eight-year period. Our hypothesis was that progression of the disease is associated with a decrease in function with time.

A total of 22 patients (44 shoulders; 17 women, 5 men, (mean age 63)) with rheumatoid arthritis were followed for eight years. All shoulders were assessed using the Constant score, anteroposterior radiographs (Larsen score, Upward-Migration-Index (UMI)) and ultrasound (US). At final follow-up, the Short Form-36, disabilities of the arm, shoulder and hand (DASH) Score, erythrocyte sedimentation rate and use of anti-rheumatic medication were determined.

The mean Constant score was 72 points (50 to 88) at baseline and 69 points (25 to 100) at final follow-up. Radiological evaluation showed progressive destruction of the peri-articular structures with time. This progression of joint and rotator cuff destruction was significantly associated with the Constant score. However, at baseline only the extent of rotator cuff disease and the UMI could predict the Constant score at final follow-up.

A plain anteroposterior radiograph of the shoulder is sufficient to assess any progression of rheumatoid disease and to predict functional outcome in the long term by using the UMI as an indicator of rotator cuff degeneration.

▶ The rheumatoid shoulder degenerates over time. The authors found a correlation between Constant Scores and rotator cuff degeneration. These findings are consistent with our current understanding of the rheumatoid shoulder.

N. C. Chen, MD

Configuration of the Shoulder Complex During the Arm-Cocking Phase in Baseball Pitching

Konda S, Yanai T, Sakurai S (Waseda Univ, Tokorozawa, Japan; Chukyo Univ, Toyota, Japan)

Am J Sports Med 43:2445-2451, 2015

Background.—The role of the scapula during high-velocity baseball pitching has been described without 3-dimensional kinematic data. It has been speculated that the scapula functions to align the humerus with the spine of the scapula on both the transverse and scapular planes at the end of the arm-cocking phase.

Hypothesis.—Two hypotheses were formulated: (1) the scapulothoracic protraction angle correlates with the humerothoracic horizontal adduction angle among participants, and (2) the scapulohumeral rhythm of the humerothoracic elevation is not the same as the normal ratio (2:1) observed widely in controlled abductions.

Study Design.—Descriptive laboratory study.

Methods.—A total of 20 Japanese professional baseball pitchers were asked to pitch 3 fastballs as they would normally during pitching practice. The 3-dimensional kinematic data of the thorax, scapulae, humeri, and pelvis were recorded using an electromagnetic tracking device operating at 240 Hz. Humerothoracic, scapulothoracic, and glenohumeral joint configurations were determined at the instant of stride-foot contact (SFC) and the end of the arm-cocking phase (MER).

Results.—The mean ($\pm$SD) glenohumeral horizontal adduction ($-6° \pm 7°$) and elevation ($85° \pm 10°$) angles at the MER indicated that the humerus was positioned almost parallel to the spine of the scapula. The mean scapulothoracic protraction angle ($15° \pm 10°$) was significantly correlated with the humerothoracic horizontal adduction angle ($10° \pm 11°$) at the MER ($r = 0.76$, $P = .001$) but not at the SFC ($r = 0.13$, $P = .58$). The scapulohumeral rhythm ($4.2 [\pm 1.9]$:1) expressed as the ratio of the glenohumeral elevation angle to the scapulothoracic upward rotation angle at the MER was significantly greater than the normal ratio (2:1) ($P < .01$).

Conclusion.—The results supported the hypotheses, providing evidence to corroborate the widely accepted concept that the scapula functions to align the humerus with the spine of the scapula so as to limit the glenohumeral joint configuration within the "safe zone" at the MER.

Clinical Relevance.—Disruption of coordination, such as abnormal patterns including "SICK" scapula (scapular malposition, inferior medial border prominence, coracoid pain, and dyskinesis) and scapular dyskinesis, may result in an abnormal configuration of the glenohumeral joint at the MER.

▶ The role of the scapula during high-velocity baseball pitching has been speculated to serve to align the humerus with the scapular spine at the end of the arm-cocking phase. This has been described but never supported by

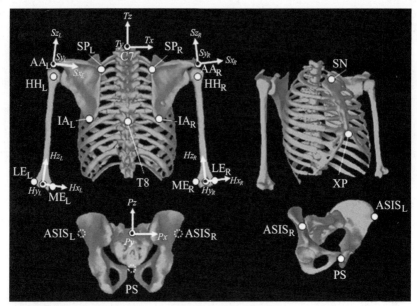

FIGURE 1.—The digitized anatomic bony landmarks and defined local coordinate system embedded to each segment. The thoracic vertical axis (Tz) was directed from the midpoint of the xiphoid process (XP) and T8 to the midpoint of the sternal notch (SN) and C7; the transverse axis (Tx) was perpendicular to the plane defined by the SN, C7, and T8; and the sagittal axis (Ty) was defined as the cross-product of Tz and Tx. The right and left scapular spine axis ($Sx_{R \text{ and } L}$) was connected between the medial border of the scapular spine ($SP_{R \text{ and } L}$) and the acromial angle ($AA_{R \text{ and } L}$); the anterior-directed axis ($Sy_{R \text{ and } L}$) was perpendicular to the plane defined by $SP_{R \text{ and } L}$, $AA_{R \text{ and } L}$, and the inferior angle ($IA_{R \text{ and } L}$); and the superior-directed axis ($Sz_{R \text{ and } L}$) was defined as the cross-product of $Sx_{R \text{ and } L}$ and $Sz_{R \text{ and } L}$. The right and left humeral longitudinal axis ($Hz_{R \text{ and } L}$) was directed from the midpoint of the medial epicondyle ($ME_{R \text{ and } L}$) and lateral epicondyle ($LE_{R \text{ and } L}$) to the humeral head ($HH_{R \text{ and } L}$); the anterior-directed axis ($Hy_{R \text{ and } L}$) was perpendicular to the plane defined by $HH_{R \text{ and } L}$, $ME_{R \text{ and } L}$, and $LE_{R \text{ and } L}$; and the lateral-directed axis ($Hx_{R \text{ and } L}$) was defined as the cross-product of $Hz_{R \text{ and } L}$ and $Hx_{R \text{ and } L}$. The pelvic vertical axis (Pz) was directed from the pubic symphysis (PS) to the midpoint of the right and left anterior superior iliac spine (ASIS); the transverse axis (Px) was perpendicular to the plane defined by $ASIS_R$, $ASIS_L$, and PS; and the sagittal axis (Py) was defined as the cross-product of Pz and Px. (Reprinted from Konda S, Yanai T, Sakurai S. Configuration of the shoulder complex during the arm-cocking phase in baseball pitching. *Am J Sports Med.* 2015;43:2445-2451, with permission from The Author(s).)

3-dimensional (3D) kinematic data. The authors designed a descriptive laboratory study using 20 professional baseball pitchers to evaluate the theory.

The shoulder complex plays a critical role in the lag of the throwing arm. Clinically, it has been recognized that the configuration of the shoulder during the arm-cocking phase plays a critical role in the development of shoulder injuries.[1,2] To prevent injury, the scapula rotates to adjust for the orientation of the glenoid in relation to the humerus. The scapula protracts and rotates in an upward direction when the humerus is positioned horizontally in adduction during arm-cocking to maintain the glenohumeral joint in the "safe zone."

A total of 20 professional Japanese baseball pitchers were included. None of the patients had shoulder complaints on the day of data collection, and none had a history of serious shoulder injury within the previous 12 months. Three-dimensional kinematic data were collected using electromagnetic

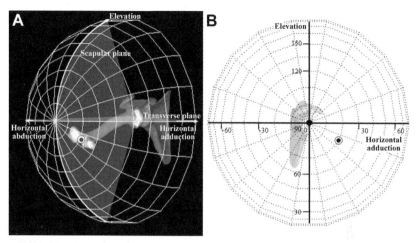

FIGURE 2.—(A) A spherical representation of the elbow position relative to the scapular glenoid. The pole of the sphere demonstrates the glenohumeral horizontal adduction/abduction angles of 0° and the glenohumeral elevation angle of 90°. (B) A projected illustration of the sphere. The plot indicates the elbow position relative to the scapular glenoid on the surface of the sphere. (Reprinted from Konda S, Yanai T, Sakurai S. Configuration of the shoulder complex during the arm-cocking phase in baseball pitching. *Am J Sports Med.* 2015;43:2445-2451, with permission from The Author(s).)

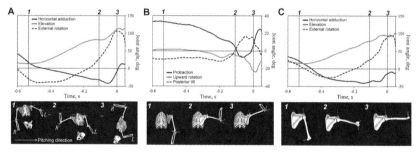

FIGURE 3.—A typical example of the time-series changes of the (A) humerothoracic, (B) scapulothoracic, and (C) glenohumeral joint configurations in baseball pitching (participant 8). Time = 0 seconds on the horizontal axis indicates the instant at which the peak value for the humerothoracic external rotation angle was recorded, and negative values on the horizontal axis indicate the stride and arm-cocking phases. (A) Side view of the body segments of a right-handed pitcher with respect to the inertial coordinate system at the initiation of humerothoracic elevation (1), the stride-foot contact point (2), and the end of the arm-cocking phase (3). "R" and "L" indicate the right and left sides of the body, respectively. (B) Back view of the right scapula, humerus, and forearm with respect to the thorax at the 3 time points. (C) Back view of the right humerus with respect to the scapula at the 3 time points. (Reprinted from Konda S, Yanai T, Sakurai S. Configuration of the shoulder complex during the arm-cocking phase in baseball pitching. *Am J Sports Med.* 2015;43:2445-2451, with permission from The Author(s).)

tracking devices. A 6-body segment model was devised, and 8 sensors were placed on the participants' skin (Fig 1). Participants pitched 3 fastballs and were instructed to throw as they normally would during practice. The anatomic coordinate system was defined by the digitized bony landmarks. The instantaneous humeral and scapular orientations with respect to the thorax and with respect to the scapula were described as Euler angles in accordance with a standard protocol from the International Society of Biomechanics (Fig 2).

The beginning of the arm-cocking phase is generally defined as the time when the stride foot contacts ground (SFC). The end was defined as the instant at which the maximum value for the humerothoracic external rotation angle (MER) was recorded. An example of the time-series changes in the humero-thoracic, scapulothoracic, and glenohumeral joints is depicted (Fig 3). Data analysis showed that at MER the scapula was protracted, upwardly rotated and tilted posteriorly, the elbow was positioned substantially posterior to the scapular plane, and the humerus was almost parallel to the spine of the scapula.

The results of the study showed that scapulothoracic protraction angle was significantly correlated with humerothoracic horizontal adduction angle at MER. An unexpected finding was that scapulohumeral rhythm was significantly greater than normal (2:1; $P < .01$). This unique rhythm serves to maintain the humerus in alignment with the scapular spine during high-velocity pitching and may be a specialized adaptation of high-velocity throwers to prevent injury.

The significance of these results provides evidence to support the widely accepted speculation that the scapula functions to align the humerus with the scapular spine to configure the glenohumeral joint within the safe zone at the MER to prevent injury.

M. O'Shaughnessy, MD

References

1. Burkhart SS, Morgan CD, Kibler WB. The disabled throwing shoulder: spectrum of pathology Part III: the SICK scapula, scapular dyskinesis, the kinetic chain, and rehabilitation. *Arthroscopy.* 2003;19:641-661.
2. Kibler WB. The role of the scapula in athletic shoulder function. *Am J Sports Med.* 1998;26:325-337.

Design and Testing of the Degree of Shoulder Involvement in Sports (DOSIS) Scale

Blonna D, Bellato E, Bonasia DE, et al (Univ of Turin, Italy; et al)
Am J Sports Med 43:2423-2430, 2015

Background.—For athletes affected by shoulder problems, the most important expectation is to resume sporting activities. The ability to return to sport is related to several parameters, including the type and level of sport played. By focusing on these parameters, the Degree of Shoulder Involvement in Sports (DOSIS) scale allows for a better assessment of the involvement of the shoulder in sports.

Purpose.—To design the DOSIS scale and test its psychometric features.

Study Design.—Cohort study; Level of evidence, 3.

Methods.—The DOSIS scale was developed as a patient self-administered scale by the Sport Committee of SIGASCOT (Società Italiana del Ginocchio Artroscopia Sport Cartilagine Tecnologie Ortopediche) to score sports activity based on 3 parameters: (1) type of sport, (2) frequency with which the sport is played, and (3) level at which the sport is played. In a subsequent phase, the psychometric features of the DOSIS scale were measured in a cohort of 85 patients who were affected by recurrent anterior shoulder instability and who underwent an open Bristow-Latarjet procedure or an arthroscopic Bankart repair. The content validity, criterion validity, construct validity, responsiveness, and test-retest reliability were measured and compared with the psychometric features of the Tegner activity scale.

Results.—Neither the DOSIS nor the Tegner activity scale showed floor or ceiling effects, but the DOSIS scale had a different distribution of scores, with a tendency toward a higher percentage of patients with high scores. The test-retest reliability analysis of the DOSIS scale revealed excellent intraobserver reliability (intraclass correlation coefficient $= 0.96$). Regarding the construct validity, 3 of the 4 hypotheses that we tested were significant. The DOSIS scale showed good criterion validity when compared with the Tegner activity scale ($\rho = 0.3$, $P = .003$), and the effect size between the preoperative and postoperative DOSIS scale was 1.1.

Conclusion.—The DOSIS scale showed acceptable psychometric features and seems to be a valid instrument for shoulder assessment in athletes.

▶ In this Level III cohort study, the authors sought to derive a new patient self-administered scoring system for the shoulder, specifically looking at high-level athletes. Current evaluation tools and outcome measurement tools available for the shoulder have problems of being not specific enough for overhead sports

1. What sports did you play before the onset of your shoulder problem? List the sports below and indicate which was the most important/predominant for you:		
List of sports	Most important/predominant	
1)	yes	no
2)	yes	no
3)	yes	no
. . .	yes	no
2. How frequently did you participate in sports?*		
Occasionally		
≥2 times a week, most of the weeks of the year		
3. What level of sport did you play?		
Recreational		
Low level of competition (regional, local)		
High level of competition (national or international or professional)		
4. Which was your dominant arm during your sports activities?		

FIGURE 1.—The Degree of Shoulder Involvement in Sports (DOSIS) scale. The scale can be completed either with respect to the sport performed at the time of the follow-up (postoperative DOSIS) or with respect to the sport performed during the period before the onset of the shoulder problem (baseline DOSIS; shown in this figure) or before surgery (preoperative DOSIS). The DOSIS scale was calculated for the most important or predominant sport. The information regarding dominant and nondominant arm was used to classify the sport according to Appendix 2, available online. *For seasonal sports, the frequency during the season was considered. (Reprinted from Blonna D, Bellato E, Bonasia DE, et al. Design and testing of the degree of shoulder involvement in sports (DOSIS) scale. *Am J Sports Med.* 2015;43:2423-2430, with permission from The Author(s).)

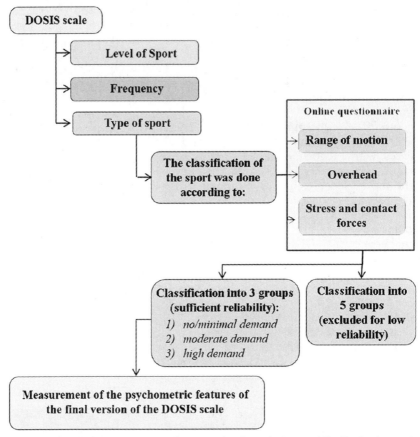

FIGURE 2.—Flow chart summarizing the steps used to design the Degree of Shoulder Involvement in Sports (DOSIS) scale. (Reprinted from Blonna D, Bellato E, Bonasia DE, et al. Design and testing of the degree of shoulder involvement in sports (DOSIS) scale. *Am J Sports Med.* 2015;43:2423-2430, with permission from The Author(s).)

nor sensitive enough to detect differences in elite athletes. The purpose of this study was to develop a new outcome measure for patients who underwent shoulder stabilization surgery.

The authors devised the DOSIS to replace the Tegner activity scale because the Tegner scale was designed for the knee. Fig 1 depicts the final DOSIS scale studied. The flow chart used to develop the scale is presented in Fig 2. In the development process, a preliminary questionnaire, including a list of 20 common sports and specific positions and roles, was sent to 7 international experts on the shoulder and elbow. It was then sent to the members of the Sport Committee of SIGASCOT (Società Italiana del Ginocchio, Artroscopia, Sport, Cartilagine e Tecnologie Ortopediche). After evaluation and further refinements, the psychometric features of the scale were then studied on subjects. A cohort of 85 patients who were affected by recurrent anterior shoulder instability and underwent open Bristow-Latarjet procedure or an arthroscopic Bankart repair were

Baseline DOSIS Scale

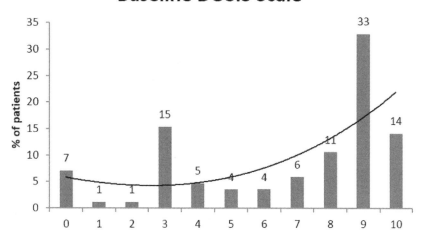

Baseline Tegner Activity Scale

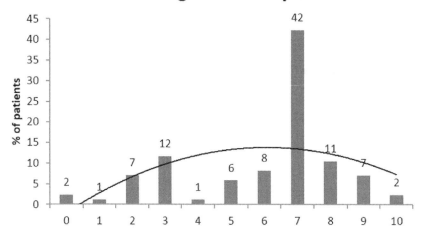

FIGURE 4.—Content validity. Neither the DOSIS nor Tegner activity scales showed a floor or ceiling effect. The DOSIS scale had a different distribution of scores, with a tendency toward a higher percentage of patients with high scores. Moreover, the graph for the DOSIS scale shows that only 7% of patients (n = 6) included in the study were not athletes. DOSIS, Degree of Shoulder Involvement in Sports. (Reprinted from Blonna D, Bellato E, Bonasia DE, et al. Design and testing of the degree of shoulder involvement in sports (DOSIS) scale. *Am J Sports Med.* 2015;43:2423-2430, with permission from The Author(s).)

queried. All but 6 patients were elite athletes. Surgery was performed in university hospitals. The test–retest reliability was measured in a subgroup of 41 patients, and during their follow-up examinations, patients were asked to complete the DOSIS scale, the Tegner activity scale, the subjective shoulder value, the Western Ontario shoulder instability index, and the Oxford shoulder score for instability. The results of content validity are presented in Fig 4.

The results of their work showed that the content validity showed no floor or ceiling effect. The test—retest validity showed no differences with an inter-class correlation of 0.97. Construct validity showed that it also met standards, as did criterion validity and responsiveness testing. The authors concluded that the DOSIS scale showed acceptable psychometric features and provided a sports-specific assessment of the shoulder compared with the Tegner activity scale.

In their concluding paragraph, the authors note that the DOSIS scale was developed in a cohort of patients with shoulder instability. Although the DOSIS scale clearly has been proven to be a valid tool, it was specifically designed, developed, and tested in patients with anterior shoulder instability who underwent either Bankart repair or Bristow-Latarjet procedures. The limitation of this assessment tool is that it was not tested and validated on patients with posterior shoulder instability, internal rotation contracture, labrum lesions, rotator cuff tears, fractures, and chondral injuries. Therefore, as a caution, if this tool is used in practice and not applied to anterior shoulder instability, its validity has not been proven.

A. B. Shafritz, MD

Deficits in Glenohumeral Passive Range of Motion Increase Risk of Shoulder Injury in Professional Baseball Pitchers: A Prospective Study

Wilk KE, Macrina LC, Fleisig GS, et al (Champion Sports Medicine, Birmingham, AL; Champion Physical Therapy & Performance, Waltham, MA; American Sports Medicine Inst, Birmingham, AL; et al)
Am J Sports Med 43:2379-2385, 2015

Background.—Shoulder injuries from repetitive baseball pitching continue to be a serious, common problem.

Purpose.—To determine whether passive range of motion of the glenohumeral joint was predictive of shoulder injury or shoulder surgery in professional baseball pitchers.

Study Design.—Cohort study; Level of evidence, 2.

Methods.—Passive range of motion of the glenohumeral joint was assessed with a bubble goniometer during spring training for all major and minor league pitchers of a single professional baseball organization over a period of 8 successive seasons (2005-2012). Investigators performed a total of 505 examinations on 296 professional pitchers. Glenohumeral external and internal rotation was assessed with the pitcher supine and the arm abducted to 90° in the scapular plane with the scapula stabilized anteriorly at the coracoid process. Total rotation was defined as the sum of internal and external glenohumeral rotation. Passive shoulder flexion was measured with the pitcher supine and the lateral border of the scapula manually stabilized. After examination, shoulder injuries and injury durations were recorded by each pitcher's respective baseball organization and reported to the league as an injury transaction as each player was placed on the disabled list.

Results.—Highly significant side-to-side differences were noted within subjects for each range of motion measurement. There were 75 shoulder injuries and 20 surgeries recorded among 51 pitchers, resulting in 5570 total days on the disabled list. Glenohumeral internal rotation deficit, total rotation deficit, and flexion deficit were not significantly related to shoulder injury or surgery. Pitchers with insufficient external rotation (<5° greater external rotation in the throwing shoulder) were 2.2 times more likely to be placed on the disabled list for a shoulder injury ($P = .014$; 95% CI, 1.2-4.1) and were 4.0 times more likely to require shoulder surgery ($P = .009$; 95% CI, 1.5-12.6).

Conclusion.—Insufficient shoulder external rotation on the throwing side increased the likelihood of shoulder injury and shoulder surgery. Sports medicine clinicians should be aware of these findings and develop a preventive plan that addresses this study's findings to reduce pitchers' risk of shoulder injury and surgery.

▶ The purpose of this article was to determine whether deficits in passive range of motion in the glenohumeral joint were predictive of shoulder injury or shoulder surgery in professional baseball pitchers (cohort study: Level II evidence). In this study, 296 professional baseball pitchers from a single professional baseball organization were studied over 8 seasons. Glenohumeral external and internal rotation was assessed using a custom bubble goniometer by 2 experienced investigators. The dominant and nondominant arms were studied and the sum of internal and external rotation of each arm was calculated and compiled into a database. The pitchers were then followed prospectively to see whether they were placed on the disabled list, developed a shoulder injury, or required shoulder surgery. The authors noted that there were significant differences in side-to-side motion and that a total of 75 shoulder injuries were reported over this time period in 51 pitchers. Twenty surgeries occurred as a result of these injuries. The study showed that glenohumeral internal rotation deficit, total rotation deficit, and forward flexion deficit were not significantly related to shoulder injury or surgery. The authors did find that pitchers with insufficient external rotation (as defined by less than 5 degrees of greater external rotation in the throwing shoulder compared with the nonthrowing shoulder) were 2 times more likely to be placed on the disabled list for shoulder injury and were 4 times more likely to require shoulder surgery. The authors conclude that insufficient external shoulder rotation on the throwing side increased the likelihood of shoulder injury and shoulder surgery in professional pitchers. They suggest that these findings be used to develop a preventative plan to address loss of external rotation in throwers. The authors cite that a thrower's shoulder exhibits less internal rotation but greater external rotation compared with nonthrowing side. Many reasons have been proposed for this passive range of motion adaptation, including osseous adaptation with increased retroversion, muscle tightness, scapular position, and capsular restrictions. Other authors have shown that glenohumeral internal rotation is associated with increased greater risk of injuries in throwers; however, this study did not correlate these findings.

There are several limitations of this study. All data entries were performed at the commencement of spring training before pitchers throwing, and these data might have changed over time during the season but were not tracked. The technique used to measure glenohumeral rotation is subjective; it was performed by 2 experienced examiners, but the technique may not be reproducible or generalizable to other practitioners.

A. B. Shafritz, MD

Correlation of Shoulder and Elbow Kinetics With Ball Velocity in Collegiate Baseball Pitchers
Post EG, Laudner KG, McLoda TA, et al (Illinois State Univ, Normal; et al)
J Athl Train 50:629-633, 2015

Context.—Throwing a baseball is a dynamic and violent act that places large magnitudes of stress on the shoulder and elbow. Specific injuries at the elbow and glenohumeral joints have been linked to several kinetic variables throughout the throwing motion. However, very little research has directly examined the relationship between these kinetic variables and ball velocity.

Objective.—To examine the correlation of peak ball velocity with elbow-valgus torque, shoulder external-rotation torque, and shoulder-distraction force in a group of collegiate baseball pitchers.

Design.—Cross-sectional study.

Setting.—Motion-analysis laboratory.

Patients or Other Participants.—Sixty-seven asymptomatic National Collegiate Athletic Association Division I baseball pitchers (age $= 19.5 \pm 1.2$ years, height $= 186.2 \pm 5.7$ cm, mass $= 86.7 \pm 7.0$ kg; 48 right handed, 19 left handed).

Main Outcome Measure(s).—We measured peak ball velocity using a radar gun and shoulder and elbow kinetics of the throwing arm using 8 electronically synchronized, high-speed digital cameras. We placed 26 reflective markers on anatomical landmarks of each participant to track 3-dimensional coordinate data. The average data from the 3 highest-velocity fastballs thrown for strikes were used for data analysis. We calculated a Pearson correlation coefficient to determine the associations between ball velocity and peak elbow-valgus torque, shoulder-distraction force, and shoulder external-rotation torque ($P < .05$).

Results.—A weak positive correlation was found between ball velocity and shoulder-distraction force ($r = 0.257$; 95% confidence interval [CI] $= 0.02, 0.47$; $r^2 = 0.066$; $P = .018$). However, no significant correlations were noted between ball velocity and elbow-valgus torque ($r = 0.199$; 95% CI $= -0.043, 0.419$; $r^2 = 0.040$; $P = .053$) or shoulder external-rotation torque ($r = 0.097$; 95% CI $= -0.147, 0.329$; $r^2 = 0.009$; $P = .217$).

TABLE 1.—Correlation of Kinetic Variables With Ball Velocity

Variable	Mean ± SD	r	r²	P Value
Elbow-valgus torque (% body weight × height)	5.7 ± 1.3	0.199	0.040	.053
Shoulder-distraction force (% body weight)	110.0 ± 16.0	0.257	0.066	.018ᵃ
Shoulder external-rotation torque (% body weight × height)	5.2 ± 1.0	0.097	0.009	.217

ᵃSignificant correlation $(P < .05)$.
Reprinted from Post EG, Laudner KG, McLoda TA, et al. Correlation of shoulder and elbow kinetics with ball velocity in collegiate baseball pitchers. *J Athl Train.* 2015;50:629-633, with permission from the National Athletic Trainers' Association, Inc.

Conclusions.—Although a weak positive correlation was present between ball velocity and shoulder-distraction force, no significant association was seen between ball velocity and elbow-valgus torque or shoulder external-rotation torque. Therefore, other factors, such as improper pitching mechanics, may contribute more to increases in joint kinetics than peak ball velocity.

▶ The identification of risk factors that predispose pitchers to shoulder and elbow ligament injury is an important pursuit in the understanding of these injuries. It is hypothesized that increased throwing velocity is associated with increased valgus elbow torque, shoulder distraction force, and shoulder external rotational torque. In this study of 67 NCAA Division 1 pitchers, motion analysis was used to measure these factors (Table 1). The authors found only weak correlation with ball velocity and shoulder distraction force. The other measured factors did not correlate with throwing velocity. The findings of this study suggest that increased throwing velocity in isolation may not be associated for injuries to the shoulder and elbow in overhead-throwing athletes and that other factors may be responsible for injuries in these injuries.

W. T. Payne, MD

High Incidence of Infraspinatus Muscle Atrophy in Elite Professional Female Tennis Players

Young SW, Dakic J, Stroia K, et al (Univ of Auckland, New Zealand; Sport Sciences and Medicine, St Petersburg, FL; et al)
Am J Sports Med 43:1989-1993, 2015

Background.—Isolated infraspinatus muscle atrophy is common in overhead athletes, who place significant and repetitive stresses across their dominant shoulders. Studies on volleyball and baseball players report infraspinatus atrophy in 4% to 34% of players; however, the prevalence of infraspinatus atrophy in professional tennis players has not been reported.

Purpose.—To investigate the incidence of isolated infraspinatus atrophy in professional tennis players and to identify any correlations with other physical examination findings, ranking performance, and concurrent shoulder injuries.

Study Design.—Cross-sectional study; Level of evidence, 3.

Methods.—A total of 125 professional female tennis players underwent a comprehensive preparticipation physical health status examination. Two orthopaedic surgeons examined the shoulders of all players and obtained digital goniometric measurements of range of motion (ROM). Infraspinatus atrophy was defined as loss of soft tissue bulk in the infraspinatus scapula fossa (and increased prominence of dorsal scapular bony anatomy) of the dominant shoulder with clear asymmetry when compared with the contralateral side. Correlations were examined between infraspinatus atrophy and concurrent shoulder disorders, clinical examination findings, ROM, glenohumeral internal rotation deficit, singles tennis ranking, and age.

Results.—There were 65 players (52%) with evidence of infraspinatus atrophy in their dominant shoulders. No wasting was noted in the nondominant shoulder of any player. No statistically significant differences were seen in mean age, left- or right-hand dominance, height, weight, or body mass index for players with or without atrophy. Of the 77 players ranked in the top 100, 58% had clinical infraspinatus atrophy, compared with 40% of players ranked outside the top 100. No associations were found with static physical examination findings (scapular dyskinesis, ROM glenohumeral internal rotation deficit, postural abnormalities), concurrent shoulder disorders, or compromised performance when measured by singles ranking.

Conclusion.—This study reports a high level of clinical infraspinatus atrophy in the dominant shoulder of elite female tennis players. Infraspinatus atrophy was associated with a higher performance ranking, and no functional deficits or associations with concurrent shoulder disorders were found. Team physicians can be reassured that infraspinatus atrophy is a common finding in high-performing tennis players and, if asymptomatic, does not appear to significantly compromise performance.

▶ This study shows a high incidence of infraspinatus muscle atrophy in elite professional female tennis players (52%). This condition does not correlate with clinical symptoms or functional deficit. In fact, it is associated with a higher performance ranking. The study's main weakness is that the clinical analysis of muscle atrophy is subjective. Its main strength is the interesting reported outcome. As long as patients are asymptomatic, the coach and team physician should be aware that this is a normal finding.

J. P. Simone, MD

What is the Best Clinical Test for Assessment of the Teres Minor in Massive Rotator Cuff Tears?

Collin P, Treseder T, Denard PJ, et al (Saint-Grégoire Private Hosp Ctr, France; Royal Melbourne Hosp, Parkville, Australia; Southern Oregon Orthopedics, Mcdford; et al)
Clin Orthop Relat Res 473:2959-2966, 2015

Background.—Few studies define the clinical signs to evaluate the integrity of teres minor in patients with massive rotator cuff tears. CT and MRI, with or without an arthrogram, can be limited by image quality, soft tissue density, motion artifact, and interobserver reliability. Additionally, the ill-defined junction between the infraspinatus and teres minor and the larger muscle-to-tendon ratio of the teres minor can contribute to error. Therefore, we wished to determine the validity of clinical testing for teres minor tears.

Question/Purposes.—The aim of this study was to determine the accuracy of commonly used clinical signs (external rotation lag sign, drop sign, and the Patte test) for diagnosing the teres minor's integrity.

Methods.—We performed a prospective evaluation of patients referred to our shoulder clinic for massive rotator cuff tears determined by CT arthrograms. The posterosuperior rotator cuff was examined clinically and correlated with CT arthrograms. We assessed interobserver reliability for CT assessment and used three different clinical tests of teres minor function (the external rotation lag sign, drop sign, and the Patte test). One hundred patients with a mean age of 68 years were available for the analysis.

Results.—The most accurate test for teres minor dysfunction was an external rotation lag sign greater than 40°, which had a sensitivity of 100% (95% CI, 80%−100%) and a specificity of 92% (95% CI, 84%−96%). External rotation lag signs greater than 10° had a sensitivity of 100% (95% CI, 80%−100%) and a specificity of 51% (95% CI, 40%−61%). The Patte sign had a sensitivity of 93% (95% CI, 70%−99%) and a specificity of 72% (95% CI, 61%−80%). The drop sign had a sensitivity of 87% (95% CI, 62%−96%) and a specificity of 88% (95% CI, 80%−93%). An external rotation lag sign greater than 40° was more specific than an external rotation lag sign greater than 10° ($p < 0.001$), and a Patte sign ($p < 0.001$), but was not more specific than the drop sign ($p < 0.47$). There was poor correlation between involvement of the teres minor and loss of active external rotation.

Conclusions.—Clinical signs can predict anatomic patterns of teres minor dysfunction with good accuracy in patients with massive rotator cuff tears. This study showed that the most accurate test for teres minor dysfunction is an external rotation lag sign and that most patients' posterior rotator cuff tears do not lose active external rotation. Because imaging is not always accurate, examination for integrity of the teres minor is important because it may be one of the most important variables affecting the outcome of reverse shoulder arthroplasty for massive rotator cuff tears, and the functional effects of tears in this muscle on day to day activities can be significant. Additionally, teres minor integrity affects the outcomes of tendon transfers, therefore knowledge of its condition is important in planning repairs.

Level of Evidence.—Level III, diagnostic study.

▶ The authors reviewed several clinical signs for the assessment of Teres minor dysfunction. These clinical tests are relevant, given the difficulty with assessing the Teres minor integrity through radiographic means. Interestingly, in this study, they chose to do a CT arthrogram rather than an MRI because of the availability of this examination method in the country of the study. The authors nicely outlined the testing of the Teres minor in relationship to type A through type E rotator cuff tears and how the clinical testing can be affected by these patterns. In testing the Teres minor, the external rotation lag sign greater than 40° appeared to be more sensitive and specific when compared with the other tests performed. These findings are clinically relevant when planning a reverse total shoulder replacement or obtaining a successful outcome from a tendon transfer for massive rotator cuff repair.

J. Brault, DO

Upper Extremity Kinematics and Muscle Activation Patterns in Subjects With Facioscapulohumeral Dystrophy

Bergsma A, Murgia A, Cup EH, et al (Radboud Univ Med Ctr, Nijmegen, The Netherlands; Univ of Groningen, The Netherlands; et al)
Arch Phys Med Rehabil 95:1731-1741, 2014

Objective.—To compare the kinematics and muscle activity of subjects with facioscapulohumeral dystrophy (FSHD) and healthy control subjects during the performance of standardized upper extremity tasks.

Design.—Exploratory case-control study

Setting.—A movement laboratory.

Participants.—Subjects (N = 19) with FSHD (n = 11) and healthy control subjects (n = 8) were measured.

Interventions.—Not applicable.

Main Outcome Measures.—Kinematic data were recorded using a 3-dimensional motion capturing system. Muscle activities, recorded using electromyography, were obtained from 6 superficial muscles around the glenohumeral joint. Shoulder elevation and elbow flexion angles, and maximum electromyographic activity during the movements as a percentage of maximum voluntary contraction (MVC) were calculated.

Results.—Kinematic differences between the FSHD group and the healthy control group were found in the shoulder elevation angle during single shoulder movements and both reaching tasks. In general, subjects with FSHD had higher percentages of muscle activation. The median activity of the trapezius was close to the MVC activity during the single shoulder movements. Moreover, deltoid and pectoralis muscles were also highly active.

Conclusions.—Higher activation of the trapezius in subjects with FSHD indicates a mechanism that could help relieve impaired shoulder muscles during arm elevation around shoulder height. Compared with healthy subjects, persons with FSHD activated their shoulder muscles to a greater extent during movements that required arm elevation.

▶ This may seem a bit esoteric, as facioscapulohumeral dystrophy is only seen in about 1 in 20,000 people in the United States. However, proximal muscular weakness is a finding in many other conditions such as proximal myopathies, upper trunk plexopathies, and upper cervical radiculopathies, to name but a few. The patterns of compensation are fairly consistent and usually involve protraction and medial rotation of the scapula. This condition leads to decrease in acromiohumeral space and likely impingement. This article describes in great detail the mechanics of the upper extremity movement in these individuals and details the muscle activation patterns of various movements. These patients are contrasted with healthy controls to highlight the differences. This description is helpful in understanding the pathomechanics of shoulder girdle weakness in general.

K. Bengston, MD

Biomechanical Consequences of Coracoclavicular Reconstruction Techniques on Clavicle Strength
Spiegl UJ, Smith SD, Euler SA, et al (Steadman Philippon Res Inst, Vail, CO; et al)
Am J Sports Med 42:1724-1730, 2014

Background.—Lateral clavicle fractures have been reported after coracoclavicular (CC) ligament reconstructions with bone tunnels through the clavicle.

Purpose.—To biomechanically compare clavicle strength following 2 common CC reconstruction techniques with different bone tunnel diameters.

Study Design.—Controlled laboratory study.

Methods.—Testing was performed on 2 groups of matched-pair cadaveric clavicles. Clavicles were prepared with either 2.4-mm tunnels and cortical fixation button (CFB) devices or 6.0-mm tunnels with hamstring tendon grafts (TGs) and tenodesis screws; contralateral clavicles were left intact. A 3-point bending load was applied to the distal clavicles at a rate of 15 mm/min until failure. Ultimate failure load and anterior-posterior width of the clavicles 45 mm medial from the lateral border were recorded. Strength reduction was determined as the percentage reduction in ultimate failure load between paired intact and surgically prepared clavicles. Relative tunnel size was determined as the quotient of tunnel diameter and clavicle width, reported as a percentage.

Results.—The TG technique significantly reduced clavicle strength relative to intact ($P=.011$) and caused significantly more strength reduction (mean, -30.7%; range, 8.1% to -62.5%) than the CFB technique (mean, -3.8%; range, 34.2% to -28.1%; $P=.031$). The CFB technique was not significantly different from intact ($P=.314$). There was a significant correlation between clavicle width and strength reduction ($\tau=-0.36$, $P=.04$) and between relative tunnel size and strength reduction ($\tau=0.51$, $P=.005$).

Conclusion.—The TG reconstruction technique with 6.0-mm tunnels, grafts, and tenodesis screws caused significantly more reduction of clavicle strength compared with the CFB technique with 2.4-mm tunnels and CFB device. Additionally, relative tunnel width correlated highly with the strength reduction.

Clinical Relevance.—This information can influence intraoperative decision making based on the individual clavicle width and might influence postoperative treatment protocols. Large bone tunnels may predispose patients to clavicle fractures after anatomic CC reconstructions.

▶ This study is cadaveric and does not represent the in vivo environment. The authors note the limitations of the study, stating that the scapula was not present and the true anatomic reconstruction was not tested in the cadaveric state. It is certainly possible that the completed reconstructed specimen may lead to different outcomes with regard to reduction in bone strength. In addition, the mechanism used to load the clavicles may not represent the biomechanical phenomenon that could cause a fracture in humans. The technique suggested for nonanatomic reconstruction in a chronic setting with cortical buttons and a looped tendon graft over the clavicle was not fully tested in this study. The key factors for the surgeon contemplating anatomic reconstruction, which can be learned from this report, are that it is important to note the diameter of the clavicle where the bone tunnels are going to be placed, especially if a 6-mm bone tunnel is going to be drilled—the clavicle must be greater than 17.4 mm; otherwise, the bone is significantly weakened and a fracture may occur intraoperatively during the placement of the interference screw and postoperatively as the bone strength is significantly weakened. The authors comment that this result is not necessarily surprising, as they cite the literature regarding impending pathologic fractures secondary to malignancy in which prophylactic fixation is recommended when 50% cortical destruction is noted radiographically.

A. B. Shafritz, MD

20 Rehabilitation

Effects of Stretching and Strengthening Exercises, With and Without Manual Therapy, on Scapular Kinematics, Function, and Pain in Individuals With Shoulder Impingement: A Randomized Controlled Trial
Camargo PR, Alburquerque-Sendín F, Avila MA, et al (Federal Univ of São Carlos, Brazil; Univ of Salamanca, Spain; et al)
J Orthop Sports Phys Ther 45:984-997, 2015

Study Design.—Randomized controlled trial.

Objective.—To evaluate the effects of an exercise protocol, with and without manual therapy, on scapular kinematics, function, pain, and mechanical sensitivity in individuals with shoulder impingement syndrome.

Background.—Stretching and strengthening exercises have been shown to effectively decrease pain and disability in individuals with shoulder impingement syndrome. There is still conflicting evidence regarding the efficacy of adding manual therapy to an exercise therapy regimen.

Methods.—Forty-six patients were assigned to 1 of 2 groups, one of which received a 4-week intervention of stretching and strengthening exercises (exercise alone) and the other the same intervention, supplemented by manual therapy targeting the shoulder and cervical spine (exercise plus manual therapy). All outcomes were measured preintervention and postintervention at 4 weeks. Outcome measures were scapular kinematics in the scapular and sagittal planes during arm elevation, function as determined through the Disabilities of the Arm, Shoulder and Hand (DASH) questionnaire, pain as assessed with a visual analog scale, and mechanical sensitivity as assessed with pressure pain threshold.

Results.—Independent of the intervention group, small, clinically irrelevant changes in scapular kinematics were observed postintervention. A significant group-by-time interaction effect ($P = .001$) was found for scapular anterior tilt during elevation in the sagittal plane, with a 3.0° increase (95% confidence interval [CI]: $-1.5°$, 7.5°) relative to baseline in the exercise-plus–manual therapy group compared to a decrease of 0.3° (95% CI: $-4.2°$, 4.8°) in the exercise-alone group. Pain, mechanical sensitivity, and the DASH score improved similarly for both groups by the end of the intervention period.

Conclusion.—Adding manual therapy to an exercise protocol did not enhance improvements in scapular kinematics, function, and pain in individuals with shoulder impingement syndrome. The noted improvements in pain and function are not likely explained by changes in scapular kinematics. The study is registered at www.clinicaltrials.gov (NCT02035618).

Level of Evidence.—Therapy, level 1b–.

▶ The authors of this study offer good additional evidence that adding manual therapy to a 4-week stretching and strengthening therapy protocol has no significant differentiating effects on outcomes with regard to pain, function, or scapular kinematics in those patients with shoulder impingement syndrome (SIS). Future additional study of a larger group of patients with similar symptom duration and activity levels would further validate evidence of the level of benefit manual therapy in the treatment of SIS. This study has added to the valuable body of literature that can help improve delivery of evidence-based quality medical care to patients.

D. Barnes, MD

Kinesio Tape and Shoulder-Joint Position Sense

Aarseth LM, Suprak DN, Chalmers GR, et al (Black Hills Surgical Hosp, Rapid City, SD; Western Washington Univ)

J Athl Train 50:785-791, 2015

Context.—Joint position sense (JPS) is a key neuromuscular factor for developing and maintaining control of muscles around a joint. It is important when performing specialized tasks, especially at the shoulder. No researchers have studied how Kinesio Tape (KT) application affects JPS.

Objective.—To investigate the effects of KT application and no tape on shoulder JPS at increasing shoulder elevations in athletes.

Design.—Cross-sectional study.

Setting.—University laboratory.

Patients or Other Participants.—A total of 27 healthy athletes who did not participate in overhead sports (age = 20.44 ± 1.05 years, height = 175.02 ± 11.67 cm, mass = 70.74 ± 9.65 kg) with no previous pathologic shoulder conditions volunteered for the study. All participants were from 1 university.

Intervention(s).—Shoulder JPS was assessed at increasing elevations with and without KT application. Participants attempted to actively replicate 3 target positions with and without the KT and without visual guidance.

Main Outcome Measure(s).—We examined absolute and variable repositioning errors at increasing shoulder-elevation levels with and without KT application.

Results.—Data revealed an interaction between tape and position for absolute error ($F_{2,52} = 4.07$, $P = .02$); simple effects revealed an increase

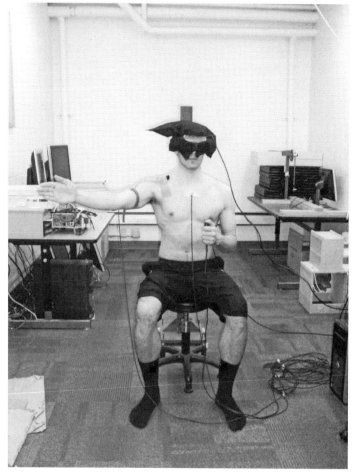

FIGURE 1.—Experimental setup showing sensors, head-mounted display, and Kinesio Tape (Kinesio Precut, Albuquerque, NM). (Reprinted from Aarseth LM, Suprak DN, Chalmers GR, et al. Kinesio tape and shoulder-joint position sense. *J Athl Train.* 2015;50:785-791, with permission from the National Athletic Trainers' Association, Inc.)

in error, with KT demonstrating a 2.65° increase in error at 90° of elevation compared with no tape ($t_{26} = 2.65$, $P = .01$). The effect size was medium ($\omega^2 = .135$). Variable error showed no interaction of tape and position ($F_{2,52} = .709$, $P = .50$). Further analysis of simple effects was not needed. However, we still calculated the effect size and observed small effect sizes for tape ($\omega^2 = .002$), position ($\omega^2 = .072$), and tape by position ($\omega^2 = .027$).

Conclusions.—At 90° of elevation, shoulder JPS was impaired by the application of KT.

▶ The utility of elastic textile taping is increasing in clinical applications. The product used in this study was Kinesio Tex Tape Gold precuts for dynamic

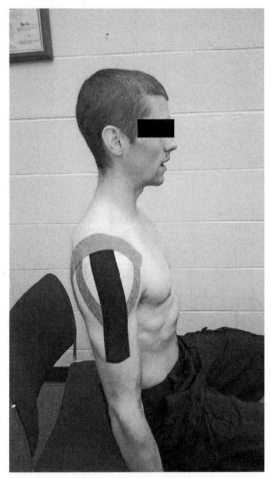

FIGURE 3.—Kinesio-Tape application (Kinesio Precut, Albuquerque, NM). (Reprinted from Aarseth LM, Suprak DN, Chalmers GR, et al. Kinesio tape and shoulder-joint position sense. *J Athl Train.* 2015;50:785-791, with permission from the National Athletic Trainers' Association, Inc.)

shoulder support (Kinesio Precut, Albuquerque, NM). However, the evidence of use of any Kinesiotape has been sparse since it appeared around 1995 in the western clinic. This study lays an additional piece of evidence for its proper application in the shoulder. Joint position sense (JPS) is used to measure the ability of the internal sense of proprioception for the shoulder. They hypothesize that the tape will enhance JPS in all shoulder ranges of motion.

A full description is given for a 1-session measurement episode. All persons included were healthy collegiate athletes and participated in a warm-up exercise and a small set of active upper extremity dynamic motions, as well as passive stretching. Kinematic data were collected via a magnetic tracking system. The participants wore a set of goggles with a digital screen that showed a gray screen with a black square in the center (Figs 1 and 3). When directed, the participant moved the dominant extremity to within 5 degrees of the desired position, with the digital screen guiding the person's arm to the desired position. They remained in that position for 1 second, their visual screen went black, and they were asked to hold that position for 5 seconds, then told to relax. After 3 seconds, they were verbally instructed to return to that same position. This return was again measured with the magnetic system. The testing consisted of 2 states: with tape and without tape. Order of the testing was randomized, and each was separated by a 10-minute break. Within each testing condition, shoulder ranges tested were forward elevation of 50, 90, and 110 degrees, 3 trials at each angle, all in the scapular plane. Appropriate statistical tests were performed and reported.

Their results found that the KT application did not affect shoulder elevation to 50 degrees and 110 degrees, but interestingly had diminished JPS acuity at 90 degrees. The differences in effect at 90 degrees were small and did not represent a clinical risk, according to the authors. The study was limited to healthy young athletes who did not participate in overhead sports, and therefore it cannot be generalized to overhead athletes or those with shoulder injuries, or to differences in the effects between sexes.

Each practitioner should be aware of the effects on the shoulder or any other part of the upper extremity. Although this is lower level evidence, it adds to the set of evidence for the use of KT in upper extremity applications.

V. H. O'Brien, OTD, OTR/L, CHT

Correlation Between American Shoulder and Elbow Surgeons and Single Assessment Numerical Evaluation Score After Rotator Cuff or SLAP Repair
Cunningham G, Lädermann A, Denard PJ, et al (Geneva Univ Hosps, Switzerland; Oregon Health & Science Univ, Portland; et al)
Arthroscopy 31:1688-1692, 2015

Purpose.—To compare the American Shoulder and Elbow Surgeons (ASES) and the Single Assessment Numerical Evaluation (SANE) scores after rotator cuff repair, rotator cuff revision, and SLAP repair.

Methods.—This study was a retrospective review of a prospectively filled database of 262 patients who underwent arthroscopic surgery for rotator cuff tears or SLAP lesions between 1999 and 2007. All patients were operated on by the same surgeon, with a minimum follow-up of 2 years. The patient database included preoperative and outcome measures, such as pain, range of motion, and notably postoperative ASES and SANE scores. Any patient with incomplete data was removed from the study.

Results.—Three groups were identified: primary rotator cuff repair (n = 135), rotator cuff revision (n = 73), and SLAP repair (n = 54). The overall mean ASES and SANE scores after surgery were 82.7 (± 20.2) and 83.3 (± 19.6), respectively. The Pearson correlation coefficient (*r*) between both scores was 0.8 (*P* < .001), demonstrating a very good correlation. In subgroup analysis, the correlation was highest in the cuff revision group ($r = 0.88$; $P < .001$) followed by the SLAP group ($r = 0.78$; $P < .001$) and primary cuff group ($r = 0.75$; $P < .001$).

Conclusions.—This study shows that there is a significant correlation between postoperative SANE and ASES rating methods in rotator cuff and SLAP repairs. We recommend the SANE score as a reliable outcome indicator for iterative follow-up, which can then be combined with a more clinically informative score such as the ASES or other process-based scores for preoperative and final workup.

Level of Evidence.—Level III, retrospective comparative study.

▶ Functional scores have become the mainstay of outcomes research. Several shoulder scales have been developed over the last few decades with the aim to obtain detailed insight into multiple domains such as pain, function, and disability. Although the utility of comprehensive functional scales cannot be understated, their routine use in the clinical setting can place a significant burden on patients and evaluators. The Single Assessment Numerical Evaluation (SANE), introduced by Williams et al in 1999, is a score based on the single question "How would you rate your shoulder today as a percentage of normal?" with possible values ranging from 0% to 100%. This simple tool for the subjective assessment of shoulder function is found to have a high correlation with multiple comprehensive shoulder scales in the setting of several shoulder conditions including rotator cuff conditions, shoulder instability, and superior labral tear from anterior to posterior (SLAP) tears. SANE thereby provides a valuable tool to obtain a quick understanding of overall shoulder function throughout a large array of conditions. The results reported by Cunningham et al again confirm the utility of SANE as a valuable tool to assess shoulder function in the setting of SLAP tears and rotator cuff repairs, both in the primary and revision setting.

P. Streubel, MD

The effectiveness of exercise for the management of musculoskeletal disorders and injuries of the elbow, forearm, wrist, and hand: a systematic review by the Ontario Protocol for Traffic Injury Management (OPTIMa) Collaboration

Menta R, Randhawa K, Côté P, et al (Canadian Memorial Chiropractic College, Toronto, Ontario; Univ of Ontario Inst of Technology, Oshawa, Canada; et al)

J Manip Physiol Ther 38:507-520, 2015

Objective.—The purpose of this systematic review was to evaluate the effectiveness of exercise compared to other interventions, placebo/sham intervention, or no intervention in improving self-rated recovery, functional recovery, clinical, and/or administrative outcomes in individuals with musculoskeletal disorders and injuries of the elbow, forearm, wrist, and hand.

Methods.—We searched MEDLINE, EMBASE, CINAHL, PsycINFO, and the Cochrane Central Register of Controlled Trials from 1990 to 2015. Paired reviewers independently screened studies for relevance and assessed the risk of bias using the Scottish Intercollegiate Guidelines Network criteria. We synthesized the evidence using the best evidence synthesis methodology.

Results.—We identified 5 studies with a low risk of bias. Our review suggests that, for patients with persistent lateral epicondylitis, (1) adding concentric or eccentric strengthening exercises to home stretching exercises provides no additional benefits; (2) a home program of either eccentric or concentric strengthening exercises leads to similar outcomes; (3) home wrist extensor strengthening exercises lead to greater short-term improvements in pain reduction compared to "wait and see"; and (4) clinic-based, supervised exercise may be more beneficial than home exercises with minimal improvements in pain and function. For hand pain of variable duration, supervised progressive strength training added to advice to continue normal physical activity provides no additional benefits.

Conclusion.—The relative effectiveness of stretching vs strengthening for the wrist extensors remains unknown for the management of persistent lateral epicondylitis. The current evidence shows that the addition of supervised progressive strength training does not provide further benefits over advice to continue normal physical activity for hand pain of variable duration.

▶ Exercise therapy (home programs and supervised therapy) is frequently recommended for a variety of musculoskeletal conditions of the upper extremity. As with any intervention, it is important to understand when and to what degree these programs are beneficial. Supervised physical therapy can be a costly and limited resource and should be used as effectively as possible.

The authors sought to limit their review to high-quality studies that investigate the use of exercise in the treatment of musculoskeletal conditions such as sprains/strains, tendinitis/tendinosis, and nerve compression syndromes. Outcomes evaluated included self-rated, clinical, and functional recovery. Although many musculoskeletal disorders were included in this review, 4 of the 5 studies selected addressed the treatment of lateral epicondylitis. The other study selected looked at the use of exercise for hand pain without major pathology. Interestingly, no studies investigated exercise therapy for other common upper extremity musculoskeletal conditions that met the inclusion criteria for this review (Fig 1, Table 4).

A high point in this report is the discussion of previous systematic reviews. The authors do a nice job of explaining their findings in the context of other systematic reviews, thereby helping the reader understand the landscape of the literature on this topic. The reader realizes that there are very few high-quality studies investigating the effectiveness of exercise therapy for upper extremity disorders; with the exception of persistent lateral epicondylitis, there is a paucity of literature with a low risk of bias to inform the use of exercise therapy.

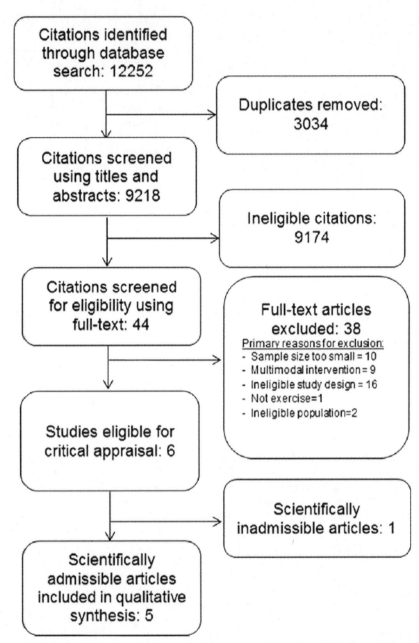

FIGURE 1.—Identification and selection of articles. (Reprinted from Menta R, Randhawa K, Côté P, et al. The effectiveness of exercise for the management of musculoskeletal disorders and injuries of the elbow, forearm, wrist, and hand: a systematic review by the Ontario Protocol for Traffic Injury Management (OPTIMa) Collaboration. *J Manip Physiol Ther.* 2015;38:507-520, with permission from National University of Health Sciences.)

TABLE 4.—Evidence Table for Randomized Controlled Trials With a Low Risk of Bias Assessing the Effectiveness of Exercise for Musculoskeletal Injuries and Neuropathies of the Elbow, Forearm, Wrist, or Hand Region

Author(s), Year	Subjects and Setting; Number (n) Enrolled	Interventions; No. (n) of Subjects	Comparisons; No. (n) of Subjects	Follow-Up	Outcomes	Key Findings
Martinez-Silvestrini et al, 2005[38]	Adult patients recruited from the Mayo Clinic and in local health clubs in Minnesota. Case definition: Pain and tenderness at lateral elbow >3 mo and pain with 2/3 tests (resisted wrist extension, resisted middle finger extension, and chair lift test); n = 94	CS: (1) Full wrist extension with resistance band (3 sets/10× daily/6 wk); (2) stretching and advice; n = 30 ES: (1) Full wrist flexion with resistance band (3 sets/10× daily/ 6 wk); (2) stretching and advice; n = 31	Stretching (S) Stretching and advice: stretches for wrist: extensors (3× for 30 s twice daily/6 wk), avoid precipitating and exacerbating activities, use of counterforce strap as needed, information sheet on ice massage; n = 33	Postintervention	Primary outcomes: PFG strength (electronic dynamometer); PRFEQ, DASH, SF-36, pain intensity (100-mm VAS).	Difference in mean change (CS − S) at 6 wk: [a] PFG (N), −1.0 (95% CI, −5.5 to 3.5); VAS, −9.0 (95% CI, −16.5 to −1.6); total PRFEQ, 0.3 (95% CI, −0.2 to 0.8); DASH, −3.0 (95% CI, −7.4 to 1.4) Difference in mean change (ES − S) at 6 wk: [a] PFG (N), −3.0 (95% CI, −1.7 to 7.7); VAS, −1.0 (95% CI, −8.2 to 6.2); total PRFEQ, −0.1 (95% CI, −0.6 to 0.4); DASH, −3.0 (95% CI, −7.5 to 1.5) Difference in mean change (ES − CS) at 6 wk: [a] PFG (N), 4.0 (95% CI, −0.0 to 8.0); VAS, 8.0 (95% CI, 0.5-15.6); total PRFEQ, −0.4 (95% CI, −1.0 to 0.2); DASH, 0.0 (95% CI, −4.5 to 4.5)

(Continued)

TABLE 4. (*continued*)

Author(s), Year	Subjects and Setting; Number (n) Enrolled	Interventions; No. (n) of Subjects	Comparisons; No. (n) of Subjects	Follow-Up	Outcomes	Key Findings
Pedersen et al, 2013[39]	Industrial workers (18-67 years old) with repetitive work tasks from Copenhagen, Denmark. Case definition: right hand pain intensity ≥3/9 on the Nordic questionnaire on trouble; n = 95	Supervised progressive strength training (wrist extension with dumbbells) at the workplace provided by staff and students trained in physical education or physiotherapy (20 min/3 times per week for 20 wk). Advice to continue their normal physical activity as usual; n = 55	Advice to continue their normal physical activity as usual; n = 40	20 wk	Primary outcome: pain intensity during the last 7 d (Nordic questionnaire on trouble 0-9)	Between-group mean differences (strength training and advice-advice): [b] No statistically significant between-group differences in pain intensity and percentage of subjects with pain reductions ≥2
Peterson et al, 2011[40]	Patients (20-75 years old) recruited from general practitioners, physiotherapist, and newspaper advertisements in Uppsala, Sweden, from 2003 to 2006 Case definition: Diagnosis of tennis elbow (>3 mo) on palpation, Mill's test loading and Maudley's middle finger test; n = 81	SE: Progressive loading exercise for extensor muscles at home (3 sets/15 repetitions/daily/3 mo) and some information as comparison group; n = 40	WS with information that condition was painful but harmless and continue ordinary daily activities; n = 41	Immediately postintervention	Primary outcomes: pain on MVC and MME (100-mm VAS); secondary outcomes: muscle strength (hand-held dynamometer); tertiary outcomes: DASH, GQL (well-being score, activity score, complaint score)	Difference in mean change (SE − WS) postintervention: [a] VAS for MVC (0-100 mm), 15.8 (95% CI, 8.3-23.4); VAS for MME (0-100 mm), 12.9 (95% CI, 5.6-20.2); muscular strength (N), 7.5 (95% CI, −5.3 to 20.3); DASH score (0-100), 4.6 (95% CI, 0.6-8.6); well-being score (0-7), 1.0 (95% CI, −0.9 to 2.9); activity score (0-2), 0.2 (95% CI, −0.2 to 0.6); complaint score, 0.0 (95% CI, −1.4 to 1.4)

| Peterson et al, 2014[41] | Patients (20-75 years old) recruited from general practitioners, physiotherapists, and newspaper advertisements in Uppsala, Sweden. Case definition: Diagnosis of tennis elbow (>3 mo) with pain on palpation, pain on stretching (Mill's test), pain on loading, and Maudley's middle finger test; n = 120 | Home-based eccentric exercise group instructed to lower weight by flexing the wrist of the affected arm downwards and to lift back up with unaffected arm (15 repetitions/ set and 3 sets daily for 3 mo). Load increased weekly by 1 hectogram; n = 60 | Home-based concentric exercise group instructed to lift the weight by extending the wrist of the affected arm upwards and lower it with unaffected arm (15 repetitions/set and 3 sets daily for 3 mo). Load increased weekly by 1 hectogram; n = 60 | 3, 6, and 12 mo after baseline assessment | Primary outcomes: pain reduction (100-mm VAS) during forearm muscle contraction, pain reduction (100-mm VAS) during forearm muscle elongation; secondary outcomes: muscle strength (N) (hand-held dynamometer); tertiary outcomes: DASH, 0-100: GQL (well-being score, 0-2; activity score, 0-7; complaint score). Adverse events | Difference in mean change (eccentric exercise − concentric exercise): [a] 3 mo: VAS for MVC (0-100 mm), 4.3 (95% CI, −1.8 to 10.4); VAS for MME (0-100 mm), 4.8 (95% CI, −1.3 to 10.9); muscle strength (N), 5.9 (95% CI, −4.8 to 16.6); DASH score (0-100), 0.1 (95% CI, −4.0 to 4.2); activity score (0-2): −1.4 (95% CI, −3.0 to 0.2); well-being score (0-7), 0 (95% CI, −0.3 to 0.3); complaint score, 0.4 (95% CI, −0.9 to 1.7) 6 mo: VAS for MVC (0-100 mm), 5.2 (95% CI, −0.7 to 11.1); VAS for MME (0-100 mm), 4.2 (95% CI −1.8 to 10.2); muscle strength (N), 5.4 ,95% CI, −5.4 to 16.2); DASH score (0-100), −0.3 (95% CI, −4.3 to 3.7); activity score (0-2), −0.6 (95% CI, −2.2 to 1.0); well-being score (0-7), −0.1 (95% CI, −0.4 to 0.2); complaint score, −0.2 (95% CI −1.4 to 1.0) 12 mo: VAS for MVC (0-100 mm), 4.8 (95% CI −1.2 to 10.8); VAS for MME (0-100 mm), 3.7 (95% CI −2.9 to 10.3); muscle strength (N), 4.3 (95% CI, −6.8 to 15.4); DASH score (0-100), 1.3 (95% CI, −2.7 to 5.3); activity score (0-2), −0.9 (95% CI, −2.6 to 0.8); well-being score (0-7), 0.1 (95% CI, −0.2 to 0.4); complaint score, 1 (95% CI, −0.3 to 2.3) No adverse events reported. |

(Continued)

TABLE 4. (*continued*)

Author(s), Year	Subjects and Setting; Number (n) Enrolled	Interventions; No. (n) of Subjects	Comparisons; No. (n) of Subjects	Follow-Up	Outcomes	Key Findings
Stasinopoulos et al, 2010[42]	Patients (18 years old) from Athens, Greece, referred by physicians and physiotherapists from 2005 to 2007. Case definition: Lateral epicondylitis (≥4 wk): (1) pain on palpation; pain with resisted elbow extension; (3) 2/4 positive tests (Tomsen, resisted middle finger, Mill's handgrip dynamometer); n = 70	CEP: slow progressive eccentric exercises of the wrist extensors and static stretching exercises of the extensor carpi radialis brevis tendon supervised by a physical therapist (5×/week/12 wk); n = 35	HEP: same exercise protocol as CEP group except performed at home (5×/week/12 wk). Visit with physical therapist 1×/week for further instructions; n = 35	12 wk postintervention, and 24 wk	Primary outcomes: pain (10-cm VAS); secondary outcomes: elbow function (10-cm VAS); tertiary outcomes: pain-free grip strength (Jamar hand-held dynamometer)	Difference in mean change (CEP − HEP): Postintervention (week 12): VAS for pain (0-10 cm), 1.54 (95% CI, 0.54-2.55); VAS for function (0-10 cm), 2.55 (95% CI, 1.72-3.38); pain-free grip strength (lb), 17.05 (95% CI, 16.03-18.07) 3 mo (week 24): VAS for pain (0-10 cm), 1.76 (95% CI, 1.03-2.50); VAS for function (0-10 cm), 2.81 (95% CI, 1.81-3.81); pain-free grip strength (lb), 17.08 (95% CI, 16.14-18.01)

Editor's Note: Please refer to original journal article for full references.
CS, concentric strengthening; CEP, clinic-based exercise program; ES, eccentric strengthening; GQL, Gothenburg Quality of Life Instrument; HEP, home exercise program; PFG, pain-free grip; PRFEQ, Patient-rated Forearm Evaluation Questionnaire; S, stretching; SE, strengthening exercises; SF-36, Short Form 36; WS, wait and see.
[a]Recalculated data from study.
[b]Data were presented in graphs; differences in mean change and 95% CIs could not be calculated.
Reprinted from Menta R, Randhawa K, Côté P, et al. The effectiveness of exercise for the management of musculoskeletal disorders and injuries of the elbow, forearm, wrist, and hand: a systematic review by the Ontario Protocol for Traffic Injury Management (OPTIMa) Collaboration. *J Manip Physiol Ther.* 2015;38:507-520, with permission from National University of Health Sciences.

The take-home message of this report is that in the setting of persistent lateral epicondylitis, exercise therapy in the clinic may be more beneficial than a home exercise program, and a home exercise program is superior to a wait-and-see approach.

E. Kinnucan, MD

Responsiveness of three Patient Report Outcome (PRO) measures in patients with hand fractures: A preliminary cohort study
Weinstock-Zlotnick G, Page C, Ghomrawi HMK, et al (Hosp for Special Surgery, NY)
J Hand Ther 28:403-411, 2015

Study Design.—Clinical measurement.

Introduction.—Few studies describe the responsiveness of functional outcomes measures in patients sustaining hand fractures.

Purpose.—1 − To explore the responsiveness of three function-oriented Patient Report Outcome (PRO) measures with a cohort of hand fracture patients. 2 − To examine patients' PRO preference.

Methods.—60 participants with 74 hand fractures at an outpatient hospital-based hand therapy clinic consented to participate in this study. They completed the Disabilities of the Arm, Shoulder, and Hand Questionnaire (DASH), Michigan Hand Outcomes Questionnaire (MHQ), and Patient-Rated Wrist/Hand Evaluation (PRWHE) at three trials: T1 (evaluation), T2 (one month later), and T3 (two months later). Participants also identified which PRO they felt best reflected their hand use and which was easiest to complete. Descriptive statistics, analyses of variance (ANOVA), effect size, and standardized response mean (SRM) were employed to describe participants, determine functional change between trials, and examine and compare PRO responsiveness. Questionnaire preference at T1 was reported.

Results.—Participants demonstrated functional improvement, as measured by the DASH, PRWHE, and MHQ. T1 scores: DASH = 41.85 (SD ± 22.78), MHQ = 50.13 (SD ± 18.36), and PRWHE = 48.18 (SD ± 22.07). T2 scores: DASH = 22.11 (SD ± 18.18), MHQ = 69.89 (SD ± 15.93), and PRWHE = 22.62 (SD ± 18.15). T3 scores: DASH = 17.56 (SD ± 18.01), MHQ = 75.37 (SD ± 19.19), and PRWHE = 22.40 (SD ± 19.04). Each PRO demonstrated significant test score differences between trials ($p < .001$). Large responsiveness ($\geq .80$) was noted between T1 and T2: (effect size: .98−1.23; SRM: 1.31−1.49) and T1 and T3 (effect size: 1.21−1.54; SRM 1.49−1.84). Smaller responsiveness effects were noted between T2 and T3 (effect size: .35−.64, SRM: .38−.81). No significant differences between questionnaire responsiveness were found. Patients reported PRWHE easiest to complete and MHQ best reflecting their hand use.

Conclusions.—DASH, MHQ, and PRWHE were each able to describe functional limitations in this cohort of patients with hand fractures. In

capturing improvement over time they demonstrated comparable responsiveness in assessing change in patients with hand fractures.
Level of Evidence.—2c.

▶ The responsiveness of many upper limb—specific patient-rated outcomes (PRO) has been well investigated across persons after distal radius fracture, carpal tunnel release, rheumatoid arthritis, and other broad categories of upper limb injuries and disorders but never specifically in persons with hand fractures. In this cross-sectional study, the responsiveness of 3 commonly used PROs, the Disabilities of the Arm, Shoulder and Hand (DASH) questionnaire,[1,2] the Michigan Hand Outcomes Questionnaire (MHQ),[3,4] and the Patient-Rated Wrist/Hand Evaluation (PRWHE)[5,6] was compared in persons with surgical and nonsurgical metacarpal and phalangeal fractures of the hand. A secondary purpose was to learn from persons of this population which outcome measure was easiest to use and which best reflected their current ability to use their affected hand. Responsiveness was measured across 3 time points: at initial therapy session, at 1 month follow-up, and then at 2 months' follow-up. Patient preferences were assessed at the time of initial evaluation.

The authors reported that no single PRO was statistically more or less responsive than another in this population; however, in 2 of 3 instances (time 2-3 and time 1-3), the MHQ trended toward yielding larger effects sizes and in 2 of 3 instances (time 1-2 and time 1-3) it also trended toward yielding larger standardized response means. In general, all tools were less responsive between months 2 and 3. Participants preferred the ease of the PRWHE over the DASH and MHQ, however, reported the MHQ to best reflect the function of their hands.

These findings support that any one of these tools will be sensitive to change in self-reported upper limb function across time but may only capture smaller to moderate changes in the latter stages of rehabilitation. This finding could be a result of the instruments failing to capture the impact of these fractures on higher-level daily activities (ie, nonwork activities in the MHQ and work/performance arts of the DASH optional modules) or rehabilitation plateau. Patient preferences show that the shortest tool (PRWHE) is preferred, likely for convenience reasons. The MHQ, however, likely because of the expansive range of survey items, best reflects patient perceptions on hand function. Given the nonsignificant differences in responsiveness, hand therapists and surgeons should consider these patient perceptions and administrative pragmatics when selecting a PRO for patients after hand fractures.

This study blends surgical and nonsurgical patients and, thus, should be interpreted with some caution. In addition, these findings reflect the responsiveness to those who discontinued from rehabilitation rather late and thus may not be generalizable to quick responders. Lastly, because patient perceptions were sought only at baseline, it is not known which tool best reflects patients' perceived changes in hand function across time. Additional study is required.

C. McGee, CHT

References

1. Hudak PL, Amadio PC, Bombardier C. Upper Extremity Collaborative Group (UECG). Development of an upper extremity outcome measure. The DASH (disabilities of the arm, shoulder, and hand). *Am J Ind Med.* 1996;29:602-608.
2. Beaton DE, Katz JN, Fossel AH, Wright JG, Tarasuk V, Bombardier C. Measuring the whole or the parts? Validity, reliability, and responsiveness of the disabilities of the arm, shoulder, and hand outcome measure in different regions of the upper extremity. *J Hand Ther.* 2001;14:128-146.
3. Chung KC, Hamill JB, Walters MR, Hayward RA. The Michigan hand outcomes questionnaire (MHQ): assessment of responsiveness to clinical change. *Ann Plast Surg.* 1999;42:619-622.
4. Chung KC, Pillsbury MS, Walters MR, Hayward RA. Reliability and validity testing of the michigan hand outcomes questionnaire. *J Hand Surg.* 1998;23A: 575-587.
5. MacDermid JC, Tottenham V. Responsiveness of the disability of the arm, shoulder, and hand (DASH) and patient-rated wrist/hand evaluation (PRWHE) in evaluating change after hand therapy. *J Hand Ther.* 2004;17:18-23.
6. MacDermid JC. Development of a scale for patient rating of wrist pain and disability. *J Hand Ther.* 1996;9:178-183.

The Minimum Clinically Important Difference of the Patient-rated Wrist Evaluation Score for Patients With Distal Radius Fractures

Walenkamp MMJ, de Muinck Keizer R-J, Goslings JC, et al (Univ of Amsterdam, The Netherlands; et al)
Clin Orthop Relat Res 473:3235-3241, 2015

Background.—The Patient-rated Wrist Evaluation (PRWE) is a commonly used instrument in upper extremity surgery and in research. However, to recognize a treatment effect expressed as a change in PRWE, it is important to be aware of the minimum clinically important difference (MCID) and the minimum detectable change (MDC). The MCID of an outcome tool like the PRWE is defined as the smallest change in a score that is likely to be appreciated by a patient as an important change, while the MDC is defined as the smallest amount of change that can be detected by an outcome measure. A numerical change in score that is less than the MCID, even when statistically significant, does not represent a true clinically relevant change. To our knowledge, the MCID and MDC of the PRWE have not been determined in patients with distal radius fractures.

Questions/Purposes.—We asked: (1) What is the MCID of the PRWE score for patients with distal radius fractures? (2) What is the MDC of the PRWE?

Methods.—Our prospective cohort study included 102 patients with a distal radius fracture and a median age of 59 years (interquartile range [IQR], 48—66 years). All patients completed the PRWE questionnaire during each of two separate visits. At the second visit, patients were asked to indicate the degree of clinical change they appreciated since the previous visit. Accordingly, patients were categorized in two groups: (1) minimally improved or (2) no change. The groups were used to anchor the changes observed in the PRWE score to patients' perspectives of what was clinically important. We determined the MCID using an anchor-based receiver operator characteristic method. In this context, the change in the PRWE score was considered a diagnostic test, and the anchor (minimally improved or no change as noted by the patients from visit to visit) was the gold standard. The optimal receiver operator characteristic cutoff point calculated with the Youden index reflected the value of the MCID.

Results.—In our study, the MCID of the PRWE was 11.5 points. The area under the curve was 0.54 (95% CI, 0.37—0.70) for the pain subscale and 0.71 (95% CI, 0.57—0.85) for the function subscale. We determined the MDC to be 11.0 points.

Conclusions.—We determined the MCID of the PRWE score for patients with distal radius fractures using the anchor-based approach and verified that the MDC of the PRWE was sufficiently small to detect our MCID.

Clinical Relevance.—We recommend using an improvement on the PRWE of more than 11.5 points as the smallest clinically relevant difference when evaluating the effects of treatments and when performing sample-size calculations on studies of distal radius fractures.

▶ This is an important study. The authors clearly outline the importance of choosing appropriate instruments to measure outcomes. This work validates the described tool and the clinical importance of that measurement in patients and providers. Significant difference is significant when it is measured consistently, interpreted appropriately by both patient and providers, and disseminated throughout the research community. This is important work with implications for practice and research.

L. Fitton, CNP

Reliability, Validity, and Responsiveness of the QuickDASH in Patients With Upper Limb Amputation
Resnik L, Borgia M (Providence Veterans Administration Med Ctr, RI)
Arch Phys Med Rehabil 96:1676-1683, 2015

Objectives.—To examine the internal consistency, test-retest reliability, validity, and responsiveness of the shortened version of the Disabilities of the Arm, Shoulder and Hand (QuickDASH) questionnaire in persons with upper limb amputation.

Design.—Cross-sectional and longitudinal.

Setting.—Three sites participating in the U.S. Department of Veterans Affairs Home Study of the DEKA Arm.

Participants.—A convenience sample of upper limb amputees (N = 44).

Interventions.—Training with a multifunction upper limb prosthesis.

Main Outcome Measures.—Multiple outcome measures including the QuickDASH were administered twice within 1 week, and for a subset of 20 persons, after completion of in-laboratory training with the DEKA Arm. Scale alphas and intraclass correlation coefficient type 3,1 (ICC3,1) were used to examine reliability. Minimum detectable change (MDC) scores were calculated. Analyses of variance, comparing Quick-DASH scores by the amount of prosthetic use and amputation level, were used for known-group validity analyses with alpha set at .05. Pairwise correlations between QuickDASH and other measures were used to examine concurrent validity. Responsiveness was measured by effect size (ES) and standardized response mean (SRM).

Results.—QuickDASH alpha was .83, and ICC was .87 (95% confidence interval, .77–.93). MDC at the 95% confidence level (MDC 95%) was 17.4. Full- or part-time prosthesis users had better QuickDASH scores compared with nonprosthesis users ($P = .021$), as did those with more distal amputations at both baseline ($P = .042$) and with the DEKA Arm ($P = .024$). The QuickDASH was correlated with concurrent measures of activity limitation as expected. The ES and SRM after training with the DEKA Arm were 0.6.

Conclusions.—This study provides evidence of reliability and validity of the QuickDASH in persons with upper limb amputation. Results provide preliminary evidence of responsiveness to prosthetic device type/training. Further research with a larger sample is needed to confirm results.

▶ The final conclusion of this study is that it "supports the use of the shortened version of the Disabilities of the Arm, Shoulder and Hand (QuickDASH) for clinical practice and research in this population." However, what we really want to know is if this is the best tool for measuring disability in this population. The DASH and the QuickDASH are convenient and generalizable for assessing disability from many etiologies. However, more specific measures are available for assessing function and disability for upper extremity amputees, specifically, the Activities Measure for Upper Limb Amputees and the University of New Brunswick Test of Prosthetic Function for Unilateral Amputees.

The DASH and the QuickDASH are useful and appropriate for comparing upper extremity disability in a population that has heterogeneous etiologies of upper extremity dysfunction. I would hope that this study does not encourage others to use the QuickDASH for the study of upper extremity amputees. It is much better to use a specific outcome measure than a generalized outcome measure.

K. Bengtson, MD

Changes in H reflex and neuromechanical properties of the trapezius muscle after 5 weeks of eccentric training: a randomized controlled trial
Vangsgaard S, Taylor JL, Hansen EA, et al (Aalborg Univ, Denmark; Univ of New South Wales, Sydney, Australia)
J Appl Physiol (1985) 116:1623-1631, 2014

Trapezius muscle Hoffman (H) reflexes were obtained to investigate the neural adaptations induced by a 5-wk strength training regimen, based solely on eccentric contractions of the shoulder muscles. Twenty-nine healthy subjects were randomized into an eccentric training group ($n = 15$) and a reference group ($n = 14$). The eccentric training program consisted of nine training sessions of eccentric exercise performed over a 5-wk period. H-reflex recruitment curves, the maximal M wave (M_{max}), maximal voluntary contraction (MVC) force, rate of force development (RFD), and electromyographic (EMG) voluntary activity were recorded before and after training. H reflexes were recorded from the middle part of the trapezius muscle by electrical stimulation of the C3/4 cervical nerves; M_{max} was measured by electrical stimulation of the accessory nerve. Eccentric strength training resulted in significant increases in the maximal trapezius muscle H reflex (H_{max}) (21.4% [5.5−37.3]; $P = 0.01$), MVC force (26.4% [15.0−37.7]; $P < 0.01$), and RFD (24.6% [3.2−46.0]; $P = 0.025$), while no significant changes were observed in the reference group. M_{max} remained unchanged in both groups. A significant positive correlation was found between the change in MVC force and the change in EMG voluntary activity in the training group ($r = 0.57$; $P = 0.03$). These results indicate that the net excitability of the trapezius muscle H-reflex pathway increased after 5 wk of eccentric training. This is the first study to investigate and document changes in the trapezius muscle H reflex following eccentric strength training.

▶ This is a challenging article to digest even for those well-versed and highly interested in neurophysiology. However, there is some gold at the end of this journey. It is well known that the first 4 to 8 weeks of strength training is largely secondary to increased muscle activation rather than the later effects of muscle hypertrophy. This study sets out to prove that this is really the case with eccentric training of the trapezius muscle and is subsequently successful in doing so. Essentially, the authors measure the net excitability of the muscle using the H reflex. This study is reassuring for those studying strengthening in various forms and certainly helpful for the building blocks of basic neurophysiology science.

K. Bengston, MD

21 Miscellaneous

Surgical Treatment Options for Glenohumeral Arthritis in Young Patients: A Systematic Review and Meta-analysis
Sayegh ET, Mascarenhas R, Chalmers PN, et al (Columbia Univ, NY; Rush Univ Med Ctr, Chicago, IL)
Arthroscopy 31:1156-1166, 2015

Purpose.—The aim of this study was to compare surgical treatment options for young patients with glenohumeral arthritis.

Methods.—A systematic review of the English-language literature was conducted by searching PubMed, EMBASE, and Scopus with the following term: "(shoulder OR glenohumeral) AND (arthritis OR osteoarthritis) AND (young OR younger)." Studies that reported clinical or radiological outcomes of nonbiologic surgical treatment of generalized glenohumeral arthritis in patients younger than 60 years of age were included. Data were extracted to include study and patient characteristics, surgical technique, outcome scores, pain relief, satisfaction, functional improvement, return to activity, health-related quality of life, complications, need for and time to revision, range of motion, and radiological outcomes. Study quality was assessed with the Modified Coleman Methodology Score.

Results.—Thirty-two studies containing a total of 1,229 shoulders met the inclusion criteria and were included in the review. Pain scores improved significantly more after total shoulder arthroplasty (TSA) than after hemiarthroplasty (HA) ($P < .001$). Patient satisfaction was similar after HA and TSA. Revision surgery was equally likely after HA, TSA, and arthroscopic debridement (AD). Complications were significantly less common after AD than after HA ($P = .0049$) and TSA ($P < .001$). AD and TSA afforded better recovery of active forward flexion and external rotation than did HA. At radiological follow-up, subluxation was similarly common after HA and TSA.

Conclusions.—According to current Level IV data, TSA provides greater improvement of pain and range of motion than does HA in the surgical treatment of young patients with glenohumeral arthritis. AD is an efficacious and particularly safe alternative in the short term for young patients with concerns about arthroplasty.

Level of Evidence.—Level IV, systematic review of Level IV studies.

▶ This systematic review evaluated case series of total shoulder arthroplasty, hemiarthroplasty, and arthroscopic debridement for young patients with glenohumeral arthritis. Unfortunately, level IV data have substantial limitations. In addition, the basic statistical treatment performed accentuates those limitations. Overall, the article provides a good summary of existing data to date.

N. C. Chen, MD

Google Glass as an Alternative to Standard Fluoroscopic Visualization for Percutaneous Fixation of Hand Fractures: A Pilot Study
Chimenti PC, Mitten DJ (Univ of Rochester, NY)
Plast Reconstr Surg 136:328-330, 2015

This pilot study investigated the feasibility of Google Glass to assist visualization of fluoroscopic images during percutaneous pinning of hand fractures. Cadavers were used to compare total time to pin each fracture and total number of radiographs per fracture from a mini C-arm. A FluoroScan monitor was used for radiographic visualization compared to projecting the images in the Google Glass display. All outcome measures significantly improved for proximal phalanx fractures (127 versus 86 seconds, $p = 0.017$; 5.3 versus 2.2 images, $p = 0.003$), and fewer images were obtained during fixation of metacarpal fractures using Google Glass compared with traditional techniques (6.4 versus 3.6, $p < 0.001$). Typical FluoroScan monitor placement may require the surgeon to alter focus away

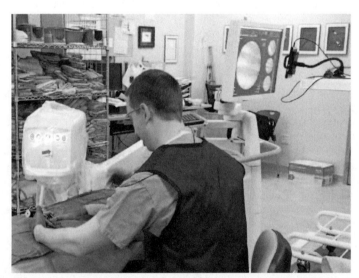

FIGURE 1.—Experimental setup. The FluoroScan monitor was alternately pointed at the cell phone when using Google Glass, or turned to face the surgeon for standard technique. (Reprinted from Chimenti PC, Mitten DJ. Google glass as an alternative to standard fluoroscopic visualization for percutaneous fixation of hand fractures: a pilot study. *Plast Reconstr Surg.* 2015;136:328-330, with permission from the American Society of Plastic Surgeons.)

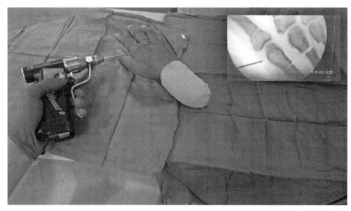

FIGURE 2.—Vignette image obtained through the Google Glass camera showing the image that appears in the user's right eye. By tilting one's head down, this image can be directly superimposed onto the operative field and give real-time feedback on pin positioning. (Reprinted from Chimenti PC, Mitten DJ. Google glass as an alternative to standard fluoroscopic visualization for percutaneous fixation of hand fractures: a pilot study. *Plast Reconstr Surg*. 2015;136:328-330, with permission from the American Society of Plastic Surgeons.)

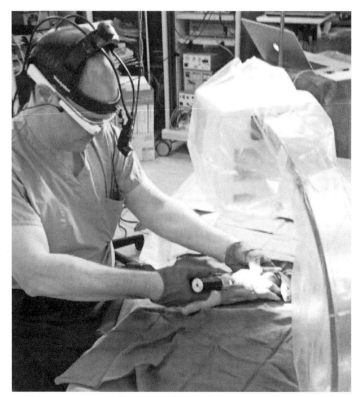

FIGURE 3.—A headlight worn in addition to the overhead lights was useful to increase the brightness of the operative field while using Google Glass. (Reprinted from Chimenti PC, Mitten DJ. Google glass as an alternative to standard fluoroscopic visualization for percutaneous fixation of hand fractures: a pilot study. *Plast Reconstr Surg*. 2015;136:328-330, with permission from the American Society of Plastic Surgeons.)

from the operative field, whereas Google Glass allows constant attention directed toward the operative field.

▶ A surgeon using fluoroscopy to percutaneously pin fractures often strains to see the monitor while visualizing the surgical field. Often the equipment used does not allow one to adequately position the screen for reasonable ergonomic use. The future may someday allow the surgeon to superimpose the fluoro-scopic image over the surgical field, a so-called augmented reality (Figs 1-3). This sort of "heads up" visualization is not yet available.

The authors used a head-mounted single-eye monitor (Google Glass) to approach the above-described augmented reality. Google Glass does not have a function to readily input video signals, so the authors improvised a system with a smart phone as an interface between the fluoroscan and the Google Glass, which required internet access.

With this system, the authors determined that their improvised image system allowed for a statistically significant improvement in percutaneous pinning of metacarpal and phalangeal fractures.

R. Papandrea, MD

Trends in incidence rate, health care consumption, and costs for patients admitted with a humeral fracture in The Netherlands between 1986 and 2012

Mahabier KC, Hartog DD, Van Veldhuizen J, et al (Univ Med Ctr Rotterdam, The Netherlands; et al)
Injury 46:1930-1937, 2015

Introduction.—This study aimed to examine long-term population-based trends in the incidence rate of patients with a humeral fracture admitted to a hospital in the Netherlands from 1986 to 2012 and to give a detailed overview of the health care consumption and productivity loss with associated costs.

Materials and Methods.—Age and gender-standardised incidence rates of hospital admissions for patients with a proximal, shaft, or distal humeral fracture were calculated for each year (1986–2012). Injury cases, length of hospital stay (LOS), trauma mechanism, and operation rate were extracted from the National Medical Registration. An incidence-based cost model was applied to calculate costs for direct health care and lost productivity in 2012.

Results.—Between 1986 and 2012 112,910 patients were admitted for a humeral fracture. The incidence rate increased from 17.8 in 1986 to 40.0 per 100,000 person years in 2012. Incidence rates of proximal fractures increased the most, especially in elderly women. Operation rates decreased in patients aged 70 years or older. The mean LOS decreased from nine days in 1997 to five days in 2012. The cumulative LOS of all patients in 2012 was 28,880 days of which 73% were caused by women and 81%

were caused by patients aged 50 years or older. Cumulative medical costs in 2012 were M55.4, of which M43.4 was spent on women. Costs increased with age. Costs for hospital care contributed most to the overall costs per case until 70 years of age. From 70 years onwards, the main cost determinants were hospital care, rehabilitation/nursing care, and home care. Cumulative costs due to lost productivity were M23.5 in 2012. Costs per case increased with age in all anatomic regions.

Conclusions.—The crude number of patients admitted for a humeral fracture increased 124% in 27 years, and was associated with age and gender. Proximal fractures in elderly women accounted most significantly for this increase and most of the costs. The main cost determinants were hospital care and productivity loss.

▶ The National Medical Registration of the Netherlands was used to identify long-term trends in the incidence rate of humeral fractures. This population-based study evaluated all patients discharged from the hospital with a primary diagnosis of a humeral fracture. In the study period from 1986 to 2012, there was a 124% increase in the number of patients admitted with a humeral fracture. The true incidence is likely higher when nonadmitted patients (emergency department only) and patients with multiple discharge diagnoses (ie, humeral fracture is not the primary discharge diagnosis) are included. The data obtained in this study are astounding. As a population, we are living longer, and the risk for osteoporosis-related fractures is increasing. Proximal humeral fractures in elderly women, in particular, have a significant economic impact. These findings underscore the importance of identifying patients at risk for fracture and counseling them on measures to promote bone health. Orthopedic surgeons should be active participants in this process.

A. T. Moeller, MD

Humeral Head Reconstruction With Osteochondral Allograft Transplantation

Saltzman BM, Riboh JC, Cole BJ, et al (Rush Univ Med Ctr, Chicago, IL)
Arthroscopy 31:1827-1834, 2015

Purpose.—To synthesize, in a systematic review, the available clinical evidence of osteochondral allograft transplants for large osteochondral defects of the humeral head.

Methods.—The Medline, Embase, and Cochrane databases were searched for studies reporting clinical or radiographic outcomes of osteochondral allograft transplantation for humeral head defects. Descriptive statistics were provided for all outcomes. After checking for data normality, we compared postoperative and preoperative values using the Student t test.

Results.—We included 12 studies (8 case reports and 4 case series) in this review. The study group consisted of 35 patients. The mean age was

35.4 ± 18.1 years; 77% of patients were male patients. Thirty-three patients had large Hill-Sachs lesions due to instability, 1 had an osteochondritis dissecans lesion, and 1 had an iatrogenic lesion after resection of synovial chondromatosis. The mean lesion size was 3 ± 1.4 cm (anteroposterior) by 2.25 ± 0.3 cm (medial-lateral), representing on average 40.5% ± 4.73% of the native articular surface. Of the 35 patients, 3 received a fresh graft, with all others receiving frozen grafts. Twenty-three femoral heads, 10 humeral heads, and 2 sets of osteochondral plugs were used. The mean length of follow-up was 57 months. Significant improvements were seen in forward flexion at 6 months (68° ± 18.1°, $P < .001$), forward flexion at 12 months (83.42° ± 18.3°, $P < .001$), and external rotation at 12 months (38.72° ± 18.8°, $P < .001$). American Shoulder and Elbow Surgeons scores improved by 14 points ($P = .02$). Radiographic studies at final follow-up showed allograft necrosis in 8.7% of cases, resorption in 36.2%, and glenohumeral arthritic changes in 35.7%. Complication rates were between 20% and 30%, and the reoperation rate was 26.67%. Although only 3 patients received fresh allografts, there were no reports of graft resorption, necrosis, or arthritic changes in these patients.

Conclusions.—Humeral head allograft—most commonly used in the setting of large Hill-Sachs lesions due to instability—has shown significant improvements in shoulder motion and American Shoulder and Elbow Surgeons scores as far as 1 year postoperatively. Return-to-work rates and satisfaction levels are high after the intervention. Complication and reoperation rates are substantial, although it is possible that use of fresh allograft tissue may result in less resorption and necrosis.

Level of Evidence.—Level V, systematic review of Level IV and V studies.

▶ The article is a systematic review of 12 studies (8 case reports and 4 small case series) with 35 patients treated for large osteochondral defects of the humeral head with osteochondral allograft transplant at a mean follow-up of 57 months. Most of the patients (33 of 35) were treated for traumatic instability, all of which had Hill-Sachs lesions, but surprisingly only 9 patients had anterior instability with the remaining patient having posterior instability. Significant outcomes included improvement in forward flexion and external rotation at 12 months postoperatively. Radiographic outcomes showed resorption in 36.2% and glenohumeral arthritic changes in 35.7% of patients. Complication rates were high, between 20% and 30% with a reoperation rate of 26.7%. The most interesting data focused on the type of allograft processing. Studies find that using fresh allograft improves cellularity and osteochondral viability compared with fresh-frozen allografts. Although only 3 patients in the 12 studies had fresh allograft implantation, there were no reports of graft resorption, necrosis, or arthritic changes.

The quality of data from a systematic review is predicated on the quality of studies from which it summarizes the data. I applaud the authors for creating a coherent manuscript with the diversity in data collection methods of the individual studies. For example, only 2 patients reported size

TABLE 2.—Grouped Summary Data of Postoperative Patient Outcomes

	No. of Patients Available for Analysis	Mean	SD	Comparison With Baseline Mean Difference ± SD	P Value
Follow-up length, mo	35	57.02	34.14	NA	NA
Return to work, %	7	100.00	0.00	NA	NA
Time to return to work, mo	7	4.29	0.76	NA	NA
FF at 6 mo, °	2	115.00	7.07	68 ± 18.1	< .001*
ER at 6 mo, °	2	37.50	10.61	19.97 ± 20.47	.20
Final postoperative FF, °	12	130.42	18.14	83.42 ± 18.3	< .001*
Final postoperative Abd, °	7	123.71	20.41	83.71 ± 23.6	< .001*
Final postoperative ER, °	12	56.25	13.71	38.72 ± 18.8	< .001*
Final postoperative IR, °	7	68.43	1.51	NA	NA
% instability at final follow-up	32	3.13	3.84	NA	NA
% with pain	28	32.11	17.62	NA	NA
% satisfied	20	90.00	8.17	NA	NA
Constant score at final follow-up	23	78.15	10.26	NA	NA
ASES score at final follow-up	5	84.84	1.03	14.72 ± 8	.02*
Intraoperative complications, %	13	38.50	0.00	NA	NA
Postoperative complications, %	9	22.22	26.35	NA	NA
Infection, %	5	0.00	0.00	NA	NA
Revision surgery, %	15	26.67	22.09	NA	NA
Allograft necrosis, %	23	8.70	8.34	NA	NA
Allograft resorption, %	30	36.23	21.71	NA	NA
Arthritic changes, %	14	35.71	23.44	NA	NA

Abd, abduction; ASES, American Shoulder and Elbow Surgeons; ER, external rotation; FF, forward flexion; IR, internal reduction; NA, not applicable.
*Statistical significance was reached ($P < .05$).

measurements of the lesion, and the number of patients available for postoperative data analysis ranged from 2 to 35 patients (Table 2). Given the inconsistent data, it is difficult to draw definitive conclusions on management of patients with large humeral defects. In fact, the authors specifically state that the results should be interpreted cautiously until higher-level research has been performed on the topic. There is still no consensus on the amount and location of humeral bone loss as well as the appropriate procedure for patients with large humeral osteochondral defects. In my practice, glenohumeral instability is common with only a small percentage of patients that cannot be treated with other stabilization procedures aimed at preventing engagement of the Hill-Sachs lesion. Stability can be achieved by increasing the surface area of the glenoid (Latarjet) or limiting external rotation (remplissage). The glenoid track concept,[1] provides a better understanding behind the rationale of why each of these procedures decreases instability episodes.

E. Gauger, MD

Reference

1. Yamamoto N. Contact between the glenoid and the humeral head in abduction, external rotation, and horizontal extension: a new concept of glenoid track. *J Shoulder Elbow Surg.* 2007;16:649-656.

Achieving the optimal epinephrine effect in wide awake hand surgery using local anesthesia without a tourniquet

Mckee DE, Lalonde DH, Thoma A, et al (McMaster Univ, Hamilton, Ontario, Canada; Saint John Regional Hosp, Saint John New Brunswick, Canada)
Hand (N Y) 10:613-615, 2015

Background.—In our experience, for all surgeries in the hand, the optimal epinephrine effect from local anesthesia—producing maximal vasoconstriction and visualization—is achieved by waiting significantly longer than the traditionally quoted 7 min from the time of injection.

Methods.—In this prospective comparative study, healthy patients undergoing unilateral carpal tunnel surgery waited either 7 min or roughly 30 min, between the time of injection of 1% lidocaine with 1:100,000 epinephrine and the time of incision. A standardized incision was made through dermis and into the subcutaneous tissue followed by exactly 60 s of measuring the quantity of blood loss using sterile micropipettes.

Results.—There was a statistically significant reduction in the mean quantity of bleeding in the group that waited roughly 30 min after injection and before incision compared to the group that waited only 7 min (95% confidence intervals of 0.06+−0.03 ml/cm of incision, compared to 0.17+−0.08 ml/cm, respectively) ($P = 0.03$).

Conclusions.—Waiting roughly 30 min after injection of local anesthesia with epinephrine as oppose to the traditionally taught 7 min, achieves an optimal epinephrine effect and vasoconstriction. In the hand, this will result in roughly a threefold reduction in bleeding—making wide awake local anesthesia without tourniquet (WALANT) possible. This knowledge has allowed our team to expand the hand procedures that we can offer using WALANT. The benefits of WALANT hand surgery include reduced cost and waste, improved patient safety, and the ability to perform active intraoperative movement examinations.

▶ The use of local anesthesia with epinephrine has been one of the single most important advances in hand surgery in recent years. Previously we were taught that epinephrine use was forbidden in the hand or other end organs ("fingers, toes, penis, nose") due to concerns about safety and digital necrosis. Don Lalonde and colleagues have dispelled this long-standing myth. Because epinephrine helps with hemostasis and provides longer acting anesthesia, tourniquet use is often not needed, and therefore use of sedation to control tourniquet pain is also frequently not needed. Use of "wide-awake local anesthesia no tourniquet" (WALANT) has many patient, surgeon and payor benefits and can reduce waste and improve surgeon productivity and patient satisfaction. One of the challenges with WALANT is performing the "block" early enough to achieve a satisfactory hemostatic effect. The authors of this article investigate the optimal time to "wait" after the block to achieve hemostasis. Waiting 30 minutes (as opposed to 7 minutes) resulted in significantly better hemostasis and less blood loss. Thus, the surgeon may optimize this effect by

considering blocking patients in the pre-procedure area well before the procedure, rather than immediately before prepping the arm.

J. E. Adams, MD

Aneurysmal Bone Cysts of the Hand, Wrist, and Forearm
Crowe MM, Houdek MT, Moran SL, et al (Mayo Clinic, Rochester, MN)
J Hand Surg Am 40:2052-2057, 2015

Purpose.—To determine the outcomes of surgical management of aneurysmal bone cysts (ABCs) in the hand, wrist, and forearm.

Methods.—The medical records of 11 patients undergoing surgical
treatment of ABCs distal to the elbow from 1994 to 2011 with at least
12 months follow-up were reviewed retrospectively. Mean follow-up
was 29 months (range, 13–56 months). There were 7 males and 4 females.
Four lesions presented in the radius, 3 in the ulna, 2 in the metacarpals,
and 2 in the phalanges.

Results.—Ten patients underwent wide unroofing and intralesional curettage with 9 undergoing associated high-speed burring. Multiple chemical
and thermal adjuvants were used. One patient underwent *en bloc* resection
with reconstruction. There was 1 recurrence in a periphyseal lesion in a 2-
year-old boy treated with curettage, burring, and adjuvant chemotherapy.
Ten patients incorporated the bone graft and healed without further surgery. One patient required revision bone grafting.

Conclusions.—The diagnosis of ABC should remain in the differential
diagnosis for cystic lesions in the upper extremity in pediatric and adult
patients. Low recurrence has been obtained predominantly with intralesional curettage and high-speed burring with and without chemical and
thermal adjuvant therapy. Appropriate healing has been obtained with
both allograft and autograft reconstructions. Periarticular and periphyseal lesions remain challenging and provide the highest chance for
incomplete resection and recurrence. Follow-up with plain radiographs
did not lead to any delay in diagnosis of recurrence in any case.

Type of Study/Level of Evidence.—Therapeutic IV.

▶ This is a retrospective review of patients treated surgically for aneurysmal
bone cyst (ABC) lesions distal to the elbow. Given that these tumors primarily
occur in the lower extremity and posterior elements of the spine, previous literature consists only of case reports and 2 small case series. The authors included
11 patients with a minimum of 1 year of follow-up and specifically reviewed
presentation, surgical methodology, and recurrence as defined by local lesion
requiring further surgery. Five patients presented with pain in the absence of
trauma, and 3 presented with pathologic fracture. Eight of 11 patients were
younger than 18 at initial presentation. Ten of 11 patients were treated with
curettage and grafting, 9 of these using high-speed burr after wide unroofing
of the lesion. Several patients also had chemical adjuvants including phenol

and full-strength hydrogen peroxide. Bone graft (allograft or autograft) was used in all patients, and cement was used in none. Overall, there was one recurrence noted 4 months after the index procedure (periphyseal lesion in the distal radius) and 1 patient who failed to incorporate the bone graft and underwent revision surgery. The 5-year disease-free survival was 92.8%. Because this is a retrospective review of only a small series of patients, the authors were unable to draw specific conclusions. However, this article suggests that intralesional treatment for ABCs is sufficient provided that the entire lesion is treated. The use of high-speed burr is important in treating microscopic disease at the periphery of the lesion. Periphyseal and periarticular lesions remain challenging, likely owing to incomplete treatment given their anatomic location. The authors also suggest that most lesions can be treated with allograft as opposed to autograft, as they had full graft incorporation in 7 of 7 patients treated in this manner. Given the relative rarity of this condition in the upper extremity, larger multicentered studies in the future would likely be the most illuminating for advancing treatment recommendations.

E. J. Gauger, MD

Recurrent Metacarpal Enchondroma Treated With Strut Allograft: 14-year Follow-up

Yalcinkaya M, Akman YE, Bagatur AE (Metin Sabanci Baltalimani Bone Diseases Training and Res Hosp, Istanbul, Turkey; Medicana International Istanbul Hosp, Turkey)
Orthopedics 38:e647-e650, 2015

Enchondroma of the hand is a common lesion with a recurrence rate of up to 13.3% after curettage and bone grafting. Pathologic fractures often occur. Although allograft bone chips are widely used in the surgical treatment of enchondroma, the use of structural allograft bone has not been reported before. This case report presents a recurrent enchondroma of the fifth metacarpal with pathologic fracture in a 13-year-old girl who had 2 previous interventions and 2 more interventions for other enchondromas in the same hand. These interventions consisted of curettage and autogenous iliac crest bone grafting. The metacarpal diaphysis was resected and reconstructed with an intercalary freeze-dried strut allograft fibular bone segment to avoid further donor graft site morbidity. At 14 years of follow-up, the patient had full range of motion of the hand, with no symptoms, and the allograft bone had been incorporated completely, with no recurrence of the tumor. With strut allograft bone, healing occurs by creeping substitution at its ends that is limited to a few millimeters. Limited vascularization also occurs on the allograft surface, leaving most of the allograft segment devoid of vascularity and leading to the complications seen in massive bone allografts. However, because of their thin cortices and decreased total volume, smaller bone allografts show higher rates of osteointegration and revascularization. In selected cases, a strut allograft bone may be considered a suitable material for long-term reconstruction of the hand after enchondroma excision, especially in young patients, who have increased healing potential compared with older patients.

▶ This article discusses an interesting treatment for a recurrent enchondroma. In this case report, Yalcinkaya et al resected the diaphysis of the fifth metacarpal and replaced the shaft with a strut allograft. This technique can be useful in the multiple recurrent, multiple operated enchondroma in which cortical integrity is an issue. In this case, the history of multiple enchondromas in different locations in the hand and multiple painful recurrences in the same location raise concern over the possible diagnosis of grade 1 chondrosarcoma, a histologic distinction that can be difficult to make. In either case, this patient was appropriately treated with a wide resection. Furthermore, there exist many different and equally effective surgical treatments for enchondromas including autograft or allograft bone draft reconstruction and simple curettage. Recurrence does, however, remain an issue, making allograft strut reconstruction attractive in situations such as this.

P. Murray, MD

Normative Values for Grip and Pinch Strength for 6- to 19-Year-Olds
McQuiddy VA, Scheerer CR, Lavalley R, et al (Cincinnati Children's Hosp Med Ctr, OH; Xavier Univ, Cincinnati, OH)
Arch Phys Med Rehabil 96:1627-1633, 2015

Objectives.—To provide current normative data for grip and pinch strength in children and young adults aged 6 to 19 years as well as to examine the effect of age, sex, and hand dominance on grip and pinch strength.
Design.—Descriptive cross-sectional.
Setting.—Two grade schools, 2 high schools, and 1 university.
Participants.—Participants (N = 1508; 741 male students and 767 female students) aged 6 to 19 years.
Interventions.—Not applicable.
Main Outcome Measures.—Means and SDs were calculated for each strength measurement (grip, tip pinch, lateral pinch, palmar pinch) and stratified by age and sex. Analysis of covariance and 2-sample t tests were used to analyze the data.
Results.—The analyses demonstrated that age and sex had a significant effect on hand strength values, as evidenced by increasing hand strength with age as well as greater hand strength in males than in females. Hand dominance was not shown to have a significant effect on hand strength. The results of this study were statistically significantly different from previously published normative values, with most hand strength values being lower than those published 28 years ago.

Conclusions.—Having updated normative data are paramount for reha-bilitation practitioners to compare the grip and pinch strength of their cli-ents with the average values to objectively assess impairment and tracking progress. The statistical significance observed for most data collected in this study as compared with those previously published supports the need for continually updating normative data.

▶ It is really difficult to make this study interesting. However, it doesn't have to be interesting to be important and useful! Normative data are used every day in clinical practice and research, and it must be current, as normal changes over time.

This article is an update of normative data collected with pristine technique measuring grip and pinch strength in children and adolescents. Interestingly, children and adolescents (in the United States) continue to show weakened pinch and grip strength over the last 30 years.

K. Bengston, MD

Forearm amputees' views of prosthesis use and sensory feedback
Wijk U, Carlsson I (Lund Univ, Malmö, Sweden)
J Hand Ther 28:269-278, 2015

Study Design.—Qualitative descriptive.
Introduction.—The lack of sensory feedback in today's hand prostheses has been in focus recently but the amputees' experiences need to be further investigated.
Purpose.—To explore forearm amputees' views of prosthesis use and sensory feedback.
Methods.—Thirteen unilateral congenital or traumatic forearm ampu-tees were interviewed. The transcribed text was subjected to content analysis.
Results.—Prostheses both facilitate and limit occupational perform-ance. Appearance is important for identity and blending into society. The feeling of agency regarding the prostheses is present but not that of body ownership. Future expectations concerned improved mobility, cos-metics, and sensory feedback.
Conclusions.—This study allows a deeper understanding of the complex relationship between a prosthetic device and the wearer. Today's pros-theses allow the wearer to feel agency concerning the artificial limb but the lack of sensory feedback seems to be an important factor still blocking the achievement of body ownership of the prosthesis.
Level of Evidence.—Not applicable.

▶ It is enjoyable to read a qualitative study to understand the patient's percep-tion of wearing a prosthesis. As a therapist, it is important to read qualitative studies to enhance knowledge and improve therapy sessions. The authors studied 7 participants with traumatic transradial amputations and 6 participants with congenital deficiency. Although sample size may appear small, no new participants were required as redundancy in answers was reached. All participants wore an esthetic or myoelectric prosthesis daily. All questions were open ended to decrease any bias.

The authors discovered that the subjects with a traumatic amputation found the prosthesis more beneficial for daily activities at work, home, and leisure. The congenital deficiency participants gave candid responses on limiting factors of wearing the prosthesis such as pinching a baby while changing a diaper. The subject who wore the myoelectric prosthesis described the frustrations of wearing the prosthesis in the cold and difficulties with the prosthesis working properly because of the cold weather. These answers offer treating clinicians an insight into client-centered values that may be relevant to future clients.

I found it fascinating that the one individual with high phantom pain had a significant decrease in his phantom pain when he tried a sensory feedback system. More research is required to understand how the phantom hand map can interact with an enabled prosthesis with sensory feedback.

Reading the future wishes of the participants to have improved cosmesis and sensory feedback for grip force, touch, and proprioception, gave me insight to help clients perform daily activities to the patient's satisfaction level. The future appears hopeful for people who wear prostheses. While reading this article, Luke Skywalker from Star Wars comes to mind. I remember the scene in The Empire Strikes Back when Luke gets his prosthesis. His new prosthetic finger is pricked, and he feels it. I hope this will soon become a reality for patients with prostheses to have a similar experience.

S. Kannas, CHT

Achieving the optimal epinephrine effect in wide awake hand surgery using local anesthesia without a tourniquet
Mckee DE, Lalonde DH, Thoma A, et al (McMaster Univ, Hamilton, Ontario, Canada; Saint John Regional Hosp, Saint John New Brunswick, Canada)
Hand (N Y) 10:613-615, 2015

Background.—In our experience, for all surgeries in the hand, the optimal epinephrine effect from local anesthesia—producing maximal vasoconstriction and visualization—is achieved by waiting significantly longer than the traditionally quoted 7 min from the time of injection.

Methods.—In this prospective comparative study, healthy patients undergoing unilateral carpal tunnel surgery waited either 7 min or roughly 30 min, between the time of injection of 1% lidocaine with 1:100,000 epinephrine and the time of incision. A standardized incision was made through dermis and into the subcutaneous tissue followed by exactly 60 s of measuring the quantity of blood loss using sterile micropipettes.

Results.—There was a statistically significant reduction in the mean quantity of bleeding in the group that waited roughly 30 min after injection and before incision compared to the group that waited only 7 min (95% confidence intervals of 0.06+−0.03 ml/cm of incision, compared to 0.17+−0.08 ml/ cm, respectively) ($P = 0.03$).

Conclusions.—Waiting roughly 30 min after injection of local anesthesia with epinephrine as oppose to the traditionally taught 7 min, achieves an optimal epinephrine effect and vasoconstriction. In the hand, this will result in roughly a threefold reduction in bleeding—making wide awake local anesthesia without tourniquet (WALANT) possible. This knowledge has allowed our team to expand the hand procedures that we can offer using WALANT. The benefits of WALANT hand surgery include reduced cost and waste, improved patient safety, and the ability to perform active intraoperative movement examinations.

▶ The authors contributed significantly to the use of local anesthesia with adrenaline in hand surgery over the last few years. The use of adrenaline reduces the need for a tourniquet in most surgeries and is well tolerated by patients. This technique is now widely accepted and has many advantages over general anesthesia. This article shows that waiting for 30 minutes seems to improve the vasoconstrictive effect. In my practice I often wait for up to 60 minutes and also obtain excellent results with a relatively bloodless field. However, additional logistical factors need to be in place using this technique. These factors include the acknowledgment and compliance with the World Health Organization preoperative checklist if the injection is performed prior to the operating room and allowing the operating room to be close to the preoperative waiting area to allow easy access for the surgeon to move between the 2 areas as the operating list proceeds.

M. Hayton, BSc(Hons) MBChB FRCS(orth) FFSEM(uk)

The Impact of Uninterrupted Warfarin on Hand and Wrist Surgery
Bogunovic L, Gelberman RH, Goldfarb CA, et al (Washington Univ School of Medicine, St. Louis, MO)
J Hand Surg Am 40:2133-2140, 2015

Purpose.—To determine the impact of uninterrupted use of warfarin on hand and wrist surgery.

Methods.—This single-center, prospective cohort trial enrolled adult patients undergoing hand and wrist surgery. Between May 2009 and August 2014, 47 surgical patients receiving uninterrupted warfarin (50 procedures) were enrolled and matched as a group by age and procedure type to 48 surgical patients (50 procedures) who were not prescribed warfarin. Complications, defined as bleeding, infection, or wound dehiscence requiring reoperation, were recorded for each group. Surgical outcome measures were composed of objective findings affected by surgical site bleeding (ie, ecchymosis extent, hematoma presence, 2-point discrimination) and standardized patient-rated assessments (*Quick*—Disabilities of the Arm, Shoulder, and Hand, and visual analog scales: pain and swelling). We collected data preoperatively and at 2 and 4 weeks postoperatively. Statistical analyses contrasted complications and outcomes data between patient groups.

Results.—One procedure (2%; 95% confidence interval, 0% to 11%) in a patient taking warfarin was complicated by hematoma requiring reoperation resulting from an elevated postoperative international normalized ratio of 5.4. There were no complications among controls (0%; 95% confidence interval, 0% to 7%). At 2 weeks postoperatively, patients receiving warfarin more frequently had hematomas (28% vs 10%) and demonstrated a greater extent of ecchymosis from the surgical incision (50 vs 19 mm). At 4 weeks, no differences existed in hematoma presence or extent of ecchymosis between groups. The incidence of transiently elevated 2-point discrimination was not different between groups (10% warfarin; 6% controls). Visual analog scores for pain and swelling were not significantly different between groups at any time. Differences in *Quick*—Disabilities of the Arm, Shoulder, and Hand scores between groups did not exceed a minimal clinically important difference.

Conclusions.—Uninterrupted use of warfarin in patients undergoing surgery of the hand and wrist was associated with an infrequent risk of bleeding complication requiring reoperation. Increased rates of hematoma and ecchymosis in patients taking warfarin normalized by 4 weeks postoperatively.

Type of Study/Level of Evidence.—Therapeutic II.

▶ The authors evaluated the impact of uninterrupted use of warfarin in 47 surgical patients undergoing 50 outpatient hand surgery procedures. Patients were matched by age and procedure type to 50 surgical procedures on patients who were not on warfarin. Only one complication required reoperation. A hematoma and acute carpal tunnel syndrome developed 4 days after a proximal row carpectomy. Of note, at the time of presentation with the hematoma, the international normalized ratio was 5.4. Overall, there was a high incidence of hematoma and ecchymosis in the warfarin group. However, this normalized by 4 weeks. There were no clinically relevant differences in patient outcomes with respect to pain, swelling, or disability as determined by Quick Disabilities of the Arm, Shoulder, and Hand scores.

Overall, this was an important study. As the risk of bleeding complications is low with minor elective hand procedures, allowing patients to continue on anticoagulation in the perioperative period reduces the risk of the patient having a stroke or other thromboembolic event in higher-risk patients. The authors discuss the limitations of the study in the Discussion section. Although the 2 groups were matched based on age and procedure, this was not a randomized, controlled trial. In addition, there were variations in management of tourniquet deflation between surgeons. Lastly, 76% of the procedures in the warfarin group were small soft tissue procedures. Of the bony procedures, 5 of 12 were small procedures involving the digits.

I currently allow patients to continue on warfarin or Plavix for minor soft tissue procedures in the hand including carpal tunnel, trigger finger, and DeQuervain's releases. Procedures are performed with a field block using 1% lidocaine with epinephrine without use of a tourniquet. This method allows for careful hemostasis throughout the procedure, with minimal risk of a hematoma. Although there was only 1 procedure requiring reoperation for a hematoma, I would recommend tourniquet deflation and careful hemostasis in all fracture cases and major bony reconstructions. I currently still recommend cessation of warfarin 5 days before any major bony procedure, with use of bridging therapy with Lovenox in the preoperative period.

J. I. Huang, MD

Hand Sensibility, Strength, and Laxity of High-Level Musicians Compared to Nonmusicians
Sims SEG, Engel L, Hammert WC, et al (Univ of Rochester, NY; Northwestern Univ, Chicago, IL; et al)
J Hand Surg Am 40:1996-2002, 2015

Purpose.—To determine whether musicians have more sensitive, stronger, and flexible hands than nonmusicians.

Methods.—A total of 100 musicians and 100 control subjects were assessed for 2-point discrimination, Semmes-Weinstein monofilament light touch, grip and pinch strength, and laxity. Musicians were included if enrolled as instrumental performance majors at a 4-year accredited conservatory of music. Nonmusician controls were university students who never or rarely engaged in playing an instrument. All subjects were between the ages of 18 and 28. The exclusion criterion was history of any hand condition, trauma, surgery, or diabetes. Statistical analyses were carried out using the *t* test, analysis of variance, and correlation coefficients as appropriate.

Results.—High-level musicians in our cohort showed the same handedness (dominance) as the general population. The musicians were weaker than the nonmusicians. Male musicians were significantly weaker in pinch and grip bilaterally than nonmusicians, whereas female musicians were significantly weaker only in grip on the right/dominant side. Two-point discrimination was significantly less in nonmusicians for the left/nondominant index, ring, and small fingers, and the right/dominant small and dominant index finger. Semmes-Weinstein testing was significantly better for the right/dominant digits, including the thumb, but not the left digits with the exception of the ring and nondominant middle and ring. There was no difference in laxity between the 2 groups.

Conclusions.—High-level musicians have, in general, more sensitive but weaker hands than nonmusicians, but the differences seem small and may not be clinically important.

Type of Study/Level of Evidence.—Diagnostic III.

▶ This study reports a surprising finding: elite, high-level performing musicians are actually weaker in overall strength as assessed by our current standard testing methodologies. On the other hand, the authors found that general sensory discrimination is better in musicians than nonmusicians, not really a surprising finding. Conjecture could lead us to conclude that musicians do not need to be strong and may lead more sedentary lives, at least with the use of the upper extremity. Alternatively, because endurance and fine coordinated movement is different from strength, we might conclude that we currently lack sensitive instruments to discern highly coordinated movement. The elite performance of playing a musical instrument may correspond similarly to the craft of cabinetmaking or hand surgery, with assessments for strength and sensibility to attain expertise currently lacking but worthy of future ventures in understanding human coordinated movement.

A. Ladd, MD

Complications Within 30 Days of Hand Surgery: An Analysis of 10,646 Patients
Lipira AB, Sood RF, Tatman PD, et al (Univ of Washington, Seattle)
J Hand Surg Am 40:1852-1859, 2015

Purpose.—The American College of Surgeons Surgical Quality Improvement Program database collects detailed and validated data on demographics, comorbidities, and 30-day postoperative outcomes of patients undergoing operations in most subspecialties. This dataset has been previously used to quantify complications and identify risk factors in other surgical subspecialties. We sought to determine the incidence of postoperative complications following hand surgery and to identify factors associated with increased risk of complications in order to focus preventive strategies.

Methods.—National Surgical Quality Improvement Program data from 2006 to 2011 were queried using 302 hand-specific Current Procedural Technology codes. Descriptive statistics were calculated for the population, and potential risk factors and patient characteristics were analyzed for their association with complications in the 30-day postoperative period using both univariate and multivariate analyses.

Results.—There were 208 hand-specific Current Procedural Technology codes represented in the data, and of these, 84 were associated with at least 1 complication. The overall incidence of complications within 30 days of hand surgery was 2.5% (95% confidence interval, 2.2%–2.8%). In univariate analysis, older age, diabetes, chronic obstructive pulmonary disease, congestive heart failure, atherosclerosis, steroids, bleeding disorder, increasing American Society of Anesthesiologists class, increasing wound class, emergency procedure, longer operative time, and preoperative transfusion were associated with significantly higher risk of complications, and local anesthesia and outpatient surgery were associated with lower risk. In the multivariate model, male sex, increasing American Society of Anesthesiologists class, wound class 4, and preoperative transfusion were associated with significantly higher risk, and outpatient surgery was associated with significantly lower risk. The most common complication was surgical-site infection (1.2%).

Conclusions.—The incidence of complications was low, with overall health status being more important than specific comorbidities in predicting complication risk. This information may be valuable in counseling patients before surgery and in identifying patients at higher risk for complications following hand surgery.

Type of Study/Level of Evidence.—Therapeutic III.

▶ In this study, the authors analyzed data over a 5-period in an attempt to determine the incidence of postoperative complications within 30 days after hand surgery and also to identify those factors associated with the increased risk of complications.

A strength of this study is the use of a large, validated database, one that has been used frequently to study 30-day postoperative complications after other procedures. One weakness of this study (which the authors also stated) is that complications that may be specific to a procedure could not be analyzed given the limited number of patients for each procedure. Another weakness is that this study looks only at complications within 30 days after a hand surgery; long-term complications such as malunion, nonunion, stiffness, and chronic pain were not included.

The authors conclude that the post-30-day complication rate after hand surgery is low (2.5%), and the most common complication was surgical-site infection (1.2%). These numbers are probably consistent with most hand surgeons' practices in the United States, including my own. They also conclude that "overall health status [is] more important than specific comorbidities in predicting complication risk." Therefore, it makes sense that they found that lower risk was associated with local anesthesia and outpatient surgery. In my practice, I try to do as many procedures under local anesthesia as possible in the outpatient ambulatory surgery setting, which obviously decreases the risk of short-term complications, as supported by this study.

S. S. Shin, MD, MMSc

Physician Empathy as a Driver of Hand Surgery Patient Satisfaction
Menendez ME, Chen NC, Mudgal CS, et al (Harvard Med School, Boston, MA)
J Hand Surg Am 40:1860-1865, 2015

Purpose.—To examine the relationship between patient-rated physician empathy and patient satisfaction after a single new hand surgery office visit.

Methods.—Directly after the office visit, 112 consecutive new patients rated their overall satisfaction with the provider and completed the Consultation and Relational Empathy Measure, the Newest Vital Sign health literacy test, a sociodemographic survey, and 3 Patient-Reported Outcomes Measurement Information System-based questionnaires: Pain Interference, Upper-Extremity Function, and Depression. We also measured the waiting time in the office to see the physician, the duration of the visit, and the time from booking until appointment. Multivariable logistic and linear regression models were used to identify factors independently associated with patient satisfaction.

Results.—Patient-rated physician empathy correlated strongly with the degree of overall satisfaction with the provider. After controlling for confounding effects, greater empathy was independently associated with patient satisfaction, and it alone accounted for 65% of the variation in satisfaction scores. Older patient age was also associated with satisfaction. There were no differences between satisfied and dissatisfied patients with regard to waiting time in the office, duration of the appointment, time from booking until appointment, and health literacy.

Conclusions.—Physician empathy was the strongest driver of patient satisfaction in the hand surgery office setting. As patient satisfaction plays a growing role in reimbursement, targeted educational programs to enhance empathic communication skills in hand surgeons merit consideration.

Type of Study/Level of Evidence.—Prognostic II.

▶ The authors sought to determine which measures correlate with patient satisfaction, completing a prospective study evaluating multiple factors. Older age was directly correlated with patient satisfaction and empathy, as tested by Consultation and Relational Empathy (CARE) Measure, accounting for 65% of the variation in satisfaction scores.

Health care reimbursement appears to be in the process of transitioning from fee for service to a value/outcomes based payment system and patient satisfaction is at the forefront of this movement. This can be challenging and frustrating for physicians. Patient satisfaction does not always equate with good medicine, as a patient may not be satisfied with the physician who does not provide opioid medications for chronic conditions or refuses to order a MRI scan when not medically indicated despite a patient's wishes. This study demonstrates that being empathetic may improve patient satisfaction notwithstanding other variables. This study did include patients with established relationships with the physicians, and one would expect higher levels of satisfaction for established patients because those unsatisfied could seek appointments elsewhere. The average wait times in the office as well as between appointment scheduling and time to being seen were not long, and variability here may change satisfaction rating even for those physicians who were more empathetic.

Even with some limitations, this article appears to give hand surgeons another tool to improving satisfaction as we move into the new performance metrics.

W. C. Hammert, MD

Google Glass as an Alternative to Standard Fluoroscopic Visualization for Percutaneous Fixation of Hand Fractures: A Pilot Study
Chimenti PC, Mitten DJ (Univ of Rochester, NY)
Plast Reconstr Surg 136:328-330, 2015

This pilot study investigated the feasibility of Google Glass to assist visualization of fluoroscopic images during percutaneous pinning of hand fractures. Cadavers were used to compare total time to pin each fracture and total number of radiographs per fracture from a mini C-arm. A FluoroScan monitor was used for radiographic visualization compared to projecting the images in the Google Glass display. All outcome measures significantly improved for proximal phalanx fractures (127 versus 86 seconds, $p = 0.017$; 5.3 versus 2.2 images, $p = 0.003$), and fewer images were obtained during fixation of metacarpal fractures using Google Glass compared with traditional techniques (6.4 versus 3.6, $p < 0.001$). Typical FluoroScan monitor placement may require the surgeon to alter focus away from the operative field, whereas Google Glass allows constant attention directed toward the operative field.

▶ Technology appears to be advancing at an ever-increasing rate. Hand surgery should be able to benefit from such developments, and this article gives interesting insight into the use of the innovative Google Glass to visualize fluoroscopic images while operating. I have no personal experience using the Google Glass but can see obvious advantages it would offer, provided the glasses are comfortable, user-friendly, and financially viable.

M. Hayton

Outcomes of Open Dorsal Wrist Ganglion Excision in Active-Duty Military Personnel

Balazs GC, Donohue MA, Drake ML, et al (Walter Reed Natl Military Med Ctr, Bethesda, MD; et al)
J Hand Surg Am 40:1739-1747, 2015

Purpose.—To examine the most common presenting complaints of active-duty service members with isolated dorsal wrist ganglions and to determine the rate of return to unrestricted duty after open excision.

Methods.—Surgical records at 2 military facilities were screened to identify male and female active duty service members undergoing isolated open excision of dorsal wrist ganglions from January 1, 2006 to January 1, 2014. Electronic medical records and service disability databases were searched to identify the most common presenting symptoms and to determine whether patients returned to unrestricted active duty after surgery. Postoperative outcomes examined were pain persisting greater than 4 weeks after surgery, stiffness requiring formal occupational therapy treatment, surgical wound complications, and recurrence.

Results.—A total of 125 active duty military personnel (Army, 54; Navy, 43; and Marine Corps, 28) met criteria for inclusion. Mean follow-up was 45 months. Fifteen percent (8 of 54) of the Army personnel were given permanent waivers from performing push-ups owing to persistent pain and stiffness. Pain persisting greater than 4 weeks after surgery was an independent predictor of eventual need for a permanent push-up waiver. The overall recurrence incidence was 9%. No demographic or perioperative factors were associated with recurrence.

Conclusions.—Patients whose occupation or activities require forceful wrist extension should be counseled on the considerable risk of residual pain and functional limitations that may occur after open dorsal wrist ganglion excision.

Type of Study/Level of Evidence.—Therapeutic IV.

▶ This article is significant in that it evaluates the effect of dorsal wrist ganglion excision on activities requiring forceful wrist extension (eg, push-ups). The authors studied a specific patient population, in this case active-duty military personnel, and found that pain present more than 4 weeks after surgery predicted the need for a "push-up waiver" in 15% of Army personnel.

Strengths of this study include the specific population of patients used and the methodical selection of the study cohort. Weaknesses of this study are its retrospective nature and the lack of use of validated functional outcome or pain scoring systems, as indicated by the authors. It would have been interesting to correlate the level of pain and function with the eventual need of a permanent waiver (in Army patients).

I commend the authors' attempt to evaluate a common concern regarding the patient's postoperative ability to bear weight on an extended wrist following dorsal ganglion excision. This is particularly concerning given society's growing fascination with yoga, where the basic plank position requires this stress on the wrist. In my practice, this is one of the most common questions from my patients, and more time is spent discussing this than the procedure itself. I believe a prospective study, with validated functional outcome and pain scores, would be worth performing and have excellent clinical relevance.

S. S. Shin, MD, MMSc

The Association of the H-Index and Academic Rank Among Full-Time Academic Hand Surgeons Affiliated With Fellowship Programs
Lopez J, Susarla SM, Swanson EW, et al (Johns Hopkins Hosp, Baltimore, MD)
J Hand Surg Am 40:1434-1441, 2015

Purpose.—To evaluate the association between the Hirsch index (a measure of publications and citations) and academic rank among hand surgeons.

Methods.—This was a cross-sectional study of full-time academic hand surgeons within Accreditation Council for Graduate Medical Education—approved hand surgery fellowship programs in the United States and Canada. The study variables were classified as bibliometric (h-index, I-10 index, total number of publications, total number of citations, maximum number of citations for a single work) and demographics (gender, training factors). The outcome was academic rank (instructor, assistant professor, associate professor, professor, endowed professor). Descriptive, bivariate, and multiple regression statistics were computed.

Results.—The sample was composed of 366 full-time academic hand surgeons; 86% were male and 98% had formal hand surgery fellowship training. The mean time since completion of surgical training was 17 ± 11 years. The distribution of primary faculty appointments was orthopedic surgery (70%) and plastic surgery (30%). Two hundred fifty surgeons (68%) were members of the American Society for Surgery of the Hand. The mean h-index was 10.2 ± 9.9 and was strongly correlated with academic rank. Gender was not associated with academic rank. Distribution of academic ranks was as follows: instructor (4%), assistant professor (28%), associate professor (40%), professor (22%), and endowed professor (5%). The h-index, years since completion of training, and American Society for Surgery of the Hand membership were associated with academic rank. The h-index had a high sensitivity and specificity for predicting academic rank.

Conclusions.—The h-index is a reliable tool for quantitatively assessing research productivity and should be considered for use in academic hand surgery.

Clinical Relevance.—When evaluating candidates for academic promotion in hand surgery, the h-index is a potentially valuable tool for assessing research productivity and impact.

▶ The authors performed a cross-sectional study of full-time academic hand surgeons within Accreditation Council for Graduate Medical Education—approved hand fellowships and analyzed the association between H-index, I-10 index, total number of publications, number of citations, and academic rank. One of the shortcomings of research productivity based on number of publications is the lack of objective assessment of quality and impact of the published research. Overall, 4% of the surgeons were instructors, 28% assistant professors, 40% associate professors, and 22% full professors. The results suggest that the H-index had the strongest correlation with academic rank. Gender was not associated with academic rank.

Many academic institutions currently offer different pathways for their clinical faculty including clinical only, clinician-educator, and clinician-scientist. Others only offer a standard academic track with promotion based on research productivity, clinical excellence, teaching, administrative responsibilities, and community service. However, research productivity is still often the most important criteria in the academic promotion process. The H-index is a useful tool to use as an objective measure of the faculty member's research productivity and impact, in addition to the number of publications.

J. I. Huang, MD

Patient education for carpal tunnel syndrome: analysis of readability
Eberlin KR, Vargas CR, Chuang DJ, et al (Harvard Med School, Boston, MA)
Hand (N Y) 10:374-380, 2015

Background.—The National Institutes of Health and American Medical Association recommend a sixth grade reading level for patient-directed content. This study aims to quantitatively evaluate the readability of the most commonly used resources for surgical treatment of carpal tunnel syndrome.

Methods.—A web search for "carpal tunnel surgery" was performed using an Internet search engine, and the 13 most popular sites were identified. Relevant, patient-directed articles immediately accessible from the main site were downloaded and formatted into plain text. A total of 102 articles were assessed for readability using ten established analyses: first overall, then by website for comparison.

Results.—Patient information about carpal tunnel surgery had an overall average reading level of 13.1. Secondary analysis by website revealed a range of mean readability from 10.8 (high school sophomore level) to 15.3 (university junior level). All sites exceeded the recommended sixth grade reading level.

Conclusions.—Online patient resources for carpal tunnel surgery uniformly exceed the recommended reading level. These are too difficult to be understood by a large portion of American adults. A better understanding of readability may be useful in tailoring more appropriate resources for average patient literacy.

▶ The authors provide an interesting evaluation of the resources available for patient education regarding carpal tunnel syndrome. The National Institutes of Health (NIH) and the American Medical Association (AMA) recommend that educational materials for patients are provided with a 6th-grade reading level. The authors evaluated the 13 most popular patient-directed sites when searching for information about carpal tunnel surgery. They then evaluated the readability of articles found on these sites with 10 well-established tests. The average reading level from these websites was 13.1, and the Flesch Reading Ease average score was 42 (0-100, with 100 being easiest to read and 60-70 considered "Plain English"). At this point in my practice, I typically direct patients to websites created by the associations that represent my medical specialties. This article specifically evaluated the websites of both the American Academy of Orthopaedic Surgery and the American Society for Surgery of the Hand. Each of these sites did not achieve the goals set forth by the NIH and the AMA. It should be a focus of ours to educate our patients in a manner that they can understand, with little jargon and technical terminology. Our patients turn to us to explain their conditions in an easy-to-understand fashion, so that they can make educated decisions regarding their care. In my practice, I try to give easy-to-understand "everyday" examples to my patients so that they are able to draw parallels between their conditions and situations they understand.

M. W. Kessler, MD, MPH

To What Degree Do Pain-coping Strategies Affect Joint Stiffness and Functional Outcomes in Patients with Hand Fractures?
Roh YH, Noh JH, Oh JH, et al (Gachon Univ School of Medicine, Incheon, Korea; Kangwon Natl Univ Hosp, Chuncheon-si, Gangwon-do, Korea; Seoul Natl Univ College of Medicine, Korea)
Clin Orthop Relat Res 473:3484-3490, 2015

Background.—Patients with hand fractures often have pain, swelling, and stiffness in the joints of the hand, which may lead them to protect their hands, resulting in more stiffness and in delayed recovery. However, the effects of pain-coping strategies and catastrophization (the tendency to expect the worst to occur when pain is present, an approach that can be thought of as the opposite of "coping") on functional recovery after hand fractures have not been investigated in depth.

Questions/Purposes.—Are preoperative catastrophization and anxiety in patients with hand fractures associated with (1) decreased grip strength; (2) decreased range of motion; and (3) increased disability at 3 and

6 months after surgical treatment for a hand fracture? Secondarily, we asked if there are other patient and injury factors that are associated with these outcomes at 3 and 6 months.

Methods.—A total of 93 patients with surgically treated hand fractures were enrolled in this prospective study. Preoperative assessments measured coping strategies evaluated by measuring catastrophic thinking with the Pain Catastrophizing Scale and pain anxiety with the Pain Anxiety Symptom Scale. At 3 and 6 months postoperatively, grip strength, total active range of motion, and disability (Quick Disabilities of the Arm, Shoulder, and Hand score) were assessed. Bivariate and multivariate analyses were performed to identify patient demographic, injury, and coping skills factors that accounted for outcomes of strength, motion, and disability.

Results.—Decreased grip strength was associated with catastrophic thinking (beta $= -1.29$ [95% confidence interval, -1.67 to -0.89], partial $R^2 = 11\%$, $p < 0.001$) and anxiety (beta $= -0.83$ [-1.16 to -0.50], partial $R^2 = 7\%$, $p = 0.007$) at 3 months, but by 6 months, only anxiety (beta $= -0.74$ [-1.04 to -0.44], partial $R^2 = 7\%$, $p = 0.010$) remained an important factor. Decreased total active range of motion was associated with pain catastrophizing (beta $= -0.63$ [-0.90 to -0.36], partial $R^2 = 6\%$, $p = 0.024$) and anxiety (beta $= -0.28$ [-0.42 to -0.14], partial $R^2 = 3\%$, $p = 0.035$) at 3 months but not at 6 months. Similarly, increased disability was associated with pain catastrophizing (beta $= 1.09$ [$1.39-0.79$], partial $R^2 = 12\%$, $p < 0.001$) and anxiety (beta $= 0.93$ [$1.21-0.65$], partial $R^2 = 11\%$, $p = 0.001$) at 3 months; these factors failed to be associated for 6-month outcomes.

Conclusions.—Preoperative poor coping skills as measured by high catastrophization and anxiety were associated with a weaker grip strength, decreased range of motion, and increased disability after surgical treatment for a hand fracture at 3 months. However, poor coping skills did not show persistent effects beyond 6 months. More research may be needed to show interventions to improve coping skills will enhance treatment outcome in patients after acute hand fractures.

Level of Evidence.—Level III, prognostic study.

▶ This is a study investigating the relationship between psychological factors such as the ability to cope with pain and postinjury outcomes in the realm of joint stiffness in the setting of hand fractures. By way of review, patients with hand fractures often have pain and swelling. However, the relationship between pain-coping strategies and outcome is not completely clear. In this study, more than 90 patients with surgically treated hand fractures were enrolled in a prospective examination. Preoperative assessments of the coping strategies were evaluated by measuring catastrophic thinking, anxiety, and pain catastrophization on standard scales. Objective and subjective outcomes were then measured at 3 and 6 months postoperatively in these patients.

The results revealed that decreased grip strength was associated with catastrophic thinking at 3 months but, by 6 months, only anxiety remained an important factor correlating with the objective and subjective measures.

Preoperative poor coping skills, as measured by high catastrophization and anxiety were, in the end, associated with weaker grip strength and decreased range of motion and increased disability after surgical treatment for hand fractures at 3 months. However, poor coping skills did not show persistent effects beyond 6 months.

In the end, most of the effect is temporary. This study seems to suggest that pain catastrophization and anxiety are more important early on after injury but not by 6 months after the injury. However, the study does not have any follow-up data on functional outcomes beyond 6 months after the surgery. The authors note that they purposely chose 6 months as the final follow-up to prevent the loss of patients during follow-up; however, this may be fortuitous because perhaps the effects of poor coping skills contribute other factors that may ramp up after that time period. They also acknowledge that they only use QuickDASH as a functional outcomes measure. These results are consistent with findings of another study, which noted that psychological makeup is important in the healthy state but less important than anxiety and negative thoughts in response to pain in the context of recovery in patients with hand fractures. The authors, in this way, are narrowing the possible sources of relationship between outcome as measured objectively or through questionnaires with psychological factors that specifically relate to pain and the ability to cope with it.

This article adds generally to a growing body of literature that relates outcomes to things other than what hand surgeons routinely strive to optimize in treatment. Here, we have a relationship between the specific psychological factors associated with the ability to cope with pain and objective outcomes including joint stiffness and functional outcomes measures. Although this study has some suboptimal features and perhaps some methodological concerns, it does add to this robust area of research. It is necessary to investigate further the relationships between psychological factors and outcomes if we are to account for the patients who do not have the best results.

J. Elfar, MD

Article Index

Chapter 1: Hand and Wrist Arthritis

Relationship between Patient Expectations and Clinical Measures in Patients Undergoing Rheumatoid Hand Surgery from the Silicone Arthroplasty in Rheumatoid Arthritis (SARA) Study ... 1

Early Osteoarthritis of the Trapeziometacarpal Joint Is Not Associated With Joint Instability During Typical Isometric Loading ... 3

Three-Corner Arthrodesis With Scaphoid and Triquetrum Excision for Wrist Arthritis ... 5

Ulnar Head Replacement: 21 Cases; Mean Follow-Up, 7.5 Years ... 7

First dorsal interosseous muscle contraction results in radiographic reduction of healthy thumb carpometacarpal joint ... 8

Joint Arthroplasty With Osteochondral Grafting From the Knee for Posttraumatic or Degenerative Hand Joint Disorders ... 9

Evaluation of Radiographic Instability of the Trapeziometacarpal Joint in Women With Carpal Tunnel Syndrome ... 11

Early Osteoarthritis of the Trapeziometacarpal Joint Is Not Associated With Joint Instability During Typical Isometric Loading ... 13

Trapeziometacarpal Arthritis: A Prospective Clinical Evaluation of the Thumb Adduction and Extension Provocative Tests ... 14

Four-Corner Arthrodesis Versus Proximal Row Carpectomy: A Retrospective Study With a Mean Follow-Up of 17 Years ... 17

Relationship between Patient Expectations and Clinical Measures in Patients Undergoing Rheumatoid Hand Surgery from the Silicone Arthroplasty in Rheumatoid Arthritis (SARA) Study ... 18

First dorsal interosseous muscle contraction results in radiographic reduction of healthy thumb carpometacarpal joint ... 21

Treatment of Digital Mucous Cysts With Intralesional Sodium Tetradecyl Sulfate Injection ... 22

Evaluation of Radiographic Instability of the Trapeziometacarpal Joint in Women With Carpal Tunnel Syndrome ... 23

What Middle Phalanx Base Fracture Characteristics are Most Reliable and Useful for Surgical Decision-making? ... 24

The Effect of a Bone Tunnel During Ligament Reconstruction for Trapeziometacarpal Osteoarthritis: A 5-Year Follow-up ... 26

Revision Proximal Interphalangeal Arthroplasty: An Outcome Analysis of 75 Consecutive Cases ... 27

Trapeziectomy With a Tendon Tie-in Implant for Osteoarthritis of the Trapeziometacarpal Joint ... 29

Distal Radioulnar Joint Reaction Force Following Ulnar Shortening: Diaphyseal Osteotomy Versus Wafer Resection ... 31

Chapter 2: Wrist Arthroscopy

Arthroscopic Skills Acquisition Tools: An Online Simulator for Arthroscopy Training   33

Chapter 3: Carpus

Force in the Scapholunate Interosseous Ligament During Active Wrist Motion   35

Accuracy of enhanced and unenhanced MRI in diagnosing scaphoid proximal pole avascular necrosis and predicting surgical outcome   36

Surgical Treatments for Scapholunate Advanced Collapse Wrist: Kinematics and Functional Performance   37

Wafer Resection of the Distal Ulna   40

Multiplanar wrist joint proprioception: The effect of anesthetic blockade of the posterior interosseous nerve or skin envelope surrounding the joint   41

Cost-Effectiveness of Diagnostic Strategies for Suspected Scaphoid Fractures   42

Midterm Outcome of Bone-Ligament-Bone Graft and Dorsal Capsulodesis for Chronic Scapholunate Instability   43

Dart-Splint: An innovative orthosis that can be integrated into a scapho-lunate and palmar midcarpal instability re-education protocol   46

The Missed Scaphoid Fracture—Outcomes of Delayed Cast Treatment   47

Results of Perilunate Dislocations and Perilunate Fracture Dislocations With a Minimum 15-Year Follow-Up   50

Delayed Avascular Necrosis and Fragmentation of the Lunate Following Perilunate Dislocation   51

The Effect of Midcarpal Versus Total Wrist Fusion on the Hand's Load Distribution During Gripping   52

Hybrid Russe Procedure for Scaphoid Waist Fracture Nonunion With Deformity   55

Results of Perilunate Dislocations and Perilunate Fracture Dislocations With a Minimum 15-Year Follow-Up   56

The Palpable Scaphoid Surface Area in Various Wrist Positions   58

Treatment of Scaphoid Nonunion: A Systematic Review of the Existing Evidence   59

Fixation and Grafting After Limited Debridement of Scaphoid Nonunions   61

Force in the Scapholunate Interosseous Ligament During Active Wrist Motion   62

A comparative study on autologous bone grafting combined with or without posterior interosseous nerve neurectomy for scaphoid nonunion treatment   64

The Missed Scaphoid Fracture –Outcomes of Delayed Cast Treatment   65

Chapter 4: Dupuytren's Contracture

Collagenase Clostridium Histolyticum versus Limited Fasciectomy for Dupuytren's Contracture: Outcomes from a Multicenter Propensity Score Matched Study   67

Factors affecting functional recovery after surgery and hand therapy in patients with Dupuytren's disease   68

Collagenase Clostridium Histolyticum versus Limited Fasciectomy for Dupuytren's Contracture: Outcomes from a Multicenter Propensity Score Matched Study   70

The Efficacy and Safety of Concurrent Collagenase Clostridium Histolyticum Injections for 2 Dupuytren Contractures in the Same Hand: A Prospective, Multicenter Study   71

Dupuytren Contracture Recurrence Following Treatment With Collagenase Clostridium Histolyticum (CORDLESS [Collagenase Option for Reduction of Dupuytren Long-Term Evaluation of Safety Study]): 5-Year Data   72

Factors affecting functional recovery after surgery and hand therapy in patients with Dupuytren's disease   74

Chapter 5: Compressive Neuropathies

Biomechanical Role of the Transverse Carpal Ligament in Carpal Tunnel Compliance   77

Longitudinal Gliding of the Median Nerve in the Carpal Tunnel: Ultrasound Cadaveric Evaluation of Conventional and Novel Concepts of Nerve Mobilization   79

Carpal Tunnel Syndrome Pathophysiology: Role of Subsynovial Connective Tissue   80

Carpal Tunnel Release: Do We Understand the Biomechanical Consequences?   83

Carpal tunnel syndrome and prediabetes: Is there a true association?   84

Multidimensional Ultrasound Imaging of the Wrist: Changes of Shape and Displacement of the Median Nerve and Tendons in Carpal Tunnel Syndrome   86

Enhanced Expression of Wnt9a in the Flexor Tenosynovium in Idiopathic Carpal Tunnel Syndrome   87

Carpal Tunnel Release: Do We Understand the Biomechanical Consequences?   88

The Effect of Moving Carpal Tunnel Releases Out of Hospitals on Reducing United States Health Care Charges   89

Pathophysiology and Etiology of Nerve Injury Following Peripheral Nerve Blockade 91

Effects of Metabolic Syndrome on the Outcome of Carpal Tunnel Release: A Matched Case-Control Study   92

Endoscopic vs Open Decompression of the Ulnar Nerve in Cubital Tunnel Syndrome: A Prospective Randomized Double-Blind Study   94

The Management of Cubital Tunnel Syndrome   96

Surgical Treatment of Cubital Tunnel Syndrome: Trends and the Influence of Patient and Surgeon Characteristics   96

Ulnar Nerve Transposition at the Elbow under Local Anesthesia: A Patient Satisfaction Study   97

Patient education for carpal tunnel syndrome: analysis of readability   100

Chapter 6: Nerve

Intraneural Ganglion in Superficial Radial Nerve Mimics de Quervain Tenosynovitis   103

Low profile radial nerve palsy orthosis with radial and ulnar deviation   104

Targeted Muscle Reinnervation of the Brachium: An Anatomic Study of Musculocutaneous and Radial Nerve Motor Points Relative to Proximal Landmarks   105

Comparative Study of Nerve Grafting versus Distal Nerve Transfer for Treatment of Proximal Injuries of the Ulnar Nerve   108

Ulnar Nerve Repair With Simultaneous Metacarpophalangeal Joint Capsulorrhaphy and Pulley Advancement   109

Targeted Muscle Reinnervation of the Brachium: An Anatomic Study of Musculocutaneous and Radial Nerve Motor Points Relative to Proximal Landmarks   111

Targeted Muscle Reinnervation in the Upper Extremity Amputee: A Technical Roadmap   112

Management of Acute Postoperative Pain in Hand Surgery: A Systematic Review   113

Comparative Study of Nerve Grafting versus Distal Nerve Transfer for Treatment of Proximal Injuries of the Ulnar Nerve   115

End-to-side neurorrhaphy for nerve repair and function rehabilitation   116

Bionic reconstruction to restore hand function after brachial plexus injury: a case series of three patients   117

Intra-articular and portal infiltration *versus* wrist block for analgesia after arthroscopy of the wrist: A prospective RCT   118

Vitamin C to Prevent Complex Regional Pain Syndrome in Patients With Distal Radius Fractures: A Meta-Analysis of Randomized Controlled Trials   119

Management of Acute Postoperative Pain in Hand Surgery: A Systematic Review   121

Effect of Time Interval Between Tumescent Local Anesthesia Infiltration and Start of Surgery on Operative Field Visibility in Hand Surgery Without Tourniquet   123

Light-Activated Sealing of Nerve Graft Coaptation Sites Improves Outcome Following Large Gap Peripheral Nerve Injury   124

Effects of a dynamic orthosis in an individual with claw deformity   126

The optimization of peripheral nerve recovery using cortical reorganization techniques: A retrospective study of wrist level nerve repairs   127

Nerve Regeneration: Is There an Alternative to Nervous Graft?   129

Light-Activated Sealing of Nerve Graft Coaptation Sites Improves Outcome Following Large Gap Peripheral Nerve Injury   130

Decellularized Nerves for Upper Limb Nerve Reconstruction: A Systematic Review of Functional Outcomes   131

Comparison of Nerve, Vessel, and Cartilage Grafts in Promoting Peripheral Nerve Regeneration   133

Chapter 7: Brachial Plexus

Spinal Accessory Nerve Transfer Outperforms Cervical Root Grafting for Suprascapular Nerve Reconstruction in Neonatal Brachial Plexus Palsy   137

Free functioning gracilis transplantation for reconstruction of elbow and hand functions in late obstetric brachial plexus palsy   138

Short-term and Long-term Clinical Results of the Surgical Correction of Thumb-in-Palm Deformity in Patients With Cerebral Palsy   139

Spinal Accessory Nerve Transfer Outperforms Cervical Root Grafting for Suprascapular Nerve Reconstruction in Neonatal Brachial Plexus Palsy   140

Chapter 8: Microsurgery

Predictors of Proximal Interphalangeal Joint Flexion Contracture After Homodigital Island Flap   143

A Comparative Study of Attitudes Regarding Digit Replantation in the United States and Japan   144

Innervated Digital Artery Perforator Propeller Flap for Reconstruction of Lateral Oblique Fingertip Defects   145

Chapter 9: Tendon

Effect of wrist and interphalangeal thumb movement on zone T2 flexor pollicis longus tendon tension in a human cadaver model   147

Stenosing flexor tenosynovitis: Validity of standard assessment tools of daily functioning and quality of life   152

Single-Stage Flexor Tendon Grafting: Refining the Steps   153

Zone III flexor tendon injuries – A proposed modification to rehabilitation   155

Biomechanical Study of the Digital Flexor Tendon Sliding Lengthening Technique   156

The Effect of 1-Ethyl-3-(3-Dimethylaminopropyl) Carbodiimide Suture Coating on Tendon Repair Strength and Cell Viability in a Canine Model   158

Biomechanical Analysis of the Modified Kessler, Lahey, Adelaide, and Becker Sutures for Flexor Tendon Repair   159

A Mechanical Evaluation of Zone II Flexor Tendon Repair Using a Knotless Barbed Suture Versus a Traditional Braided Suture   160

Single-Stage Flexor Tendon Grafting: Refining the Steps   162

Comparison of Flexor Tendon Suture Techniques Including 1 Using 10 Strands   163

Risk Assessment of Tendon Attrition Following Treatment of Distal Radius Fractures With Volar Locking Plates Using Audible Crepitus and Placement of the Plate: A Prospective Clinical Cohort Study   164

The Effect of the Epitendinous Suture on Gliding in a Cadaveric Model of Zone II Flexor Tendon Repair   165

Ultrasound-Guided Hyaluronic Acid Injections for Trigger Finger: A Double-Blinded, Randomized Controlled Trial   167

Self-regulated frequent power pinch exercises: A non-orthotic technique for the treatment of old mallet deformity 168

Conservative treatment of mallet finger: A systematic review 168

Stenosing flexor tenosynovitis: Validity of standard assessment tools of daily functioning and quality of life 169

The Dorsal Triangular Fibrocartilage of the Metacarpophalangeal Joint: A Cadaveric Study 170

Chapter 10: Trauma

Reduction of Fifth Metacarpal Neck Fractures With a Kirschner Wire 173

Distal Oblique Bundle Reinforcement for Treatment of DRUJ Instability 174

Impact of Joint Position and Joint Morphology on Assessment of Thumb Metacarpophalangeal Joint Radial Collateral Ligament Integrity 175

A Comparison of K-Wire Versus Screw Fixation on the Outcomes of Distal Phalanx Fractures 176

A Comparative Study of Attitudes Regarding Digit Replantation in the United States and Japan 177

The Epidemiology of Upper Extremity Fractures in the United States, 2009 178

Early Versus Delayed Fourth Ray Amputation With Fifth Ray Transposition for Management of Mutilating Ring Finger Injuries 180

Two Versus 3 Lag Screws for Fixation of Long Oblique Proximal Phalanx Fractures of the Fingers: A Cadaver Study 181

A review of phalangeal neck fractures in children 182

A Systematic Review of Outcomes after Revision Amputation for Treatment of Traumatic Finger Amputation 183

A Comparison of K-Wire Versus Screw Fixation on the Outcomes of Distal Phalanx Fractures 184

The Effect of Timing on the Treatment and Outcome of Combined Fourth and Fifth Carpometacarpal Fracture Dislocations 186

Dorsal Screw Penetration With the Use of Volar Plating of Distal Radius Fractures: How Can You Best Detect? 187

The Effect of Closed Reduction of Small Finger Metacarpal Neck Fractures on the Ultimate Angular Deformity 188

What Middle Phalanx Base Fracture Characteristics are Most Reliable and Useful for Surgical Decision-making? 189

Extension Block Pinning Versus Hook Plate Fixation for Treatment of Mallet Fractures 191

Management of the Acutely Burned Hand 192

Early Versus Delayed Fourth Ray Amputation With Fifth Ray Transposition for Management of Mutilating Ring Finger Injuries 193

Biomechanical Comparison of 2 Methods of Intramedullary K-Wire Fixation of Transverse Metacarpal Shaft Fractures 194

Anatomic Considerations for Plating of the Distal Ulna   196

Chapter 11: Distal Radius Fractures

In Vivo Contact Characteristics of Distal Radioulnar Joint With Malunited Distal Radius During Wrist Motion   199

Volar, Intramedullary, and Percutaneous Fixation of Distal Radius Fractures   201

The Unstable Distal Radius Fracture—How Do We Define It? A Systematic Review   202

Catastrophic Thinking Is Associated With Finger Stiffness After Distal Radius Fracture Surgery   203

Is Bone Grafting Necessary in the Treatment of Malunited Distal Radius Fractures?   205

The Effect of Elbow Extension on the Biomechanics of the Osseoligamentous Structures of the Forearm   206

Arthroscopic assistance does not improve the functional or radiographic outcome of unstable intra-articular distal radial fractures treated with a volar locking plate: a randomised controlled trial   207

Vitamin C to Prevent Complex Regional Pain Syndrome in Patients With Distal Radius Fractures: A Meta-Analysis of Randomized Controlled Trials   208

Functional Outcomes Following Bridge Plate Fixation for Distal Radius Fractures   210

Are Volar Locking Plates Superior to Percutaneous K-wires for Distal Radius Fractures? A Meta-analysis   212

Acute Median Nerve Problems in the Setting of a Distal Radius Fracture   213

External Fixation and Adjuvant Pins Versus Volar Locking Plate Fixation in Unstable Distal Radius Fractures: A Randomized, Controlled Study With a 5-Year Follow-Up   215

Utility and Cost Analysis of Radiographs Taken 2 Weeks Following Plate Fixation of Distal Radius Fractures   217

Coronal Shift of Distal Radius Fractures: Influence of the Distal Interosseous Membrane on Distal Radioulnar Joint Instability   218

Volar Subluxation of the Ulnar Head in Dorsal Translation Deformities of Distal Radius Fractures: An In Vitro Biomechanical Study   221

Distal Radioulnar Joint Reaction Force Following Ulnar Shortening: Diaphyseal Osteotomy Versus Wafer Resection   221

In Vivo Contact Characteristics of Distal Radioulnar Joint With Malunited Distal Radius During Wrist Motion   223

Reconstruction of the Distal Oblique Bundle of the Interosseous Membrane: A Technique to Restore Distal Radioulnar Joint Stability   224

The Unstable Distal Radius Fracture—How Do We Define It? A Systematic Review   225

Effect of Volarly Angulated Distal Radius Fractures on Forearm Rotation and Distal Radioulnar Joint Kinematics   226

No Difference in Adverse Events Between Surgically Treated Reduced and Unreduced Distal Radius Fractures   227

Wrist Fracture and Risk of Subsequent Fracture: Findings from the Women's Health Initiative Study   229

Catastrophic Thinking Is Associated With Finger Stiffness After Distal Radius
Fracture Surgery   230

Hemiarthroplasty for Complex Distal Radius Fractures in Elderly Patients   231

Biomechanical Comparison of Volar Fixed-Angle Locking Plates for AO C3 Distal
Radius Fractures: Titanium Versus Stainless Steel With Compression   233

Volar Marginal Rim Fracture Fixation With Volar Fragment-Specific Hook Plate
Fixation   234

Functional Outcomes of the Aptis-Scheker Distal Radioulnar Joint Replacement in
Patients Under 40 Years Old   236

Arthroscopic assistance does not improve the functional or radiographic outcome
of unstable intra-articular distal radial fractures treated with a volar locking
plate: a randomised controlled trial   237

Is it time to revisit the AO classification of fractures of the distal radius? Inter- and
intra-observer reliability of the AO classification   239

Functional Outcomes Following Bridge Plate Fixation for Distal Radius Fractures   240

The Utility of the Fluoroscopic Skyline View During Volar Locking Plate Fixation
of Distal Radius Fractures   241

Are Volar Locking Plates Superior to Percutaneous K-wires for Distal Radius
Fractures? A Meta-analysis   242

The Minimum Clinically Important Difference of the Patient-rated Wrist
Evaluation Score for Patients With Distal Radius Fractures   244

External Fixation and Adjuvant Pins Versus Volar Locking Plate Fixation in
Unstable Distal Radius Fractures: A Randomized, Controlled Study With a 5-Year
Follow-Up   245

A novel computational method for evaluating osteochondral autografts in distal
radius reconstruction   247

Wrist Fracture and Risk of Subsequent Fracture: Findings from the Women's
Health Initiative Study   248

Chapter 12: Diagnostic Imaging

Efficacy of Magnetic Resonance Imaging and Clinical Tests in Diagnostics of Wrist
Ligament Injuries: A Systematic Review   249

Approach to the Swollen Arm With Chronic Dialysis Access: It's Not Just Deep
Vein Thrombosis   250

Calcific tendinopathy of the rotator cuff: the correlation between pain and imaging
features in symptomatic and asymptomatic female shoulders   251

The Reliability of Ultrasound Measurements of the Median Nerve at the Carpal
Tunnel Inlet   253

Routine Imaging after Operatively Repaired Distal Radius and Scaphoid Fractures:
A Survey of Hand Surgeons   254

Advanced imaging of the scapholunate ligamentous complex   255

Cine MRI: a new approach to the diagnosis of scapholunate dissociation   257

Elbow US: Anatomy, Variants, and Scanning Technique   258

Chapter 13: Elbow: Trauma

An Expedited Care Pathway with Ambulatory Brachial Plexus Analgesia Is a
Cost-effective Alternative to Standard Inpatient Care after Complex Arthroscopic
Elbow Surgery: A Randomized, Single-blinded Study 259

A survey of current practices and preferences for internal fixation of displaced
olecranon fractures 260

What Factors are Associated With a Surgical Site Infection After Operative
Treatment of an Elbow Fracture? 261

Distal Biceps Tendon Ruptures: An Epidemiological Analysis Using a Large
Population Database 262

Revisiting the 'bag of bones': functional outcome after the conservative
management of a fracture of the distal humerus 264

Clinical and functional outcomes and treatment options for paediatric elbow
dislocations: Experiences of three trauma centres 265

The frequency and risk factors for subsequent surgery after a simple elbow
dislocation 267

Current Treatment Concepts for "Terrible Triad" Injuries of the Elbow 270

Incarcerated Medial Epicondyle Fracture Following Pediatric Elbow Dislocation:
11 Cases 270

Extension Test and Ossal Point Tenderness Cannot Accurately Exclude Significant
Injury in Acute Elbow Trauma 272

Chapter 14: Elbow: Miscellaneous

Total elbow joint replacement for fractures in the elderly—Functional and
radiological outcomes 275

Corticosteroid and platelet-rich plasma injection therapy in tennis elbow (lateral
epicondylalgia): a survey of current UK specialist practice and a call for clinical
guidelines 276

Factors Associated With Failure of Nonoperative Treatment in Lateral
Epicondylitis 277

Plate and Screw Fixation of Bicolumnar Distal Humerus Fractures: Factors
Associated With Loosening or Breakage of Implants or Nonunion 278

Subcutaneous Versus Submuscular Anterior Transposition of the Ulnar Nerve for
Cubital Tunnel Syndrome: A Systematic Review and Meta-Analysis of Randomized
Controlled Trials and Observational Studies 279

Outcomes After Ulnar Nerve *In Situ* Release During Total Elbow Arthroplasty 280

Elbow Positioning and Joint Insufflation Substantially Influence Median and
Radial Nerve Locations 281

Trends in Medial Ulnar Collateral Ligament Reconstruction in the United States:
A Retrospective Review of a Large Private-Payer Database From 2007 to 2011 283

Prognostic Factors of Arthroscopic Extensor Carpi Radialis Brevis Release for
Lateral Epicondylitis 284

Impact of Ulnar Collateral Ligament Tear on Posteromedial Elbow Biomechanics 287

Restoring Isometry in Lateral Ulnar Collateral Ligament Reconstruction   288

Radial head dislocation due to gigantic solitary osteochondroma of the proximal ulna: case report and literature review   289

Cold Hyperalgesia Associated with Poorer Prognosis in Lateral Epicondylalgia: A 1-Year Prognostic Study of Physical and Psychological Factors   290

Trends in Revision Elbow Ulnar Collateral Ligament Reconstruction in Professional Baseball Pitchers   291

Elbow Positioning and Joint Insufflation Substantially Influence Median and Radial Nerve Locations   293

Restoring Isometry in Lateral Ulnar Collateral Ligament Reconstruction   295

Repair of distal biceps brachii tendon assessed with 3-T magnetic resonance imaging and correlation with functional outcome   296

Chapter 15: Pediatric Trauma

Common medial elbow injuries in the adolescent athlete   299

Biomechanical Analysis of Screws Versus K-Wires for Lateral Humeral Condyle Fractures   300

Screw Fixation of Lateral Condyle Fractures: Results of Treatment   303

Intra-articular Radial Head Fractures In the Skeletally Immature Patient: Complications and Management   305

Outcome of Displaced Fractures of the Distal Metaphyseal-Diaphyseal Junction of the Humerus in Children Treated With Elastic Stable Intramedullary Nails   307

A Swollen Hand With Blisters: A Case of Compartment Syndrome in a Child   309

Imaging of the elbow in children with wrist fracture: an unnecessary source of radiation and use of resources?   310

Fishtail deformity — a delayed complication of distal humeral fractures in children   312

Intra-articular Radial Head Fractures in the Skeletally Immature Patient: Complications and Management   317

Chapter 16: Congenital

Soft-Tissue Surgery for Camptodactyly Corrects Skeletal Changes   321

Pediatric Trigger Digits   323

Safety and Efficacy of Derotational Osteotomy for Congenital Radioulnar Synostosis   324

Results of Treatment of Delta Triphalangeal Thumbs by Excision of the Extra Phalanx   326

Applying the Patient-Reported Outcomes Measurement Information System to Assess Upper Extremity Function among Children with Congenital Hand Differences   327

Bone lengthening of the radius with temporary external fixation of the wrist for mild radial club hand   329

Addressing muscle performance impairments in cerebral palsy: Implications for
upper extremity resistance training   331

Congenital Radial Nerve Palsy   332

Syndactyly Web Space Reconstruction Using the Tapered M-to-V Flap:
A Single-Surgeon, 30-Year Experience   334

Stability of the Basal Joints of the New Thumb After Pollicization for Thumb
Hypoplasia   336

Use of an Axial Flap to Increase the Girth of Wassel IV Thumb Reconstructions   337

Short-term and Long-term Clinical Results of the Surgical Correction of
Thumb-in-Palm Deformity in Patients With Cerebral Palsy   338

Chapter 17: Shoulder: Rotator Cuff

A Randomized, Double-Blinded, Placebo-Controlled Clinical Trial Evaluating the
Effectiveness of Daily Vibration After Arthroscopic Rotator Cuff Repair   341

Preoperative Deltoid Size and Fatty Infiltration of the Deltoid and Rotator Cuff
Correlate to Outcomes After Reverse Total Shoulder Arthroplasty   343

Which patients do not recover from shoulder impingement syndrome, either with
operative treatment or with nonoperative treatment? Subgroup analysis involving
140 patients at 2 and 5 years in a randomized study   345

Chronic Degeneration Leads to Poor Healing of Repaired Massive Rotator Cuff
Tears in Rats   346

A Systematic Review of the Psychometric Properties of Patient-Reported Outcome
Instruments for Use in Patients with Rotator Cuff Disease   350

The Optimum Tension for Bridging Sutures in Transosseous-Equivalent Rotator
Cuff Repair: A Cadaveric Biomechanical Study   351

Prolotherapy for Refractory Rotator Cuff Disease: Retrospective Case-Control
Study of 1-Year Follow-Up   353

Arthroscopic Partial Repair of Irreparable Rotator Cuff Tears: Preoperative
Factors Associated with Outcome Deterioration over 2 Years   354

Effectiveness of Botulinum Toxin for Shoulder Pain Treatment: A Systematic
Review and Meta-Analysis   357

Early mobilisation following mini-open rotator cuff repair: a randomised control
trial   359

Clinical Outcomes of Modified Mason-Allen Single-Row Repair for Bursal-Sided
Partial-Thickness Rotator Cuff Tears: Comparison With the Double-Row
Suture-Bridge Technique   361

Early Versus Delayed Passive Range of Motion after Rotator Cuff Repair:
A Systematic Review and Meta-analysis   363

Smoking Predisposes to Rotator Cuff Pathology and Shoulder Dysfunction:
A Systematic Review   364

Outcome of Large to Massive Rotator Cuff Tears Repaired With and Without
Extracellular Matrix Augmentation: A Prospective Comparative Study   368

Low Serum Vitamin D Is Not Correlated With the Severity of a Rotator Cuff Tear
or Retear After Arthroscopic Repair   370

Traumatic Supraspinatus Tears in Patients Younger Than 25 Years — 371

Botulinum Toxin is Detrimental to Repair of a Chronic Rotator Cuff Tear in a Rabbit Model — 372

Does Rotator Cuff Repair Improve Psychologic Status and Quality of Life in Patients With Rotator Cuff Tear? — 373

What Is the Prevalence of Senior-athlete Rotator Cuff Injuries and Are They Associated With Pain and Dysfunction? — 375

Fluoroquinolones Impair Tendon Healing in a Rat Rotator Cuff Repair Model: A Preliminary Study — 376

Platelet-Rich Plasma for Arthroscopic Repair of Medium to Large Rotator Cuff Tears: A Randomized Controlled Trial — 378

Early Versus Delayed Passive Range of Motion After Rotator Cuff Repair: A Systematic Review and Meta-analysis — 380

Chapter 18: Shoulder: Trauma

Long stem reverse shoulder arthroplasty and cerclage for treatment of complex long segment proximal humeral fractures with diaphyseal extension in patients more than 65 years old — 383

Multicenter Randomized Clinical Trial of Nonoperative Versus Operative Treatment of Acute Acromio-Clavicular Joint Dislocation — 384

A Comparison of the Charlson and Elixhauser Comorbidity Measures to Predict Inpatient Mortality After Proximal Humerus Fracture — 387

The Interrater and Intrarater Agreement of a Modified Neer Classification System and Associated Treatment Choice for Lateral Clavicle Fractures — 388

Surgical Versus Conservative Treatments for Displaced Midshaft Clavicular Fractures: A Systematic Review of Overlapping Meta-Analyses — 390

Bilateral weighted radiographs are required for accurate classification of acromioclavicular separation: An observational study of 59 cases — 391

Reverse shoulder arthroplasty as a salvage procedure after failed internal fixation of fractures of the proximal humerus: outcomes and complications — 393

Midterm outcome and complications after minimally invasive treatment of displaced proximal humeral fractures in patients younger than 70 years using the Humerusblock — 394

Deltoid Tuberosity Index: A Simple Radiographic Tool to Assess Local Bone Quality in Proximal Humerus Fractures — 396

Transosseous braided-tape and double-row fixations are better than tension band for avulsion-type greater tuberosity fractures — 402

Outcomes After Hemiarthroplasty for Proximal Humerus Fracture Are Significantly Affected by Hand Dominance — 405

Chapter 19: Shoulder: Miscellaneous

The Effect of Cartilage Injury After Arthroscopic Stabilization for Shoulder Instability — 409

Arthroscopic Capsulolabral Reconstruction for Posterior Shoulder Instability in
Patients 18 Years Old or Younger   412

Operative Management Options for Traumatic Anterior Shoulder Instability in
Patients Younger Than 30 Years   413

Does External Rotation Bracing for Anterior Shoulder Dislocation Actually Result
in Reduction of the Labrum? A Systematic Review   416

A Qualitative Investigation of Return to Sport After Arthroscopic Bankart Repair:
Beyond Stability   417

Complications Associated With Arthroscopic Labral Repair Implants: A Case
Series   419

Arthroscopic Stabilization of Posterior Shoulder Instability Is Successful in
American Football Players   419

Anterior Shoulder Instability Is Associated with an Underlying Deficiency of the
Bony Glenoid Concavity   420

Posterior Instability of the Shoulder: A Systematic Review and Meta-analysis of
Clinical Outcomes   424

Arm Abduction Provides a Better Reduction of the Bankart Lesion During
Immobilization in External Rotation After an Initial Shoulder Dislocation   428

Comparison of 3-Dimensional Computed Tomography–Based Measurement of
Glenoid Bone Loss With Arthroscopic Defect Size Estimation in Patients with
Anterior Shoulder Instability   430

The Effect of a Combined Glenoid and Hill-Sachs Defect on Glenohumeral
Stability: A Biomechanical Cadaveric Study Using 3-Dimensional Modeling of 142
Patients   434

Sporting Activity After Arthroscopic Bankart Repair for Chronic Glenohumeral
Instability   436

External Rotation Immobilization for Primary Shoulder Dislocation:
A Randomized Controlled Trial   437

Latissimus Dorsi and Teres Major Transfer With Reverse Shoulder Arthroplasty
Restores Active Motion and Reduces Pain for Posterosuperior Cuff Dysfunction   438

The Impact of Rotator Cuff Deficiency on Structure, Mechanical Properties, and
Gene Expression Profiles of the Long Head of the Biceps Tendon (LHBT):
Implications for Management of the LHBT During Primary Shoulder Arthroplasty   441

Arthroscopic Tissue Culture for the Evaluation of Periprosthetic Shoulder Infection   442

Conversion of Stemmed Hemi- or Total to Reverse Total Shoulder Arthroplasty:
Advantages of a Modular Stem Design   443

Preoperative Deltoid Size and Fatty Infiltration of the Deltoid and Rotator Cuff
Correlate to Outcomes After Reverse Total Shoulder Arthroplasty   445

A novel osteotomy in shoulder joint replacement based on analysis of the cartilage/
metaphyseal interface   446

Glenohumeral Pressure With Surface Replacement Arthroplasty Versus
Hemiarthroplasty   448

Outcomes After Hemiarthroplasty for Proximal Humerus Fracture Are
Significantly Affected by Hand Dominance   449

The Incidence of *Propionibacterium acnes* in Shoulder Arthroscopy   451

Expert Surgeons Can Be Distinguished From Trainees, and Surgical Proficiency
Can Be Defined, Using Validated Metrics and Shoulder Models 452

Utility of the Instability Severity Index Score in Predicting Failure After
Arthroscopic Anterior Stabilization of the Shoulder 452

Assessment of the Postoperative Appearance of the Rotator Cuff Tendon Using
Serial Sonography After Arthroscopic Repair of a Rotator Cuff Tear 453

Outcome After Arthroscopic Decompression of Inferior Labral Cysts Combined
With Labral Repair 454

Demographic Analysis of Open and Arthroscopic Distal Clavicle Excision in a
Private Insurance Database 458

The natural history of the rheumatoid shoulder: a prospective long-term follow-up
study 460

Configuration of the Shoulder Complex During the Arm-Cocking Phase in Baseball
Pitching 461

Design and Testing of the Degree of Shoulder Involvement in Sports (DOSIS) Scale 464

Deficits in Glenohumeral Passive Range of Motion Increase Risk of Shoulder Injury
in Professional Baseball Pitchers: A Prospective Study 468

Correlation of Shoulder and Elbow Kinetics With Ball Velocity in Collegiate
Baseball Pitchers 470

High Incidence of Infraspinatus Muscle Atrophy in Elite Professional Female
Tennis Players 471

What is the Best Clinical Test for Assessment of the Teres Minor in Massive
Rotator Cuff Tears? 473

Upper Extremity Kinematics and Muscle Activation Patterns in Subjects With
Facioscapulohumeral Dystrophy 474

Biomechanical Consequences of Coracoclavicular Reconstruction Techniques on
Clavicle Strength 475

Chapter 20: Rehabilitation

Effects of Stretching and Strengthening Exercises, With and Without Manual
Therapy, on Scapular Kinematics, Function, and Pain in Individuals With Shoulder
Impingement: A Randomized Controlled Trial 477

Kinesio Tape and Shoulder-Joint Position Sense 478

Correlation Between American Shoulder and Elbow Surgeons and Single
Assessment Numerical Evaluation Score After Rotator Cuff or SLAP Repair 481

The effectiveness of exercise for the management of musculoskeletal disorders and
injuries of the elbow, forearm, wrist, and hand: a systematic review by the Ontario
Protocol for Traffic Injury Management (OPTIMa) Collaboration 482

Responsiveness of three Patient Report Outcome (PRO) measures in patients with
hand fractures: A preliminary cohort study 489

The Minimum Clinically Important Difference of the Patient-rated Wrist
Evaluation Score for Patients With Distal Radius Fractures 491

Reliability, Validity, and Responsiveness of the QuickDASH in Patients With Upper
Limb Amputation 492

Changes in H reflex and neuromechanical properties of the trapezius muscle after
5 weeks of eccentric training: a randomized controlled trial — 494

Chapter 21: Miscellaneous

Surgical Treatment Options for Glenohumeral Arthritis in Young Patients:
A Systematic Review and Meta-analysis — 495

Google Glass as an Alternative to Standard Fluoroscopic Visualization for
Percutaneous Fixation of Hand Fractures: A Pilot Study — 496

Trends in incidence rate, health care consumption, and costs for patients admitted
with a humeral fracture in The Netherlands between 1986 and 2012 — 498

Humeral Head Reconstruction With Osteochondral Allograft Transplantation — 499

Achieving the optimal epinephrine effect in wide awake hand surgery using local
anesthesia without a tourniquet — 502

Aneurysmal Bone Cysts of the Hand, Wrist, and Forearm — 503

Recurrent Metacarpal Enchondroma Treated With Strut Allograft: 14-year Follow-
up — 504

Normative Values for Grip and Pinch Strength for 6- to 19-Year-Olds — 505

Forearm amputees' views of prosthesis use and sensory feedback — 506

Achieving the optimal epinephrine effect in wide awake hand surgery using local
anesthesia without a tourniquet — 507

The Impact of Uninterrupted Warfarin on Hand and Wrist Surgery — 508

Hand Sensibility, Strength, and Laxity of High-Level Musicians Compared to
Nonmusicians — 510

Complications Within 30 Days of Hand Surgery: An Analysis of 10,646 Patients — 511

Physician Empathy as a Driver of Hand Surgery Patient Satisfaction — 513

Google Glass as an Alternative to Standard Fluoroscopic Visualization for
Percutaneous Fixation of Hand Fractures: A Pilot Study — 514

Outcomes of Open Dorsal Wrist Ganglion Excision in Active-Duty Military
Personnel — 515

The Association of the H-Index and Academic Rank Among Full-Time Academic
Hand Surgeons Affiliated With Fellowship Programs — 516

Patient education for carpal tunnel syndrome: analysis of readability — 517

To What Degree Do Pain-coping Strategies Affect Joint Stiffness and Functional
Outcomes in Patients with Hand Fractures? — 518

Author Index

A

Aarseth LM, 478
Abboud JA, 413
Ablove RH, 262
Abzug JM, 332
Ackerson R, 305, 317
Adikrishna A, 131
Adkinson JM, 96
Agnew S, 210, 240
Agrawal Y, 118
Agur A, 155
Ahn J, 309
Aitken SA, 264
Akman YE, 504
Al-Qattan AM, 182
Al-Qattan MM, 182
Alaia MJ, 288, 295
Alburquerque-Sendín F, 477
Alemann G, 296
Alewijnse JV, 139, 338
Algar L, 168
Aliu O, 96
Alluri R, 201
Alluri RK, 458
Alvarez-Pinzon AM, 368
An K-N, 80, 158
Anand P, 287
Andernord D, 249
Anderson M, 303
Andersson JK, 249
Anderton MJ, 33
Appy-Fedida B, 50, 56
Arciero RA, 434
Arner JW, 419
Arnold C, 452
Aszmann OC, 117
Atiyya AN, 109
Atzei A, 46
Avila MA, 477
Avisar E, 29
Axelsson P, 7
Ayalon O, 175
Aytekin AH, 133

B

Bachour Y, 17
Bae DS, 323
Bagatur AE, 504
Bakri K, 210, 240
Bakshi NK, 430
Balazs GC, 515

Bar-Haim Erez A, 152, 169
Barcksdale L, 368
Bashir MM, 123
Bauer AS, 323
Begonia MT, 194
Beikircher R, 79
Bellato E, 464
Benninger E, 396
Bergsma A, 474
Berkhout MJL, 17
Berkow K, 58
Bernhardson AS, 434
Bhamber NS, 276
Bignotti B, 258
Bindra R, 196
Bishop JY, 364
Bisset L, 290
Black JS, 334
Blazar P, 72
Blazar PE, 213
Blonna D, 464
Bogunovic L, 508
Bohl DD, 254, 270
Bohn K, 270
Bonasia DE, 464
Booker SJ, 276
Boone S, 14, 96
Borbas P, 443
Borgia M, 492
Boros MC, 250
Bosch HG, 86
Bot AGJ, 203, 230
Bouliane M, 359
Brabender RC, 160, 217
Bradley JP, 419, 424
Braidotti F, 46
Brais G, 402
Brand JC, 452
Braun Y, 261, 278
Brink PRG, 174
Brkljac M, 59
Brock G, 236
Brull R, 91
Bulut M, 265
Burkhart KJ, 281, 293
Burns PB, 1, 18
Byun DJ, 55

C

Cahill KE, 438
Calfee RP, 96, 277
Camargo PR, 477

Campbell ST, 351
Canavese F, 307
Canham CD, 31, 221
Cannada LK, 187
Carlozzi N, 327
Carlsson I, 506
Carry PM, 305, 317
Castagna A, 383
Cauley JA, 229, 248
Cavalcanti MF, 84
Cavinatto LM, 346
Chakrabarti I, 118
Chalmers GR, 478
Chalmers PN, 495
Chaudhry H, 212, 242
Chen NC, 513
Chen RE, 277
Chen YR, 199, 223
Chhabra AB, 36
Chimenti PC, 496, 514
Chinchalkar SJ, 155
Chivers DA, 280
Cho C-H, 373, 388
Choi J-Y, 453
Christen T, 97
Christian M, 372
Chuang DJ, 100, 517
Chuang MJ, 451
Chung KC, 1, 18, 113, 121
Chung SW, 284
Claessen FMAP, 261, 278
Cole BJ, 499
Coleman S, 72
Collin P, 473
Consonni O, 251
Cooley J, 206
Coombes BK, 290
Côté P, 482
Crandall CJ, 229, 248
Cravino M, 307
Crowe MM, 503
Cruz Eng H, 259
Cuénod P, 43
Cunningham G, 481
Cup EH, 474

D

Dachs RP, 280
Dakic J, 471
Dautel G, 337
Davis DE, 413
de Macêdo MP, 126

de Muinck Keizer R-J, 244, 491
De Rizzo LALM, 129
Delattre O, 5
Dell PC, 224
DeLong JM, 424
Denard PJ, 473, 481
Deslivia MF, 131
Devitt BM, 417
Dietsch E, 296
Dilisio MF, 371, 442
Dimitris C, 35, 62
Disseldorp DJG, 205
Dodds SD, 270
Donohue MA, 515
Drake ML, 515
Dumanian GA, 112

E

Earp BE, 213
Eberhardt A, 233
Eberhardt AW, 300
Eberlin KR, 100, 517
Eisenschenk A, 257
Ek ET, 438, 443
El-Gammal TA, 138
El-Sayed A, 138
Elliott MP, 419
Elmorsy A, 452
Elvey M, 29
Engel L, 510
English C, 165
Engstrand C, 68, 74
Erickson BJ, 283
Ernstbrunner L, 420
Euler SA, 475
Evaniew N, 119, 208
Evans PJ, 77

F

Faber KJ, 405, 449
Fairbairn NG, 124, 130
Fairplay T, 46
Farrokhyar F, 260
Felder JJ, 419
Feldon P, 40
Fernandes M, 129
Feucht MJ, 436
Filius A, 86
Firat C, 133
Fischer S, 257
Flanagin B, 383

Flanagin BA, 270
Fleisig GS, 468
Fletcher DR, 153, 162
Flores LP, 108, 115
Floyd WE IV, 213
Fouly EH, 180, 193
Fowler JR, 253
Fox AJS, 376
Fox MG, 36
Francis KA, 375
Franzblau LE, 327
Freitas Paiva AM, 84
Fu Y, 357
Funk L, 33
Fuzzard S, 137, 140

G

Gallinet D, 296
Gammon B, 221, 226
Gandhi MJ, 33
Ganley T, 299
Gannotti ME, 331
Gao W, 116
Garg R, 37
Garofalo R, 383
Gart MS, 112
Gaston RG, 71
Gelberman RH, 14, 96, 508
Gendelberg D, 188
Geyik Y, 133
Gharb BB, 236
Ghomrawi HMK, 489
Giladi AM, 183
Gilot GJ, 368
Gilotra M, 372
Giuffre JL, 61
Giugale JM, 58
Goldfarb CA, 508
Golding LP, 310
Gong HS, 11, 23
Gong K-T, 42
Goslings JC, 244, 491
Goulon G, 5
Grant JA, 350
Gray A, 43
Grewal R, 47, 65
Griska A, 40
Grottkau BE, 312

H

Hackl M, 281, 293
Hadzic A, 91

Halilaj E, 3, 13
Haller JM, 103
Hamada Y, 289
Hamilton KL, 321
Hammert WC, 510
Hannemann PFW, 174, 205
Hansen EA, 494
Hansen K, 341
Hardy J, 231
Harhaus L, 64
Harris A, 83, 88
Harrold F, 446
Hartog DD, 498
Hashimoto K, 156
Hassan MY, 180, 193
Hassan SE, 287
Hay RA, 176
Hay RAS, 184
Hayes AG, 181
Hazel A, 196
Hedley H, 239
Heffinger C, 64
Hellund JC, 215, 245
Hendriks S, 241
Hernandez-Boussard T, 89
Hiatt SV, 194
Hibino N, 289
Hickson C, 239
Hill BW, 187
Hirsch D, 253
Hirzinger C, 394
Hitachi S, 428
Hiwatari R, 158
Hoffelner T, 394
Hong SH, 453
Horii E, 289
Horrow MM, 250
Houdek MT, 27, 503
Hovey KM, 229, 248
Hovius SER, 67, 70
Hsu JW, 247
Huang H, 350
Huang JI, 247
Huang X, 173
Hunter-Smith DJ, 170
Husby T, 215, 245
Hussey MM, 393
Hussey SE, 393
Hutchinson DT, 326
Hwang I, 373

I

Ichihara S, 241
Iida A, 143

Ipaktchi K, 270
Isik M, 265
Itoi E, 428

J

Jacobson JA, 430
Jancosko JJ, 451
Jansen H, 159
Janssen SJ, 24, 189
Jenkins PJ, 264
Jeong J-J, 454
Jiang K, 424
Jie KE, 272
Jo CH, 378
Jordan MC, 159
Jordan RW, 416
Joyce DA, 35, 62
Jung G-H, 388

K

Kaestle N, 396
Kakar S, 51, 234
Kalliainen L, 127
Karl JW, 178
Karlsson J, 249
Kärrholm J, 7
Ke X-B, 279
Kedilioglu MA, 26
Keighley G, 341
Kelley BP, 113, 121
Kelly MP, 262
Ketola S, 345
Killian ML, 346
Kim BH, 370
Kim JH, 11, 23
Kim SS, 22
Kim TH, 163
Kim YH, 11, 23
King AH, 409
Kitamura T, 428
Kleinlugtenbelt YV, 119,
  208, 212, 242
Kleist Welch-Guerra W, 94
Kluczynski MA, 363, 380
Knutsen EJ, 277
Kodama N, 9
Koh KH, 354
Kollitz KM, 247
Komatsu M, 164, 207, 237

Konda S, 461
Kook S-H, 361
Kotb MM, 138
Koueiter DM, 343, 445
Kraszewski AP, 37
Kremenic IJ, 288, 295
Kreulen M, 139, 338
Krevers B, 68, 74
Krief E, 50, 56
Kroonen LT, 105, 111
Kruse K, 253
Krych AJ, 409, 412
Kuniyoshi K, 156
Kupperman AI, 458
Kurdziel MD, 441
Kvist J, 68, 74
Kwack K-S, 353

L

Lädermann A, 481
Lalonde DH, 502, 507
Lam PH, 341
Langer D, 152, 169
Langner I, 257
Lappen S, 281, 293
Larsen SE, 71
Lauder A, 210, 240
Laudner KG, 470
Lavalley R, 505
Leahy I, 299
LeBlanc JEM, 405, 449
Lee BK, 92
Lee D-H, 353
Lee H-J, 131
Lee HI, 163
Lee JS, 163
Lee SK, 55
Lee Y, 370
Lehtinen J, 345
Leigey D, 58
Lese AB, 254
Li S, 116
Li Z-M, 77
Liang C, 186
Lim TK, 354
Lin S-H, 167
Lipira AB, 511
Liu C-H, 279
Liu D-H, 167
Liu Q, 116
Liu S, 175
Livermore M, 270

Long L, 390
Longacre M, 201
Lopez J, 516
Lubowitz JH, 452
Luo TD, 27
Luria S, 152, 169

M

Mabit C, 231
MacDermid JC, 47, 65,
  405, 449
Macionis V, 168
Macrina LC, 468
Maerz T, 343, 445
Mahabier KC, 498
Maiorano E, 251
Mair SD, 419
Malhas A, 446
Malone PSC, 206
Maqsoodi N, 31, 221
Marengo L, 307
Marquardt TL, 77
Marshall T, 233
Martinoli C, 258
Marzo JM, 363, 380
Mascarenhas R, 495
Matthes M, 94
Mayne IP, 267
McCarthy C, 119, 208
McClincy MP, 419
McClinton MA, 153, 162
McGarry MH, 351
McGee C, 8, 21
McGlinn EP, 183
McInnes CW, 61
Mckee DE, 502, 507
McLoda TA, 470
McMahon PJ, 375
McQuiddy VA, 505
Ménard J, 402
Mendoza V, 451
Menendez ME, 387, 513
Meng S, 79
Menta R, 482
Menuki K, 87
Meppelink AM, 124, 130
Mericli AF, 334
Meyer VM, 41
Mi JY, 145
Mighell MA, 393
Miller BS, 350
Miller LR, 442

Milstein A, 89
Mitten DJ, 496, 514
Mochida J, 329
Modi CS, 267
Momaya A, 233
Montgomery SR, 458
Moore DC, 3, 13
Moran SL, 503
Moravek JE, 441
Moreau NG, 331
Morgan RF, 334
Moroder P, 420
Morrell NT, 83, 88, 291
Mudgal CS, 513
Mühldorfer-Fodor M, 52
Mulder F, 227
Mundi R, 212, 242
Murgia A, 474
Murnaghan ML, 417
Mutch J, 402

N

Nakanishi A, 143
Narayanan S, 312
Nassar WAM, 109
Naughton N, 168
Nayak AN, 160
Nayyar S, 363, 380
Neal K, 303
Nemeth N, 196
Netscher DT, 321
Ng-Glazier J, 124, 130
Nguyen A, 305, 317
Nguyen C, 89
Nguyen D-V, 160
Nguyen T, 372
Nishiwaki M, 221, 226
Nishizuka T, 144, 177
Noble JS, 371
Noel CR, 371
Noh JH, 92, 518
Nota SP, 227
Nwachukwu BU, 283

O

O'Brien V, 8, 21
Oh JH, 388, 518
Old J, 416
Ollason J, 104
Olson PR, 178
Omokawa S, 143
Orbay JL, 218

Osei DA, 14
O'Shaughnessy MA, 234

P

Pace GI, 188
Page C, 489
Pan BS, 192
Panchal K, 454
Pannell W, 201
Papaloïzos MY, 43
Park EJ, 22
Park JS, 351
Park S-E, 454
Park SE, 22
Parks BG, 181, 287
Parrino A, 434
Patel I, 430
Patel TK, 3, 13
Patterson JT, 254
Paz L, 321
Peck J, 104
Peimer CA, 72
Pekince O, 191
Perkinson SG, 262
Perrin P, 337
Pess GM, 71
Peters RM, 278
Petraglia CA, 448
Phadnis J, 452
Pidgeon TS, 291
Pijls BG, 460
Pinder RM, 59
Pipicelli JG, 155
Plant CE, 239
Plath JE, 436
Poeze M, 205
Pomwenger W, 420
Pooley J, 275
Post EG, 470
Potter MQ, 103
Prasad A, 375
Provencher MT, 452

Q

Qayyum R, 123

R

Raffoul W, 97
Rah UW, 353

Ramirez MA, 448
Rampazzo A, 236
Randhawa K, 482
Rao N, 361
Rappaport PO, 147
Reddy SN, 250
Reger A, 52
Reina MA, 91
Reissig LF, 79
Renninger CH, 105, 111
Resnik L, 492
Riazi S, 259
Riboh JC, 499
Riggenbach MD, 224
Rimmke N, 364
Ring D, 387
Rios-Alba T, 309
Rix L, 59
Rizzitelli A, 170
Roberti del Vecchio PM, 97
Rocchi VJ, 105, 111
Roche AD, 117
Roh YH, 92, 518
Roman-Deynes JL, 55
Rosas S, 283
Rosenwasser MP, 178
Rotari V, 50, 56
Rousi T, 345
Russon K, 118
Rymaszewski L, 264
Ryu KJ, 370

S

Sabongi RG, 129
Sadek AF, 180, 193
Saier T, 436
Saithna A, 416
Sakurai S, 461
Saleem MH, 123
Salminger S, 117
Saltzman BM, 499
Salvador Carreno J, 275
Sansone V, 251
Santiago-Torres JE, 364
Sayegh ET, 495
Schär MO, 376
Scheerer CR, 505
Scheltens M, 86
Schleck CD, 412
Schlitz RS, 300
Schmidt S, 94
Schmitt V, 159
Schoonhoven Jv, 52
Schorpion M, 299

Schreck MJ, 31, 221
Schwertz JM, 300
Sears ED, 1, 18
Seki A, 329
Seruya M, 137, 140
Shaftel ND, 175
Shah AS, 324
Shahabpour M, 255
Shailam R, 312
Shakir I, 187
Shao X, 173
Shauver MJ, 113, 121,
    144, 177
Shearin JW, 288, 295
Shen SH, 137, 140
Shen XF, 145
Sheps DM, 359
Shi LL, 438
Shin AY, 234
Shin JS, 378
Shin S-J, 361
Shin WH, 378
Shirley E, 303
Shon MS, 354
Simcock X, 324
Sims SEG, 510
Sinclair M, 103
Singh J, 310
Skjong C, 83, 88
Slattery PG, 170
Slijper HP, 67, 70
Smeulders MJC, 139, 338
Smith LB, 41
Smith SD, 475
Sollerman C, 7
Song HX, 357
Song K-S, 373
Song X, 332
Sood RF, 511
Sousa GGQ, 126
Sousa PL, 409
Sousa Vasconcelos JT, 84
Souza JM, 112
Spekreijse KR, 26
Spiegel UJ, 475
Spross C, 396
Staelens B, 255
Stanbury SJ, 165
Stone JD, 217
Strackee SD, 202, 225
Stroia K, 471
Styles-Tripp F, 359
Subasi M, 265
Suh N, 47, 65

Suprak DN, 478
Susarla SM, 516
Suzuki T, 156
Swanson EW, 516

T

Tagliafico AS, 258
Takagi T, 329
Takemura Y, 9
Tatman PD, 511
Tauber M, 394
Tay SC, 176, 184
Taylor JL, 494
Taylor KF, 41, 188
Terenghi G, 206
Teunis T, 203, 227, 230
Thiagarajan G, 194
Thoma A, 502, 507
Thomas K, 260
Thomassen BJW, 460
Thoreson AR, 147, 158
Thornton ER, 203, 230
Titchener AG, 276
Tjong VK, 417
Toker S, 191
Tonkin MA, 336
Trehan SK, 218
Treseder T, 473
Trist ND, 336
Tsai M-W, 167
Tsai MA, 448
Türkmen F, 191
Tzang C, 29

U

Uchiyama S, 164, 207, 237
Ueba H, 9

V

Vaccaro LM, 217
Vaiss L, 241
Valdes K, 168
van Dam LF, 272
van der Spuy DJ, 336
van der Zwaal P, 460
van Leeuwen WF, 261

Van Nortwick S, 8, 21
Van Overstraeten L, 255
Van Veldhuizen J, 498
Vangsgaard S, 494
Vargas CR, 100, 517
Veillette C, 259
Vergnenègre G, 231
Verhagen TF, 272
Vermeulen GM, 26
Vicenzino B, 290
Vogels J, 5
Vos LM, 202, 225
Vrettos BC, 280
Vu AT, 192

W

Wagner ER, 27
Walbruch B, 127
Walenkamp MMJ, 202,
    225, 244, 491
Waljee JF, 327
Wang AA, 326
Wang DT, 36
Wang H, 186
Wang J, 390
Wanivenhaus F, 376
Ward SR, 346
Warner JJP, 442
Wasserstein D, 267
Waters PM, 324
Weinstock-Zlotnick G, 489
Welsh M, 221
Welsh MF, 226
Werner FW, 35, 62
Werthel J-DR, 80
Whelan DB, 437
Wiater BP, 343, 441, 445
Wieser K, 443
Wigderowitz C, 446
Wijk U, 506
Wilk KE, 468
Wilke B, 51
Williksen JH, 215, 245
Wilson AT, 291
Wolfe SW, 218
Wolff AL, 37
Wood T, 260
Wooten CJ, 412
Wright TW, 224
Wu S-Q, 279
Wu T, 357

X

Xie RG, 199, 223
Xing SG, 199, 223
Xiong L, 64
Xue MY, 145

Y

Yakuboff KP, 192
Yalcinkaya M, 504

Yamanaka Y, 87
Yamazaki H, 164, 207, 237
Yanai T, 461
Yang T-H, 147
Yaseen Z, 165
Yasin Y, 310
Yi JH, 284
Yin Z-G, 42
Yoo HJ, 453
Yoon JP, 284
Young SW, 471
Yuan F, 183

Z

Zelken JA, 181
Zenke Y, 87
Zhang C, 186
Zhang J-B, 42
Zhang X, 173
Zhao C, 80
Zhao J-G, 390
Zheng KH, 17
Zhong L, 96, 144, 177
Zhou C, 67, 70